T0338110

Clinical Reproductive Science

Clinical Reproductive Science

Edited by Michael Carroll

Manchester Metropolitan University
Manchester
UK

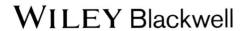

Registered Offices
John Wiley & Sons, Inc., 111 River Street, Hoboken, NJ 07030, USA
John Wiley & Sons Ltd, The Atrium, Southern Gate, Chichester, West Sussex, PO19 8SQ, UK

Editorial Office
The Atrium, Southern Gate, Chichester, West Sussex, PO19 8SQ, UK

For details of our global editorial offices, customer services, and more information about Wiley products visit us at www.wiley.com.

Wiley also publishes its books in a variety of electronic formats and by print-on-demand. Some content that appears in standard print versions of this book may not be available in other formats.

Library of Congress Cataloging-in-Publication Data

Names: Carroll, Michael, 1974– editor.
Title: Clinical reproductive science / [edited by] Michael Carroll.
Description: Hoboken, NJ : Wiley-Blackwell, 2018. | Includes bibliographical references and index. |
Identifiers: LCCN 2018023658 (print) | LCCN 2018024515 (ebook) | ISBN 9781118977255 (Adobe PDF) |
    ISBN 9781118977248 (ePub) | ISBN 9781118975954 (hbk.)
Subjects: | MESH: Infertility–therapy | Reproductive Techniques, Assisted | Embryonic Development
Classification: LCC RG133.5 (ebook) | LCC RG133.5 (print) | NLM WP 570 | DDC 616.6/9206–dc23
LC record available at https://lccn.loc.gov/2018023658

Cover design: Wiley
Cover image: © Dabarti CGI/Shutterstock

Set in 10/12pt Warnock by SPi Global, Pondicherry, India
Printed and bound in Singapore by Markono Print Media Pte Ltd

10 9 8 7 6 5 4 3 2 1

I dedicate this book to my Mother (always in my thoughts), and to my children Isabelle, Darwin, and Leo.

Contents

List of Contributors

Omar Abdel-Mannan
Population Policy and Practice
Institute of Child Health
London
UK

Tope Adeniyi
Department of Reproductive Medicine
Old St Mary's Hospital
Manchester University NHS Foundation Trust
Manchester
UK

Muhammad A. Akhtar
Department of Reproductive Medicine
Old St Mary's Hospital
Manchester University NHS Foundation Trust
Manchester
UK

Ruth Arnesen
Reproductive Health Group,
Centre for Reproductive Health
Daresbury Park
Daresbury
UK

Brendan Ball
Bourn Hall Fertility Centre
Al Hudaiba Awards Building
Jumeirah
Dubai
UAE

Stéphane Berneau
School of Healthcare Science
Manchester Metropolitan University
John Dalton Building
Manchester
UK

Daniel R. Brison
Maternal and Fetal Health Research Centre
Division of Developmental Biology and Medicine
School of Medicine, Faculty of Biology, Medicine and Health
University of Manchester
Manchester
UK

and

Department of Reproductive Medicine
Old St Mary's Hospital
Manchester University NHS Foundation Trust
Manchester
UK

Michael Carroll
School of Healthcare Science
Manchester Metropolitan University
Manchester
UK

James Coey
Department of Anatomical Sciences
St Georges' University School of Medicine
KBT Global Scholar's Program
Newcastle upon Tyne
UK

J. Diane Critchlow
Department of Reproductive Medicine
Old St Mary's Hospital
Manchester University NHS Foundation Trust
Manchester
UK

Rachel Cutting
Jessop Fertility
The Jessop Wing
Sheffield
UK

Emma Derbyshire
Nutritional Insight Ltd
Surrey
UK

Derrick Ebot
Department of Anatomical Sciences
St Georges' University School of Medicine
KBT Global Scholar's Program
Newcastle upon Tyne
UK

Edmond Edi-Osagie
Department of Reproductive Medicine
Old St Mary's Hospital
Manchester University NHS Foundation Trust
Manchester
UK

Val Edwards Jones
School of Healthcare Science
Manchester Metropolitan University
John Dalton Building
Manchester
UK

Cheryl T. Fitzgerald
Department of Reproductive Medicine
Old St Mary's Hospital
Manchester University NHS Foundation Trust
Manchester
UK

Tom P. Fleming
Biological Sciences
University of Southampton
Southampton General Hospital
Southampton
UK

Jacques Gilloteaux
Unité de Recherche en Physiologie Moléculaire
(URPhyM)
Faculté de Médecine
Université de Namur
Namur
Belgium

Stephen Harbottle
Cambridge IVF
Cambridge University Hospitals, NHS Foundation
Trust
Cambridge
UK

Mary Herbert
Newcastle Fertility Centre
Centre for Life, Times Square
Newcastle upon Tyne
UK
and
Wellcome Trust Centre for Mitochondrial
Research
Institute of Genetic Medicine
Newcastle University
Newcastle upon Tyne
UK

Elizabeth Hester
Faculty of Biology, Medicine and Health
The University of Manchester
Manchester
UK

Haider Hilal
Department of Anatomical Sciences
St Georges' University School of
Medicine
KBT Global Scholar's Program
Newcastle upon Tyne
UK

Louise Hyslop
Newcastle Fertility Centre
International Centre for Life
Newcastle upon Tyne
UK

Narmada Katakam
Reproductive Health Group
Centre for Reproductive Health
Daresbury Park
Daresbury
UK

Robbie Kerr
GCRM-Belfast Ltd
Edgewater House
Belfast
UK

Henry J. Leese
Hull York Medical School
University of Hull
Hull
UK

Colleen Lynch
Cooper Genomics
MediCity Nottingham
Nottingham

Luciano G. Nardo
Reproductive Health Group
Centre for Reproductive Health
Daresbury Park
Daresbury
UK

Mahshid Nickkho-Amiry
Department of Reproductive Medicine
Old St Mary's Hospital
Manchester University NHS Foundation Trust
Manchester
UK

Allan Pacey
Department of Oncology & Metabolism Academic
Unit of Reproductive and Developmental Medicine
The Jessop Wing
Sheffield
UK

Rebecca M. Perrett
Nuffield Department of Clinical Neurosciences
John Radcliffe Hospital
Oxford
UK

Aarush Sajjad
Sofia Medical University
Sofia
Bulgaria

Solmaz Gul Sajjad
Sofia Medical University
Sofia
Bulgaria

Yasmin Sajjad
Burjeel Center for Reproductive Medicine
Burjeel Hospital
Abu Dhabi
UAE

Bert Stewart
Reproductive Health Group
Centre for Reproductive Health
Daresbury Park
Daresbury
UK

Sara Sulaiman
Department of Anatomical Sciences
St Georges' University School of Medicine
KBT Global Scholar's Program
Newcastle upon Tyne
UK

Congshan Sun
Biological Sciences
University of Southampton
Southampton General Hospital
Southampton
UK

Alastair G. Sutcliffe
Population Policy and Practice
Institute of Child Health
London
UK

Mathew Tomlinson
Fertility Unit
Nottingham University Hospital
Nottingham
UK

Ana-Maria Tomova
School of Healthcare Science
Manchester Metropolitan University
John Dalton Building
Manchester
UK

Rosa Trigas
Department of Reproductive Medicine
Old St Mary's Hospital
Manchester University NHS Foundation Trust
Manchester
UK

Nikolaos Tsampras
Department of Reproductive Medicine
Old St Mary's Hospital
Manchester University NHS Foundation Trust
Manchester
UK

Caroline Watkins
Reproductive Health Group
Centre for Reproductive Health
Daresbury Park
Daresbury
UK

Katrina Williams
Department of Oncology and Metabolism
Academic Unit of Reproductive and Developmental
Medicine
The Jessop Wing
Sheffield
UK

Bryan Woodward
X&Y Fertility
Leicester
UK

Dawn Yell
Complete Fertility Centre Southampton
Princess Anne Hospital
Southampton
UK

Kenneth Ma Kin Yue
Department of Gynaecology
Central Manchester University Hospitals
NHS Trust
Manchester
UK

About the Editor

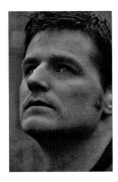

Dr Michael Carroll is a Senior Lecturer in Reproductive Science and the Course Director for the MSc in Clinical Science/Cellular Science. This is the academic component for the Scientist Training Program (STP), which is part of the Department of Health's Modernising Science Careers (MSC). The MSC is a UK-wide government initiative to address the training and education needs of the whole healthcare science workforce in the National Health Service (NHS). The Cellular Science STP is designed to train and educate clinical embryologists, andrologists, histopathologists, and cytopathologists for the UK clinical workforce.

Michael studied Toxicology (Athlone Institute of Technology, Eire) and Biomedical Science (University of Bradford). After completing a PhD in Reproductive Cellular Physiology from the University of Newcastle he went on to postdoctoral positions at the Howard Hughes Medical Institute, UT Southwestern, Dallas, The CNRS, Station Zollogique, VileFranceh sur Mer, France, and at Southampton University. After his time in research Michael trained as a Clinical Embryologist (obtaining the ACE Postgraduate Certificate in Clinical Embryology) and worked in a busy IVF clinic before being appointed as a Lecturer in Reproductive Science at Manchester Metropolitan University. Michael's research interests includes reproductive cell biology, andrology, investigating lifestyle and environmental effects on human sperm, and evolutionary biology.

Preface

Infertility is defined as a disease of the reproductive system that can result in the inability to achieve a pregnancy within 12 months of trying. Assisted reproductive technology (ART) is in its fortieth year, and since the birth of Louise Brown – the first IVF baby – over 6.5 million babies have been born through ART.

The field of ART has expanded in terms of what we understand about human reproduction, the causes of infertility, and how ART has developed as a field of medicine to treat infertility.

The training of Clinical Embryologists in the UK is intensive. Trainees are selected through a very competitive recruitment process and those who are successful are enrolled on to the Scientist Training Programme (STP). As part the STP, trainees must enrol on an MSc in Clinical Science and undertake their clinical training in an IVF clinic. The MSc and training is carried out over three years, and after successful completion of both elements, the trainee can then register as a Clinical Scientist.

As the Programme Director for the MSc, I believed a textbook containing all the elements of the Clinical Reproductive Science Academic Programme would be a useful learning source. Therefore, the aim of this book is to provide a concise text to support the Clinical Embryologists and Andrologists in training. The format and style of this book also makes it a good source for Doctors, Nurses and Scientists with an interest in clinical reproductive science, and for both undergraduate and postgraduate students studying reproductive science. The authors of each chapter are leading Clinicians, Clinical Embryologists, Andrologists, and Scientists in the UK and abroad.

Areas such as ethics and regulation have been intentionally omitted so an international readership can appreciate the science and clinical practice of reproductive science. As ethics and regulation will vary in each country, such readers are encouraged to seek alternative sources for this information.

This book is divided into three sections. *Section 1* outlines the fundamentals of human reproduction from the development of the gonads and external genitals to embryo development and how the Fallopian tube influences embryo development and health. Some chapters on basic anatomy and physiology are present as a source of reference to support chapters in Sections 2 and 3. Other chapters are detailed reviews of the areas of development and reproduction, which will give the reader a more in-depth knowledge base. *Section 2* concerns infertility. There are chapters covering disorders of male and female reproductive endocrinology, and pathologies of both the male and female reproductive system, which can affect reproduction. The effect of maternal age on oocyte quality is included as well as chapters describing how lifestyle, environment,and infections can affect fertility. *Section 3* covers the practical and clinical aspects of clinical reproductive science, including patient consultation and assessment, ovarian stimulation, gamete retrieval and preparation, *in vitro* insemination and intracytoplasmic sperm injection, embryo culture, embryo transfer, and cryopreservation. There is also a chapter on preimplantation genetic screening and on the long-term follow-up of children conceived through ART.

Overall, this book offers the reader a complete up-to date volume on clinical reproductive science and will be an invaluable concise source for this field.

Manchester, 2018   *Michael Carroll PhD, CBiol,*
FRSB, FIBMS, FHEA, FLS

Acknowledgements

A book of this nature and size would not be possible to accomplish without the willingness and hard work of all the contributors. Thank you all for giving your time to write the chapters that make this book what it is.

I would like to thank Henry Leese for reviewing some of the chapters and his constant encouragement during this process. Thanks also goes to Phoebe Ingram, Keith Carroll, Mahdi Lamb, and Ana-Maria Tomova for providing the illustrations presented in some chapters.

And finally, thank you Sarah for your patience and taking the burden of parenthood during this process.

About the Companion Website

Don't forget to visit the companion website for this book:

www.wiley.com/go/carroll/clinicalreproductivescience

There you will find valuable material designed to enhance your learning, including:

- Figures from the book (colour images)

Section One

Reproductive Science

Fundamentals of Human Reproductive Biology

1

Sexual Differentiation, Gonadal Development, and Development of the External Genitalia: A Review of The Regulation of Sexual Differentiation

Rebecca M. Perrett

Introduction

The development of one's sex comprises 'sex determination' – the development of the undifferentiated gonad into testis or ovaries during embryogenesis, followed by 'sex differentiation' – the determination of phenotypic sex induced by factors produced by the differentiated gonad. This chapter will highlight the molecular mechanisms underpinning these two processes.

During the first 2 weeks of human embryonic development, the only difference between XX and XY embryos is their karyotype. At the two-cell stage of the XX zygote, X chromosome inactivation occurs, enabling males and females to have equal transcript levels from the X chromosome (Huynh and Lee 2001). In developing germ cells, the X is reactivated in the female, so both X chromosomes contribute to oogenesis (Sugimoto and Abe 2007).

The Bipotential Gonad

During the fourth week of human development, the urogenital ridges develop as a thickening of the mesodermic mesonephros covered by coelomic epithelium (CE); it is from this structure that the urogenital system and adrenal cortex originate. In the fifth week, or mouse embryonic day (E) 9.5–10.5, the urogenital ridge divides into a urinary and adrenogonadal ridge the latter of which forms the gonads and adrenal gland (Swain and Lovell-Badge 1999). Until the sixth week of human development, or mouse E11.5, the undifferentiated gonads of XX and XY individuals are identical and have the potential to form either ovary or testes (bipotential).

Molecular Determinants of Gonadal Development

A number of factors have been shown to be required for the development of the undifferentiated gonad, as illustrated in Figure 1.1. However, due to the limited studies in human development, mouse studies have revealed several more important factors involved in gonadal development, and these are outlined below.

Empty spiracles homeobox 2 (Emx2)

Emx2 encodes a homeodomain transcription factor expressed in urogenital epithelial cells. Knockout mice completely lack kidneys, gonads, ureters and genital tracts, but the adrenal glands and bladder are normal (Miyamoto et al. 1997), indicating *Emx2* acts after division of the urogenital ridge. It may regulate tight junction assembly, allowing migration of the gonadal epithelia to the mesenchyme (Kusaka et al. 2010).

Paired box gene 2 (Pax2)

Pax2 is a transcriptional regulator expressed within the urogenital system during development, in both ductal and mesenchymal components (Torres et al. 1995). Null mice lack kidneys, ureters, and genital tracts, and the Wolffian and Müllerian tracts degenerate.

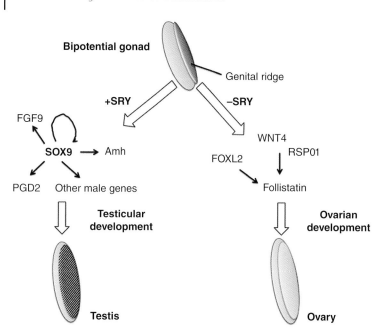

Figure 1.1 Simplistic illustration of the molecular determinants for gonadal differentiation. In the presence of SRY, SOX9 is upregulated and is responsible for the regulation for testicular development. In the absence of SRY, pro-ovarian factors regulate ovarian development (see text for more detail).

Transcription factor 2 (Tcf2)

The POU domain containing *Tcf2* gene functions in epithelial differentiation (Coffinier et al. 1999; Kolatsi-Joannou et al. 2001). It is essential for urogenital development, as patients harbouring mutations exhibit genital malformations (Lindner et al. 1999; Bingham et al. 2002).

Steroidogenic factor 1 (Sf1)/Nr5a1

The transcription factor Sf1 is expressed in the hypothalamus, pituitary, gonads, and adrenal glands (Luo et al. 1994; Val et al. 2003). Null mice lack gonads and adrenal glands (Luo et al. 1994; Shinoda et al. 1995). Sf1 also functions later in testis development.

Wilms' tumour 1 *(Wt1)*

Wt1 encodes multiple isoforms of a zinc finger protein, which act as transcriptional repressors (Menke et al. 1998) or activators (Lee et al. 1999). The –KTS variant promotes cell survival and proliferation in the indifferent gonad, whereas the +KTS isoform functions in testes differentiation (Hammes et al. 2001). The –KTS isoform activates the *sex-determining region Y (Sry)* and *Sf1* promoters (Hossain and Saunders 2001; Wilhelm and Englert 2002). *Wt1* is expressed in urogenital ridges (Pritchard-Jones et al. 1990) where it maintains the identity of adreno-gonadal primordium (AGP) the precursor to the gonads and adrenal primordia

(Bandiera et al. 2013). Accordingly, null mice lack kidneys and gonads (Kreidberg et al. 1993).

LIM homeobox 9 (Lhx9)

Knockout of Lhx9, a homeobox protein, causes failure of gonadal development (Birk et al. 2000) and synergizes with Wt1 to regulate Sf1 expression (Birk et al. 2000; Wilhelm and Englert 2002).

Chromobox homologue 2 *(Cbx2)*

Cbx2 is the mouse homologue of the Drosophila polycomb gene and regulates transcription by altering chromatin structure. Knockout XX mice have small or absent ovaries and XY mice show male–female sex reversal (Katoh-Fukui et al. 1998). *Cbx2* may regulate Sf1 expression in the gonad, as it does in the adrenal gland (Katoh-Fukui et al. 2005), or it may alter Sry expression directly (Katoh-Fukui et al. 2012).

CBP/p300 interacting transactivator, with glu/asp-rich c-terminal domain, 2 (Cited2)

Cited2 is a transcriptional regulator expressed in the AGP, and later in the CE and underlying mesenchyme of the genital ridge (Bhattacharya et al. 1999; Braganca et al. 2003). It cooperates with Wt1 to stimulate *Sf1* expression in the AGP (Val et al. 2007; Buaas et al. 2009), and also ensures Sry levels are sufficient to trigger testis determination.

Gata binding protein 4 (Gata4)

Gata4 is a transcription factor first detected at E11.5 in somatic cells of XX and XY gonads; at E13.5 it is upregulated in XY Sertoli cells and downregulated in interstitial cells and XX gonads (Viger et al. 1998). It is required for gonadal ridge formation (Hu et al. 2013), along with later functions in testicular and ovarian development.

Primordial Germ Cells

Specification

Primordial germ cells (PGCs), the founder cells of the germ cell lineage, are typically established early during embryonic development. Germ cell specification can either occur through the inheritance of germ cell determinants already present in the egg (preformation), as in *Drosophila melanogaster* and *Caenorhabditis elegans*, or in response to inductive signals, as for mice and probably all mammals (epigenesis) (Extavour and Akam 2003; Saitou and Yamaji 2012).

Mouse PGCs (mPGCs) originate in the pluripotent proximal epiblast at about E6.0 when they respond to signals from extraembryonic tissues and express Fragilis/Interferon-induced transmembrane protein 3 (Ifitm3) (Saitou et al. 2002). Bone morphogenetic protein 4 (Bmp4) and 8b from the extraembryonic ectoderm and Bmp2 and wingless-type MMTV integration site family, member 3 (Wnt3) from the visceral endoderm are critical for specification (Lawson et al. 1999; Ying et al. 2000; Ying and Zhao, 2001; Ohinata et al. 2009). At E6.25, about six of these cells express B-lymphocyte-induced maturation protein 1 (Blimp1, also known as PR domain-containing 1, Prdm1): these cells are PGC precursors (Ohinata et al. 2005), although further cells are recruited to become PGCs before E7.25 (Saitou et al. 2002; McLaren and Lawson 2005; Ohinata et al. 2005). Wnt3 acts via β-catenin to activate the mesodermal factor T (brachyury), which in turn induces Blimp1 and Prdm14 expression (Aramaki et al. 2013); these are transcriptional repressors which suppress the somatic program while allowing establishment of germ cell character (Saitou et al. 2002; Saitou et al. 2005; Ohinata et al. 2005; Vincent et al. 2005; Yabuta et al. 2006; Seki et al. 2007; Kurimoto et al. 2008; Yamaji et al. 2008). The expression of genes which establish/maintain pluripotency are retained via the epiblast, including *Sox2, Nanog, Oct4,* and Embryonal stem cell gene 1 *(Esg1)* (Scholer et al. 1990; Ohinata et al. 2005; Western et al. 2005; Yamaguchi et al. 2005; Yabuta et al. 2006; Chambers et al. 2007).

Following establishment of the germ cell lineage, extensive reprogramming of the genome occurs, i.e. erasure of epigenetic marks such as DNA methylation and establishment of new marks (Surani 2001; Hajkova et al. 2002). Imprinting must be reprogrammed in the germ line, as a maternal allele in one generation may be a paternal allele in the next. PGCs do initially acquire genome wide *de novo* methylation; however, following entry into the gonadal ridge, there is rapid demethylation, simultaneously in male and females, prior to their sex-specific differentiation. The timing of erasure in humans is not known, but in mice it begins between E10.5 and E11.5, i.e. after arrival in the gonadal ridge (Lee et al. 2002). Remethylation occurs in XY germ cells once they have committed to the spermatogenic fate, and in XX germ cells just before ovulation (Hajkova 2011).

Human PGCs (hPGCs) are first identified in the wall of the yolk sac at 23–26 days postfertilization (Witschi 1946). The process of hPGC specification is thought to be similar to that in mPGCs, given the conserved expression of key regulatory genes, including that of *OCT4, NANOG, BLIMP1, TFAP2C* and *cKIT* (Anderson et al. 2007; Eckert et al. 2008; Kerr et al. 2008a; Kerr et al. 2008b). Human PGCs also undergo extensive epigenetic reprogramming (Gkountela et al. 2013). However, in contrast to mPGCs, hPGCs do not express the key pluripotency transcription factor SOX2 (Perrett et al. 2008), hinting towards fundamental differences between human and mouse PGC specification.

Migration

At approximately E10.5 in the mouse and between weeks 5 and 8 of human gestation, PGCs actively migrate from the allantois through the gut mesentery to the genital ridges of the developing gonad (Figure 1.2), exhibiting polarized morphology and extending cytoplasmic protrusions (Fujimoto et al. 1977; Anderson et al. 2000; Molyneaux et al. 2001). Again, studies in the mouse have revealed the involvement of a number of key molecules, which are also implicated hPGC migration. Thus, the c-Kit

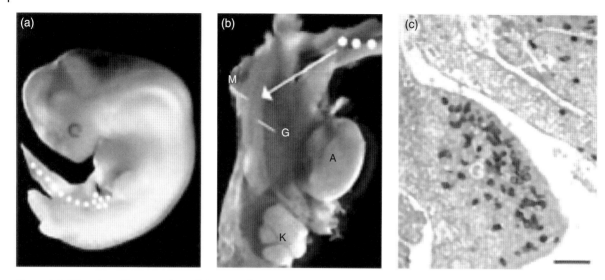

Figure 1.2 Migration of human primordial germ cells. Representation of human primordial germ cell (PGC) migration from the allantois to the gonadal ridge in the intact embryo (a) and through the gut mesentery within the dissected abdomen (b) at approximately 6 weeks after conception. The gonadal ridge (G) has developed on the medial surface of the mesonephros (M) adjacent to the adrenal gland (A) and superior to the kidney (K). (c) Human embryo section corresponding to (b) showing PGCs darkly stained for alkaline phosphatase activity in the gonad (G) and throughout the folds of the gut mesentery (arrow). Bar = 250 µm. Reproduced with permission of Wiley.

receptor tyrosine kinase on PGCs, and its ligand, stem cell factor (Scf), expressed by somatic cells along the migratory route, are required (McCoshen and McCallion 1975; Buehr et al. 1993b; Merkwitz et al. 2011) as well as the chemokine stromal-cell derived factor 1 (Sdf1) which is released from somatic cells and acts on the chemokine (C-X-C motif), receptor 4b (Cxcr4b), on the PGC surface (Ara et al. 2003; Molyneaux et al. 2003).

In addition, the following all interfere with PGC migration: knockout/mutation of *β1 integrin* (Anderson et al. 1999), *E-cadherin* (Bendel-Stenzel et al. 2000; Di Carlo and De Felici, 2000), *Fgf8* (Sun et al. 1999), *Forkhead box c1 (Foxc1)* (Mattiske et al. 2006), *Lhx1* (Tanaka et al. 2010), *Wnt5a* (Chawengsaksophak et al. 2012), Receptor tyrosine kinase-like orphan receptor 2 (*Ror2*) (Laird et al. 2011), and the germ cell deficient (GCD) locus (Pellas et al. 1991). Extracellular matrix (ECM) proteins, including fibronectin and laminin, also play a role (Ffrench-Constant et al. 1991; Garcia-Castro et al. 1997). Inhibition of 3-hydroxy-3-methylglutaryl-coenzyme A reductase (HMGCR), involved in cholesterol synthesis, reduces PGC migration (Ding et al. 2008). Hindgut endoderm expansion is essential for

mPGC migration (Hara et al. 2009), and the long and narrow genital ridge structure helps capture migrating germ cells (Harikae et al. 2013a).

Human PGC migration is less well understood. During the fifth week of human embryonic development, PGCs are apparent in the genital ridges and gut mesentery. They migrate along nerve fibres and Schwann cells to reach the gonadal ridge, indicating that these nerve/Schwann cells release germ cell chemoattractants (Mollgard et al. 2010).

Upon arrival in the genital ridge, germ cells (now termed gonocytes) lose their motility and polarized morphology and associate with somatic cells (Baillie 1964; Donovan et al. 1986). Studies in *Drosophila* and zebrafish indicate that PGCs stop migrating at the site of highest chemoattractant expression (Van Doren et al. 1998; Reichman-Fried et al. 2004), and that somatic–germ cell interactions are also required (Jenkins et al. 2003; Van Doren et al. 2003; Mathews et al. 2006).

Proliferation

A number of factors are involved in mPGC proliferation, which when ablated, cause PGC loss. Bcl-x, an anti-apoptotic B-cell leukemia/lymphoma 2 (Bcl2) family member maintains the survival of mPGCs (Rucker et al. 2000), Fgf2 and Fgf4 promote mPGC proliferation in vitro (Matsui et al. 1992, Resnick et al. 1998, Kawase et al. 2004), and PGC numbers are reduced in Fgfr2-IIIb knockout embryos (Takeuchi et al. 2005).

As well as being required for migration, Kit signalling is required for germ cell growth, maturation and survival (Merkwitz et al. 2011). Loss of β-catenin, a member of the Wnt signalling pathway, and follistatin (Fst), a Tgfβ family member, cause germ cell loss in the ovary (Yao et al. 2004; Liu et al. 2009).In addition, co-expression of Wnt4 and Rspo1 is required for proliferation in the undifferentiated gonad (Chassot et al. 2012), as well as being involved later in ovarian development.

The Internal Reproductive Tract

As well as forming the gonad, the mesonephros and CE also give rise to components of the internal reproductive tract and urinary system, including the Wolffian ducts (WDs) which form the epididymides,

vasa deferentia, and seminal vesicles in the male, and the Müllerian ducts (MDs) which generate the Fallopian tubes, uterus, and upper vagina in the female (Hashimoto 2003). In the human embryo, the internal reproductive tract is similar in both sexes up to 8 weeks postconception (WPC) (the indifferent stage).

The precursor of the WD (also known as the mesonephric duct) is the pronephric duct (Jirasek 1971; Hashimoto 2003), which regresses at 4 WPC and is replaced by the mesonephros (Seville et al. 2002). The precursor of the MD, the paramesonephric duct, develops in parallel (Sobel et al. 2004). The WD first appears as a single uteric bud, and then develops as a continuous tube along the urogenital ridge, which reaches the caudal part of the hindgut, the cloaca. The WD develops by mesenchymal cell rearrangement, rather than by cell proliferation (Keller et al. 1985), involving Gata3 (Grote et al. 2006), Ret signalling (a receptor tyrosine kinase involved in glial derived neurotrophic factor signalling) (Hoshi et al. 2012), Gremlin1, Bmp4 and Bmp7 (Goncalves and Zeller 2011). The mature WD drains the primitive kidney, the mesonephros, to the cloaca. In males and females it develops into the trigone of the bladder, part of the bladder wall (Figure 1.3).

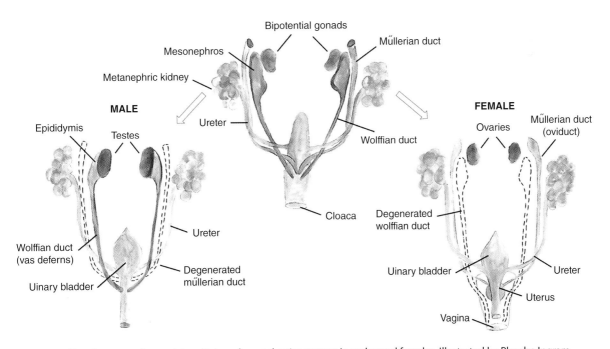

Figure 1.3 Development of gonadal and internal reproductive system in males and females. Illustrated by Phoebe Ingram.

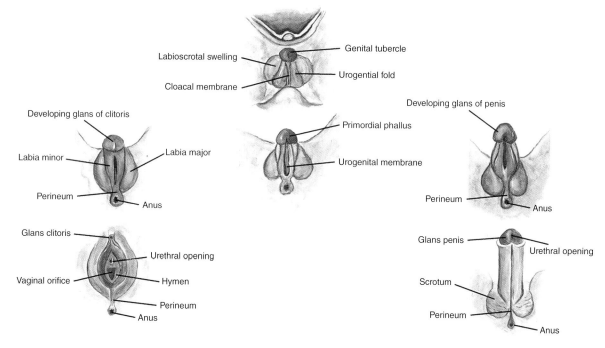

Figure 1.4 Development of external genitalia in both males and females. Illustrated by Phoebe Ingram.

The MDs are paired ducts, which run down the side of the urogenital ridge. They arise as a thickening of CE cells (Zhan et al. 2006; Arango et al. 2008), which migrate to the WD, proliferate and elongate at the tip (Guioli et al. 2007; Orvis and Behringer 2007). The Wolffian epithelium secretes Wnt9b, required for Müllerian growth (Carroll et al. 2005). MD development also requires retinoic acid (RA) (Mendelsohn et al. 1994), Wnt4 (Vainio et al. 1999; Heikkila et al. 2005), and Wnt7 which induces anti-Müllerian receptor-II (Amhr-II) expression (Parr and McMahon 1998). Lim1 and Wnt7 expression is regulated by members of the Dachsung gene family (Davis et al. 2008). Knockout of Discs large homolog 1, involved in epithelial polarization and adhesion, causes defective MD development (Iizuka-Kogo et al. 2007).

The External Genitalia

During the third week of human development, the cloacal membrane is formed; this shifts caudally during the fourth week, and by the fifth week cloacal folds form on either side, joining at the anterior end, the genital tubercle. At 7 WPC, the urorectal septum divides the cloacal membrane, forming the urogenital membrane and urethral folds at the ventral section (urogenital sinus), and anal membrane and folds at the dorsal section. The urogenital membrane then dissolves leaving the urogenital sinus opening (ostium) surrounded by labioscrotal swellings (Figure 1.4).

A number of signalling molecules are involved in the early patterning of the indifferent external genitalia. Fgf8, activated in the urethra by β-catenin, and Bmps are required for genital tubercle growth and differentiation (Suzuki et al. 2003, Lin et al. 2008, Haraguchi et al. 2000), while Fgf10 is required for glans penis and clitoridis development (Haraguchi et al. 2000). Sonic hedgehog (Shh) signalling plays a central role (Perriton et al. 2002; Klonisch et al. 2004), as do various homeotic (Hox) genes (Mortlock and Innis 1997; Warot et al. 1997; Post and Innis 1999).

Testis Differentiation

Molecular Determinants of Testis Differentiation

Testis development is triggered by Sry (Lovell-Badge and Robertson 1990; Koopman et al. 1991), a member of the *SOX* gene family of HMG transcription factors encoded on the Y chromosome. Sry is first detected in supporting cell precursors in the XY gonad from E10.75 (Albrecht and Eicher 2001; Bullejos and Koopman 2001; Sekido et al. 2004; Wilhelm et al. 2005). Expression is transient (approximately 4 h in each cell precursor), reaching a peak at E11.5 and being extinguished shortly after E12.5 (Koopman et al. 1990; Lee and Taketo 1994; Hacker et al. 1995; Jeske et al. 1995; Sekido et al. 2004), its function being to activate transcription of Sox9, the so-called master regulator of testis determination, approximately 10 h after Sry expression (Bullejos and Koopman 2005).

Regulation of Sry Expression

Gata4 activates the mouse, but not the human, Sry promoter (Miyamoto et al. 2008); this activation is enhanced via mitogen-activated protein 3 kinase 4 (Map3k4) activation of p38 kinase, which phosphorylates Gata4 (Gierl et al. 2012; Warr et al. 2012). This activation requires interaction of Gata4 with its cofactor, Friend of Gata4 (Fog2) (Tevosian et al. 2002; Manuylov et al. 2011). Fog2 expression is in turn regulated by the transcription factors Six homeobox 1 (Six1) and Six4 (Fujimoto et al. 2013), which also regulate Sf1 expression. Map3k4 is activated by Growth arrest and DNA-damage-inducible protein (Gadd45g) (Miyake et al. 2007; Gierl et al. 2012) with null XY mice showing sex reversal (Warr et al. 2012; Johnen et al. 2013). Gata6 is co-expressed with Gata4 in the testis (Ketola et al. 1999), with double knockout mice having smaller testes (Padua et al. 2015). Mouse Gata6 has 85% homology with Gata4 (Molkentin 2000) and the two are postulated to carry overlapping functions (Robert et al. 2006; Bennett et al. 2012).

Sf1 activates the Sry promoter (de Santa Barbara et al. 2001; Pilon et al. 2003) and null XY gonads degenerate with due to lack of Sry expression (Luo et al. 1994). Lhx9 and Cbx2 regulate Sry expression indirectly via Sf1 upregulation, and Cited2 interacts with Sf1 and Wt1 to increase Sry expression to initiate testis development. Additionally, Wt1 directly activates the Sry promoter (Shimamura et al. 1997; Hossain and Saunders 2001; Miyamoto et al. 2008), synergizes with Gata4 on the Sry promoter (Miyamoto et al. 2008) and may stabilize Sry mRNA (Polanco and Koopman 2007). The

transcription factor Sp1 also transactivates the Sry promoter (Desclozeaux et al. 1998; Assumpcao et al. 2005).

Methylation of lysine 9 of histone H3 on the Sry promoter represses gene transcription (Barski et al. 2007), and is demethylated by lysine-specific demethylase 3A (encoded by the Jmjd1a gene) (Kuroki et al. 2013). Jmjd1a-null mice show XY sex reversal.

Sry Targets
Sox9

A threshold level of Sry expression is required to activate Sox9 expression in Sertoli cells (SCs), but only within a specific window; if this does not occur, either ovotestes or ovaries form (Hiramatsu et al. 2009; Wilhelm et al. 2009). In addition, the level of Sox9 expression must also reach a threshold level. Once expression is initiated within SCs, however, it remains throughout their lifetime.

Sry and Sf1 bind directly to several sites within the Sox9 promoter, within a 3.2 kb testis-specific enhancer (TES) or 1.4 kb of its core element (TESCO), present approximately 14 kb upstream (Sekido and Lovell-Badge 2008). Sox9 also binds to this region with Sf1 to maintain its own expression. Sox9 is the only critical direct target of Sry, as Sox9 expression in the XX gonad leads to male sex reversal (Bishop et al. 2000; Vidal et al. 2001). Deletion of Sox9 interferes with sex cord development and the activation of male specific markers (Chaboissier et al. 2004). In humans, heterozygous mutations cause campomelic dysplasia, with XY sex reversal (Foster et al. 1994; Wagner et al. 1994), and gain of function mutations cause XX sex reversal (Huang et al. 1999). There are also more distal regulatory regions of Sox9 (Bagheri-Fam et al. 2006), mutation of which cause XY gonadal dysgenesis (White et al. 2011). Interestingly, mouse Sry can activate Sox9 directly, through its C terminal polyglutamine tract, but this has been lost in the human, which relies on Sry partner protein(s) to activate Sox9 transcription (Zhao et al. 2014).

Pod1 (Transcription factor 21, Tcf21)

The promoter of Pod1, a basic helix-loop-helix (bHLH) transcription factor, contains Sry binding sites, and Pod1 promotes sex reversal of ovarian cells to Sertoli precursors (Bhandari et al. 2011).

Null XY mice demonstrate defects in testis formation (Cui et al. 2004), indicating that Pod1 might be an Sry target; however it is expressed prior to Sry, and Pod1 knockout increases apoptosis. Its sex reversal effect may therefore occur because it represses Sf1 expression leading to Leydig cell and SC differentiation (Luo et al. 1994; Tamura et al. 2001).

Neurotrophin 3 (Ntf3)

In the mouse testis, Sertoli-secreted Ntf3 acts on its receptor Tropomyosin receptor kinase C (TrkC) to promote mesonephric cell migration (Cupp et al. 2003), and Sry activates the Ntf3 promoter (Clement et al. 2011). TrkC-null mice show defective testis cord formation (Cupp et al. 2002).

Cerebellin 4 precursor gene (Cbln4)

Another direct target of Sry and Sox9 is Cbln4 (Bradford et al. 2009), although the function of this secreted protein is unknown.

Sox9 Targets

Fgf9 and Prostaglandin D2 (Pgd2)

As well as acting on its own promoter, Sox9 upregulates the expression of Fgf9 and prostaglandin D2 (Pgd2) synthase, creating feedforward loops which also maintain Sox9 expression. Pgd2 induces Sox9 expression and nuclear import in neighbouring cells (Wilhelm et al. 2005; Malki et al. 2005; Wilhelm et al. 2007; Moniot et al. 2009). Via interaction with its receptor Fgfr2, Fgf9 maintains Sox9 and downregulates Wnt4 expression (Kim et al. 2006; Kim et al. 2007). Fgf9- or Fgfr2-null XY mice demonstrate complete or partial sex reversal, respectively (Colvin et al. 2001; Kim et al. 2007; Bagheri-Fam et al. 2008), and Fgf9 causes proliferation of SC precursors (Schmahl et al. 2004; Kim et al. 2006).

Anti-Müllerian hormone (AMH)

Sox9 upregulates the expression of AMH, secreted from SCs and involved in the development of the internal reproductive tract (Arango et al. 1999; Lasala et al. 2011).

Sox Family Members

Sox8 is upregulated by Sox9 (Chaboissier et al. 2004) and cooperates with Sf1 to activate AMH transcription (Schepers et al. 2003). In addition, Sox3 and Sox10 are expressed in the mouse testis, and all three Sox proteins interact with Sf1 to maintain Sox9 expression (Sutton et al. 2011; Sekido and Lovell-Badge, 2013). Later in development Sox8 and Sox9 synergize to promote basal lamina integrity of testis cords and suppress Forkhead box L2 (Foxl2) expression (Georg et al. 2012).

Other Factors Involved in Testis Differentiation

The chromatin remodeler ATRX (α-thalassemia and mental retardation associated with the X chromosome) functions in human sexual differentiation (Tang et al. 2004), with mutations causing gonadal and urogenital defects (Reardon et al. 1995). Mutations in testis-specific protein Y-like-1 (TSPYL1), another chromatin modifier, cause sudden infant death with dysgenesis of the testis in males (SIDDT) (Puffenberger et al. 2004), along with other disorders of testicular development (Vinci et al. 2009). The transcription factor Mamld1 (Mastermind-Like Domain-Containing Protein 1) activates the transcription of a noncanonical Notch target gene hairy/enhancer of split 3 (Hes3) and augments testosterone production, likely regulated by Sf1 (Fukami et al. 2008).

Dmrt1 (Doublesex and mab-3 related transcription factor 1) maintains mammalian testis differentiation throughout development and postnatally (Matson et al. 2011; Minkina et al. 2014). It determines sex in a number of nonmammalian vertebrates (Matsuda et al. 2002; Yoshimoto et al. 2008; Smith et al. 2009), but is dispensable in mammals, in which it has been replaced by Sry (Raymond et al. 2000). However, overexpression in mouse XX gonads causes sex reversal (Zhao et al. 2015), indicating it has retained its ability to trigger testis differentiation.

Duplication of the dosage sensitive sex reversal region on the X chromosome, encoding the transcription factor Dax1, causes sex reversal in XY patients (Bardoni et al. 1994; Swain et al. 1998). However, mutation in XX gonads does not prevent ovary development (Yu et al. 1998), and further investigations indicate that Dax1 is required for development of both the ovary and testis (Ludbrook and Harley 2004).

As well as transcription factors, signalling molecules are involved in initiating the early stages of testis differentiation. Loss of function mutations in the insulin receptor, the insulin-like growth factor receptor (Igf1r), and the insulin-related receptor result in reduced Sry expression (Nef et al. 2003; Pitetti et al. 2013). However, these factors affect cell proliferation, which can cause XY ovary formation (Schmahl and Capel 2003). Male Desert Hedgehog (Dhh)-null mice are sterile with reduced spermatogenesis (Bitgood and McMahon 1995), possibly due to decreased germ cell survival (Makela et al. 2011; Sahin et al. 2014). Dhh is secreted by SCs and its receptor Patched homologue 1 (Ptch1) is expressed by the interstitium, and also positively regulates fetal Leydig cell differentiation (Yao et al. 2002). In addition, palmitoyl-transferase hedgehog acyl-transferase (Hhat) is involved in testis cord formation and fetal Leydig cell differentiation (Callier et al. 2014).

Cord Formation

Testis cord formation is initiated by the clustering of pre-SCs around germ cells, first evident as 'proto-cords' in the mouse testis at 12 days post-conception (DPC) and 7 WPC in the human (Francavilla et al. 1990; Heyn et al. 2001). Within 24 h in the mouse, definitive cords have formed (Nel-Themaat et al. 2009; Combes et al. 2009a), made up of germ cells surrounded by epithelialized SCs (Nel-Themaat et al. 2011), encased by peritubular myoid cells (PMCs, smooth muscle) and ECM (Maekawa et al. 1996; Skinner et al. 1985). This boundary tissue is termed lamina propria, and also contains myofibroblasts in humans (Davidoff et al. 1990; Dym 1994; Holstein et al. 1996). The cords elongate, causing expansion of the gonad, eventually forming the 'spaghetti'-like network of tubules seen in the mature adult testes (Combes et al. 2009a; Nel-Themaat et al. 2009). A protective layer of fibrous tissue surrounds the testes. The main component is the tunica albuginea, formed due to basement membrane deposition just beneath the CE (Carmona et al. 2009), plus smooth muscle (Langford and Heller 1973) and contractile cells (Middendorff et al. 2002). Its rhythmic contractions regulate blood flow, sperm movement, and intertesticular pressure (Ohanian et al. 1979; Banks et al. 2006).

Pre-SCs originate from the CE and express Sry, which induces their differentiation to primitive SCs (Karl and Capel 1998; Albrecht and Eicher 2001; Bullejos and Koopman 2001), which are Sox9, Amh and Dhh positive (Josso et al. 1993; Morais da Silva et al. 1996; Park et al. 2005). The molecular mechanisms underpinning cord formation are not clearly understood, but involve Sertoli-derived nerve growth factor 3 and its receptors Ntrk1 and Ntrk3 (Russo et al. 1999; Cupp et al. 2000; Levine et al. 2000), involved in forming adhesive cell contacts (Cupp et al. 2002,; Gassei et al. 2008), and Fgf9 diffusion (Hiramatsu et al. 2010). Tgfβ, activin, and inhibin b signalling also play a role (Yao et al. 2006; Memon et al. 2008; Sarraj et al. 2010; Liu et al. 2010; Miles et al. 2013). Germ cells themselves do not provide the trigger for cord formation, as cords develop normally in XY gonads without germ cells (Merchant 1975; McCoshen 1982; McCoshen 1983; Escalante-Alcalde and Merchant-Larios 1992). In contrast, germ cell progression through meiosis is essential for ovarian development (Adams and McLaren 2002).

Vascularization of the gonadal ridge, the formation of the major coelomic vessel and interstitial microvasculature, is crucial for cord formation (Cool et al. 2008; Coveney et al. 2008; Brennan et al. 2002; Combes et al. 2009b). Migration of vascular endothelial cells requires endothelial expressed platelet-derived growth factor B (PDGF-B) and mesenchymal expressed vascular endothelial growth factor A (VEGF-A) (Brennan et al. 2003; Bott et al. 2006; Cool et al. 2011). Yolk sac derived macrophages also mediate vascular reorganization (DeFalco et al. 2014).

Mesonephric cell migration into the gonad is also necessary for cord formation (Buehr et al. 1993a; Martineau et al. 1997; Tilmann and Capel 1999), the cells of which contribute to the Leydig and endothelial cell populations (Martineau et al. 1997; Merchant-Larios and Moreno-Mendoza 1998). Cell migration requires pre-SCs lying beneath the CE (Tilmann and Capel 2002) and Fgf9 (Colvin et al. 2001).

Germ Cells

Human PGC number increases rapidly in the testis from ~3000 at 6 WPC to ~30 000 at 9 WPC (Bendsen et al. 2003). At around 41–44 days postconception, between E12.5 and E14.5 in the mouse, PGCs begin to enter mitotic arrest in G0/G1 as prospermatogonia, associated with SC differentiation and testicular cord formation (Gondos and Hobel 1971; Western et al. 2008), resuming mitosis after birth (McLaren 1984), with meiosis delayed until well after birth (McLaren 1988). Mitotic arrest is induced by expression of the cell cycle regulator retinoblastoma 1 (Spiller et al. 2010).

Somatic Factors Acting on XY Germ Cells

The chromosomal make-up of germ cells does not influence their sex differentiation, XX germ cells in the testis will differentiate to spermatogonia, whereas XY germ cells in the ovary develop into oogonia (McLaren 2000), demonstrating that somatic secreted factors play a determining role.

RA is secreted from the mesonephros in XX and XY gonads (Bowles et al. 2006), and somatic cells in the testis (Bowles et al. 2009) due to expression of retinaldehyde dehydrogenases (ALDHs). Meiosis in the fetal testis is antagonized by Fgf9 expression, which reduces the responsiveness of germ cells to RA (Barrios et al. 2010; Bowles et al. 2010) and Sox9/Sry-induced expression of Cyp26b1 (Bowles et al. 2006; MacLean et al. 2007; Kashimada et al. 2011b), a P450 enzyme that degrades RA. The human fetal testis, however, may respond to RA, as RA receptors are present but *CYP26B1* is absent (Cupp et al. 1999; Childs et al. 2011). Fgf9 also prolongs germ cell pluripotency by stimulating the expression of the Nodal coreceptor Cripto (Bowles and Koopman 2010; Spiller et al. 2012). Fsh promotes the survival of germ cells (Meachem et al. 2005), and Tgfβ and Activin A regulate quiescence (Moreno et al. 2010; Mendis et al. 2011).

Leydig Cells

The androgen producing cells of the testis, the Leydig cells, are found within the interstitial compartment at around 8 WPC in the human testis (Codesal et al. 1990). However, their origin is unknown (Griswold and Behringer 2009; DeFalco et al. 2011; Barsoum et al. 2013). Their initial differentiation is induced by SC-derived PDGF binding to the PDGFRα (Brennan et al. 2003), the paracrine action of Dhh (Barsoum et al. 2009; Huang and Yao 2010) and Notch signalling (Tang et al. 2008). Human fetal testosterone production is detectable by 9 weeks, peaks between weeks 15 and 16, before dropping sharply (Reyes et al. 1974). Initial androgen production does not require gonadotrophin stimulation (Word et al. 1989) but placental-derived human chorionic gonadotrophin (hCG) and, in the third trimester, fetal pituitary luteinizing hormone (LH), regulate final differentiation and androgen production (Rabinovici and Jaffe 1990; Mendis-Handagama 1997).

Male Differentiation of the Internal Reproductive Tract

Leydig cell-derived testosterone and insulin-like growth factor 3 (Insl3) cause WD stabilization and differentiation into the epididymis, vas deferens, and seminal vesicle, masculization of the external genitalia, and testicular descent (Nef and Parada 1999; Klonisch et al. 2004; Hannema and Hughes 2007; Feng et al. 2009; Ivell and Anand-Ivell 2011). Insl3 controls the first, transabdominal phase of testicular descent, by stimulating gubernaculums testis development (Kumagai et al. 2002). Testosterone is converted to dihydrotestosterone (DHT) by 5α-reductase, which has a higher affinity for the androgen receptor (AR) and thus is a more potent driver of external genitalia and prostate development (Wilson et al. 1981; Imperato-McGinley and Zhu 2002). In addition, the testis itself produces DHT via a testosterone-independent pathway (Wilson et al. 2002). The AR translocates to the nucleus upon stimulation and binds to androgen response elements to regulate gene transcription (Roche et al. 1992; Jenster et al. 1993). androgens are responsible for the inguinoscrotal phase of testicular descent (Su et al. 2012) and the disappearance of the cranial suspensory ligament (van der Schoot and Elger 1992).

The MDs regress at around 8 WPC due to apoptosis (Roberts et al. 1999; Allard et al. 2000), in turn, due to Sertoli-derived AMH (Josso et al. 2006, Josso et al. 2012). AMH is a member of the Tgfβ family (Cate et al. 1986), whose expression is triggered by Sox9 (Arango et al. 1999), increased by Sf1, Gata4, and Wt1 (Watanabe et al. 2000; Hossain and Saunders 2003; Viger et al. 2008), and stimulated by

Fsh postnatally (Al-Attar et al. 1997; Lukas-Croisier et al. 2003; Young et al. 2005).

Male Differentiation of the External Genitalia

Up to around 9 WPC, the external genitalia remain undifferentiated (Jirasek 1977). The genital tubercle elongates to form the penis in males, beginning around 9 WPC by lengthening of the angogenital distance (Jirasek 1977). Part of the cloacal folds form the urogenital folds, which surround the urogenital ostium laterally. Fusion of the labioscrotal folds occurs, forming the epithelial seam of the scrotum (Baskin et al. 2001). The proximal urethra forms by fusion of the urethral folds around the urethral plate, and the distal urethra arises from an invagination of the apical ectoderm. The urethral folds fuse in the midline converting the urethral groove into the penile urethra, which is formed by 14 WPC; however, there is no difference in penile and clitoral size until 14 WPC (Feldman and Smith 1975; Zalel et al. 2001). The third trimester sees maximal phallic growth, curiously at a time when testosterone levels are declining (Winter et al. 1977; O'Shaughnessy et al. 2007)

The urogenital sinus is the precursor to the bladder, urethra, and prostate and is formed in response to androgens on E13.5 (approx. 6 WPC) as cylindrical gut endoderm surrounded by mesenchyme (Goldstein and Wilson 1975; Cunha and Lung 1978). Up to around 9 WPC, it remains undifferentiated. Solid epithelial outgrowths (prostatic buds) form by E16.5 in the mouse, or 10 WPC in the human (Cunha et al. 1987). There is a period of quiescence in the human, until puberty, when increased androgen levels promote prostatic growth, forming the complex ductal network of the prostatic gland (Glenister 1962; Berry et al. 1984). The prostatic utricle forms – the male equivalent of the vagina, as an epithelial-lined diverticulum of the prostatic urethra – it serves no function (Glenister 1962).

Ovarian Differentiation

Ovarian development is generally considered to be the default pathway (Jost 1947; Burgoyne 1988; Goodfellow and Darling 1988), occurring in the absence of *Sry* expression and the presence of Wnt4, Fst, and Foxl2 (Tevosian 2013). Ovarian development involves germ cell meiosis and apoptosis, granulosa cell differentiation, and primordial follicle formation.

Germ Cells

Survival and Proliferation
Deleted in AZoospermia (Dazl)
The RNA-binding protein Dazl is one of the first factors expressed by PGCs required for ovarian development. It is detected shortly after PGC migration (Cooke et al. 1996) and knockout causes oocyte loss at the time of meiotic entry (McNeilly et al. 2000). It is thought to enable the gonads to respond to ovarian cues (Gill et al. 2011).

Factor in Germ Line α *(Figlα)*
Figlα is a transcription factor expressed by oocytes from E13 (Liang et al. 1997), required for germ cell survival and primordial follicle formation (Soyal et al. 2000; Lei et al. 2006).

Wnt4
In the absence of Sry, Wnt4 is expressed in the female gonad from E12.5 (Heikkila et al. 2005) and represses Fgf9 and Sox9 expression and stabilizes β-catenin (Kim et al. 2006), as well as upregulating Dax1, which antagonizes Sf1 and thereby inhibits steroidogenic enzymes (Jordan et al. 2001). Wnt4 is required for female germ cell survival (Yao et al. 2004) and null XX embryos exhibit masculinized gonads (Vainio et al. 1999). It prevents the production of steroids and the formation of the male-specific coelomic blood vessels by preventing the binding of β-catenin to Sf1 sites on steroidogenic genes (Jeays-Ward et al. 2003; Jordan et al. 2003).

R-spondin1 (Rspo1)
Rspo1 is essential for ovarian development in several vertebrate species, and upregulates Wnt4 in a cooperative manner to increase β-catenin and Fst levels (Yao et al. 2004; Parma et al. 2006; Chassot et al. 2008; Kim et al. 2008; Smith et al. 2008; Tomizuka et al. 2008). β-catenin then activates Wnt4 expression in a positive feedback loop (Chang et al. 2008). Rspo1 knockout impairs ovarian development, but does not cause sex reversal (Chassot et al. 2008; Tomizuka et al. 2008), and overexpression does not perturb testis

differentiation (Buscara et al. 2009). Rspo1 stimulates germ cell proliferation, and with Wnt4 regulates germ cell entry into meiosis (Naillat et al. 2010; Chassot et al. 2011) and maintains pregranulosa cell quiescence (Maatouk et al. 2013). Human RSPO1 is upregulated between 6 and 9 WPC, and augments β-catenin signalling (Tomaselli et al. 2011).

β-catenin regulates germ cell fate, possibly by regulating cell–cell adhesion (Fleming et al. 2012) along with Wnt4 (Naillat et al. 2010). It prevents Sf1 binding to the Sox9 TESCO enhancer, inhibiting Sox9 expression and SC differentiation (Bernard et al. 2012). It also induces Fst expression, which represses Activin B thus inhibiting endothelial cell migration and coelomic vessel formation (Yao et al. 2004; Yao et al. 2006).

Ablation of Rspo1, Wnt4 and β-catenin causes development of seminiferous tubules in XX gonads (Chassot et al. 2008), indicating that the three genes together are required to suppress the male pathway.

Fst

Fst acts downstream of Wnt4 to promote germ cell survival (Yao et al. 2004), and knockout causes infertility (Kimura et al. 2010; Kimura et al. 2011). Wnt4 is required to initiate, but not maintain, Fst expression; this requires Bmp2 and Foxl2 (Kashimada et al. 2011a). Bmp2 is expressed in the gonad at E12.5 (Yao et al. 2004), but its role in ovarian development is unknown.

Gata4-Fog2 interaction

The Gata4 and Fog2 interaction, required for testis formation, is also required for early ovarian differentiation, with knockout resulting in multiple defects including reduced Fst, Wnt4, and Foxl2 expression (expression of Sf1 is not affected) (Manuylov et al. 2008). The Gata4-Fog2 complex serves as a repressor of Dickkopf Wnt signalling pathway inhibitor 1 (Dkk1), which inhibits β-catenin signalling.

Meiosis

Between 10.5 and 13.5 DPC in the mouse ovary, mitotic germ cells (oogonia) develop as clusters of interconnected cells, termed germ cell cysts (Pepling and Spradling 1998). Cyst formation occurs due to incomplete mitosis, with daughter germ cells remaining connected to one another by intercellular bridges (McKearin and Ohlstein 1995). Whilst within these cysts, germ cells lose expression of Oct4 (Pesce et al. 1998) and enter meiosis, at around E13.5 in the mouse, and approximately 12 WPC in the human (Gondos and Hobel 1971). The intercellular bridges breakdown and the oocytes become enclosed within ovigerous cords, forming 'pregranulosa cells' surrounded by a basal lamina (Odor and Blandau 1969; Gondos 1987; Pepling and Spradling 1998). There are two waves of pregranulosa cell recruitment from the surface epithelium; one just before sexual differentiation and the second immediately postbirth during follicle formation (Harikae et al. 2013b).

RA binding to its receptor causes meiotic entry of germ cells, stimulated by retinoic acid gene 8 (Stra8) gene expression (Baltus et al. 2006; Koubova et al. 2006; Childs et al. 2011). Stra8 functions in premeiotic DNA replication and chromosome cohesion and synapsis (Baltus et al. 2006). Sycp1 (Synaptonemal complex protein 1) (de Vries et al. 2005), Sycp3 (Di Carlo et al. 2000; Yuan et al. 2002) and Rec8 (yeast meiotic recombination protein Rec8 homologue) (Prieto et al. 2004) are then expressed, which are involved in the formation of the meiotic synaptonemal and cohesion complexes respectively, marking the beginning of prophase I. Germ cells that do not undergo cell death progress through leptonema, zygonema, pachynema, and diplonema, entering a prolonged arrest stage termed dictyate around the time of birth (Borum 1961; Borum 1967; Speed 1982). They remain in this stage until just before ovulation, when they complete the first meiotic division, begin the second, and arrest again; meiosis is completed only at fertilization.

Germ cells enter meiotic prophase at about the same time even if outside the genital ridge (Zamboni and Upadhyay 1983; McLaren 1995; Chuma and Nakatsuji 2001); thus the default pathway for a germ cell is to develop as an oocyte, unless it is within the male genital ridge.

Apoptosis

At around 20 WPC, germ cell cysts break down forming primordial follicles, i.e. individual oocytes surrounded by a layer of squamous granulosa (follicular) cells with an underlying layer of basement membrane (Pepling and Spradling 2001; Hummitzsch et al. 2013). Only one third of oocytes form primordial follicles, the rest die (McGee et al. 1998; Pepling et al. 2010), either by Bcl2-dependent apoptosis (Felici et al. 1999; Yan et al. 2000) or autophagy (Rodrigues et al. 2009). There are two waves of apoptosis in the fetal mouse; the first coincides with entry to meiosis (E13.5-15.5) and the second with primordial follicle assembly (E17.5 to postnatal day 1) (Coucouvanis et al. 1993; Ratts et al. 1995).

In the human, apoptosis occurs primarily between 14 and 28 WPC (Vaskivuo et al. 2001). Human females are unable to produce oocytes beyond 34 WPC. The fetus is born with two million oocytes, which declines to 400 000 at puberty and 400 by ovulation. Only a few follicles develop to preovulatory follicles, and thus only a few oocytes undergo ovulation, with the majority of follicles and oocytes degenerating before ovulation (Baker 1963). Primary follicles are first detected around 15–16 weeks, and Graafian follicles around 23–24 weeks (Pryse-Davies and Dewhurst 1971; Reynaud et al. 2004).

Granulosa Cell Differentiation and Primordial Follicle Formation

Transcription Factors

Forkhead box L2 (Foxl2) is a member of the forkhead box gene family, whose expression is stimulated by Rspo1 and β-catenin (Manuylov et al. 2008; Auguste et al. 2011). It is one of the earliest granulosa cell markers, detected around E11.5 (Wilhelm et al. 2009), and required for granulosa cell differentiation and the development of primary follicles (Schmidt et al. 2004; Uda et al. 2004; Ottolenghi et al. 2005). Foxl2 directly acts on the Sox9 TESCO enhancer to repress Sox9 expression (Uhlenhaut et al. 2009) and represses Sf1 expression by antagonizing Wt1-KTS (Takasawa et al. 2014). It also promotes germ cell survival (Uhlenhaut et al. 2009). While Rspo1 and Wnt4 regulate ovarian development cooperatively, Wnt4 and Foxl2 operate through independent, but complementary, pathways (Ottolenghi et al. 2007; Schlessinger et al. 2010). When Wnt4 or Foxl2 is knocked-down, the other is still expressed (Ottolenghi et al. 2007; Chassot et al. 2008; Manuylov et al. 2008), and each regulate distinct sets of genes (Garcia-Ortiz et al. 2009). Ablation of both Foxl2 and Wnt4 causes testis differentiation in XX mice. However, the reversal

is incomplete, with ovarian somatic cells and oocytes remaining (Ottolenghi et al. 2007).

Despite the complicated interplay between Rspo1, Wnt4, β-catenin, and Foxl2 in establishing and maintaining the ovary, the gonad is surprisingly plastic. Loss of Dmrt1 expression in SCs activates Foxl2 and reprograms them to granulosa cells (Matson et al. 2011). In contrast, Dmrt1 expression in the ovary silences Foxl2 and reprograms granulosa cells to SCs (Lindeman et al. 2015).

Both Gata4 and Gata6 are required later, independently of the Fog2 interaction for granulosa cell proliferation and differentiation, and thus primordial follicular development (Bennett et al. 2012; Padua et al. 2014). Gata4 granulosa cell-specific knockout mice are subfertile, whereas Gata6 knockouts have no reproductive defects (Kyronlahti et al. 2011; Bennett et al. 2012), indicating that Gata4 plays a more substantial role (Bennett et al. 2013).

Newborn ovary homeobox protein (Nobox), spermatogenesis, and oogenesis specific bHLH 1 (Sohlh1) and Sohlh2 are critical transcription factors required for the primordial to primary follicle transition (Rajkovic et al. 2004; Choi et al. 2008b; Bouilly et al. 2014). Nobox is expressed in the oocyte and granulosa cells; it inhibits Foxl2 activation of its own promoter (Bouilly et al. 2014), and upregulates the Growth differentiation factor 9 (Gdf9) promoter (Bayne et al. 2015). Sohlh1 and 2 are expressed in oocytes (Ballow et al. 2006; Pangas et al. 2006), and knockout reduces Nobox and Lhx8 expression (Pangas et al. 2006; Choi et al. 2008b). Lhx8 is also expressed in oocytes and involved in folliculogenesis (Choi et al. 2008a).

Signalling Molecules

Tgfβ and Notch signalling are involved in cyst breakdown and primordial follicle formation. Bmp15 and Gdf9 play a synergistic role in stimulating primary follicle development (Yan et al. 2001), and Activin A increases germ and granulosa cell proliferation (Bristol-Gould et al. 2006). In addition, Fst is required for germ cell cyst breakdown and primordial follicle formation (Kimura et al. 2011). Finally, AMH is expressed in postnatal granulosa cells and inhibits primordial follicle growth (Baarends et al. 1995; Durlinger et al. 2002; Nilsson et al. 2011). Mutation of the Notch signalling regulator, lunatic fringe, causes aberrant folliculogenesis (Hahn et al. 2005), and suppression of Notch signalling decreases primordial follicle formation (Trombly et al. 2009).

Neurotrophins (Ntfs) are also involved in follicle formation. Nerve growth factor and the neurotrophin tyrosine kinase receptors 1 and 2 (Ntrk1 and 2) are required for the primordial follicle growth (Dissen et al. 2001; Kerr et al. 2009), and Ntf4 and Brain-derived neurotrophic factor (Bdnf) promote oocyte survival (Spears et al. 2003).

Female Differentiation of the Internal Reproductive Tract

Female differentiation of the internal reproductive tract involves the loss of the WDs at 13 WPC, due to the absence of androgens, and persistence of the MDs, in the presence of oestrogen. The proximal part of the ducts form the Fallopian tubes and the distal portion forms the uterus, cervix, and upper vagina (Orvis and Behringer 2007). The uterine endometrium develops as an epithelial tube and the myometrium develops from surrounding mesenchyme; both are fully differentiated by 20 WPC (Arango et al. 2008). The uterovaginal canal is formed by 22 WPC, and the vaginal epithelium is formed from the vaginal plate, which originates from the urogenital sinus, over the next 2 months (Fritsch et al. 2013).

Female Differentiation of the External Genitalia

The genital tubercle lengthens and then retracts, and after 14 WPC, the clitoris becomes visible. The lower end of the vagina opens onto the perineum surface at 22 WPC. The remainder of external genitalia development in the female is fairly benign, unlike the male. The genital swellings do not fuse, forming the labia majora, fusing at the front (mons pubis) and the rear (commissure of the labia), and the urogenital sinus remains wide open, with the urethra in the anterior part and the vagina in the posterior part. The urethral folds do not fuse, but form the labia minora.

Genetic and Hormonal Control of Female Differentiation

The use of knockout mice has revealed a number of factors essential for female development. Vaginal and cervical development requires Wnt5A (Suzuki et al. 2003; Mericskay et al. 2004), Pax8-null mice lack a vaginal opening or uterus (Mittag et al. 2007) and Van Gogh-like 2 (Vangl2), a protein involved in regulating cell polarity, also regulates vaginal opening (Kibar et al. 2001). The development of the female reproductive tract is regulated by oestrogens, acting on ERα and ERβ. ERα is expressed in the uterus, vagina, and thecal cells, whereas ERβ is expressed in granulosa cells (Couse and Korach 1999; Muramatsu and Inoue 2000).

Conclusion

This chapter has described sexual development and determination during embryogenesis, highlighting the key regulatory genes and molecules involved in the process. While much of this information has been gleaned from the mouse, and is likely to be applicable to the human, a number of key differences between the species exist, for example the absence of SOX2 in hPGCs and the lack of CYP26B1 expression and Gata4 Sry regulation in the human testis, highlighting the need for further work before these processes in humans are fully elucidated.

References

Adams, I.R. and McLaren, A. (2002). Sexually dimorphic development of mouse primordial germ cells: switching from oogenesis to spermatogenesis. Development 129: 1155–1164.

Agoulnik, A.I., Lu, B., Zhu, Q. et al. (2002). A novel gene, Pog, is necessary for primordial germ cell proliferation in the mouse and underlies the germ cell deficient mutation, gcd. Hum Mol Genet 11: 3047–3053.

Al-Attar, L., Noel, K., Dutertre, M. et al. (1997). Hormonal and cellular regulation of Sertoli cell anti-Mullerian hormone production in the postnatal mouse. J Clin Invest 100: 1335–1343.

Albrecht, K.H. and Eicher, E.M. (2001). Evidence that *Sry* is expressed in pre-Sertoli cells and Sertoli and granulosa cells have a common precursor. Dev Biol 240: 92–107.

Allard, S., Adin, P., Gouedard, L. et al. (2000). Molecular mechanisms of hormone-mediated Mullerian duct regression: involvement of beta-catenin. Development 127: 3349–3360.

Anderson, R., Copeland, T.K., Scholer, H. et al. (2000). The onset of germ cell migration in the mouse embryo. Mech Dev 91: 61–68.

Anderson, R., Fassler, R., Georges-Labouesse, E. et al. (1999). Mouse primordial germ cells lacking beta1 integrins enter the germline but fail to migrate normally to the gonads. Development 126: 1655–1664.

Anderson, R. A., Fulton, N., Cowan, G. et al. (2007). Conserved and divergent patterns of expression of DAZL, VASA and OCT4 in the germ cells of the human fetal ovary and testis. BMC Dev Biol 7: 136.

Ara, T., Nakamura, Y., Egawa, T. et al. (2003). Impaired colonization of the gonads by primordial germ cells in mice lacking a chemokine, stromal cell-derived factor-1 (SDF-1). Proc Natl Acad Sci USA 100: 5319–5323.

Aramaki, S., Hayashi, K., Kurimoto, K. et al. (2013). A mesodermal factor, T, specifies mouse germ cell fate by directly activating germline determinants. Dev Cell 27: 516–529.

Arango, N.A., Kobayashi, A., Wang, Y. et al. (2008). A mesenchymal perspective of Mullerian duct differentiation and regression in *Amhr2-lacZ* mice. Mol Reprod Dev 75: 1154–1162.

Arango, N.A., Lovell-Badge, R. and Behringer, R.R. (1999). Targeted mutagenesis of the endogenous mouse *Mis* gene promoter: in vivo definition of genetic pathways of vertebrate sexual development. Cell 99: 409–419.

Assumpcao, J.G., Ferraz, L.F., Benedetti, C.E. et al. (2005). A naturally occurring deletion in the SRY promoter region affecting the Sp1 binding site is associated with sex reversal. J Endocrinol Invest 28: 651–656.

Auguste, A., Chassot, A.A., Gregoire, E.P. et al. (2011). Loss of *R-spondin1* and *Foxl2* amplifies female-to-male sex reversal in XX mice. Sex Dev 5: 304–317.

Baarends, W.M., Uilenbroek, J.T., Kramer, P. et al. (1995). Anti-mullerian hormone and anti-mullerian hormone type II receptor messenger ribonucleic acid expression in rat ovaries during postnatal development, the estrous cycle, and gonadotropin-induced follicle growth. Endocrinology 136: 4951–4962.

Bagheri-Fam, S., Barrionuevo, F., Dohrmann, U. et al. (2006). Long-range upstream and downstream enhancers control distinct subsets of the complex spatiotemporal *Sox9* expression pattern. Dev Biol 291: 382–397.

Bagheri-Fam, S., Sim, H., Bernard, P. et al. (2008). Loss of *Fgfr2* leads to partial XY sex reversal. Dev Biol 314: 71–83.

Baillie, A. H. (1964). The histochemistry and ultrastructure of the genocyte. J Anat 98: 641–645.

Baker, T.G. (1963). A quantitative and cytological study of germ cells in human ovaries. Proc R Soc Lond B Biol Sci 158: 417–433.

Ballow, D.J., Xin, Y., Choi, Y. et al. (2006). *Sohlh2* is a germ cell-specific bHLH transcription factor. Gene Expr Patterns 6: 1014–1018.

Baltus, A.E., Menke, D.B., Hu, Y.C. et al. (2006). In germ cells of mouse embryonic ovaries, the decision to enter meiosis precedes premeiotic DNA replication. Nat Genet 38: 1430–1434.

Bandiera, R., Vidal, V.P., Motamedi, F.J. et al. (2013). WT1 maintains adrenal-gonadal primordium identity and marks a population of AGP-like progenitors within the adrenal gland. Dev Cell 27: 5–18.

Banks, F.C., Knight, G.E., Calvert, R.C. et al. (2006). Smooth muscle and purinergic contraction of the human, rabbit, rat, and mouse testicular capsule. Biol Reprod 74: 473–480.

Bardoni, B., Zanaria, E., Guioli, S. et al. (1994). A dosage sensitive locus at chromosome Xp21 is involved in male to female sex reversal. Nat Genet 7: 497–501.

Barrios, F., Filipponi, D., Pellegrini, M. et al. (2010). Opposing effects of retinoic acid and FGF9 on *Nanos2* expression and meiotic entry of mouse germ cells. J Cell Sci 123: 871–880.

Barski, A., Cuddapah, S., Cui, K. et al. (2007). High-resolution profiling of histone methylations in the human genome. Cell 129: 823–837.

Barsoum, I.B., Bingham, N.C., Parker, K.L. et al. (2009). Activation of the Hedgehog pathway in the mouse fetal ovary leads to ectopic appearance of fetal Leydig cells and female pseudohermaphroditism. Dev Biol 329: 96–103.

Barsoum, I.B., Kaur, J., Ge, R.S. et al. (2013). Dynamic changes in fetal Leydig cell populations influence adult Leydig cell populations in mice. FASEB J 27: 2657–2666.

Baskin, L.S., Erol, A., Jegatheesan, P. et al. (2001). Urethral seam formation and hypospadias. Cell Tissue Res 305: 379–387.

Bayne, R.A., Kinnell, H.L., Coutts, S.M. et al. (2015). GDF9 is transiently expressed in oocytes before follicle formation in the human fetal ovary and is regulated by a Novel NOBOX Transcript. PLoS One 10: e0119819.

Bendel-Stenzel, M.R., Gomperts, M., Anderson, R. et al. (2000). The role of cadherins during primordial germ cell migration and early gonad formation in the mouse. Mech Dev 91: 143–152.

Bendsen, E., Byskov, A.G., Laursen, S.B. et al. (2003). Number of germ cells and somatic cells in human fetal testes during the first weeks after sex differentiation. Hum Reprod 18: 13–18.

Bennett, J., Baumgarten, S.C. and Stocco, C. (2013). GATA4 and GATA6 silencing in ovarian granulosa cells affects levels of mRNAs involved in steroidogenesis, extracellular structure organization, IGF-I activity, and apoptosis. Endocrinology 154: 4845–4858.

Bennett, J., Wu, Y.G., Gossen, J. et al. (2012). Loss of GATA-6 and GATA-4 in granulosa cells blocks folliculogenesis, ovulation, and follicle stimulating hormone receptor expression leading to female infertility. Endocrinology 153: 2474–2485.

Bernard, P., Ryan, J., Sim, H. et al. (2012). Wnt signaling in ovarian development inhibits Sf1 activation of *Sox9* via the *Tesco* enhancer. Endocrinology 153: 901–912.

Berry, S.J., Coffey, D.S., Walsh, P.C. et al. (1984). The development of human benign prostatic hyperplasia with age. J Urol 132: 474–479.

Bhandari, R.K., Sadler-Riggleman, I., Clement, T.M. et al. (2011). Basic helix-loop-helix transcription factor TCF21 is a downstream target of the male sex determining gene SRY. PLoS One 6: e19935.

Bhattacharya, S., Michels, C.L., Leung, M.K. et al. (1999). Functional role of p35srj, a novel p300/CBP binding protein, during transactivation by HIF-1. Genes Dev 13: 64–75.

Bingham, C., Ellard, S., Cole, T.R. et al. (2002). Solitary functioning kidney and diverse genital tract malformations associated with hepatocyte nuclear factor-1beta mutations. Kidney Int 61: 1243–1251.

Birk, O.S., Casiano, D.E., Wassif, C.A. et al. (2000). The LIM homeobox gene *Lhx9* is essential for mouse gonad formation. Nature 403: 909–913.

Bishop, C.E., Whitworth, D.J., Qin, Y. et al. (2000). A transgenic insertion upstream of *Sox9* is associated with dominant XX sex reversal in the mouse. Nat Genet 26: 490–494.

Bitgood, M.J. and McMahon, A.P. (1995). *Hedgehog* and *Bmp* genes are coexpressed at many diverse sites of cell-cell interaction in the mouse embryo. Dev Bio, 172: 126–138.

Borum, K. (1961). Oogenesis in the mouse. A study of the meiotic prophase. Exp Cell Res 24: 495–507.

Borum, K. (1967). Oogenesis in the mouse. A study of the origin of the mature ova. Exp Cell Res 45: 39–47.

Bott, R.C., Mcfee, R.M., Clopton, D.T. et al. (2006). Vascular endothelial growth factor and kinase domain region receptor are involved in both seminiferous cord formation and vascular development during testis morphogenesis in the rat. Biol Reprod 75: 56–67.

Bouilly, J., Veitia, R.A. and Binart, N. (2014). NOBOX is a key FOXL2 partner involved in ovarian folliculogenesis. J Mol Cell Biol 6: 175–177.

Bowles, J., Feng, C.W., Knight, D. et al. (2009). Male-specific expression of *Aldh1a1* in mouse and chicken fetal testes: implications for retinoid balance in gonad development. Dev Dyn 238: 2073–2080.

Bowles, J., Feng, C.W., Spiller, C. et al. (2010). FGF9 suppresses meiosis and promotes male germ cell fate in mice. Dev Cell 19: 440–449.

Bowles, J., Knight, D., Smith, C. et al. (2006). Retinoid signaling determines germ cell fate in mice. Science 312: 596–600.

Bowles, J. and Koopman, P. (2010). Sex determination in mammalian germ cells: extrinsic versus intrinsic factors. Reproduction 139: 943–958.

Bradford, S.T., Hiramatsu, R., Maddugoda, M.P. et al. (2009). The cerebellin 4 precursor gene is a direct target of SRY and SOX9 in mice. Biol Reprod 80: 1178–1188.

Braganca, J., Eloranta, J.J., Bamforth, S.D. et al. (2003). Physical and functional interactions among AP-2 transcription factors, p300/CREB-binding protein, and CITED2. J Biol Chem 278: 16021–16029.

Brennan, J., Karl, J. and Capel, B. (2002). Divergent vascular mechanisms downstream of Sry establish the arterial system in the XY gonad. Dev Biol 244: 418–428.

Brennan, J., Tilmann, C. and Capel, B. (2003). *Pdgfr-alpha* mediates testis cord organization and fetal Leydig cell development in the XY gonad. Genes Dev 17: 800–10.

Bristol-Gould, S.K., Kreeger, P.K., Selkirk, C.G. et al. (2006). Postnatal regulation of germ cells by activin: the establishment of the initial follicle pool. Dev Biol 298: 132–148.

Buaas, F.W., Val, P. and Swain, A. (2009). The transcription co-factor CITED2 functions during sex determination and early gonad development. Hum Mol Genet 18: 2989–3001.

Buehr, M., Gu, S. and McLaren, A. (1993a). Mesonephric contribution to testis differentiation in the fetal mouse. Development 117: 273–281.

Buehr, M., Mclaren, A., Bartley, A. et al. (1993b). Proliferation and migration of primordial germ cells in W^e/W^e mouse embryos. Dev Dyn 198: 182–189.

Bullejos, M. and Koopman, P. (2001). Spatially dynamic expression of *Sry* in mouse genital ridges. Dev Dyn 221: 201–205.

Bullejos, M. and Koopman, P. (2005). Delayed *Sry* and *Sox9* expression in developing mouse gonads underlies B6-Y(DOM) sex reversal. Dev Biol 278: 473–481.

Burgoyne, P.S. (1988). Role of mammalian Y chromosome in sex determination. Philos Trans R Soc Lond B Biol Sci 322: 63–72.

Buscara, L., Montazer-Torbati, F., Chadi, S. et al. (2009. Goat *RSPO1* over-expression rescues sex-reversal in *Rspo1*-knockout XX mice but does not perturb testis differentiation in XY or sex-reversed XX mice. Transgenic Res 18: 649–654.

Callier, P., Calvel, P., Matevossian, A. et al. (2014). Loss of function mutation in the palmitoyl-transferase HHAT leads to syndromic 46,XY disorder of sex development by impeding Hedgehog protein palmitoylation and signaling. PLoS Genet 10: e1004340.

Carmona, F.D., Lupianez, D.G., Martin, J.E. et al. (2009). The spatio-temporal pattern of testis organogenesis in mammals – insights from the mole. Int J Dev Biol 53: 1035–1044.

Carroll, T.J., Park, J.S., Hayashi, S. et al. (2005). Wnt9b plays a central role in the regulation of mesenchymal to epithelial transitions underlying organogenesis of the mammalian urogenital system. Dev Cell 9: 283–292.

Cate, R.L., Mattaliano, R.J., Hession, C. et al. (1986). Isolation of the bovine and human genes for Mullerian inhibiting substance and expression of the human gene in animal cells. Cell 45: 685–698.

Chaboissier, M.C., Kobayashi, A., Vidal, V.I. et al. (2004). Functional analysis of *Sox8* and *Sox9* during sex determination in the mouse. Development 131: 1891–1901.

Chambers, I., Silva, J., Colby, D. et al. (2007). Nanog safeguards pluripotency and mediates germline development. Nature 450: 1230–1234.

Chang, H., Gao, F., Guillou, F. et al. (2008). *Wt1* negatively regulates beta-catenin signaling during testis development. Development 135: 1875–1885.

Chassot, A.A., Bradford, S.T., Auguste, A. et al. (2012). WNT4 and RSPO1 together are required for cell proliferation in the early mouse gonad. Development 139: 4461–4472.

Chassot, A.A., Gregoire, E.P., Lavery, R., et al. (2011). RSPO1/beta-catenin signaling pathway regulates oogonia differentiation and entry into meiosis in the mouse fetal ovary. PLoS One 6: e25641.

Chassot, A.A., Ranc, F., Gregoire, E.P. et al. (2008). Activation of beta-catenin signaling by Rspo1 controls differentiation of the mammalian ovary. Hum Mol Genet 17: 1264–1277.

Chawengsaksophak, K., Svingen, T., Ng, E.T. et al. (2012). Loss of *Wnt5a* disrupts primordial germ cell migration and male sexual development in mice. Biol Reprod 86: 1–12.

Childs, A.J., Cowan, G., Kinnell, H.L. et al. (2011). Retinoic acid signalling and the control of meiotic entry in the human fetal gonad. PLoS One 6: e20249.

Choi, Y., Ballow, D.J., Xin, Y et al. (2008a). Lim homeobox gene, *Lhx8*, is essential for mouse oocyte differentiation and survival. Biol Reprod 79: 442–449.

Choi, Y., Yuan, D. and Rajkovic, A. (2008b). Germ cell-specific transcriptional regulator *Sohlh2* is essential for early mouse folliculogenesis and oocyte-specific gene expression. Biol Reprod 79: 1176–1182.

Chuma, S. and Nakatsuji, N. (2001). Autonomous transition into meiosis of mouse fetal germ cells in vitro and its inhibition by gp130-mediated signaling. Dev Biol 229: 468–479.

Clement, T.M., Bhandari, R.K., Sadler-Riggleman, I. et al. (2011). SRY directly regulates the neurotrophin 3 promoter during male sex determination and testis development in rats. Biol Reprod 85: 277–284.

Codesal, J., Regadera, J., Nistal, M. et al. (1990). Involution of human fetal Leydig cells. An immunohistochemical, ultrastructural and quantitative study. J Anat 172: 103–114.

Coffinier, C., Barra, J., Babinet, C. et al. (1999). Expression of the vHNF1/HNF1beta homeoprotein gene during mouse organogenesis. Mech Dev 89: 211–213.

Colvin, J.S., Green, R.P., Schmahl, J. et al. (2001). Male-to-female sex reversal in mice lacking fibroblast growth factor 9. Cell 104: 875–889.

Combes, A.N., Lesieur, E., Harley, V.R. et al. (2009a). Three-dimensional visualization of testis cord morphogenesis, a novel tubulogenic mechanism in development. Dev Dyn 238: 1033–1041.

Combes, A.N., Wilhelm, D., Davidson, T. et al. (2009b). Endothelial cell migration directs testis cord formation. Dev Biol 326: 112–120.

Cooke, H.J., Lee, M., Kerr, S. et al. (1996). A murine homologue of the human DAZ gene is autosomal and expressed only in male and female gonads. Hum Mol Genet 5: 513–516.

Cool, J., Carmona, F.D., Szucsik, J.C. et al. (2008). Peritubular myoid cells are not the migrating population required for testis cord formation in the XY gonad. Sex Dev 2: 128–133.

Cool, J., Defalco, T.J. and Capel, B. (2011). Vascular-mesenchymal cross-talk through Vegf and Pdgf drives organ patterning. Proc Natl Acad Sci USA 108: 167–172.

Coucouvanis, E.C., Sherwood, S.W., Carswell-Crumpton, C. et al. (1993). Evidence that the mechanism of prenatal germ cell death in the mouse is apoptosis. Exp Cell Res 209: 238–247.

Couse, J.F. and Korach, K.S. (1999). Estrogen receptor null mice: what have we learned and where will they lead us? Endocr Rev 20: 358–417.

Coveney, D., Cool, J., Oliver, T. et al. (2008). Four-dimensional analysis of vascularization during primary development of an organ, the gonad. Proc Natl Acad Sci USA 105: 7212–7217.

Cui, S., Ross, A., Stallings, N. et al. (2004). Disrupted gonadogenesis and male-to-female sex reversal in *Pod1* knockout mice. Development 131: 4095–4105.

Cunha, G.R., Donjacour, A.A., Cooke, P.S. et al. (1987). The endocrinology and developmental biology of the prostate. Endocr Rev 8: 338–362.

Cunha, G.R. and Lung, B. (1978). The possible influence of temporal factors in androgenic responsiveness of urogenital tissue recombinants from wild-type and androgen-insensitive (Tfm) mice. J Exp Zool 205: 181–193.

Cupp, A.S., Dufour, J.M., Kim, G. et al. (1999). Action of retinoids on embryonic and early postnatal testis development. Endocrinology 140: 2343–2352.

Cupp, A.S., Kim, G.H. and Skinner, M.K. (2000). Expression and action of neurotropin-3 and nerve growth factor in embryonic and early postnatal rat testis development. Biol Reprod 63: 1617–1628.

Cupp, A.S., Tessarollo, L. and Skinner, M.K. (2002). Testis developmental phenotypes in neurotropin receptor trkA and trkC null mutations: role in formation of seminiferous cords and germ cell survival. Biol Reprod 66: 1838–1845.

Cupp, A.S., Uzumcu, M. and Skinner, M.K. (2003). Chemotactic role of neurotropin 3 in the embryonic testis that facilitates male sex determination. Biol Reprod 68: 2033–2037.

Davidoff, M.S., Breucker, H., Holstein, A.F. et al. (1990). Cellular architecture of the lamina propria of human seminiferous tubules. Cell Tissue Res 262: 253–261.

Davis, R.J., Harding, M., Moayedi, Y. et al. (2008). Mouse *Dach1* and *Dach2* are redundantly required for Mullerian duct development. Genesis 46: 205–213.

De Santa Barbara, P., Mejean, C., Moniot, B. et al. (2001). Steroidogenic factor-1 contributes to the cyclic-adenosine monophosphate down-regulation of human SRY gene expression. Biol Reprod 64: 775–783.

De Vries, F.A., De Boer, E., Van Den Bosch, M. et al. (2005). Mouse *Sycp1* functions in synaptonemal complex assembly, meiotic recombination, and XY body formation. Genes Dev 19: 1376–1389.

Defalco, T., Bhattacharya, I., Williams, A. V. et al. (2014). Yolk-sac-derived macrophages regulate fetal testis vascularization and morphogenesis. Proc Natl Acad Sci USA 111: E2384–2393.

Defalco, T., Takahashi, S. and Capel, B. (2011). Two distinct origins for Leydig cell progenitors in the fetal testis. Dev Biol 352: 14–26.

Desclozeaux, M., Poulat, F., De Santa Barbara, P. et al. (1998). Characterization of two Sp1 binding sites of the human sex determining SRY promoter. Biochim Biophys Acta 1397: 247–252.

Di Carlo, A. and De Felici, M. (2000). A role for E-cadherin in mouse primordial germ cell development. Dev Biol 226: 209–219.

Di Carlo, A.D., Travia, G. and De Felici, M. (2000). The meiotic specific synaptonemal complex protein SCP3 is expressed by female and male primordial germ cells of the mouse embryo. Int J Dev Biol 44: 241–244.

Ding, J., Jiang, D., Kurczy, M. et al. (2008). Inhibition of HMG CoA reductase reveals an unexpected role for cholesterol during PGC migration in the mouse. BMC Dev Biol 8: 120.

Dissen, G.A., Romero, C., Hirshfield, A.N. et al. (2001). Nerve growth factor is required for early follicular development in the mammalian ovary. Endocrinology 142: 2078–2086.

Donovan, P.J., Stott, D., Cairns, L.A. et al. (1986). Migratory and postmigratory mouse primordial germ cells behave differently in culture. Cell 44: 831–838.

Durlinger, A.L., Gruijters, M.J., Kramer, P. et al. (2002). Anti-Mullerian hormone inhibits initiation of primordial follicle growth in the mouse ovary. Endocrinology 143: 1076–1084.

Dym, M. (1994). Basement membrane regulation of Sertoli cells. Endocr Rev 15: 102–115.

Eckert, D., Biermann, K., Nettersheim, D. et al. (2008). Expression of *BLIMP1/PRMT5* and concurrent histone H2A/H4 arginine 3 dimethylation in fetal germ cells, CIS/IGCNU and germ cell tumors. BMC Dev Biol 8: 106.

Escalante-Alcalde, D. and Merchant-Larios, H. (1992). Somatic and germ cell interactions during histogenetic aggregation of mouse fetal testes. Exp Cell Res 198: 150–158.

Extavour, C.G. and Akam, M. (2003). Mechanisms of germ cell specification across the metazoans: epigenesis and preformation. Development 130: 5869–5884.

Feldman, K.W. and Smith, D.W. (1975). Fetal phallic growth and penile standards for newborn male infants. J Pediatr 86: 395–398.

Felici, M.D., Carlo, A.D., Pesce, M. et al. (1999). Bcl-2 and Bax regulation of apoptosis in germ cells during prenatal oogenesis in the mouse embryo. Cell Death Differ 6: 908–915.

Feng, S., Ferlin, A., Truong, A. et al. (2009). INSL3/ RXFP2 signaling in testicular descent. Ann N Y Acad Sci 1160: 197–204.

Ffrench-Constant, C., Hollingsworth, A., Heasman, J. et al. (1991). Response to fibronectin of mouse primordial germ cells before, during and after migration. Development 113: 1365–1373.

Fleming, A., Ghahramani, N., Zhu, M.X. et al. (2012). Membrane beta-catenin and adherens junctions in early gonadal patterning. Dev Dyn 241: 1782–1798.

Foster, J.W., Dominguez-Steglich, M.A., Guioli, S. et al. (1994). Campomelic dysplasia and autosomal sex reversal caused by mutations in an *SRY*-related gene. Nature 372: 525–530.

Francavilla, S., Cordeschi, G., Properzi, G., et al. (1990). Ultrastructure of fetal human gonad before sexual differentiation and during early testicular and ovarian development. J Submicrosc Cytol Pathol 22: 389–400.

Fritsch, H., Hoermann, R., Bitsche, M. et al. (2013). Development of epithelial and mesenchymal regionalization of the human fetal utero-vaginal anlagen. J Anat 222: 462–472.

Fujimoto, T., Miyayama, Y. and Fuyuta, M. (1977). The origin, migration and fine morphology of human primordial germ cells. Anat Rec 188: 315–330.

Fujimoto, Y., Tanaka, S.S., Yamaguchi, Y.L. et al. (2013). Homeoproteins Six1 and Six4 regulate male sex determination and mouse gonadal development. Dev Cell 26: 416–430.

Fukami, M., Wada, Y., Okada, M. et al. (2008). Mastermind-like domain-containing 1 (*MAMLD1* or *CXorf6*) transactivates the *Hes3* promoter, augments testosterone production, and contains the SF1 target sequence. J Biol Chem 283,: 5525–5532.

Garcia-Castro, M.I., Anderson, R., Heasman, J. et al. (1997). Interactions between germ cells and extracellular matrix glycoproteins during migration and gonad assembly in the mouse embryo. J Cell Biol 138: 471–480.

Garcia-Ortiz, J.E., Pelosi, E., Omari, S. et al. (2009). *Foxl2* functions in sex determination and histogenesis throughout mouse ovary development. BMC Dev Biol 9: 36.

Gassei, K., Ehmcke, J. and Schlatt, S. (2008). Initiation of testicular tubulogenesis is controlled by neurotrophic tyrosine receptor kinases in a three-dimensional Sertoli cell aggregation assay. Reproduction 136: 459–469.

Georg, I., Barrionuevo, F., Wiech, T. et al. (2012). *Sox9* and *Sox8* are required for basal lamina integrity of testis cords and for suppression of FOXL2 during embryonic testis development in mice. Biol Reprod 87: 99.

Gierl, M.S., Gruhn, W.H., Von Seggern, A. et al. (2012). GADD45G functions in male sex determination by promoting p38 signaling and *Sry* expression. Dev Cell 23: 1032–1042.

Gill, M.E., Hu, Y.C., Lin, Y. et al. (2011). Licensing of gametogenesis, dependent on RNA binding protein DAZL, as a gateway to sexual differentiation of fetal germ cells. Proc Natl Acad Sci USA 108: 7443–7448.

Gkountela, S., Li, Z., Vincent, J.J., et al. (2013). The ontogeny of cKIT+ human primordial germ cells proves to be a resource for human germ line reprogramming, imprint erasure and in vitro differentiation. Nat Cell Biol 15: 113–122.

Glenister, T.W. (1962). The development of the utricle and of the so-called 'middle' or 'median' lobe of the human prostate. J Anat 96: 443–455.

Goldstein, J.L. and Wilson, J.D. (1975). Genetic and hormonal control of male sexual differentiation. J Cell Physiol 85: 365–377.

Goncalves, A. and Zeller, R. (2011). Genetic analysis reveals an unexpected role of BMP7 in initiation of ureteric bud outgrowth in mouse embryos. PLoS One 6: e19370.

Gondos, B. (1987). Comparative studies of normal and neoplastic ovarian germ cells: 2. Ultrastructure and pathogenesis of dysgerminoma. Int J Gynecol Pathol 6: 124–131.

Gondos, B. and Hobel, C.J. (1971). Ultrastructure of germ cell development in the human fetal testis. Z Zellforsch Mikrosk Anat 119: 1–20.

Goodfellow, P.N. and Darling, S.M. (1988). Genetics of sex determination in man and mouse. Development 102: 251–258.

Griswold, S.L. and Behringer, R.R. (2009). Fetal Leydig cell origin and development. Sex Dev 3: 1–15.

Grote, D., Souabni, A., Busslinger, M. et al. (2006). Pax 2/8-regulated Gata 3 expression is necessary for morphogenesis and guidance of the nephric duct in the developing kidney. Development 133: 53–61.

Guioli, S., Sekido, R. and Lovell-Badge, R. (2007). The origin of the Mullerian duct in chick and mouse. Dev Biol 302: 389–398.

Hacker, A., Capel, B., Goodfellow, P. et al. (1995). Expression of *Sry*, the mouse sex determining gene. Development 121: 1603–1614.

Hahn, K.L., Johnson, J., Beres, B.J. et al. (2005). Lunatic fringe null female mice are infertile due to defects in meiotic maturation. Development 132: 817–828.

Hajkova, P. (2011). Epigenetic reprogramming in the germline: towards the ground state of the epigenome. Philos Trans R Soc Lond B Biol Sci 366: 2266–2273.

Hajkova, P., Erhardt, S., Lane, N. et al. (2002). Epigenetic reprogramming in mouse primordial germ cells. Mech Dev 117: 15–23.

Hammes, A., Guo, J.K., Lutsch, G. et al. (2001). Two splice variants of the Wilms' tumor 1 gene have distinct functions during sex determination and nephron formation. Cell 106: 319–329.

Hannema, S.E. and Hughes, I.A. (2007). Regulation of Wolffian duct development. Horm Res 67: 142–151.

Hara, K., Kanai-Azuma, M., Uemura, M. et al. (2009). Evidence for crucial role of hindgut expansion in directing proper migration of primordial germ cells in mouse early embryogenesis. Dev Biol 330: 427–439.

Haraguchi, R., Suzuki, K., Murakami, R. et al. (2000). Molecular analysis of external genitalia formation: the role of fibroblast growth factor (Fgf) genes during genital tubercle formation. Development 127: 2471–2479.

Harikae, K., Miura, K. and Kanai, Y. (2013a). Early gonadogenesis in mammals: significance of long and narrow gonadal structure. Dev Dyn 242: 330–338.

Harikae, K., Miura, K., Shinomura, M. et al. (2013b). Heterogeneity in sexual bipotentiality and plasticity of granulosa cells in developing mouse ovaries. J Cell Sci 126: 2834–2844.

Hashimoto, R. (2003). Development of the human Mullerian duct in the sexually undifferentiated stage. Anat Rec A Discov Mol Cell Evol Biol 272: 514–519.

Heikkila, M., Prunskaite, R., Naillat, F. et al. (2005). The partial female to male sex reversal in *Wnt-4*-deficient females involves induced expression of testosterone biosynthetic genes and testosterone production, and depends on androgen action. Endocrinology 146: 4016–4023.

Heyn, R., Makabe, S. and Motta, P.M. (2001). Ultrastructural morphodynamics of human Sertoli cells during testicular differentiation. Ital J Anat Embryol 106: 163–171.

Hiramatsu, R., Harikae, K., Tsunekawa, N. et al. (2010). FGF signaling directs a center-to-pole expansion of tubulogenesis in mouse testis differentiation. Development 137: 303–312.

Hiramatsu, R., Matoba, S., Kanai-Azuma, M. et al. (2009). A critical time window of *Sry* action in gonadal sex determination in mice. Development 136: 129–138.

Holstein, A.F., Maekawa, M., Nagano, T. et al. (1996). Myofibroblasts in the lamina propria of human seminiferous tubules are dynamic structures of heterogeneous phenotype. Arch Histol Cytol 59: 109–125.

Hoshi, M., Batourina, E., Mendelsohn, C. et al. (2012). Novel mechanisms of early upper and lower urinary tract patterning regulated by RetY1015 docking tyrosine in mice. Development 139: 2405–2415.

Hossain, A. and Saunders, G. F. (2001). The human sex-determining gene *SRY* is a direct target of *WT1*. J Biol Chem 276: 16817–16823.

Hossain, A. and Saunders, G. F. (2003). Synergistic cooperation between the beta-catenin signaling pathway and steroidogenic factor 1 in the activation of the Mullerian inhibiting substance type II receptor. J Biol Chem 278: 26511–26516.

Hu, Y.C., Okumura, L.M. and Page, D.C. (2013). *Gata4* is required for formation of the genital ridge in mice. PLoS Genet 9: e1003629.

Huang, B., Wang, S., Ning, Y. et al. (1999). Autosomal XX sex reversal caused by duplication of SOX9. Am J Med Genet 87: 349–353.

Huang, C.C. and Yao, H.H. (2010). Diverse functions of Hedgehog signaling in formation and physiology of steroidogenic organs. Mol Reprod Dev 77: 489–496.

Hummitzsch, K., Irving-Rodgers, H.F., Hatzirodos, N. et al. (2013). A new model of development of the mammalian ovary and follicles. PLoS One 8: e55578.

Huynh, K.D. and Lee, J.T. (2001). Imprinted X inactivation in eutherians: a model of gametic execution and zygotic relaxation. Curr Opin Cell Biol 13, 690–7.

Iizuka-Kogo, A., Ishidao, T., Akiyama, T. et al. (2007). Abnormal development of urogenital organs in Dlgh1-deficient mice. Development 134: 1799–1807.

Imperato-Mcginley, J. and Zhu, Y.S. (2002). Androgens and male physiology the syndrome of 5alpha-reductase-2 deficiency. Mol Cell Endocrinol 198: 51–59.

Ivell, R. and Anand-Ivell, R. (2011). Biological role and clinical significance of insulin-like peptide 3. Curr Opin Endocrinol Diabetes Obes 18: 210–216.

Jeays-Ward, K., Hoyle, C., Brennan, J. et al. (2003). Endothelial and steroidogenic cell migration are regulated by WNT4 in the developing mammalian gonad. Development 130: 3663–3670.

Jenkins, A.B., Mccaffery, J.M. and Van Doren, M. (2003). Drosophila E-cadherin is essential for proper germ cell-soma interaction during gonad morphogenesis. Development 130: 4417–4426.

Jenster, G., Trapman, J. and Brinkmann, A.O. (1993). Nuclear import of the human androgen receptor. Biochem J 293 (Pt 3): 761–768.

Jeske, Y.W., Bowles, J., Greenfield, A. et al. (1995). Expression of a linear *Sry* transcript in the mouse genital ridge. Nat Genet 10: 480–482.

Jirasek, J.E. (1971). Genital ducts and external genitalia: development and anomalies. Birth Defects Orig Artic Ser 7: 131–139.

Jirasek, J.E. (1977). Morphogenesis of the genital system in the human. Birth Defects Orig Artic Ser 13: 13–39.

Johnen, H., Gonzalez-Silva, L., Carramolino, L. et al. (2013). Gadd45g is essential for primary sex determination, male fertility and testis development. PLoS One 8, e58751.

Jordan, B.K., Mohammed, M., Ching, S.T. et al. (2001). Up-regulation of WNT-4 signaling and dosage-sensitive sex reversal in humans. Am J Hum Genet 68: 1102–1109.

Jordan, B.K., Shen, J.H., Olaso, R., et al. (2003). Wnt4 overexpression disrupts normal testicular vasculature and inhibits testosterone synthesis by repressing steroidogenic factor 1/beta-catenin synergy. Proc Natl Acad Sci USA 100: 10866–108671.

Josso, N., Lamarre, I., Picard, J.Y. et al. (1993). Anti-mullerian hormone in early human development. Early Hum Dev 33: 91–99.

Josso, N., Picard, J.Y., Rey, R. et al. (2006). Testicular anti-Mullerian hormone: history, genetics, regulation and clinical applications. Pediatr Endocrinol Rev 3: 347–358.

Josso, N., Rey, R. and Picard, J.Y. (2012). Testicular anti-Mullerian hormone: clinical applications in DSD. Semin Reprod Med 30: 364–373.

Jost, A. (1947). Recherches Sur La Differenciation Sexuelle De Lembryon De Lapin. Archives D Anatomie Microscopique Et De Morphologie Experimentale 36: 151–315.

Karl, J. and Capel, B. (1998). Sertoli cells of the mouse testis originate from the coelomic epithelium. Dev Biol 203: 323–333.

Kashimada, K., Pelosi, E., Chen, H. et al. (2011a). FOXL2 and BMP2 act cooperatively to regulate *Follistatin* gene expression during ovarian development. Endocrinology 152: 272–280.

Kashimada, K., Svingen, T., Feng, C.W. et al. (2011b). Antagonistic regulation of *Cyp26b1* by transcription factors SOX9/SF1 and FOXL2 during gonadal development in mice. FASEB J 25: 3561–3569.

Katoh-Fukui, Y., Miyabayashi, K., Komatsu, T. et al. (2012). *Cbx2*, a polycomb group gene, is required for *Sry* gene expression in mice. Endocrinology 153: 913–924.

Katoh-Fukui, Y., Owaki, A., Toyama, Y. et al. (2005). Mouse Polycomb M33 is required for splenic vascular and adrenal gland formation through regulating *Ad4BP/SF1* expression. Blood 106: 1612–1620.

Katoh-Fukui, Y., Tsuchiya, R., Shiroishi, T. et al. (1998). Male-to-female sex reversal in M33 mutant mice. Nature 393: 688–692.

Kawase, E., Hashimoto, K. and Pedersen, R.A. (2004). Autocrine and paracrine mechanisms regulating primordial germ cell proliferation. Mol Reprod Dev 68: 5–16.

Keller, R.E., Danilchik, M., Gimlich, R. et al. (1985). The function and mechanism of convergent extension during gastrulation of Xenopus laevis. J Embryol Exp Morphol 89 Suppl: 185–209.

Kerr, B., Garcia-Rudaz, C., Dorfman, M. et al. (2009). NTRK1 and NTRK2 receptors facilitate follicle assembly and early follicular development in the mouse ovary. Reproduction 138: 131–140.

Kerr, C.L., Hill, C.M., Blumenthal, P.D. et al. (2008a). Expression of pluripotent stem cell markers in the human fetal ovary. Hum Reprod 23: 589–599.

Kerr, C.L., Hill, C.M., Blumenthal, P.D. et al. (2008b). Expression of pluripotent stem cell markers in the human fetal testis. Stem Cells 26: 412–421.

Ketola, I., Rahman, N., Toppari, J. et al. (1999). Expression and regulation of transcription factors GATA-4 and GATA-6 in developing mouse testis. Endocrinology 140: 1470–1480.

Kibar, Z., Vogan, K.J., Groulx, N. et al. (2001). *Ltap*, a mammalian homolog of *Drosophila Strabismus/Van Gogh*, is altered in the mouse neural tube mutant Loop-tail. Nat Genet 28: 251–255.

Kim, K.A., Wagle, M., Tran, K. et al. (2008). R-Spondin family members regulate the Wnt pathway by a common mechanism. Mol Biol Cell 19: 2588–2596.

Kim, Y., Bingham, N., Sekido, R. et al. (2007). Fibroblast growth factor receptor 2 regulates proliferation and Sertoli differentiation during male sex determination. Proc Natl Acad Sci USA 104: 16558–16563.

Kim, Y., Kobayashi, A., Sekido, R. et al. (2006). *Fgf9* and *Wnt4* act as antagonistic signals to regulate mammalian sex determination. PLoS Biol 4: e187.

Kimura, F., Bonomi, L.M. and Schneyer, A.L. (2011). Follistatin regulates germ cell nest breakdown and primordial follicle formation. Endocrinology 152: 697–706.

Kimura, F., Sidis, Y., Bonomi, L., Xia, Y. et al. (2010.) The follistatin-288 isoform alone is sufficient for survival but not for normal fertility in mice. Endocrinology 151: 1310–1319.

Klonisch, T., Fowler, P.A. and Hombach-Klonisch, S. (2004). Molecular and genetic regulation of testis descent and external genitalia development. Dev Biol 270: 1–18.

Kolatsi-Joannou, M., Bingham, C., Ellard, S. et al. (2001). Hepatocyte nuclear factor-1beta: a new kindred with renal cysts and diabetes and gene expression in normal human development. J Am Soc Nephrol 12: 2175–2180.

Koopman, P., Gubbay, J., Vivian, N. et al. (1991). Male development of chromosomally female mice transgenic for Sry. Nature 351: 117–121.

Koopman, P., Munsterberg, A., Capel, B. et al. (1990). Expression of a candidate sex-determining gene during mouse testis differentiation. Nature 348: 450–452.

Koubova, J., Menke, D. B., Zhou, Q. et al. (2006). Retinoic acid regulates sex-specific timing of meiotic initiation in mice. Proc Natl Acad Sci USA 103: 2474–2479.

Kreidberg, J.A., Sariola, H., Loring, J.M. et al. (1993). WT-1 is required for early kidney development. Cell 74: 679–691.

Kumagai, J., Hsu, S.Y., Matsumi, H. et al. (2002). INSL3/Leydig insulin-like peptide activates the LGR8 receptor important in testis descent. J Biol Chem 277: 31283–31286.

Kurimoto, K., Yamaji, M., Seki, Y. et al. (2008). Specification of the germ cell lineage in mice: a process orchestrated by the PR-domain proteins, Blimp1 and Prdm14. Cell Cycle 7: 3514–3518.

Kuroki, S., Matoba, S., Akiyoshi, M. et al. (2013). Epigenetic regulation of mouse sex determination by the histone demethylase Jmjd1a. Science 341: 1106–1109.

Kusaka, M., Katoh-Fukui, Y., Ogawa, H. et al. (2010). Abnormal epithelial cell polarity and ectopic epidermal growth factor receptor (EGFR) expression induced in Emx2 KO embryonic gonads. Endocrinology 151: 5893–5904.

Kyronlahti, A., Vetter, M., Euler, R. et al. (2011). GATA4 deficiency impairs ovarian function in adult mice. Biol Reprod 84: 1033–1044.

Laird, D.J., Altshuler-Keylin, S., Kissner, M.D. et al. (2011). Ror2 enhances polarity and directional migration of primordial germ cells. PLoS Genet 7: e1002428.

Langford, G.A. and Heller, C.G. (1973). Fine structure of muscle cells of the human testicular capsule: basis of testicular contractions. Science 179: 573–575.

Lasala, C., Schteingart, H.F., Arouche, N. et al. (2011). SOX9 and SF1 are involved in cyclic AMP-mediated upregulation of anti-Mullerian gene expression in the testicular prepubertal Sertoli cell line SMAT1. Am J Physiol Endocrinol Metab 301: E539–E547.

Lawson, K.A., Dunn, N.R., Roelen, B.A. et al. (1999). *Bmp4* is required for the generation of primordial germ cells in the mouse embryo. Genes Dev 13: 424–436.

Lee, C.H. and Taketo, T. (1994). Normal onset, but prolonged expression, of *Sry* gene in the B6.YDOM sex-reversed mouse gonad. Dev Biol 165: 442–452.

Lee, J., Inoue, K., Ono, R. et al. (2002). Erasing genomic imprinting memory in mouse clone embryos produced from day 11.5 primordial germ cells. Development 129: 1807–1817.

Lee, S.B., Huang, K., Palmer, R. et al. (1999). The Wilms tumor suppressor *WT1* encodes a transcriptional activator of *amphiregulin*. Cell 98: 663–673.

Lei, L., Zhang, H., Jin, S. et al. (2006). Stage-specific germ-somatic cell interaction directs the primordial folliculogenesis in mouse fetal ovaries. J Cell Physiol 208: 640–647.

Levine, E., Cupp, A.S. and Skinner, M.K. (2000). Role of neurotropins in rat embryonic testis morphogenesis (cord formation). Biol Reprod 62: 132–142.

Liang, L., Soyal, S.M. and Dean, J. (1997). FIGalpha, a germ cell specific transcription factor involved in the coordinate expression of the zona pellucida genes. Development 124: 4939–4947.

Lin, C., Yin, Y., Long, F. and Ma, L. (2008). Tissue-specific requirements of beta-catenin in external genitalia development. Development 135: 2815–2825.

Lindeman, R.E., Gearhart, M.D., Minkina, A. et al. (2015). Sexual cell-fate reprogramming in the ovary by DMRT1. Curr Biol 25: 764–771.

Lindner, T.H., Njolstad, P.R., Horikawa, Y. et al. (1999). A novel syndrome of diabetes mellitus, renal dysfunction and genital malformation associated with a partial deletion of the pseudo-POU domain of hepatocyte nuclear factor-1beta. Hum Mol Genet 8: 2001–2008.

Liu, C.F., Bingham, N., Parker, K. et al. (2009). Sex-specific roles of beta-catenin in mouse gonadal development. Hum Mol Genet 18: 405–417.

Liu, C.F., Parker, K. and Yao, H.H. (2010). WNT4/beta-catenin pathway maintains female germ cell survival by inhibiting activin betaB in the mouse fetal ovary. PLoS One 5: e10382.

Lovell-Badge, R. and Robertson, E. (1990). XY female mice resulting from a heritable mutation in the primary testis-determining gene, *Tdy*. Development 109: 635–646.

Ludbrook, L.M. and Harley, V.R. (2004). Sex determination: a 'window' of DAX1 activity. Trends Endocrinol Metab 15: 116–21.

Lukas-Croisier, C., Lasala, C., Nicaud, J. et al. (2003). Follicle-stimulating hormone increases testicular Anti-Mullerian hormone (AMH) production through sertoli cell proliferation and a nonclassical cyclic adenosine 5′-monophosphate-mediated activation of the AMH Gene. Mol Endocrinol 17: 550–561.

Luo, X., Ikeda, Y. and Parker, K. L. (1994). A cell-specific nuclear receptor is essential for adrenal and gonadal development and sexual differentiation. Cell 77: 481–490.

Maatouk, D.M., Mork, L., Chassot, A.A. et al. (2013). Disruption of mitotic arrest precedes precocious differentiation and transdifferentiation of pregranulosa cells in the perinatal *Wnt4* mutant ovary. Dev Biol 383: 295–306.

Maclean, G., Li, H., Metzger, D., Chambon, P. et al. (2007). Apoptotic extinction of germ cells in testes of *Cyp26b1* knockout mice. Endocrinology 148: 4560–4567.

Maekawa, M., Kamimura, K. and Nagano, T. (1996). Peritubular myoid cells in the testis: their structure and function. Arch Histol Cytol 59: 1–13.

Makela, J.A., Saario, V., Bourguiba-Hachemi, S. et al. (2011). Hedgehog signalling promotes germ cell survival in the rat testis. Reproduction 142: 711–721.

Malki, S., Nef, S., Notarnicola, C. et al. (2005). Prostaglandin D2 induces nuclear import of the sex-determining factor SOX9 via its cAMP-PKA phosphorylation. EMBO J 24: 1798–1809.

Manuylov, N.L., Smagulova, F.O., Leach, L. et al. (2008). Ovarian development in mice requires the GATA4-FOG2 transcription complex. Development 135: 3731–3743.

Manuylov, N.L., Zhou, B., Ma, Q. et al. (2011). Conditional ablation of *Gata4* and *Fog2* genes in mice reveals their distinct roles in mammalian sexual differentiation. Dev Biol 353, 229–241.

Martineau, J., Nordqvist, K., Tilmann, C. et al. (1997). Male-specific cell migration into the developing gonad. Curr Biol 7: 958–968.

Mathews, W.R., Ong, D., Milutinovich, A.B. et al. (2006). Zinc transport activity of Fear of Intimacy is essential for proper gonad morphogenesis and DE-cadherin expression. Development 133: 1143–1153.

Matson, C.K., Murphy, M.W., Sarver, A.L. et al. (2011). DMRT1 prevents female reprogramming in the postnatal mammalian testis. Nature 476: 101–104.

Matsuda, M., Nagahama, Y., Shinomiya, A. et al. (2002). DMY is a Y-specific DM-domain gene required for male development in the medaka fish. Nature 417: 559–563.

Matsui, Y., Zsebo, K. and Hogan, B.L. (1992). Derivation of pluripotential embryonic stem cells from murine primordial germ cells in culture. Cell 70: 841–847.

Mattiske, D., Kume, T. and Hogan, B. L. (2006). The mouse forkhead gene *Foxc1* is required for primordial germ cell migration and antral follicle development. Dev Biol 290: 447–458.

McCoshen, J.A. (1982). In vivo sex differentiation of congeneic germinal cell aplastic gonads. Am J Obstet Gynecol 142: 83–88.

McCoshen, J.A. (1983). Quantitation of sex chromosomal influence(s) on the somatic growth of fetal gonads in vivo. Am J Obstet Gynecol 145: 469–473.

McCoshen, J.A. and McCallion, D.J. (1975). A study of the primordial germ cells during their migratory phase in Steel mutant mice. Experientia 31: 589–590.

McGee, E.A., Hsu, S.Y., Kaipia, A. et al. (1998). Cell death and survival during ovarian follicle development. Mol Cell Endocrinol 140: 15–18.

McKearin, D. and Ohlstein, B. (1995). A role for the Drosophila bag-of-marbles protein in the differentiation of cystoblasts from germline stem cells. Development 121: 2937–2947.

McLaren, A. (1984). Meiosis and differentiation of mouse germ cells. Symp Soc Exp Biol 38: 7–23.

McLaren, A. (1988). Somatic and germ-cell sex in mammals. Philos Trans R Soc Lond B Biol Sci 322: 3–9.

McLaren, A. (1995). Germ cells and germ cell sex. Philos Trans R Soc Lond B Biol Sci 350: 229–233.

McLaren, A. (2000). Germ and somatic cell lineages in the developing gonad. Mol Cell Endocrinol 163: 3–9.

McLaren, A. and Lawson, K.A. (2005). How is the mouse germ-cell lineage established? Differentiation 73: 435–437.

McNeilly, J.R., Saunders, P.T., Taggart, M. et al. (2000). Loss of oocytes in Dazl knockout mice results in maintained ovarian steroidogenic function but altered gonadotropin secretion in adult animals. Endocrinology 141: 4284–4294.

Meachem, S.J., Ruwanpura, S.M., Ziolkowski, J. et al. (2005). Developmentally distinct in vivo effects of FSH on proliferation and apoptosis during testis maturation. J Endocrinol 186: 429–446.

Memon, M.A., Anway, M.D., Covert, T.R. et al. (2008). Transforming growth factor beta (TGFbeta1, TGFbeta2 and TGFbeta3) null-mutant phenotypes in embryonic gonadal development. Mol Cell Endocrinol 294: 70–80.

Mendelsohn, C., Lohnes, D., Decimo, D. et al. (1994). Function of the retinoic acid receptors (RARs) during development (II). Multiple abnormalities at various stages of organogenesis in RAR double mutants. Development 120: 2749–2771.

Mendis, S.H., Meachem, S.J., Sarraj, M.A. et al. (2011). Activin A balances Sertoli and germ cell proliferation in the fetal mouse testis. Biol Reprod 84: 379–391.

Mendis-Handagama, S.M. (1997). Luteinizing hormone on Leydig cell structure and function. Histol Histopathol 12: 869–882.

Menke, A.L., Van Der Eb, A.J. and Jochemsen, A.G. (1998). The Wilms' tumor 1 gene: oncogene or tumor suppressor gene? Int Rev Cytol 181: 151–212.

Merchant, H. (1975). Rat gonadal and ovarioan organogenesis with and without germ cells. An ultrastructural study. Dev Biol 44: 1–21.

Merchant-Larios, H. and Moreno-Mendoza, N. (1998). Mesonephric stromal cells differentiate into Leydig cells in the mouse fetal testis. Exp Cell Res 244: 230–238.

Mericskay, M., Kitajewski, J. and Sassoon, D. (2004). *Wnt5a* is required for proper epithelial-mesenchymal interactions in the uterus. Development 131: 2061–2072.

Merkwitz, C., Lochhead, P., Tsikolia, N. et al. (2011). Expression of KIT in the ovary, and the role of somatic precursor cells. Prog Histochem Cytochem 46: 131–814.

Middendorff, R., Muller, D., Mewe, M. et al. (2002). The tunica albuginea of the human testis is characterized by complex contraction and relaxation activities regulated by cyclic GMP. J Clin Endocrinol Metab 87: 3486–3499.

Miles, D.C., Wakeling, S.I., Stringer, J.M. et al. (2013). Signaling through the TGF beta-activin receptors ALK4/5/7 regulates testis formation and male germ cell development. PLoS One 8: e54606.

Minkina, A., Matson, C.K., Lindeman, R.E. et al. (2014). DMRT1 protects male gonadal cells from retinoid-dependent sexual transdifferentiation. Dev Cell 29: 511–520.

Mittag, J., Winterhager, E., Bauer, K. et al. (2007). Congenital hypothyroid female pax8-deficient mice are infertile despite thyroid hormone replacement therapy. Endocrinology 148: 719–725.

Miyake, Z., Takekawa, M., Ge, Q. et al. (2007). Activation of MTK1/MEKK4 by GADD45 through induced N-C dissociation and dimerization-mediated *trans* autophosphorylation of the MTK1 kinase domain. Mol Cell Biol 27: 2765–2776.

Miyamoto, N., Yoshida, M., Kuratani, S. et al. (1997). Defects of urogenital development in mice lacking Emx2. Development 124: 1653–1664.

Miyamoto, Y., Taniguchi, H., Hamel, F. et al. (2008). A GATA4/WT1 cooperation regulates transcription of genes required for mammalian sex determination and differentiation. BMC Mol Biol 9: 44.

Molkentin, J.D. (2000). The zinc finger-containing transcription factors GATA-4, -5, and -6. Ubiquitously expressed regulators of tissue-specific gene expression. J Biol Chem 275: 38949–38952.

Mollgard, K., Jespersen, A., Lutterodt, M.C. et al. (2010). Human primordial germ cells migrate along nerve fibers and Schwann cells from the dorsal hind gut mesentery to the gonadal ridge. Mol Hum Reprod 16: 621–631.

Molyneaux, K.A., Stallock, J., Schaible, K. et al. (2001). Time-lapse analysis of living mouse germ cell migration. Dev Biol 240: 488–498.

Molyneaux, K.A., Zinszner, H., Kunwar, P.S. et al. (2003). The chemokine SDF1/CXCL12 and its receptor CXCR4 regulate mouse germ cell migration and survival. Development 130: 4279–4286.

Moniot, B., Declosmenil, F., Barrionuevo, F. et al. (2009). The PGD2 pathway, independently of FGF9, amplifies SOX9 activity in Sertoli cells during male sexual differentiation. Development 136: 1813–1821.

Morais Da Silva, S., Hacker, A., Harley, V. et al. (1996). *Sox9* expression during gonadal development implies a conserved role for the gene in testis differentiation in mammals and birds. Nat Genet 14: 62–68.

Moreno, S.G., Attali, M., Allemand, I. et al. (2010). TGFbeta signaling in male germ cells regulates gonocyte quiescence and fertility in mice. Dev Biol 342: 74–84.

Mortlock, D.P. and Innis, J.W. (1997). Mutation of *HOXA13* in hand-foot-genital syndrome. Nat Genet 15: 179–180.

Muramatsu, M. and Inoue, S. (2000). Estrogen receptors: how do they control reproductive and nonreproductive functions? Biochem Biophys Res Commun 270: 1–10.

Naillat, F., Prunskaite-Hyyrylainen, R., Pietila, I. et al. (2010). Wnt4/5a signalling coordinates cell adhesion and entry into meiosis during presumptive ovarian follicle development. Hum Mol Genet 19: 1539–1550.

Nef, S. and Parada, L.F. (1999). Cryptorchidism in mice mutant for *Insl3*. Nat Genet 22: 295–299.

Nef, S., Verma-Kurvari, S., Merenmies, J. et al. (2003). Testis determination requires insulin receptor family function in mice. Nature 426: 291–295.

Nel-Themaat, L., Jang, C.W., Stewart, M.D. et al. (2011). Sertoli cell behaviors in developing testis cords and postnatal seminiferous tubules of the mouse. Biol Reprod 84: 342–350.

Nel-Themaat, L., Vadakkan, T.J., Wang, Y. et al. (2009). Morphometric analysis of testis cord formation in *Sox9-EGFP* mice. Dev Dyn 238: 1100–1110.

Nilsson, E.E., Schindler, R., Savenkova, M.I. et al. (2011). Inhibitory actions of Anti-Mullerian Hormone (AMH) on ovarian primordial follicle assembly. PLoS One 6: e20087.

O'Shaughnessy, P.J., Baker, P. J., Monteiro, A. et al. (2007). Developmental changes in human fetal testicular cell numbers and messenger ribonucleic acid levels during the second trimester. J Clin Endocrinol Metab 92: 4792–4801.

Odor, D.L. and Blandau, R.J. (1969). Ultrastructural studies on fetal and early postnatal mouse ovaries. II. Cytodifferentiation. Am J Anat 125: 177–215.

Ohanian, C., Rodriguez, H., Piriz, H. et al. (1979). Studies on the contractile activity and ultrastructure of the boar testicular capsule. J Reprod Fertil 57: 79–85.

Ohinata, Y., Ohta, H., Shigeta, M. et al. (2009). A signaling principle for the specification of the germ cell lineage in mice. Cell 137: 571–584.

Ohinata, Y., Payer, B., O'Carroll, D. et al. (2005). Blimp1 is a critical determinant of the germ cell lineage in mice. Nature 436: 207–213.

Orvis, G.D. and Behringer, R.R. (2007). Cellular mechanisms of Mullerian duct formation in the mouse. Dev Biol 306: 493–504.

Ottolenghi, C., Omari, S., Garcia-Ortiz, J.E. et al. (2005.) *Foxl2* is required for commitment to ovary differentiation. Hum Mol Genet 14: 2053–2062.

Ottolenghi, C., Pelosi, E., Tran, J. et al. (2007). Loss of *Wnt4* and *Foxl2* leads to female-to-male sex reversal extending to germ cells. Hum Mol Genet 16: 2795–2804.

Padua, M.B., Fox, S.C., Jiang, T. et al. (2014. Simultaneous gene deletion of *gata4* and *gata6* leads to early disruption of follicular development and germ cell loss in the murine ovary. Biol Reprod 91: 24.

Padua, M.B., Jiang, T., Morse, D.A. et al. (2015). Combined Loss of the GATA4 and GATA6 Transcription Factors in Male Mice Disrupts Testicular Development and Confers Adrenal-Like Function in the Testes. Endocrinology en20141907.

Pangas, S.A., Choi, Y., Ballow, D.J. et al. (2006). Oogenesis requires germ cell-specific transcriptional regulators *Sohlh1* and *Lhx8*. Proc Natl Acad Sci USA 103: 8090–8095.

Park, S.Y., Meeks, J.J., Raverot, G. et al. (2005). Nuclear receptors Sf1 and Dax1 function cooperatively to mediate somatic cell differentiation during testis development. Development 132: 2415–2423.

Parma, P., Radi, O., Vidal, V. et al. (2006). R-spondin1 is essential in sex determination, skin differentiation and malignancy. Nat Genet 38: 1304–1309.

Parr, B.A. and McMahon, A.P. (1998). Sexually dimorphic development of the mammalian reproductive tract requires Wnt-7a. Nature 395: 707–710.

Pellas, T.C., Ramachandran, B., Duncan, M. et al. (1991). Germ-cell deficient (gcd), an insertional mutation manifested as infertility in transgenic mice. Proc Natl Acad Sci USA 88: 8787–8791.

Pepling, M.E. and Spradling, A.C. (1998). Female mouse germ cells form synchronously dividing cysts. Development 125: 3323–3328.

Pepling, M.E. and Spradling, A.C. (2001). Mouse ovarian germ cell cysts undergo programmed breakdown to form primordial follicles. Dev Biol 234: 339–351.

Pepling, M.E., Sundman, E.A., Patterson, N.L. et al. (2010). Differences in oocyte development and estradiol sensitivity among mouse strains. Reproduction 139: 349–357.

Perrett, R.M., Turnpenny, L., Eckert, J.J. et al. (2008). The early human germ cell lineage does not express SOX2 during in vivo development or upon in vitro culture. Biol Reprod 78: 852–858.

Perriton, C. L., Powles, N., Chiang, C. et al. (2002). Sonic hedgehog signaling from the urethral epithelium controls external genital development. Dev Biol 247: 26–46.

Pesce, M., Wang, X., Wolgemuth, D.J. et al. (1998). Differential expression of the Oct-4 transcription factor during mouse germ cell differentiation. Mech Dev 71: 89–98.

Pilon, N., Daneau, I., Paradis, V. et al. (2003). Porcine *SRY* promoter is a target for steroidogenic factor 1. Biol Reprod 68: 1098–1106.

Pitetti, J.L., Calvel, P., Romero, Y. et al. (2013). Insulin and IGF1 receptors are essential for XX and XY gonadal differentiation and adrenal development in mice. PLoS Genet 9: e1003160.

Polanco, J.C. and Koopman, P. (2007). *Sry* and the hesitant beginnings of male development. Dev Biol 302: 13–24.

Post, L.C. and Innis, J.W. (1999). Infertility in adult hypodactyly mice is associated with hypoplasia of distal reproductive structures. Biol Reprod 61: 1402–1408.

Prieto, I., Tease, C., Pezzi, N. et al. (2004). Cohesin component dynamics during meiotic prophase I in mammalian oocytes. Chromosome Res 12: 197–213.

Pritchard-Jones, K., Fleming, S., Davidson, D. et al. (1990). The candidate Wilms' tumour gene is involved in genitourinary development. Nature 346: 194–17.

Pryse-Davies, J. and Dewhurst, C. J. (1971). The development of the ovary and uterus in the foetus, newborn and infant: a morphological and enzyme histochemical study. J Pathol 103: 5–25.

Puffenberger, E.G., Hu-Lince, D., Parod, J.M. et al. (2004). Mapping of sudden infant death with dysgenesis of the testes syndrome (SIDDT) by a SNP genome scan and identification of TSPYL loss of function. Proc Natl Acad Sci USA 101: 11689–11694.

Rabinovici, J. and Jaffe, R.B. (1990). Development and regulation of growth and differentiated function in human and subhuman primate fetal gonads. Endocr Rev 11: 532–557.

Rajkovic, A., Pangas, S.A., Ballow, D. et al. (2004). NOBOX deficiency disrupts early folliculogenesis and oocyte-specific gene expression. Science 305: 1157–1159.

Ratts, V.S., Flaws, J.A., Kolp, R. et al. (1995). Ablation of *bcl-2* gene expression decreases the numbers of oocytes and primordial follicles established in the post-natal female mouse gonad. Endocrinology 136: 3665–3668.

Raymond, C.S., Murphy, M.W., O'Sullivan, M.G. et al. (2000). *Dmrt1*, a gene related to worm and fly sexual regulators, is required for mammalian testis differentiation. Genes Dev 14: 2587–2595.

Reardon, W., Gibbons, R.J., Winter, R.M. et al. (1995). Male pseudohermaphroditism in sibs with the alpha-thalassemia/mental retardation (ATR-X) syndrome. Am J Med Genet 55: 285–287.

Reichman-Fried, M., Minina, S. and Raz, E. (2004). Autonomous modes of behavior in primordial germ cell migration. Dev Cell 6: 589–596.

Resnick, J.L., Ortiz, M., Keller, J.R. et al. (1998). Role of fibroblast growth factors and their receptors in mouse primordial germ cell growth. Biol Reprod 59: 1224–1229.

Reyes, F.I., Boroditsky, R.S., Winter, J.S. et al. (1974). Studies on human sexual development. II. Fetal and maternal serum gonadotropin and sex steroid concentrations. J Clin Endocrinol Metab 38: 612–617.

Reynaud, K., Cortvrindt, R., Verlinde, F. et al. (2004). Number of ovarian follicles in human fetuses with the 45,X karyotype. Fertil Steril 81: 1112–1119.

Robert, N.M., Miyamoto, Y., Taniguchi, H. et al. (2006). LRH-1/NR5A2 cooperates with GATA factors to regulate inhibin alpha-subunit promoter activity. Mol Cell Endocrinol 257–258, 65–74.

Roberts, L.M., Hirokawa, Y., Nachtigal, M.W. et al. (1999). Paracrine-mediated apoptosis in reproductive tract development. Dev Biol 208: 110–122.

Roche, P.J., Hoare, S.A. and Parker, M.G. (1992). A consensus DNA-binding site for the androgen receptor. Mol Endocrinol 6: 2229–2235.

Rodrigues, P., Limback, D., McGinnis, L.K. et al. (2009). Multiple mechanisms of germ cell loss in the perinatal mouse ovary. Reproduction 137: 709–720.

Rucker, E.B., 3rd, Dierisseau, P., Wagner, K.U. et al. (2000). Bcl-x and Bax regulate mouse primordial germ cell survival and apoptosis during embryogenesis. Mol Endocrinol 14: 1038–1052.

Russo, M.A., Giustizieri, M.L., Favale, A. et al. (1999). Spatiotemporal patterns of expression of neurotrophins and neurotrophin receptors in mice suggest functional roles in testicular and epididymal morphogenesis. Biol Reprod 61, 1123–1132.

Sahin, Z., Szczepny, A., Mclaughlin, E. A. et al. (2014). Dynamic Hedgehog signalling pathway activity in germline stem cells. Andrology 2: 267–274.

Saitou, M., Barton, S.C. and Surani, M.A. (2002). A molecular programme for the specification of germ cell fate in mice. Nature 418: 293–300.

Saitou, M., Payer, B., O'Carroll, D. et al. (2005). Blimp1 and the emergence of the germ line during development in the mouse. Cell Cycle 4: 1736–1740.

Saitou, M. and Yamaji, M. (2012). Primordial germ cells in mice. Cold Spring Harb Perspect Biol 4.

Sarraj, M.A., Escalona, R.M., Umbers, A. et al. (2010). Fetal testis dysgenesis and compromised Leydig cell function in *Tgfbr3* (beta glycan) knockout mice. Biol Reprod 82: 153–162.

Schepers, G., Wilson, M., Wilhelm, D. et al. (2003). SOX8 is expressed during testis differentiation in mice and synergizes with SF1 to activate the *Amh* promoter *in vitro*. J Biol Chem 278: 28101–28108.

Schlessinger, D., Garcia-Ortiz, J.E., Forabosco, A. et al. (2010). Determination and stability of gonadal sex. J Androl 31: 16–25.

Schmahl, J. and Capel, B. (2003). Cell proliferation is necessary for the determination of male fate in the gonad. Dev Biol 258: 264–276.

Schmahl, J., Kim, Y., Colvin, J.S. et al. (2004). *Fgf9* induces proliferation and nuclear localization of FGFR2 in Sertoli precursors during male sex determination. Development 131: 3627–3636.

Schmidt, D., Ovitt, C.E., Anlag, K. et al. (2004). The murine winged-helix transcription factor Foxl2 is required for granulosa cell differentiation and ovary maintenance. Development 131: 933–942.

Scholer, H.R., Dressler, G.R., Balling, R. et al. (1990). Oct-4: a germline-specific transcription factor mapping to the mouse t-complex. EMBO J 9: 2185–2195.

Seki, Y., Yamaji, M., Yabuta, Y. et al. (2007). Cellular dynamics associated with the genome-wide epigenetic reprogramming in migrating primordial germ cells in mice. Development 134: 2627–2638.

Sekido, R., Bar, I., Narvaez, V. et al. (2004). SOX9 is up-regulated by the transient expression of SRY specifically in Sertoli cell precursors. Dev Biol 274: 271–279.

Sekido, R. and Lovell-Badge, R. (2008). Sex determination involves synergistic action of SRY and SF1 on a specific *Sox9* enhancer. Nature 453: 930–934.

Sekido, R. and Lovell-Badge, R. (2013). Genetic control of testis development. Sex Dev 7: 21–32.

Seville, R.A., Nijjar, S., Barnett, M.W. et al. (2002.) Annexin IV (Xanx-4) has a functional role in the formation of pronephric tubules. Development 129: 1693–1704.

Shimamura, R., Fraizer, G.C., Trapman, J. et al. (1997). The Wilms' tumor gene WT1 can regulate genes involved in sex determination and differentiation: SRY, Mullerian-inhibiting substance, and the androgen receptor. Clin Cancer Res 3: 2571–2580.

Shinoda, K., Lei, H., Yoshii, H. et al. (1995). Developmental defects of the ventromedial hypothalamic nucleus and pituitary gonadotroph in the *Ftz-F1* disrupted mice. Dev Dyn 204: 22–29.

Skinner, M.K., Tung, P.S. and Fritz, I.B. (1985). Cooperativity between Sertoli cells and testicular peritubular cells in the production and deposition of extracellular matrix components. J Cell Biol 100: 1941–1947.

Smith, C.A., Roeszler, K.N., Ohnesorg, T. et al. (2009). The avian Z-linked gene *DMRT1* is required for male sex determination in the chicken. Nature 461: 267–271.

Smith, C.A., Shoemaker, C.M., Roeszler, K.N. et al. (2008). Cloning and expression of *R-Spondin1* in different vertebrates suggests a conserved role in ovarian development. BMC Dev Biol 8: 72.

Sobel, V., Zhu, Y.S. and Imperato-Mcginley, J. (2004). Fetal hormones and sexual differentiation. Obstet Gynecol Clin North Am 31: 837–856, x–xi.

Soyal, S. M., Amleh, A. and Dean, J. (2000). FIGalpha, a germ cell-specific transcription factor required for ovarian follicle formation. Development 127: 4645–4654.

Spears, N., Molinek, M.D., Robinson, L.L. et al. (2003). The role of neurotrophin receptors in female germ-cell survival in mouse and human. Development 130: 5481–5491.

Speed, R.M. (1982). Meiosis in the foetal mouse ovary. I. An analysis at the light microscope level using surface-spreading. Chromosoma 85: 427–437.

Spiller, C.M., Feng, C.W., Jackson, A. et al. (2012). Endogenous Nodal signaling regulates germ cell potency during mammalian testis development. Development 139: 4123–4132.

Spiller, C.M., Wilhelm, D. and Koopman, P. (2010). Retinoblastoma 1 protein modulates XY germ cell entry into G1/G0 arrest during fetal development in mice. Biol Reprod 82: 433–443.

Su, S., Farmer, P.J., Li, R. et al. (2012). Regression of the mammary branch of the genitofemoral nerve may be necessary for testicular descent in rats. J Urol 188: 1443–1448.

Sugimoto, M. and Abe, K. (2007). X chromosome reactivation initiates in nascent primordial germ cells in mice. PLoS Genet 3: e116.

Sun, X., Meyers, E.N., Lewandoski, M. et al. (1999). Targeted disruption of *Fgf8* causes failure of cell migration in the gastrulating mouse embryo. Genes Dev 13: 1834–1846.

Surani, M.A. (2001). Reprogramming of genome function through epigenetic inheritance. Nature 414: 122–128.

Sutton, E., Hughes, J., White, S. et al. (2011). Identification of *SOX3* as an XX male sex reversal gene in mice and humans. J Clin Invest 121: 328–341.

Suzuki, K., Bachiller, D., Chen, Y.P. et al. (2003). Regulation of outgrowth and apoptosis for the terminal appendage: external genitalia development by concerted actions of BMP signaling [corrected]. Development 130: 6209–6220.

Swain, A. and Lovell-Badge, R. (1999). Mammalian sex determination: a molecular drama. Genes Dev 13: 755–767.

Swain, A., Narvaez, V., Burgoyne, P. et al. (1998). *Dax1* antagonizes *Sry* action in mammalian sex determination. Nature 391: 761–767.

Takasawa, K., Kashimada, K., Pelosi, E. et al. (2014). FOXL2 transcriptionally represses *Sf1* expression by antagonizing WT1 during ovarian development in mice. FASEB J 28: 2020–2028.

Takeuchi, Y., Molyneaux, K., Runyan, C. et al. (2005). The roles of FGF signaling in germ cell migration in the mouse. Development 132: 5399–53409.

Tamura, M., Kanno, Y., Chuma, S. et al. (2001). *Pod-1/ Capsulin* shows a sex- and stage-dependent expression pattern in the mouse gonad development and represses expression of *Ad4BP/SF-1*. Mech Dev 102: 135–144.

Tanaka, S. S., Yamaguchi, Y. L., Steiner, K. A. et al. (2010). Loss of *Lhx1* activity impacts on the localization of primordial germ cells in the mouse. Dev Dyn 239: 2851–2859.

Tang, H., Brennan, J., Karl, J. et al. (2008). Notch signaling maintains Leydig progenitor cells in the mouse testis. Development 135: 3745–3753.

Tang, P., Park, D.J., Marshall Graves, J.A. et al. (2004). ATRX and sex differentiation. Trends Endocrinol Metab 15: 339–344.

Tevosian, S.G. (2013). Genetic control of ovarian development. Sex Dev 7: 33–45.

Tevosian, S.G., Albrecht, K.H., Crispino, J.D. et al. (2002). Gonadal differentiation, sex determination and normal *Sry* expression in mice require direct interaction between transcription partners GATA4 and FOG2. Development 129: 4627–4634.

Tilmann, C. and Capel, B. (1999). Mesonephric cell migration induces testis cord formation and Sertoli cell differentiation in the mammalian gonad. Development 126: 2883–2890.

Tilmann, C. and Capel, B. (2002). Cellular and molecular pathways regulating mammalian sex determination. Recent Prog Horm Res 57: 1–18.

Tomaselli, S., Megiorni, F., Lin, L. et al. (2011). Human *RSPO1/*R-spondin1 is expressed during early ovary development and augments beta-catenin signaling. PLoS One 6: e16366.

Tomizuka, K., Horikoshi, K., Kitada, R. et al. (2008). R-spondin1 plays an essential role in ovarian development through positively regulating Wnt-4 signaling. Hum Mol Genet 17: 1278–1291.

Torres, M., Gomez-Pardo, E., Dressler, G.R. et al. (1995). Pax-2 controls multiple steps of urogenital development. Development 121: 4057–4065.

Trombly, D.J., Woodruff, T.K. and Mayo, K.E. (2009). Suppression of Notch signaling in the neonatal mouse ovary decreases primordial follicle formation. Endocrinology 150: 1014–1024.

Turnpenny L, Spalluto CM, Perrett RM et al. (2006) Evaluating human embryonic germ cells: concord and conflict as pluripotent stem cells. Stem Cells 24: 212–220.

Uda, M., Ottolenghi, C., CrisponI, L. et al. (2004). *Foxl2* disruption causes mouse ovarian failure by pervasive blockage of follicle development. Hum Mol Genet 13: 1171–1181.

Uhlenhaut, N.H., Jakob, S., Anlag, K. et al. (2009). Somatic sex reprogramming of adult ovaries to testes by FOXL2 ablation. Cell 139: 1130–1142.

Vainio, S., Heikkila, M., Kispert, A. et al. (1999). Female development in mammals is regulated by Wnt-4 signalling. Nature 397, 405–9.

Val, P., Lefrancois-Martinez, A.M., Veyssiere, G. et al. (2003). SF-1 a key player in the development and differentiation of steroidogenic tissues. Nucl Recept 1: 8.

Val, P., Martinez-Barbera, J.P. and Swain, A. (2007). Adrenal development is initiated by Cited2 and Wt1 through modulation of Sf-1 dosage. Development 134: 2349–2358.

Van Der Schoot, P. and Elger, W. (1992). androgen-induced prevention of the outgrowth of cranial gonadal suspensory ligaments in fetal rats. J Androl 13: 534–542.

Van Doren, M., Broihier, H.T., Moore, L.A. et al. (1998). HMG-CoA reductase guides migrating primordial germ cells. Nature 396: 466–469.

Van Doren, M., Mathews, W.R., Samuels, M. et al. (2003). fear of intimacy encodes a novel transmembrane protein required for gonad morphogenesis in Drosophila. Development 130: 2355–2364.

Vaskivuo, T.E., Anttonen, M., Herva, R. et al. (2001). Survival of human ovarian follicles from fetal to adult life: apoptosis, apoptosis-related proteins, and transcription factor GATA-4. J Clin Endocrinol Metab 86: 3421–3429.

Vidal, V.P., Chaboissier, M.C., De Rooij, D.G et al. (2001). Sox9 induces testis development in XX transgenic mice. Nat Genet 28: 216–217.

Viger, R.S., Guittot, S.M., Anttonen, M. et al. (2008). Role of the GATA family of transcription factors in endocrine development, function, and disease. Mol Endocrinol 22: 781–798.

Viger, R.S., Mertineit, C., Trasler, J.M. et al. (1998). Transcription factor GATA-4 is expressed in a sexually dimorphic pattern during mouse gonadal development and is a potent activator of the Mullerian inhibiting substance promoter. Development 125: 2665–2675.

Vincent, S.D., Dunn, N.R., Sciammas, R. et al. (2005). The zinc finger transcriptional repressor Blimp1/Prdm1 is dispensable for early axis formation but is required for specification of primordial germ cells in the mouse. Development 132: 1315–1325.

Vinci, G., Brauner, R., Tar, A. et al. (2009). Mutations in the *TSPYL1* gene associated with 46,XY disorder of sex development and male infertility. Fertil Steril 92: 1347–1350.

Wagner, T., Wirth, J., Meyer, J. et al. (1994). Autosomal sex reversal and campomelic dysplasia are caused by mutations in and around the *SRY*-related gene *SOX9*. Cell 79: 1111–1120.

Warot, X., Fromental-Ramain, C., Fraulob, V. et al. (1997). Gene dosage-dependent effects of the Hoxa-13 and Hoxd-13 mutations on morphogenesis of the terminal parts of the digestive and urogenital tracts. Development 124: 4781–4791.

Warr, N., Carre, G.A., Siggers, P. et al. (2012). *Gadd45gamma* and Map3k4 interactions regulate mouse testis determination via p38 MAPK-mediated control of *Sry* expression. Dev Cell 23: 1020–1031.

Watanabe, K., Clarke, T.R., Lane, A.H. et al. (2000). Endogenous expression of Mullerian inhibiting substance in early postnatal rat sertoli cells requires multiple steroidogenic factor-1 and GATA-4-binding sites. Proc Natl Acad Sci USA 97: 1624–1629.

Western, P., Maldonado-Saldivia, J., Van Den Bergen, J. et al. (2005). Analysis of *Esg1* expression in pluripotent cells and the germline reveals similarities with *Oct4* and *Sox2* and differences between human pluripotent cell lines. Stem Cells 23: 1436–1442.

Western, P.S., Miles, D.C., Van Den Bergen, J.A. et al. (2008). Dynamic regulation of mitotic arrest in fetal male germ cells. Stem Cells 26: 339–347.

White, S., Ohnesorg, T., Notini, A. et al. (2011). Copy number variation in patients with disorders of sex development due to 46,XY gonadal dysgenesis. PLoS One 6: e17793.

Wilhelm, D. and Englert, C. (2002). The Wilms tumor suppressor WT1 regulates early gonad development by activation of *Sf1*. Genes Dev 16: 1839–1851.

Wilhelm, D., Hiramatsu, R., Mizusaki, H. et al. (2007). SOX9 regulates prostaglandin D synthase gene transcription in vivo to ensure testis development. J Biol Chem 282: 10553–10560.

Wilhelm, D., Martinson, F., Bradford, S. et al. (2005). Sertoli cell differentiation is induced both cell-autonomously and through prostaglandin signaling during mammalian sex determination. Dev Biol 287: 111–124.

Wilhelm, D., Washburn, L.L., Truong, V. et al. (2009). Antagonism of the testis- and ovary-determining pathways during ovotestis development in mice. Mech Dev 126: 324–336.

Wilson, J.D., Griffin, J.E., Leshin, M. et al. (1981). Role of gonadal hormones in development of the sexual phenotypes. Hum Genet 58: 78–84.

Wilson, J.D., Shaw, G., Leihy, M.L. et al. (2002). The marsupial model for male phenotypic development. Trends Endocrinol Metab 13: 78–83.

Winter, J.S., Faiman, C. and Reyes, F.I. (1977). Sex steroid production by the human fetus: its role in morphogenesis and control by gonadotropins. Birth Defects Orig Artic Ser 13: 41–58.

Witschi, E. (1946). Early history of the human germ cells. Anat Rec 94: 506.

Word, R.A., George, F.W., Wilson, J.D. et al. (1989). Testosterone synthesis and adenylate cyclase activity in the early human fetal testis appear to be independent of human chorionic gonadotropin control. J Clin Endocrinol Metab 69: 204–208.

Yabuta, Y., Kurimoto, K., Ohinata, Y. et al. (2006). Gene expression dynamics during germline specification in mice identified by quantitative single-cell gene expression profiling. Biol Reprod 75: 705–716.

Yamaguchi, S., Kimura, H., Tada, M. et al. (2005). Nanog expression in mouse germ cell development. Gene Expr Patterns 5: 639–646.

Yamaji, M., Seki, Y., Kurimoto, K. et al. (2008). Critical function of *Prdm14* for the establishment of the germ cell lineage in mice. Nat Genet 40: 1016–1022.

Yan, C., Wang, P., Demayo, J. et al. (2001). Synergistic roles of bone morphogenetic protein 15 and growth differentiation factor 9 in ovarian function. Mol Endocrinol 15: 854–866.

Yan, W., Suominen, J., Samson, M. et al. (2000). Involvement of Bcl-2 family proteins in germ cell apoptosis during testicular development in the rat and pro-survival effect of stem cell factor on germ cells in vitro. Mol Cell Endocrinol 165: 115–129.

Yao, H.H., Aardema, J. and Holthusen, K. (2006). Sexually dimorphic regulation of inhibin beta B in establishing gonadal vasculature in mice. Biol Reprod 74: 978–983.

Yao, H.H., Matzuk, M.M., Jorgez, C.J. et al. (2004). *Follistatin* operates downstream of *Wnt4* in mammalian ovary organogenesis. Dev Dyn 230: 210–215.

Yao, H.H., Whoriskey, W. and Capel, B. (2002). Desert Hedgehog/Patched 1 signaling specifies fetal Leydig cell fate in testis organogenesis. Genes Dev 16: 1433–1440.

Ying, Y., Liu, X.M., Marble, A., Lawson, K.A. et al. (2000). Requirement of *Bmp8b* for the generation of primordial germ cells in the mouse. Mol Endocrinol 14: 1053–1063.

Ying, Y. and Zhao, G. Q. (2001). Cooperation of endoderm-derived BMP2 and extraembryonic ectoderm-derived BMP4 in primordial germ cell generation in the mouse. Dev Biol 232: 484–492.

Yoshimoto, S., Okada, E., Umemoto, H. et al. (2008). A W-linked DM-domain gene, DM-W, participates in primary ovary development in Xenopus laevis. Proc Natl Acad Sci USA 105: 2469–2474.

Young, J., Chanson, P., Salenave, S. et al. (2005). Testicular anti-mullerian hormone secretion is stimulated by recombinant human FSH in patients with congenital hypogonadotropic hypogonadism. J Clin Endocrinol Metab 90: 724–748.

Yu, R.N., Ito, M., Saunders, T.L. et al. (1998). Role of Ahch in gonadal development and gametogenesis. Nat Genet 20: 353–357.

Yuan, L., Liu, J.G., Hoja, M.R. et al. (2002). Female germ cell aneuploidy and embryo death in mice lacking the meiosis-specific protein SCP3. Science 296: 1115–1118.

Zalel, Y., Pinhas-Hamiel, O., Lipitz, S. et al. (2001). The development of the fetal penis–an in utero sonographic evaluation. Ultrasound Obstet Gynecol 17: 129–131.

Zamboni, L. and Upadhyay, S. (1983). Germ cell differentiation in mouse adrenal glands. J Exp Zool 228: 173–193.

Zhan, Y., Fujino, A., Maclaughlin, D.T. et al. (2006). Mullerian inhibiting substance regulates its receptor/SMAD signaling and causes mesenchymal transition of the coelomic epithelial cells early in Mullerian duct regression. Development 133: 2359–2369.

Zhao, L., Ng, E.T., Davidson, T.L. et al. (2014). Structure-function analysis of mouse Sry reveals dual essential roles of the C-terminal polyglutamine tract in sex determination. Proc Natl Acad Sci USA 111: 11768–11773.

Zhao, L., Svingen, T., Ng, E.T. et al. (2015). Female-to-male sex reversal in mice caused by transgenic overexpression of *Dmrt1*. Development 142: 1083–1088.

2

Male and Female Reproductive Anatomy

Sara Sulaiman and James Coey

Female Reproductive System (Figure 2.1)

The primary organs of the female reproductive system are the two ovaries (gonads), which produce the oocytes and sex hormones. Other structures, termed the accessory sex organs, include the internal and external organs responsible for transporting the oocyte and transmitting the spermatozoa to the site of fertilization. After implantation the female reproductive system provides a suitable environment for the developing fetus and delivers it to the outside world through labour or parturition.

Ovaries

The two ovaries are solid ovoid/almond-shaped structures, about 3 cm long, 2 cm wide, and 1 cm thick whose size and shape differs throughout life. Before puberty, they are smooth, dull white, and solid in consistency. During the reproductive years, the ovaries increase in size and have an irregular surface. Postmenopausally, they shrink and are covered with scar tissue (see Chapter 4 for more detail on ovarian anatomy, the oocyte, and folliculogenesis).

The ovaries develop on the posterior abdominal wall and descend to the level of the pelvic brim at the end of the fimbriae of the uterine tubes. As ovoid structures the ovaries have two poles:

1) The superior pole: receiving the ovarian vessels, nerves, and lymphatics through a peritoneal fold called the suspensory ligament of the ovary.

2) The inferior pole: attached to a fibromuscular band, the ligament of the ovary; continuous with the round ligament of the uterus as it crosses the uterine horns.

The anterior border of the ovary is covered by a double fold of the broad ligament called the mesovarium. The lateral surface is related to the internal and external iliac vessels and separated from the obturator nerve by the parietal peritoneum. The medial surface is closely approximated to the fimbriae of the uterine tubes.

- *Blood supply:* from the gonadal or ovarian arteries originating from the anterolateral side of the abdominal aorta. Each artery descends on the posterior abdominal wall, anterior to psoas muscle where it crosses the ureter obliquely. As it descends over the pelvic brim the ovarian artery passes over the external iliac vessels and enters the suspensory ligament. Approaching the lateral side of the ovary, the ovarian artery gives a branch to the uterine tube, which anastomoses with the uterine artery before reaching the ovary.
- *Venous drainage:* through ovarian plexuses found in the suspensory ligaments that accompany the ovarian arteries. The plexuses join on each side to form ovarian veins that drain asymmetrically into the interior vena cava: directly on the right and via the left renal vein on the left.
- *Lymphatic drainage:* towards the para-aortic nodes in the lumbar region around the origin of the ovarian arteries.
- *Innervation:* sympathetic innervation from T10 and 11 spinal segments via the ovarian plexus is

Clinical Reproductive Science, First Edition. Edited by Michael Carroll.
© 2019 John Wiley & Sons Ltd. Published 2019 by John Wiley & Sons Ltd.
Companion website: www.wiley.com/go/carroll/clinicalreproductivescience

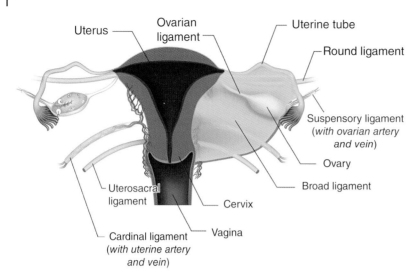

Uterus — Ovarian ligament — Uterine tube — Round ligament — Suspensory ligament (*with ovarian artery and vein*) — Ovary — Broad ligament — Cervix — Vagina — Cardinal ligament (*with uterine artery and vein*) — Uterosacral ligament

Figure 2.1 Female reproductive organs (posterior view). Reproduced with permission of Alila Medical Media/shutterstock.com.

carried along the ovarian arteries. As sensory fibres travel with the sympathetics, ovarian pain is referred to the periumbilical region. Parasympathetic fibres can reach the ovaries via the inferior hypogastric plexus and bring about vasodilation.

Fallopian Tubes

Their function is to carry the expelled oocyte from the ovary to the uterus and provide the site of fertilization and early embryo development (Chapter 8 discusses the role of the Fallopian tubes in early embryo development in more detail). Fallopian tubes are about 10 cm in length and extend posterolaterally from the uterine horns to open into the peritoneal cavity near the medial surface of the ovary. They are suspended bilaterally in the free anterosuperior edge of the broad ligament, called the mesosalpinx. The uterine tube has four parts from lateral to medial:

1) Infundibulum: the lateral/distal end of the tube also known as the fimbriated portion of the uterine tube. It is characterized by finger-like projections surrounding the opening into the peritoneal cavity (abdominal ostium). The fimbriae surround the medial surface of the ovary; one large fimbria usually extends and is closely related to the superior pole of the ovary.

2) Ampulla: the normal site of fertilization. It is the widest and longest part, forming more than half of the length of the uterine tube.

3) Isthmus: a thick-walled, narrow and straight portion of the tube, about 2.5 cm in length that enters into the uterine horn. Functions as a reservoir for spermatozoa.

4) Uterine: the most medial part, which is also known as the intramural segment. It is about 1–2.5 cm long and passes through the wall of the uterus to open into the cavity via the uterine ostium.

- *Blood supply:* from tubal branches of the ovarian artery and the uterine artery, originating from the abdominal aorta and internal iliac artery respectively. Branches from both arteries supply the tube from opposite ends and anastomose with each other.
- *Venous drainage:* through the ovarian and uterine venous plexuses.
- *Lymphatic drainage:* towards the para-aortic lymph nodes of the abdomen.
- *Innervation:* by the ovarian and uterine plexuses.

Uterus

The uterus is a hollow pear-shaped muscular structure, about 7.5 cm long, 5 cm wide, and 2.5 cm thick, that lies in the true pelvis during the nonpregnant phase. Like the ovaries the uterus changes size over the course of life, growing during puberty and atrophying postmenopausally. The position of the uterus changes relative to fullness of the urinary bladder/rectum, and the stage of pregnancy. It is typically positioned on top of the urinary bladder, angled anterosuperiorly relative to the axis of the vagina (anteverted), and flexed anteriorly relative to the cervix (anteflexed). The uterus has two surfaces:

1) A superior surface: related to the intestines.
2) An inferior surface: separated from the urinary bladder by the vesicouterine fascia.

The uterus can be considered as three anatomically distinct regions named from superior to inferior:

1) Fundus: the rounded part that lies superior to the level of the uterine ostia (openings of the uterine tubes). Pelvic peritoneum covers the fundus and extends inferiorly toward the body.
2) Body: extending from the fundus above to the cervix inferiorly; it receives the openings of the uterine tube at the junction between the fundus and the body in a region termed the cornua or uterine horn. The body narrows inferiorly within a segment called the isthmus demarcating where the cervix begins. The body is enveloped in peritoneum that extends laterally as the mesometrium of the broad ligament
3) Cervix: the inferior third of the uterus can be further subdivided into two parts:
   - Supravaginal part: extending from the isthmus to the vagina.
   - Vaginal part: protruding into the vagina and is surrounded by a sulcus. The sulcus is termed a fornix and is deepest posteriorly.

An anterior wall of the cervix is located posterior to the urinary bladder and is attached above the bladder trigone by dense connective tissue. It is related to ureters that pass laterally then anterior to the anterior fornix. The posterior wall is covered by peritoneum forming the anterior wall of the rectouterine pouch.

The cervical canal is continuous with the cavity of the body through the internal os and with the vagina through the external os. The external os is normally at the level of the ischial spines.

Many ligaments and muscles support the uterus and keep it centred in the pelvic cavity. They also prevent the uterus from being pushed through the vagina and act as passageway for vessels, lymphatics and nerves to get to pelvic organs:

- The broad ligament of the uterus: a double layer of peritoneum enveloping the uterus and extending laterally to pelvic wall and floor, it comprises:
  - Mesosalpinx: the upper border covering the uterine tubes.
  - Mesovarium: the small posterior extension of mesentery holding the ovaries.
  - Mesometrium: the extension that spans over the body of the uterus inferior to mesosalpinx.
- Suspensory ligament of the ovary (infundibular ligament): the upper lateral part of the broad ligament covering the ovarian vessels and nerves. It extends laterally as a fold over the iliac vessels on its way to the superior pole of the ovary.
- The round ligament of the ovary: extends from the inferior pole of the ovary to the junction between the uterus and the uterine tubes.
- The round ligament of the uterus: continuous with the ligament of the ovary, this ligament extends from the junction between the uterus and the uterine tubes to the deep inguinal ring. It passes through the inguinal canal and ends as fibrous tissue blending with the subcutaneous tissue in the labia majora. This ligament contributes to the uterus position in an anteflexed–anteverted position.
- The transverse cervical (cardinal) ligament: a thickening of connective tissue at the base of the broad ligament extending laterally to the pelvic wall. It is key to the support of the the cervix and uterus.
- The uterosacral ligaments: fibrous tissue that extends from the cervix to the sacrum. It maintains the cervix and positions the uterus in an anteverted state against the forward pull of the round ligament.
- Pubovaginalis muscle: a part of levator ani (pelvic diaphragm) that plays an important role in supporting the vagina and positioning the cervix.

- *Blood supply*: from branches of the uterine arteries. As the ovarian arteries anastomose with the uterine arteries, there is also contribution from the ovarian arteries to the blood supply of the uterus.
- *Venous drainage:* the uterine veins converge to form a uterine venous plexus around the cervix and drain through the internal iliac veins.

- *Lymphatic drainage:* follows the arterial supply to four sets of lymph nodes:
  - The fundus and upper part of the uterine body drain towards para-aortic lymph nodes.
  - The lower part of the uterine body and small part of the cervix drain towards the external iliac nodes.
  - The cervix mainly drains towards the internal iliac and sacral lymph nodes.
  - A small region of the uterine horns drain toward the superficial inguinal nodes along with the round ligament of the uterus.
- *Innervation:* the uterovaginal nerve plexus from the inferior hypogastric plexus carries sympathetic, parasympathetic, and visceral afferents fibres to the uterus. Sympathetic fibres originate from T10-L1 spinal segments and parasympathetic fibres from S2-S4. Visceral afferents conducting pain from the fundus, body, and upper cervix follow the sympathetic pathway and are carried back to the inferior thoracic/superior lumbar ganglia. Visceral afferents conducting pain from the cervix follow the parasympathetic fibres pathway and are carried back toward S2-S4 spinal ganglia.

Vagina

The vagina is a 7–10 cm long, fibromuscular collapsible tube between the cervix of the uterus and the vaginal orifice. The vaginal orifice opens into the vestibule of the vagina, a cleft between the labia minora. The cervix projects into the vagina forming a circular groove termed the fornix: it is subdivided into anterior, posterior, and lateral forniciesfor descriptive purposes. The vagina is located anterior to the rectum, anal canal, and perineal body, separated from the rectum by a rectovaginal septum. The posterior fornix is covered by peritoneum and lies anterior to the rectouterine pouch. The anterior wall of the vagina is closely related to the base of the urinary bladder and urethra that pass anterior to the anterior fornix, embedded within the vaginal wall. Inferiorly, the vagina is related to pubovaginalis parts of levator ani muscle. The urethra passes through the urogenital diaphragm, perineal membrane, and into the superficial perineal space where it opens into the vestibule of the vagina. The hymen or remnants thereof can be seen internally at the junction between the vagina and the vestibule. The ducts of greater vestibular glands open posteriorlaterally in the vestibule just inferior to the hymen whereas the urethra opens anterior to the vaginal orifice.

- *Blood supply:* from the vaginal artery, a branch of the internal iliac artery. The uterine, inferior vesicle, and middle rectal arteries supplement the vaginal artery and create an anastomotic network around the vagina.
- *Venous drainage:* through the uterovaginal venous plexus which drains into the internal iliac veins and anastasmoses with the vesical and rectal plexuses.
- *Lymphatic drainage:* like the uterus, lymphatic drainage of the vagina follows the arterial supply to four scts of nodes:
  - The superior part; towards the internal and external lymph nodes,
  - The middle part; towards the internal iliac nodes.
  - The inferior part; towards sacral and common iliac nodes.
  - The external orifice; below the level of the hymen, drains towards the superficial inguinal lymph nodes.
- *Innervation:* by visceral fibres to the superior three quarters and somatic fibres to the inferior quarter:
  - Somatic innervation of the vagina is supplied by the deep perineal nerve, a branch from the pudendal nerve, carrying both sympathetic and visceral afferents. The inferior quarter of the vagina is sensitive to touch and temperature.
  - Visceral innervation is supplied by the uterovaginal nerve plexus which descend from the inferior hypogastric plexus. The upper three quarters of the vagina is sensitive only to stretch.

Female External Genitalia

The female external genitalia include the mons pubis, labia majora, labia minora, clitoris, bulbs of vestibule, and vestibular glands:

1) The mons pubis: the fatty eminence which continues with the anterior abdominal wall superiorly. It is situated anterior to the pubic symphysis, pubic tubercles, and the superior pubic rami. After puberty, the amount of fat in

the mons pubis increases and skin is covered with coarse pubic hair.

2) Labia majora: the mons pubis extends backwards as the labia majora which are the lateral folds of the pudendal cleft. The round ligaments of the uterus terminate at the anterior part of each labium. The labia majora join anteriorly as the anterior commissure and join posteriorly in a less prominent ridge called the posterior commissure overlying the perineal body.

3) Labia minora: between the labia majora, surrounding the vaginal vestibule are the hairless cutaneous folds termed the labia minora. Anteriorly the labia minora join forming the frenulum and the prepuce of the clitoris (which usually overlies the clitoris). Posteriorly they join by the frenulum of the labia.

4) The clitoris: an erectile organ formed by the paired bulbs and crura of the superficial perineal pouch that continue as the corpora cavernosae (body) and glans clitoris respectively.

5) The vestibule: the space between the two labia minora that receives the urethra, vagina, and the ducts of the vestibular glands. The external urethral opening is located posteroinferior to the glans and anterior to the vaginal opening. Paraurethral glands open laterally on each side of the urethral opening. In infancy the vaginal opening is partially occluded by a mucosal fold of variable thickness called the hymen. After it ruptures, remnants form tags (hymenal caruncles).

6) The greater vestibular glands: oval or round-shaped glands, about 1 cm in diameter and are located posterolateral to the vaginal opening. Each gland opens by a single duct into the vestibule, in the grove between the hymen (or its remnants) and labium minora. The greater vestibular glands are homologous with the male bulbourethral glands and secrete mucus into the vestibule during sexual arousal. Smaller mucus glands with minute openings between the urethra and the vaginal openings are called lesser vestibular glands.

Alongside of the vaginal opening are the bulbs of the vestibule, which are elongated erectile masses covered by bulbospongiosus muscles.

- *Blood supply:* from branches of the internal pudendal artery.

- *Venous drainage:* through the internal pudendal veins.

- *Lymphatic drainage:* the skin of the perineum including the inferior vagina, vaginal opening, and the vestibule drains initially toward the superficial inguinal nodes. The clitoris, vestibular bulb, and anterior labia minora drain toward the deep inguinal nodes or internal iliac nodes.

- *Innervation:* the mons pubis and anterior labia are innervated by the ilioinguinal nerve and genital branch of the genitofemoral nerve. The posterior aspects of the female external genitalia are supplied by the perineal branch of the posterior cutaneous nerve of the thigh laterally and the pudendal nerve medially. The erectile tissue in the bulb of the vestibule and the clitoris receive parasympathetic fibres from the uterovaginal nerve plexus known as the cavernous nerves.

Female Arousal and Orgasm

Parasympathetic stimulation relaxes the blood vessels feeding the erectile tissue leading to engorgement of the vulva, mainly the bulbs of the vestibule and the glans clitoris. In addition, vascular engorgement of the vagina, which increases lubrication, also occurs upon sexual arousal. Sympathetic innervation is responsible for the rhythmic contraction leading to orgasm.

Male Reproductive System (Figure 2.2)

In terms of function, the organs of the male reproductive system can be divided into primary and accessory organs. The primary sex organs (testes) are the site of spermatogenesis and the production of the male sex hormone, testosterone. The accessory sex organs are responsible for the production of the majority of the ejaculate and its delivery to the female reproductive tract through erection and ejaculation during sexual intercourse.

Testis (Testes)

After developing on the posterior abdominal wall, the testes normally descend towards the scrotum in the latter stages of gestation. Optimal

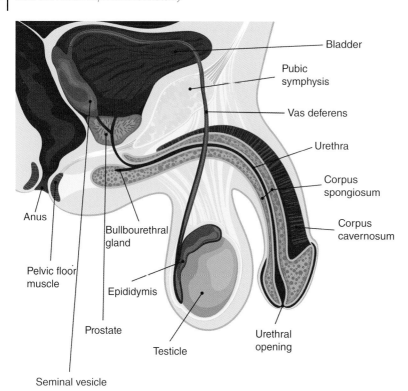

Bladder

Pubic symphysis

Vas deferens

Urethra

Corpus spongiosum

Corpus cavernosum

Anus

Bullbourethral gland

Pelvic floor muscle

Epididymis

Prostate

Urethral opening

Testicle

Seminal vesicle

Figure 2.2 Male reproductive organs. Reproduced with permission of logika600/shutterstock.com.

spermatogenesis occurs at a 1–8 °C (1.8–14.4 °F) below the normal body temperature of 37 °C (98.6 °F). Failure of one or both testes to descend (cryptorchidism), is a well-recognized cause of male infertility.

The testes are white ovoid structures, about 4 cm long, 2.5 cm wide and 3 cm thick. Suspended in the scrotum by the spermatic cords, the left testis is usually lower than the right. Each testis is covered by the tunica vaginalis, an embryological derivative of the out-pouching of peritoneum (process vaginalis) that guided them through the inguinal canal into the scrotum. The tunica vaginalis consists of two layers:

1) A visceral layer: closely related to the testes and deficient at the point of attachment between the testis and the epididymis/spermatic cord.
2) A parietal layer: extending to the distal part of the spermatic cord.

A cavity containing a small amount of fluid between the two layers allows for the free movement of the testis in the scrotum. Deep in to tunica vaginalis is a tough fibrous layer, the tunica albuginea, a protective capsule around the testis continuous with

the mediastinum testis. Numerous thin fibrous layers, or septa, extend from the mediastinum testis internally, dividing it into lobules that contain the seminiferous tubules.

Seminiferous tubules are highly coiled and convoluted tubes reaching up to 70 cm in length when uncoiled. They are the site of spermatogenesis. Tubules converge posteriorly to form a network in the mediastinum of the testis called the rete testis. Multiple efferent ductules (ductus efferentes) extend from the rete testis to meet the head of the epididymis.

- *Blood supply:* the testes are supplied by symmetrical testicular arteries that originate directly from the abdominal aorta, just distal to the renal arteries and pass over the anterior surface of the psoas major muscles, crossing the ureters and external iliac artery to enter the deep inguinal ring. In doing so the arteries enter the inguinal canals within the spermatic cord before reaching the scrotum.
- *Venous drainage:* through the pampiniform venous plexus – networks of veins that surround the testicular artery in the spermatic cord that

drain the testis and the epididymis. The veins of the pampiniform plexus join on each side to form testicular veins that drain asymmetrically into the interior vena cava; directly on the right side and via the renal vein on the left.

- *Lymphatic drainage:* towards lumbar and preaortic nodes.
- *Innervation:* by testicular plexuses of nerves carrying vagal parasympathetic, visceral afferent, and sympathetic fibres from the T7 spinal segment carried on the testicular arteries.

Epididymis (Epididymides)

Towards the posterior aspect of the testes are the fine convoluted networks of tubules connecting the testes and the ductuli (vasa) deferentes (deferentia). The epididymides allow spermatozoa to mature and acquire motility. They are also the site of storage of spermatozoa prior to intercourse. Each epididymis can be divided into three anatomically distinct regions:

1) A head: situated on the superior posterior pole of the testis and formed by the ends of the efferent ductules.
2) A body: known as the true epididymis it extends inferiorly on the posteriolateral border of the testis as a single long coiled duct.
3) A tail: continuous with the ductus (vas) deferens at the inferior pole of the testis.

Ductuli (Vasa) Deferentes (Deferentia)

Muscular tubes spanning 30–45 cm from the tail of the epididymides to the base of the bladder where they join the seminal vesicles to form the ejaculatory ducts of the prostate. The ductuli (vasa) deferentes (deferentia) ascend posterior to the testes, medial to the epididymides and continue within the spermatic cords. They pass through the superficial inguinal rings into the inguinal canals penetrating the abdominal wall through the deep inguinal rings. Once in the abdominopelvic cavity, the ductuli (vasa) deferentes (deferentia) pass lateral to the inferior epigastric vessels before turning medially to cross the external iliac vessels. They continue medially, deep to the parietal peritoneum passing over the ureters posterior to the urinary bladder.

Continuing in an inferomedial direction at the base of the urinary bladder and anterior to the rectum, they enlarge to form the ampullae of the ductuli (vasa) deferentes (deferentia). The ampullae merge with the ducts of the seminal vesicles to form the ejaculatory ducts that penetrate the prostate gland to join the prostatic urethra.

- *Blood supply:* arterial supply is from the arteries to ductuli (vasa) deferentes (deferentia) arising from the superior or inferior vesical arteries which in turn are typically branches of the anterior trunks of the internal iliac arteries. There are anastomoses with the testicular arteries posterior to the testis.
- *Venous drainage:* most of the venous drainage of the ductuli (vasa) deferentes (deferentia) is into testicular veins. The pelvic portion drains into the vesicular and prostatic venous plexuses.
- *Lymphatic drainage:* mainly towards the external iliac lymph nodes.
- *Innervation:* sympathetic nerve innervation (mainly from the first lumbar ganglion) is derived from the inferior hypogastric plexus.

Seminal Vesicles

Lying between the bladder and the rectum, the elongated seminal vesicles secrete a thick-yellowish-alkaline fluid. This fluid nourishes the spermatozoa and contributes to about 60% of the volume of the ejaculate. The superior aspect of the vesicles are covered by peritoneum and separated from the rectum by the rectovesical pouch. Below this point they are closely related to the rectum and separated from it by only the rectovesical fascia. Each vesicle can be found lateral to the ampulla of the ductus (vas) deferens and at its lower end join it to form the ejaculatory duct.

- *Blood supply:* the seminal vesicles are supplied by the inferior vesicle and middle rectal arteries, typically branches from the anterior trunk of internal iliac arteries.
- *Venous drainage:* veins have similar names and accompany arteries.
- *Lymphatic drainage:* the superior part of the seminal vesicles drains mainly towards the internal iliac nodes but may also drain toward the sacral nodes. The inferior part of the seminal vesicle drain towards the external iliac nodes.

Ejaculatory Ducts

The paired ejaculatory ducts are formed by the union of the ducts of the ductus (vas) deferens and seminal vesicles. They are about 2.5 cm long and pass close together in an anteroinferior direction through the posterior prostate to open into the prostatic utricle.

- *Blood supply:* from the artery of ductus (vas) deferens.
- *Venous drainage:* through the prostatic and vesicle plexuses.
- *Lymphatic drainage:* toward the external iliac nodes.

Prostate Gland

The prostate gland is normally about 3 cm long, 4 cm wide and 2 cm deep. It has a glandular component, comprising two-thirds of the prostate, and a fibromuscular component which makes up the remaining third. It contributes about 30% of the volume of the ejaculate.

The prostate gland is surrounded by a dense fibrous capsule containing the prostatic plexuses of veins and nerves. Pelvic fascia condenses and surrounds the capsule forming a fibrous prostatic sheath, known as the false capsule. The fibrous sheath is continuous anterolaterally with the puboprostatic ligaments and blends posteriorly with the rectovesical fascia.

The prostate gland is located inferior to the bladder, posterior to the pubic symphysis and anterior to the rectum. It has a base and an apex in addition to anterior, posterior, and inferiolateral surfaces:

- The base: surrounds and fuses with the neck of the urinary bladder.
- The apex: the most inferior part of the prostate is closely/directly related to the superior aspect of the fascia surrounding the sphincter urethrae and deep perineal muscles. The prostatic urethra, extending from the neck of the urinary bladder to the apex of the prostate gland, passes through the perineum and becomes the membranous urethra.
- The anterior surface, related to the retropubic space, is connected to the pubic bones by the puboprostatic ligaments.
- The posterior surface, anterior to the ampulla of the rectum, is separated from it by the rectovesical fascia.
- The inferolateral surfaces are in contact with the puborectalis part of the levator ani.

The ejaculatory ducts pierce the posterior surface of the prostate, just inferior to the urinary bladder, and pass inferomedially for about 2 cm to empty into the prostatic urethra. The prostate gland also empties into the prostatic urethra through several duct openings.

The prostate gland can be divided into three zones:

1) The transitional zone: 5% of the glandular substance; surrounds the prostatic urethra.
2) The central zone: 20% of the glandular substance; is wedged-shaped and surrounds the ejaculatory ducts as they course into the gland.
3) The peripheral zone: 70% of the glandular substance; extends around the central zone surrounding it posteriorly and inferiorly. It also extends inferiorly forming the base of the prostate gland.

In addition to the three zones, a fibromuscular portion, positioned anterior to the prostatic urethra can also be noted. It is closely related to the bladder detrusor muscle superiorly and the external urethral sphincter inferiorly.

- *Blood supply:* from the inferior vesicle, internal pudendal, and middle rectal arteries which are all branches of the internal iliac artery.
- *Venous drainage:* veins around and at the base of the prostate join to form plexuses draining into the internal iliac vein. Prostatic venous plexuses also communicate with the internal vertebral venous plexuses.
- *Lymphatic drainage:* towards the internal iliac nodes. However, there is some drainage to the sacral nodes.
- *Innervation:* sympathetic fibres from the T12-L2 spinal segment reach the prostate through the hypogastric and pelvic plexuses.

Bulbo-Urethral Glands

The paired bulbo-urethral glands are pea-shaped mucus secreting glands located within the deep perineal pouch, posterolateral to the membranous urethra. Their ducts (3 cm long) pass inferomedially to penetrate the deep perineal membrane and open into the bulb of the spongy urethra at the root of the penis. Secretions enter the urethra during sexual arousal lubricating the penis and facilitating its entry into the vagina. Lymph is drained toward the internal iliac nodes.

Penis

The penis is a common outlet for urine and semen that can be considered as three anatomically distinct regions: a root, body, and glans. It is composed of three cylindrical erectile bodies: two paired corpora cavernosa and one corpus spongiosum. The erectile bodies are continuous with the crura and bulb of the root of the penis in the superficial perineal pouch:

- The crura are attached to the margins of the ischiopubic ramus and inferior surface of the perineal membrane. The crura fuse to form the two corpora cavernosa of the body of the penis distally and receive the helicine arteries proximally.
- The bulb, attached to the inferior surface of the perineal membrane, extends to form the corpus spongiosum of the body of the penis. The proximal part of the bulb is penetrated by the urethra which continues through the corpus spongiosum to form the external urethral orifice of the glans. The bulb receives the bulbourethral glands and the arteries of the bulb.

The crura and the bulb together form the root of the penis. The body of the penis is formed as the two corpora cavernosa extend distally fusing with each other along with the corpus spongiosum ventrally. It is suspended from the pubic symphysis by the suspensory ligament of the penis. Distally the corpora cavernosa expands overlapping the distal ends of the corpora cavernosa forming the glans penis. A double layer of skin, the prepuce, covers the glans to a variable extent if uncircumcised.

- *Blood supply:* the penis is mainly supplied by three branches of the internal pudendal arteries:
  - The artery of the bulb of the penis: supplying the corpus spongiosum including the glans penis.
  - The deep artery of the penis: supplying the crura and corpora cavernosa via the helicine arteries.
  - The dorsal artery of the penis: courses on the dorsal surface supplying the glans and superficial fascia.
  - The artery of the bulb and the dorsal arteries of the penis anastomose. Branches of the external pudendal arteries also supply the penile skin.
- *Venous drainage:* through the deep dorsal vein of the penis which drains into the prostatic plexus. The skin and subcutaneous tissue of the penis is drained by the superficial dorsal vein into the superficial external pudendal vein.
- *Lymphatic drainage:* toward internal iliac and deep inguinal lymph nodes. Lymphatic drainage from the glans and the distal corpus spongiosum including the distal urethra is toward the deep inguinal nodes, whereas the cavernous bodies and the proximal parts of the urethra drain to the internal iliac nodes.
- *Innervation:* is derived from various sources:
  - The skin of the penis is innervated by the pudendal nerve with contribution from the ilioinguinal nerve to a small region of the proximal dorsal penile skin.
  - The ischiocavernosus and bulbocavernosus muscles surrounding the erectile tissue are supplied by the perineal nerve, a branch of the pudendal nerve.
  - Parasympathetic fibres, originating from the S2 and S3 spinal segments, are supplied by the pelvic splanchnic nerves.
  - Sympathetic fibres, originating from the L1 spinal segment, are supplied by the superior and inferior hypogastric plexuses.

Scrotum

The scrotum is a cutaneous fibromuscular pouch that contains the testes and associated structures. It is located posteroinferiorly to the penis and inferior to the pubis. It develops bilaterally and fuses at a midline raphe from which a septum extends internally separating the scrotum into two compartments.

- *Blood supply:* branches of the internal and external pudendal arteries supply posterior and anterior aspects of the scrotum respectively.
- *Venous drainage:* through the external pudendal veins.

- *Lymphatic drainage:* towards the superficial lymph nodes.
- *Innervation:* the anterior aspect of the scrotum is innervated by the ilioinguinal and the genital branch of the genitofemoral nerve. The posterior aspect is innervated by branches of the pudendal nerve and the posterior cutaneous nerve of the thigh.

Semen (Seminal Fluid)

The alkaline cloudy white fluid (pH 7–7.5) that is expelled to the outside during ejaculation is called semen. It is comprised of spermatozoa and the secretions of the seminal vesicles, prostate, and the bulbourethral glands. Semen contains prostaglandins, citric acid, amino acids, fructose, protein-splitting enzymes, phosphorylcholine, potassium, and zinc. The volume of ejaculate varies from 2 to 5 mL with an average of 120 million sperm per millilitre. Spermatozoa can live up to 6 days in the female reproductive tract.

Erection and Ejaculation

Output from the autonomic nervous system increases during sexual arousal resulting in erection and subsequent ejaculation. Erection is under parasympathetic control while ejaculation is controlled by the sympathetic system and somatic fibres:

- Parasympathetic innervation (S2-S4) brings about vasodilation of the helicine arteries supplying the corpora cavernosa. The resulting engorgement of erectile tissue brings about erection that is maintained by compression of venular plexuses by bulbospongiosus and ischiocavernosus muscles.
- Sympathetic innervation (L1-L2) causes the contraction of the smooth muscles in the epididymis, ductus (vas) deferens, seminal vesicle, ejaculatory ducts, prostate, and the internal urethral sphincter at the neck of the bladder. This contraction moves seminal fluid to the prostatic urethra and prevents its retrograde flow into the urinary bladder. The rhythmic contraction of bulbospongiosus muscle compresses the spongy urethra and expels the fluid.

After ejaculation, the bulbospongiosus and ischiocavernosus muscles relax allowing more blood to be drained into the deep dorsal vein returning the penis to the flaccid state. The smooth muscles of the arteries feeding the erectile tissue constrict, decreasing the amount of blood going into the erectile tissue.

Further Reading

Coad, J. and Dunstall, M. (2001). *Anatomy and Physiology for Midwives*. London: Mosby.

Graaff, V.D. (2001). *Human Anatomy*, 6th edition. New York: McGraw Hill Higher Education.

Gray, H., Standring, S., Ellis, H., Berkovitz, B.K. (2005). *Gray's Anatomy: The Anatomical Basis of Clinical Practice*, 39th edition. Edinburgh: Churchill Livingstone. pp. 1305–1355.

Heffner, L.J. and Schust D.J. (2010). *The Reproductive System at a Glance*. Chichester: Wiley.

Moore, K.L., Dalley, A.F. and Agur A.M. (2013). *Clinically Oriented Anatomy*. Baltimore: Lippincott Williams & Wilkins.

Sinnatamby, C. (2006). *Last's Anatomy: Regional and Applied*. 11th edition. Edinburgh: Churchill Livingstone.

Verralls, S. (1993). *Anatomy and Physiology Applied to Obstetrics*. 3rd edition. Edinburgh: Churchill Livingstone.

3

Fundamentals of Reproductive Endocrinology

Derrick Ebot, Haider Hilal, Michael Carroll, and James Coey

Introduction

After the development and differentiation of the gonads and external genitalia (see Chapter 1), the nascent reproductive organs remain in relative quiescence until the onset of puberty. Puberty is marked by the maturation of the genital organs, development of the secondary sex characteristics, acceleration of growth, and the occurrence of menarche in the female. The age at onset of puberty and the cadence at which puberty develops is dependent on many factors. In girls, increased ovarian and adrenal sex steroid secretion leads to the indicators of puberty such as breast development (thelarche) and appearance of pubic hair (pubarche). Usually these changes occur between 8 and 13 years of age. The mean age at menarche among different ethnic groups is between 12 and 13 years. In boys, the earliest physical appearance of puberty is an increase in testicular volume, usually occurring between 9 and 14 years of age. This early sexual development in both sexes is mostly due to the activity of the adrenal cortical steroids dehydroepiandrosterone (DHEA), dehydroepiandrosterone sulfate (DHEAS), and androstenedione, and is referred to as adrenadarche.

Adrenadarche is distinct from hypothalamic pituitary gonadal regulation of reproductive physiology (gonadarche). Increased gonadal steroidogenesis and the completion of gametogenesis during gonadarche are stimulated by enhanced secretion of the gonadotropins: luteinizing hormone (LH) and follicle-stimulating hormone (FSH). The production of gonadal steroidogenesis is regulated by the hypothalamic gonadotropin-releasing hormone (GnRH).

GnRH is a 10-amino-acid peptide that is synthesized in specialized neuronal bodies of the arcuate nucleus of the medial basal hypothalamus. These GnRH-producing neurons are limited in number (approximately 1000 to 2000). Normal gonadotropin secretion requires pulsatile release of GnRH. This pulsatile, rhythmic activity is an inherent property of GnRH neurons (termed the GnRH-pulse generator), and various hormones and neurotransmitters can temper this rhythm. GnRH is transported to the anterior pituitary via the hypophyseal portal circulation where it activates gonadotropin secretion. Enhanced secretion of the gonadotropins, LH and FSH, stimulate increased gonadal steroidogenesis and the completion of gametogenesis during gonadarche (see Figure 3.1 for an outline of steroidogenesis).

The timing of puberty is precisely controlled by a plethora of endogenous signals and environmental cues that impinge at different levels of the hypothalamic–pituitary–gonadal axis. The role of leptin and kisspeptin are key regulators of GnRH release and are important in the timing of puberty, where they act directly on the GnRH pulse generator. Furthermore, metabolic conditions and the amount of energy reserves play an essential role in the modulation the GnRH-pulse generator and hence the timing of puberty. This makes good biological sense, especially in the female, so that the reproductive capacity, which implies the potential metabolic drainage of pregnancy and lactation, is only acquired when threshold energy stores and optimal metabolic conditions are achieved. Successful reproduction requires intact, healthy reproductive anatomy and functional endocrine signalling.

Clinical Reproductive Science, First Edition. Edited by Michael Carroll.
© 2019 John Wiley & Sons Ltd. Published 2019 by John Wiley & Sons Ltd.
Companion website: www.wiley.com/go/carroll/clinicalreproductivescience

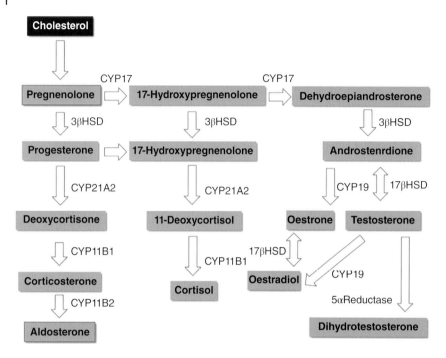

Figure 3.1 Steroidogenesis. A simplified scheme of steroidogenesis showing the various pathways and associated enzymes involved in the synthesis of the adrenal and gonadal steroid hormones.

This chapter will give an overview of the control of female and male reproductive endocrinology.

Female Reproductive Endocrinology

The female reproductive system is responsible for the production and release of oocytes (oogenesis and ovulation), fertilization, embryo implantation and gestation, parturition (expelling the fetus from the uterus), and lactation (provision of milk during nursing). Reproduction function in the female is characterized by cycles of follicular development, ovulation and endometrial receptivity, and menstruation.

The Ovaries and Ovarian Cycle

From birth the ovaries contain a number of immature, primordial follicles. These follicles each contain similarly immature primary oocytes. The start of puberty in females is associated with the start of

folliculogenesis and the onset of regular ovulatory and menstrual cycles. These cycles represent complex hormonal changes involving the hypothalamic–pituitary–ovarian axis (Figure 3.2).

This section will give a brief overview of the ovary and ovarian control. See Chapter 4 for more detail on the ovarian anatomy, the oocyte, and folliculogenesis. The ovary constantly alternates between two phases:

1) The follicular phase: dominated by the presence of maturing follicles that will secrete oestrogen when mature.
2) The luteal phase: characterized by the presence of the corpus luteum (CL), secreting predominantly progesterone.

Folliculogenesis

1) Primitive germ cells (oogonia) undergo cellular division in meiosis 1 to become a primary oocyte within the ovary.
2) At 18–22 weeks postconception the oocyte becomes surrounded by a single layer of flat granulosa cells forming the primordial follicle.

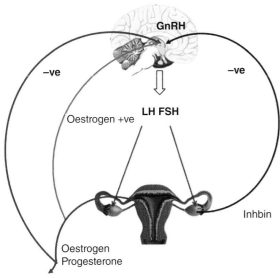

GnRH

−ve   −ve

Oestrogen +ve   **LH FSH**

                     Inhbin

Oestrogen
Progesterone

Hormonal function

Figure 3.2 Female reproductive endocrinology. GnRH released from the hypothalamus stimulates the release of luteinizing hormone (LH) and follicle-stimulating hormone (FSH) from the anterior pituitary. These gonadotropins stimulate the synthesis of the ovarian reproductive hormones. Oestrogen and progesterone are released into the circulation where they exert various hormonal responses including preparing the endometrium for implantation. They also have a negative effect, where increasing levels decrease gonadotropin release. Mid cycle, increasing oestrogen levels stimulates a surge of LH release. Inhibin, an ovarian peptide hormone, downregulates FSH release.

3) Under the influence of local paracrine signalling the zona pellucida forms and granulosa cells become cuboidal forming the primary (preantral) follicle. The oocyte genome is activated and gene transcription starts. Granulosa cells will eventually become responsive to FSH.

4) Stroma-like thecal cells are recruited through oocyte-secreted signals and undergo differentiation to become the theca externa and theca interna of the secondary (preantral) follicle.

5) An oestrogen-rich antrum starts to form, demarcating the early tertiary (developing antral or Graafian) follicle. Thecal cells will become responsive to LH causing oestrogen levels to rise.

6) Follicles of a certain size (2–5 mm) at the beginning of the follicular phase are referred to as recruitable antral follicles, the rest undergo atresia (follicular death).

7) After 2 weeks of growth under the influence of FSH the recruited follicle has developed into a late tertiary (dominant/mature) follicle.

Control of the Ovarian Cycle

The early stages of preantral follicular growth that precede the follicular phase do not require GnRH. Hormonal support from LH and FSH is required for further follicular development and antral formation. GnRH acts directly on the pituitary regulating the synthesis and release of these gonadotropins. Under the influence of FSH and LH, granulosa cells secret high levels of oestrogen along with inhibins that exert negative feedback on the pituitary.

LH stimulates the theca interna cells to convert cholesterol to androgens (androstenedione), which is converted by FSH-stimulated granulosa cells to oestrogen (estradiol). Oestrogen contributes to antral formation locally whilst rising; circulating levels have effects throughout the body. The marked increase in circulating levels that occur around mid-cycle act on the pituitary and the hypothalamus through positive feedback causing a sudden surge in LH levels. This LH surge triggers the onset of ovulation.

Control of Ovulation

Ovulation is the process by which the oocyte is expelled from a bulge on the ovarian surface of the late tertiary (dominant or mature) follicle. This process is facilitated by a release of enzymes from follicular cells that digest connective tissue in the follicular wall, in turn triggered by the aforementioned burst in LH secretion. Just before ovulation the oocyte completes its first meiotic division. The resulting secondary oocyte, surrounded by the zona pellucida and granulosa cells (corona radiata), is expelled into the abdominal cavity. A rise in basal temperature occurs about 2 days prior to ovulation.

Control of the Corpus Luteum

Following ovulation, the remaining granulosa and surrounding capsule differentiate to form the CL. LH maintains the CL, which secretes large amounts of progesterone and smaller amounts of oestrogen and inhibin. Progesterone and inhibin exert negative feedback on the anterior pituitary preventing a further LH surge. The CL functions for approximately 2 weeks before degenerating to form corpus albicans if fertilization does not occur, otherwise the CL will become the CL of pregnancy. The placenta will then continue to secret the oestrogens and progesterone for the maintenance of pregnancy. The mechanisms that govern the degeneration of the CL have yet to be fully elucidated but are thought to involve a complex interplay between declining levels of LH along with prostaglandins and oestrogen released from the luteal cells. The demise of the CL marks the end of the luteal phase and the start of a new follicular phase as a result of a fall in plasma progesterone and oestrogen levels. Withdrawal of the inhibitory effect of these hormones on the anterior pituitary stimulates the production of LH and FSH.

The Uterus and Menstrual Cycle

Fluctuations in circulating levels of oestrogen and progesterone during the ovarian cycle bring about a menstrual cycle of a similar, 28-day duration. The most obvious manifestation is menstrual bleeding over 3–5 days in a fertile female, although less obvious changes take place throughout the cycle. The uterus is comprised of two main layers: (1) the myometrium – an outer smooth muscle layer and (2) the endometrium – an inner lining containing numerous blood vessels and glands.

Raised oestrogen levels from during the follicular phase of the ovarian cycle stimulates the growth of both the endometrium and myometrium. The hypertrophic effect on the cells of the endometrium (proliferative phase of menstrual cycle) brings about a two- to threefold increase in thickness by the time ovulation takes place. It also induces the synthesis of progesterone receptors; thus progesterone can only have an effect on the endometrium after being primed by oestrogen. Progesterone facilitates the endometrial implantation of a fertilized ovum through the accumulation of electrolytes, water, and the glandular secretion of large amounts of glycogen. The menstrual cycle consists of three phases: menstrual, proliferative, and secretory or progestational phases.

Menstrual Phase

The most overt phase of the menstrual cycle typically lasts for about 5–7 days after the degeneration of the CL. Convention dictates that the first day of menstruation is the start of new ovarian and menstrual cycles. It coincides with the end of the ovarian luteal phase and the onset of a new follicular phase. In the absence of fertilization, the CL degenerates resulting in a drop in circulating levels of oestrogen and progesterone. This fall in hormonal support for the endometrium stimulates the release of uterine prostaglandins bringing about vasoconstriction of the spiral arteries supplying the functional layer of the endometrium. The resulting hypoxia brings about the death of the endometrium and supporting arteries resulting in bleeding and flushing of sloughed off endometrial tissue. The same local uterine prostaglandins also stimulate mild rhythmic contractions of the uterine myometrium that help to expel blood and endometrial debris (menstrual flow) from the uterus through the vagina.

Proliferative Phase

After 5–7 days of menstruation the influence of FSH and LH enable the newly recruited antral follicles to secrete sufficient oestrogen to promote repair and growth of the endometrium. The ensuing proliferative phase coincides with the last portion of the ovarian follicular phase. Oestrogen stimulates once again the proliferation of epithelial cells, glands, and blood vessels. The oestrogen-dominant proliferative phase spans from the end of menstruation to ovulation, triggered by the oestrogen-induced LH surge.

Secretory or Progestational Phase

Following ovulation the uterus enters the secretory or progestational phase that coincides with the ovarian luteal phase. Large amounts of oestrogen and progesterone secreted by the CL transform the endometrium into a richly vascularized, glycogen-secreting lining capable of supporting the embryo after implantation. If fertilization and implantation do not occur a new menstrual/follicular phase will ensue (see Figure 3.3 – a summary of the menstrual cycle).

Pregnancy

Fertilization is followed by implantation of the embryo (blastocyst) into the endometrium. The CL persists and with it the production of progesterone and oestrogen. On implantation the blastocyst

MENSTRUAL CYCLE

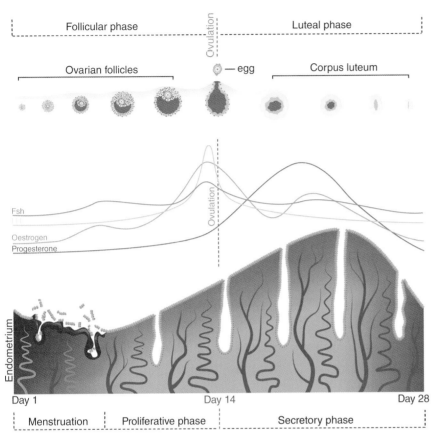

Figure 3.3 Ovarian and menstrual cycle. Changes in the ovarian follicle, endometrial thickness, and serum hormone levels during a typical 28-day menstrual cycle. *Source:* Marochkina Anastasiia/shutterstock.com.

becomes surrounded by an inner layer of cells, the cytotrophoblast, and an outer layer, the syncytiotrophoblast. The later erodes through the endometrium anchoring the implantation site. The placenta develops and becomes associated with the trophoblastic covering of the developing embryo.

At approximately 9 days following implantation the syncytiotrophoblast begins to secrete human chorionic gonadotropin (hCG). hCG is a glycoprotein that promotes the persistence of the CL and, therefore, the continuous secretion of oestrogen and progesterone. hCG has an effect very similar to LH and not only prevents the degeneration of the CL but also strongly stimulates its steroid secretion, reaching a peak at 60–80 days. Its presence in urine

enables a routine laboratory test for confirming pregnancy and is detectable approximately 2 weeks postconception. The developing placenta further supplements the production of hCG and progressively begins to produce oestrogen and progesterone through the first trimester. Low levels of hCG during pregnancy is indicative of placental insufficiency, as hCG is produced in proportion to the size of the placenta.

Throughout pregnancy, plasma concentrations of oestrogen and progesterone continually increase. Oestrogen stimulates the growth of the uterine myometrium. Progesterone inhibits uterine contractility so that the fetus is not expelled prematurely. Almost all the oestrogen and progesterone is supplied by the

CL during the first 2 months of pregnancy. Once the CL degenerates, the placenta becomes the main source of oestrogen and progesterone. The syncytiotrophoblast also secrets large amounts of another hormone – human placental lactogen (hPL) or chorionic somatomammotropin (hCS). hPL is thought to have a similar effect as human growth hormone, causing retention of electrolytes (nitrogen, potassium, and calcium). Other purported functions include promoting lipolysis, inhibiting free glucose uptake by the mother in order to divert a larger amount to the developing fetus, and encouraging mammary gland development in preparation for lactation.

Parturition

Mechanisms that Control the Events of Parturition

1) The smooth muscle cells of the myometrium have inherent rhythmicity and are capable of autonomous contractions, propagated as the muscle is stretched by the growing fetus.
2) The near-term uterus secretes several prostaglandins (PGE_2 and $PGF_2\alpha$) that are potent stimulators of uterine smooth muscle contraction.
3) Oxytocin, from the posterior pituitary gland, is a potent uterine muscle stimulant, acting not only directly on uterine smooth muscle but also stimulating the synthesis of prostaglandins. Oxytocin is released in response to uterine stretch, particularly the cervix. The number of oxytocin receptors in the uterus increases during the last few weeks of pregnancy. Therefore, the contractile response to any given plasma concentration of oxytocin is greatly increased at parturition.

Parturition, the process of giving birth, usually occurs about 9 months after fertilization. It involves relaxation/dilation of the cervical canal to allow easy passage of the fetus as well as contraction of the uterine myometrium providing a propulsive force to expel the fetus out of the mother. It is preceded by a month of irregular uterine contractions in the third trimester. These contractions (Braxton Hicks contractions) increase in intensity and become more regular as birth approaches. Due to their regularity and increase in intensity they are sometimes mistaken for the onset of labour and thus sometimes called 'false labour'. The exact mechanism that dictates the onset of labour is not fully understood. It involves interplay of various hormones as follows:

- DHEA-derived oestrogens increase the excitability of the uterine myometrium causing an increase in secretion of prostaglandins. Prostaglandins promote softening of the cervix by stimulating cervical enzymes that degrade collagen around the birth canal.
- Oestrogen enhances the formation of gap junctions (with connexons) between adjacent myometrial cells to encourage communication and synchrony between the muscle fibres during contraction. Oestrogens promote a significant increase in receptors within the myometrium and endometrium on which oxytocin and prostaglandins act, promoting uterine contraction.
- Oxytocin is produced by the paraventricular nucleus of the hypothalamus and stored within the posterior pituitary. There is a significant increase in oxytocin receptors within the myometrium and endometrium, on which oxytocin and prostaglandins act, promoting uterine contraction.
- Relaxin produced by the placenta also plays a part in parturition. As its name suggests, this polypeptide plays a vital role in the relaxation of the cervix/ birth canal and the connective tissue around pelvic bones once labour is initiated.

Some studies indicate that the fetus/baby may dictate its own time of birth. This is due to an increase in secretion of corticotropin-releasing hormone (CRH) mainly from the placenta into maternal and fetal circulation. A smaller amount of CRH also comes from the fetal hypothalamus, which increases the production of adrenocorticotrophic hormone (ACTH) from the pituitary. This results in an increase in circulating cortisol and DHEA from the adrenal cortex. Cortisol hastens maturation of the fetal lungs by promoting surfactant secretion and facilitating lung expansion prior to parturition. The increase in fetal cortisol (supplemented by maternal ACTH) also favours a high oestrogen to progesterone ratio from the placenta and thus an increase in prostaglandin secretion leading to relaxation of the birth canal. This mechanism explains why fetal stress induces premature labour and why levels of placenta-produced CRH has now been well

Table 3.1 Hormones involved in pregnancy.

Organ	Hormonal Effect
Placenta	▲ Oestrogen, progesterone, hCG, inhibin, hPL
Anterior pituitary gland	▲ Prolactin ▼ FSH and LH
Posterior pituitary gland	▲ Vasopressin
Adrenal cortex	▲ Aldosterone and cortisol
Parathyroids	▲ Parathyroid hormone
Kidneys	▲ Renin, erythropoietin, and 1,25-dihydroxyvitamin D

FSH, follicle-stimulating hormone; hCG, human chorionic gonadotrophin; hPL, human placental lactogen; LH, luteinizing hormone.

established as a predictor of timing for parturition (see Table 3.1 for a summary of hormones and organs of origin involved during pregnancy).

Lactation

Breast development (thelarche) involves the interplay of various hormones. Oestrogen and progesterone in general promote development of the mammary duct and of the lobules respectively as the female matures. The lobules (containing alveoli) synthesize the milk that is then conducted through a ductal system to the nipple ready for ejection after parturition.

During pregnancy, full maturation of the glands and milk production is achieved under the influence of prolactin. Rising levels of oestrogen stimulate an increase in prolactin release from the anterior pituitary. Together with hCS coming from the placenta, these hormones upregulate the production of enzymes taking part in milk synthesis. Although breast development during pregnancy is largely controlled by the increasing levels of prolactin, its actual milk secretory function is limited by the antagonism of oestrogen. After parturition, the drop in oestrogen levels produces a surge in prolactin and thus an increase in milk production/secretion. Prolactin also enhances the production of activated vitamin D (calcitriol), which may maintain calcium levels during pregnancy.

The ejection of milk from the mammary glands usually occurs after parturition and is controlled by oxytocin, which is released by the pituitary gland. The release of this hormone and maintenance of prolactin secretion is induced by the suckling of the newborn. Suckling stimulates nerve fibres in the nipple that release action potentials that travel to the hypothalamus. The activated hypothalamus thus potentiates a massive release of oxytocin from the posterior pituitary.

Suckling enhances the release of prolactin by inhibiting the release of the prolactin inhibitory factor dopamine from the hypothalamus and enhancing the release of prolactin-stimulating factors like thyrotropin-releasing hormone (TRH) and vasoactive intestinal peptide (VIP). The absence of inhibition and an increase in stimulating peptides on the pituitary leads to an increased prolactin release and thus milk secretion in the nursing breast.

In turn, production of prolactin causes a decrease in levels of gonadotropins. This is achieved by inhibiting GnRH from the hypothalamus, which leads to a decreased pituitary release of LH and FSH, and a subsequent decrease in the levels of oestrogens and progesterone from the ovary. This inhibitory property of prolactin on the gonadotropins is attributed to the lack of ovulation that occurs during nursing. As such, nursing women have been found to have significantly longer periods of amenorrhea when compared to their non-nursing counterparts. In the absence of nursing there is a decrease in prolactin levels and thus limited milk production.

Male Reproductive Endocrinology

Overview and Development

Chapter 1 details the sexual differentiation of the male reproductive gonads and sexual organs. Briefly, at approximately 7 weeks gestation, the human embryo remains sexually ambiguous. In males, testis-inducing factors cause differentiation from the default female phenotype. During formation of the testes, testosterone and other androgens bring about the formation of the external genitalia and internal male reproductive structures, whilst other testicular factors cause regression of female reproductive organ precursors. Androgens also play a role in the descent of the testicles from their origin in the upper abdomen. Germ cells enter an arrested phase of maturation in the first trimester. A surge of testosterone in the neonatal period plays a role in testicular development, but it is not until the largest androgen surge during puberty that gonadarche occurs, with the onset of spermatogenesis.

The Testes and Testosterone

The testes are the site of spermatogenesis and the production of testosterone, the male sex hormone, which along with other androgens including dihydrotestosterone (DHT) has wide ranging effects (Figure 3.4):

1) Male genital tract:
   – Growth of accessory organs of reproduction.
   – Maintaining normal reproductive function in adult males.
2) Secondary sexual characteristics: testosterone affects a variety of other organs in the human body, producing the overall male pattern in humans:

– Pubic hair: during the early stages of adolescence, sex hormones from the adrenals and testis are responsible for growth of pubic hair. Hair follicles on other parts of the body are also stimulated, with the exception of those on the scalp. Dihydrotestosterone is thought to be responsible for loss of scalp hair (causing male pattern baldness) in later life and stimulation of sebaceous glands.
– Voice: over the course of puberty, growth of the larynx and vocal cord occurs in response to testosterone and other androgens, and results in the characteristic deep voice of the male.
– Growth: growth hormones affect growing long bones, where oestradiol plays a vital role in closure of epiphyseal plates. Additionally, testosterone promotes muscle mass along with physical vigour.

Males are thought to have higher cellular enzymatic activity than females. These activities are seen in mitochondrial cytochrome C oxidase

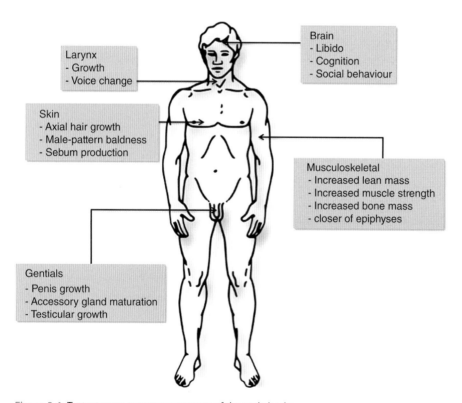

Figure 3.4 Testosterone targets many parts of the male body.

and lysosomal hydroxylase inside the cells. Cellular patterns specific to males can be induced by administration of testosterone in castrated male rats.

Testosterone levels decline with age. Throughout the life cycle, testosterone maintains libido, develops secondary sexual characteristics, and affects behaviour in males. Men with low levels of testosterone (hypogonadism) typically complain of low energy levels, libido, and muscle.

Control of Testosterone Production

Role of Leydig Cells

Leydig cells, present in the interstitial area of the testes, are responsible for synthesis and secretion of testosterone. This function occurs in response to stimulation by LH, which is the main hormone required for the maintenance and growth of Leydig cells. High affinity surface LH receptors are present on Leydig cells and trigger the formation of cyclic adenosine monophosphate (cAMP) and activation of protein kinase A. This ultimately leads to increased synthesis of enzymes specific for testosterone production. Testosterone regulates both intratesticular and extratesticular functions through its release from Leydig cells into surrounding capillaries or diffusion into the seminiferous tubules, the site of spermatogenesis.

During fetal development, placental chorionic gonadotropin (hCG) controls growth and differentiation of Leydig cells as well as secretion of testosterone. As the pituitary gland develops subsequently, LH becomes the principal hormone regulating Leydig cell activity.

Testicular oestrogens, also produced by Leydig cells, contribute to normal sperm formation.

Role of Sertoli cells

Sertoli cells are found between spermatogonia and vasculature within the germinal epithelium. Their primary function is to provide nourishment to developing sperm. FSH stimulates these cells by acting on specific FSH surface receptors. FSH causes proliferation and differentiation of Sertoli cells prior to puberty and maintains production of functional Sertoli cells in the adult. FSH also indirectly regulates sperm development by preventing germ cell death.

In response to FSH the following proteins are synthesized:

- Androgen binding protein:
  - Helps in development of sperm cells.
  - Helps maintain high levels of testosterone.
- Inhibin:
  - Has both endocrine and paracrine function.
  - Member of transforming growth factor B (TGF beta) family and locally acts on Leydig cells.
  - Important role in hypothalamic–pituitary–testicular axis (HPT).
- Aromatase:
  - Converts testosterone, secreted from Leydig cells, into oestradiol, responsible for negative feedback in brain, regulation of fertility, and sealing of epiphyseal plates during growth.
- Growth factors:
  - Supports spermatogenesis.
  - Increases motility of sperm and thus fertility.

Control of Testicular Function

The HPT axis in males controls production of sperm within the germinal epithelium and synthesis of testosterone in the Leydig cells of testes. The HTP axis is controlled by positive and negative feedback loops – where inhibition of LH and FSH is accomplished by increased testosterone, inhibin, and other hormones. Additionally, other factors can influence the activity of the HPT (Figure 3.5).

Hypothalamus

As in the female, GnRH stimulates the production and release of gonadotropins FSH and LH, secreted from the pituitary gland. The limbic system is thought to be an additional site of production of GnRH, with a role in regulation of sexual behaviour.

- GnRH takes hypothalamic–pituitary portal channels to reach the anterior pituitary gland.
- GnRH acts on high affinity surface receptors on anterior pituitary gland cells, causing activation of protein kinase C and thus synthesis/release of FSH and LH.
- Secretion of GnRH into the portal system is pulsatile thus making secretion of FSH and LH episodic.
- Continuous influx of GnRH or GnRH analogues causes suppression of release of the gonadotropins (FSH and LH).

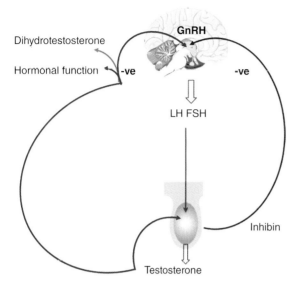

Dihydrotestosterone

Hormonal function

GnRH

-ve   -ve

LH FSH

Inhibin

Testosterone

Figure 3.5 Male reproductive endocrinology. The testis is controlled by classic positive feed-forward and negative feedback mechanisms. As in the female, gonadotropin-releasing hormone (GnRH) released from the hypothalamus stimulates the release of luteinizing hormone (LH) and follicle-stimulating hormone (FSH) from the anterior pituitary. LH stimulates the testicular Leydig cells to produce testosterone. Testosterone is converted to dihydrotestosterone. Both testosterone and dihydrotestosterone are responsible for the induction and maintenance of secondary sexual characteristics. Testosterone and inhibin both control the hypothalamic–pituitary–testicular axis through negative feedback.

Pituitary

FSH and LH are the principal regulatory hormones required for testicular function. Release of these glycoprotein hormones from cells of the pituitary gland depends on stages of development of a male human. By the end of the first trimester, the male fetus has a considerable amount of functional gonadotropins in the pituitary gland. This level rises towards a plateau and then decreases by the end of pregnancy, with an ultimate surge after birth.

Testicular

Testosterone and inhibin control the HPT axis through negative feedback:

1) Testosterone inhibits LH and GnRH production while maintaining relatively constant secretion of LH and FSH.
2) Testosterone can be converted to DHT, which inhibits LH secretion. Inhibin exerts its negative feedback by inhibiting FSH secretion.
3) Aromatase enzyme also has an effective negative feedback role by producing oestradiol in the brain.

There is a reciprocal relationship between FSH and inhibin hormone. Inhibin, produced by Sertoli cells, exerts negative feedback action over FSH secretion from pituitary gland cells. Conversely, FSH stimulates secretion of inhibin causing its level to rise in blood.

Inhibin is a nonsteroidal hormone and belongs to the transforming growth factor beta (TGF-beta) family of hormones. Its concentration in blood is indicative of the number of functional Sertoli cells. Inhibin B is considered to be the most important functional form secreted by human testes. In addition to inhibin, another member of same family, activin (2 beta units), stimulates FSH secretion.

Other Hormones Involved in Male Reproductive Behaviour

Sex hormones are usually thought to be the principal hormones for sexual behaviour. However, in some animals, peptide hormones, in addition to prolactin and GnRH, could play a regulatory role in testicular function. Peptide hormones shown to have a role in male sexual behaviour include: oxytocin, CRH, vasopressin, cholecystokinin, vasoactive intestinal peptides, neuropeptide Y, and galanin.

Further Reading

Barrett, K., Boitano, S. and Barman, S. (2010). *Ganong's Review of Medical Physiology*. 23rd Edition. New York: McGraw-Hill Professional Publishing.

Boron, W.F. and Boulpaep, E.L. (2012). *Medical Physiology*. 2nd Edition. Philadelphia: Elsevier.

Goodman, H.M. (2009). *Basic Medical Endocrinology*. 4th Edition. Oxford: Academic Press.

Hadley, M.E. and Levine, J.E. (2007). *Endocrinology*. 6th Edition. New Jersey: Pearson Education.

Nelson, R.J. (2011). *Behavioral Endocrinology*. 4th Edition. Massachusetts: Sinauer.

McLaughlin, D., Stamford, J. and White, D. (2007). *Human Physiology*. (Bios Instant notes) London: Routledge.

Strauss, J.F. and Barbieri, R.L. (2009). *Yen & Jaffe's Reproductive Endocrinology: Physiology, Pathophysiology, and Clinical Management*. 6th edition. Philadelphia: Elsevier.

4

The Ovaries, Oocytes, and Folliculogenesis

Jacques Gilloteaux and James Coey

Introduction

A pair of ovaries are attached to the lateral, right and left pelvic cavities, by the suspensory ligaments covered by the peritoneum. The ovaries are ellipsoid-shaped, 4 cm long, 2 cm wide, and about 1 cm thick, with some variations according to age, time of the reproductive cycle, and whether pregnancy is present. An old ovary is often covered with scars left by previous ovulations and pregnancies. The ovary is subdivided into a central medulla and a peripheral cortex delimited by a capsule of a dense irregular connective tissue layer or tunica albuginea (Figure 4.1). Their functions are: (1) as endocrine organs making and secreting the female steroids controlling the reproductive cycle, all reproductive tissues, especially those adapted to an eventual pregnancy, the mammary glands, and hence, maintenance of the female phenotype; and (2) producing female gametes.

Development of Ovaries

Gonadogenesis is covered in more detail in Chapter 1; this section will give a brief overview. The ovaries, like the testes (gonads), derive from three embryonic tissues and cells:

1) Mesodermal epithelium lining the posterior abdominal wall.
2) The underlying mesenchyme (embryonic connective tissue).
3) The primordial germ cells.

At first, each gonad develops during the fifth week when a mesothelial thickening grows in the medial side of the mesonephros. Covered by an actively proliferating epithelium both tissues make an elongated bulge: the gonadal ridge. This structure is also named an indifferent gonad made of an external cortex (epithelium) and an internal medulla (mesenchyme). The embryos with a pair of XX sex chromosomes grow the cortex to differentiate into an ovary while the medulla regresses.

Out of the wall of the umbilical vesicle, primordial germ cells migrate along the dorsal mesentery of the gut to the gonadal ridges. During the sixth week, these primordial germ cells penetrate the mesenchyme and parts of the gonadal cords. These cells become the oogonia. Follicular/granulosa cells derive from the surface epithelium of the primitive ovaries; this original population of surface cells also produce the germinative epithelium or mesothelium.

Sex Determination

Fertilization with a combination of two gametes with X sex chromosomes establish the female sex. However, before the seventh week, the gonads of the two sexes are identical in appearance as indifferent gonads. Both XX chromosomes are required for the development of the female phenotype. There is at least one autosomal gene (*Rspo1*) that plays a role in ovarian organogenesis. It is only by the tenth week that ovaries are identifiable histologically. When the gonadal cord extensions in the medulla form primitive rete ovarii, this structure undergoes

Clinical Reproductive Science, First Edition. Edited by Michael Carroll.
© 2019 John Wiley & Sons Ltd. Published 2019 by John Wiley & Sons Ltd.
Companion website: www.wiley.com/go/carroll/clinicalreproductivescience

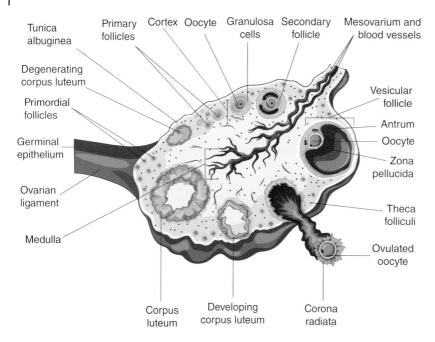

Figure 4.1 Human ovary. Reproduced with permission of Vecton/shutterstock.com.

degeneration about 5 weeks later. The cortical cords extending out of the surface epithelium increase in size and the primordial germ cells merge with them. Around the sixteenth week the cortical cords fragment into isolated cell clusters, now called primordial follicles. These structures, covered by flat cells, that derive from the surface or germinal epithelium and the primordial germ cells, constitute the primordial follicles each containing one oogonium.

The ovary surface epithelium makes its basal lamina and the basement membrane with the capsule, a dense irregular connective tissue or tunica albuginea, are formed by the mesenchymal tissue and maintained by the cortical stroma later.

Endocrine Organs

The ovaries are the organs that secrete the female, cholesterol-derived steroid hormones (oestrogens and progesterone) under the control of the gonadotropin-releasing hormones (GnRH) (from the hypothalamus) and the gonadotropins (see Chapter 3) during reproductive life. Thus, the ovaries not only provide ova but also support sexual differentiation, fetal development, growth with sexual maturation, and maintenance of the female phenotype.

Gametogenesis

The female germ cells issued from ootids maturing into ova are highly specialized cells that contain half the chromosomes of any other cells of the body, i.e. haploid cells. Each cell has 23 chromosomes (22 autosomes and 1 sex chromosome X). This number is required in order to unite with the male gamete to form a new living being (diploid) which carries either an X or Y sex chromosome, which determines the gender of the fertilized ovum. This then develops into either a male XY or female XX embryo. Distributed in the main cortical ovarian zone, oogonia (plural of oogonium) undergo gametogenesis, which in females is called oogenesis.

The Ovarian Epithelium

The ovaries are completely enveloped by the mesothelium. This envelope appears histologically as a simple epithelium of flat cuboidal to low columnar cells called germinal epithelium. These cells are more keratinized after menopause. Like most mesothelial cells their surfaces are decorated by numerous microvilli and rare cilia. Numerous pinocytotic vesicles and mitochondria can be seen. Even though the term germinal epithelium is often taught to be a misnomer, it has a developmental relationship with the covering of the oogonia and several ovarian pathologies. Its basal membrane extends on a stroma of a dense irregular connective tissue layer: the ovary capsule or tunica albuginea.

The Hilum and Medulla

Near its attachment with the aforementioned ligament, each ovary has a hilum or structure containing the mesovarium, the ovarian blood vessels, lymphatics, and nerves. This hilum continues into the medulla, at first showing twisted tracts that decrease in diameter, while branching into fine capillaries and nerves into a stroma of dense to loose connective tissue. This stroma extends into the cortex and reaches the capsule. Amongst the initial parts of these vessels, especially in the hilum, vestiges of Wolffian ducts can appear as flat to cuboidal tubular remnants, along with aggregates of hilar cells. These hilar cells can be numerous and display a morphology similar to the interstitial Leydig cells of the testes, which probably also originated from modified, smooth muscle cells from the walls of arterioles. They have a round to oval shape, lots of endoplasmic reticulum, mitochondria with tubular cristae, and lipid and lipofuscin deposits. Some contain Reinke crystals and hyaline bodies. These hilar cells (also called hilus cells) distribute in the aforementioned medullar stroma constituting, after some local replication, the theca interna cells of the growing follicles, producing androgens (testosterone and metabolites).

The Cortex

The cortical region encompasses:

- Gamete-producing and growing structures and their supporting cells (described later).
- A supportive stroma of loose to dense irregular connective tissue with irregularly distributed fibroblast-like cells and diverse collagens, especially condensed in the outer cortex. With aging and especially menopause, the aggregation and amount of dense collagen increases, initially in the same outer stromal region as if this region becomes an extension of the capsule. Some hilar cells, disseminated from the hilus, or as remnants

of theca cells during early gonadal development, can increase and distribute into clusters after menopause resulting in increased androgen production.

Female gametes and cyclically released hormones are produced from the ovarian cortex. Each month, these hormones control and stimulate oogenesis.

Oogenesis or Gamete Production

The term oogenesis encompasses a series of events that makes each stem cell or oogonium an ootid, then an ovum or oocyte (haploid female sex cells). In order to become female gametes, oogonia, have to undergo meiosis. During this dynamic activity, these cells undergo morphological changes, reduce the nucleus DNA content by half (becoming haploid), and mature to permit fertilization. This differentiation process, initiated during the fetal period of development, is not completed until after puberty or for some, oogonia only, 40 years later.

During follicular maturation, the following histological types can be recognized:

- Primordial follicle (15–20 μm)
- Growing follicles:
  - Primary follicle (25–80 μm)
  - Secondary or antral follicle (±80–200 μm)
  - Tertiary, mature, or Graafian follicle (±200–1500 μm)
- Corpus haemorrhagicum
- Corpus luteum (of the reproductive cycle) and of pregnancy
- Corpus albicans
- Dying or dead follicles: atretic follicles (occurring in primary to mature follicles).

Each follicle encompasses an epithelium of variable thickness consisting of flattened to cuboidal cells according to their stage of maturation; this epithelium encloses a differentiating oocyte or gamete. From several dozen maturing each reproductive cycle (± every 28-day cycle), one is destined to ovulate. Not every cycle results in ovulation and, sometimes, more than one ovum is shed during a cycle (resulting in dizygotic twins). In most normal women, a single ovum is produced each month, alternately from the two ovaries, for about 40 years, i.e. between menarche (±12 years of age) and menopause (±53 years of age), depending upon latitude or ethnic origin.

During each cycle, many follicles undergo the late stages of development but only one ovary releases a mature ovum. The other follicles degenerate or perish by atresia.

Primordial Follicles to Primary Follicles

During the earliest stage, oogonia replicate abundantly by mitotic activity and enlarge to form primary oocytes. At birth, these primary oocytes are locked in the prophase of the first meiotic division until puberty or later. They are numerous and mainly observed in the ovarian superficial cortex surrounded by a thin layer of squamous cells and are called primordial follicles (15–20 μm in diameter). At this stage of maturation, the layer of flat, squamous cells encaging the oocyte enlarges, become cuboidal cells and replicate, making one or more layers; this complex structure is the primary follicle (25–30 μm) in which each oocyte enlarges and develops a ooplasm with more evident organelles, such as the Balbiani body made of a perinuclear accumulation of annulate lamellae (nuclear envelope precursors), mitochondria, endoplasmic reticulum, Golgi apparatus, and lysosomes (Figure 4.2). A primary follicle shows that both oocytes and granulosa cells secrete an intercellular layer of acidophilic glycoproteins, the zona pellucida. Through this added structure, fine extensions of the tips of both cells connect with tiny gap junctions. Several layers of follicular or granulosa cells (stratum granulosum) around the oocyte make the overall structure a late primary follicle (±80–90 μm in diameter). At the base of the primary follicles, the granulosa cells form a basal lamina or membrana granulosa. The loose connective tissue or stroma surrounding the growing follicles forms the theca folliculi in which some myofibroblasts, and blood and lymph supply is located.

The primary oocytes are arrested in the prophase of the first meiotic division, from 12 to 50 years, so possible defects can occur, i.e. aneuploidy of chromosome 21 in women older than 40 years of age (Down syndrome or trisomy 21). Other rare defects caused by nondisjunction are associated with fragility of chromosome 22. Many spermatozoa in an ejaculate can carry abnormal morphology (two or more heads, more than one flagella, etc.) but do not fertilize a female gamete.

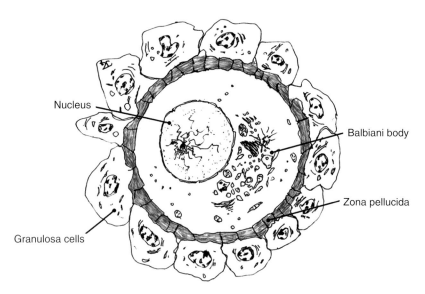

Figure 4.2 Primary follicle enlarged as if in transmission electron microscopy. From inside to outside: the primary oocyte with nucleus displaying prophase of meiosis I (chromosomal structures evident); the Balbiani body corresponds to the crescentic organization of organelles in the perikaryon. A blue belt-like is the zona pellucida built by the interacting oocyte and the connected layer of granulosa or follicular cells (contacts with fine extensions of both cells with gap junctions).

The secondary follicle or antral follicle can be recognized when spaces (Call-Exner bodies) are interrupting contacts between the proliferating granulosa cells and, in so doing, disrupting the closely associated follicle cells by coalescing and forming one, then several spaces filled by a viscous, glycoprotein-rich fluid, containing much hyaluronic acid – the liquor folliculi. These viscous, fluidic spaces eventually fuse into a single, eccentric large 'lake-like' space or antrum, while the primary oocyte and the overall follicle further enlarges. The increased number and layers of granulosa cells along with their antrum also are accompanied by an increased number of surrounding theca interna cells, organized in layers, circumferentially around the membrana granulosa.

Further growth of at least one follicle creates a mature, tertiary, or Graafian follicle, which can be as large as 2000 μm and can form a blister the size of the entire width of the ovary. Sometimes called the preovulatory follicle, this structure grows a large antrum that forces the oocyte and its surrounding granulosa cells, the cumulus oophorus, to one side of the follicle. During the same period the granulosa cell layer is formed, the corona radiata, which is directly attached to the zona pellucida.

At this stage of growth, meiosis continues from the prophase of the first meiotic division, induced by a maturation promoting factor (MPF), which facilitates a first meiotic division. The new secondary oocyte liberates a first polar body. The second meiotic division is initiated and halts at the metaphase. Meiosis only resumes if this selected secondary oocyte is fertilized. At this point of maturation, using the transmission electron microscope, the granulosa cells display abundant mitochondria and rough endoplasmic reticulum, free (poly)ribosomes, and a large Golgi apparatus, which are important for the secretion of the liquor folliculi. In comparison, theca interna cells have mitochondria with tubular cristae, smooth endoplasmic reticulum with scattered lipid deposits, which is suggested to be important in the production of testosterone and related steroids. Both cell types are involved in producing the ovarian steroid hormones that act on other body tissues with responsive receptors, such as those of the endometrium, myometrium, and mammary glands. In addition, these ovarian steroid hormones exert both positive and negative feedback to the hypothalamo-pituitary axis, thus influencing the production of gonadotropins and gonadotrophs.

Preovulatory Follicle

On further maturation of the follicle, the secondary oocyte with a single layer of granulosa cells containing its zona pellucida, detaches from the cumulus and 'floats' on the upper fluidic zone of the large antrum. The lining made by the membrana granulosa and the ovarian capsule are left with the germinal epithelium (mesothelium) to cover the preovulatory follicle, growing to reach the entire width of the ovarian cortex (>1500 μm). Before ovulation, each oocyte further undergoes the second meiotic division that stops at the metaphase. Bulging from the ovary, within a day following a huge LH surge, the swollen follicle is squeezed by the theca externa cells where the remaining follicular cells fold, and fluid pressure amputates the protruded edge caused by the mature follicle. At this stage, the antrum contains a viscous fluid, in addition to the contractile cells of the theca externa. The pressure increases on the follicle wall, producing a weakened area, called the stigma. The stigma ruptures due the thinning of cortex and the activities of lysosomal enzymes. The oocyte along with its corona radiata (referred to as cumulous cells), antrum fluid and small amounts of blood is evacuated in the local abdominal space. The oocyte–cumulous complex is captured by uterine aspiration caused by the fimbriae ciliated cells of the oviduct infundibulum. During ovulation, the presence of the liquor folliculi and blood can provoke a transient lower abdominal pain in some women, known as mittelschmerz or ovulatory pain. The remaining ruptured follicle, containing blood originating from ruptured theca interna vessels of the follicle, eventually forms a corpus hemorrhagicum. During ovulation, the basal body temperature rises by between 0.4 and 0.7 °C.

Corpus Luteum

As a result of ovulation, the remaining follicular structure collapses and is invaded by connective cells with some blood from the stroma/theca externa components. The former theca interna and granulosa cells acquire fatty reserves and become theca lutein cells and granulosa lutein cells, containing connective cells and blood vessels. This follicle becomes yellowish to the naked eye, hence its name: corpus luteum (latin for yellow body). This corpus or 'body' appears mid-cycle (about day 14) and remains only until the end of the reproductive cycle (about another 14 days). If the ovulated oocyte has not been fertilized after 12 h from expulsion/ovulation, this secondary oocyte with its corona dies in the oviduct ampulla. In this case, the corpus luteum regresses into a hyaline mass endowed with collagen-like material, by undergoing degradative, necrotic changes caused by a lack of nutritional vascular and hormonal supports. Both granulosa and theca lutein undergo fatty degeneration in a sort of saponification-like, oncotic death. Thus, from a yellowish body, it becomes a whitish body or corpus albicans. This body remnant may also undertake some calcification, then is progressively and slowly removed by ovarian macrophages, leaving scar tissue that may never disappear (see Figure 4.3 for stages of folliculogenesis).

Fertilization: A Short-Lived Female Gamete

This event occurs when the corona and zona pellucida of the ovulated oocyte is reached by a few spermatozoa and the penetration of one male gamete occurs, facilitated by the zona pellucida (see Chapter 6 for more detail). This penetration triggers:

- Calcium transients in the oocyte.
- A 'cortical reaction' in the oocyte causing circumferentially located cortical vesicles to be released. The entire zona pellucida then becomes immediately impermeable to any other male gamete.
- The liberation of the block on the second meiotic division of a maturation inhibitor. This causes the second anaphase and telophase producing the final haploid female precursor gamete or ootid and liberation of a second polar body under the zona pellucida that in some cases, divides itself but degenerates.

Fertilization usually takes place in the ampulla region of one oviduct.

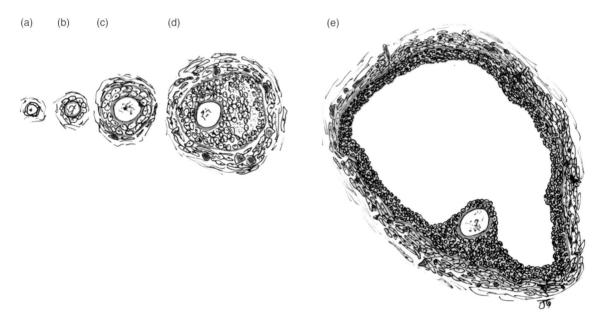

Figure 4.3 Stages of follicular growth during oogenesis. (a) Primordial follicle. (b) Primary follicle. (c) Late primary follicle (more than two layers of granulosa cells). (d) Secondary follicle. (e) Tertiary, mature or Graafian follicle. Green: membrane granulosa; blue, zona pellucida; red, vascularization in theca interna layer. Scales are not respected, i.e. structure in (b) is approximately 20 μm and (e) is 1500–1800 μm.

When fertilization has occurred, the zona pellucida is maintained while the slowly dividing embryo migrates to reach its uterine implantation site.

The corpus luteum supports the normal continuation of embryo growth and early fetal development for a few months. The syncytiotrophoblast layer of the placenta gives additional hormonal and other metabolic support until delivery. Ultimately, after delivery or any interruption of pregnancy, the corpus luteum degrades into an enormous corpus albicans and is progressively removed from the ovary described previously.

Loss of Follicles

From an estimated population of 7 million primordial follicles, there are around 1.5–2.5 million follicles at birth, decreasing further in infancy and childhood due to ovarian follicle atresia. At puberty around 400 000 primordial follicles remain. This process continues during reproductive life when about 400–500 finally ovulate. Typically, about 20 follicles mature each month and only a single follicle ovulates. The rest undergo atresia: this process of involution and disappearance through the process of follicular death occurs while or even before completing their stages of growth. Microscopically, primary and secondary follicles are left without scars, but a collapsed or crumpled zona pellucida squeezed in a narrow, emptied space can be seen. Larger follicles, such as those in the mature (tertiary) stage undergo degradation and leave hyaline fibrous tissue with a degenerated zona pellucida.

Atresia is a hormonally controlled apoptotic process which depends mainly on granulosa cell apoptosis triggered by: (i) the lack of oestrogens – this triggers their apoptotic death; (ii) a reduction in the level of receptors; or (iii) a combination of (i) and (ii) with other external factors. Moreover, a single dominant follicle could diffuse enough inhibitory signals to the 'competitors'. To date, at least five cell-death ligand and receptor systems have been reported in granulosa cells that play a role in atresia regulation. They are: tumor necrosis factor alpha (TNF alpha); Fas ligand; TNF-related apoptosis-inducing ligand (TRAIL, called APO-2); APO-3 ligand; PFG-5 ligand. In addition, two intracellular inhibitor proteins, FLICE-like inhibitory protein short form (cFLIPS) and long form (cFLIPL), which are strongly expressed in granulosa cells, may act as antiapoptotic factors.

As the formation of new follicles is impossible during women's lives, the phenomenon of follicular atresia gradually leads to the depletion of the female gonads. This is completed around the age of 50, culminating with menopause, when the organs of the female endocrine and reproductive centres undergo ageing depletion. As a result of this postmenopausal oestrogenic deficiency, the female reproductive organs and tissues undergo atrophy.

The Hormonal Changes

The reproductive hormones responsible for ovarian maturity, follicular growth, maturity, and ovulation include the GnRH of the hypothalamic region, which in turn stimulates the production and release of follicle-stimulating hormone (FSH) and luteinizing hormone (LH) from the anterior pituitary gland. LH stimulates the production of androgens (i.e. androstenedione) by the theca interna cells which diffuses in the granulosa/follicular cells to be aromatized into oestrogens (mainly oestradiol or E2). Primary follicles develop receptors to FSH, but they are gonadotropin-independent until the antral stage (see Figure 3.3, Chapter 3).

Follicular Phase

With more theca cell formation in the tertiary follicle, the amount of oestrogens increases abruptly due to aromatization of theca-derived androgen into oestrogens by the granulosa cells. At low concentration, oestrogens inhibit the gonadotropins, but a high concentration of oestrogens stimulates them. In addition, the more oestrogens that are made and diffused, the more LH receptors are made by the theca cells. As a result, theca cells produce more androgen that will become oestrogens downstream. This positive feedback loop causes LH to spike sharply, around the fourteenth day of the cycle and it is this spike that causes ovulation. This is the end of the follicular phase in the ovary, i.e. growth and a successful ovulation has occurred, while several other less mature follicles undergo atresia.

Luteal Phase

Following ovulation, LH stimulates the formation of the corpus luteum. Oestrogens drop to negative stimulatory levels after ovulation and only serve to maintain the concentration of FSH and LH. The main endocrine secretion of the corpus luteum are gestagens (mainly progesterone). Inhibin, which is also secreted by the corpus luteum, contributes to FSH inhibition. The depression of both female sex steroids (oestrogens and gestagens – mainly E2 and progesterone) coincides with the end of the luteal phase or luteolysis and the initiation of menstruation if no fertilization has occurred.

Conclusion

The ovary is a complex organ essential for the production of oocytes and reproductive hormones. Healthy functioning ovaries and female reproductive physiology is dependent on stringent communication along the hypothalamic–pituitary–ovarian (HPO) axis. Female factor infertility is associated closely with perturbations of HPO; therefore, understanding the functioning of the ovaries is essential to understanding any pathologies that can impede reproduction (see Chapters 10–12 for more details).

Further Reading

Bukovsky, A., Svetlikova, M. and Caudle, M.R. (2005). Oogenesis in cultures derived from adult human ovaries. Reprod Biol Endocrinol 3: 1–13.

Chassot, A.A. Gregoire EP, Magliano M, et al. (2008). Genetics of ovarian differentiation: Rspo1, a major player. Sex Dev 2: 219–227.

FICAT (2008). *Terminologia Histologica and Cytologica.* Philadelphia: Wolter Kluwer/Lippincott Williams & Wilkins.

Johnson, K.E. (1982). *Histology: Microscopic Anatomy and Embryology.* Hobeken, NJ: Wiley.

Kaipia, A. and Hsueh, A.J. (1997). Regulation of ovarian follicle atresia. Ann Rev Physiol 59: 349–363.

Kierszenbaum, A.L. (2005). *Histology and Cell Biology.* St Louis: CV Mosby/Elsevier Co.

Manabe, N. Goto Y, Matsuda-Minehata F, et al. (2004). Regulation mechanism of selective atresia in porcine follicles: regulation of granulosa cell apoptosis during atresia. J Reprod Dev 50: 493–514.

Matsuda, F. Inoue N, Goto Y, et al. (2008). cFLIP regulates death receptor-mediated apoptosis in an ovarian granulosa cell line by inhibiting procaspase-8 cleavage. J Reprod Dev 54: 314–320.

Moore, K.L. and Persaud, T.V.N. (2008). *Before We Are Born*, 7th edn. Philadelphia: Saunders Elsevier.

Nishida, T. and Nishida, N. (2006). Reinstatement of 'germinal epithelium' of the ovary Reprod Biol Endocrinol 4: 42.

Rolaki, A., Drakakis, P., Millingos, S., et al. (2005). Novel trends in follicular development, atresia and corpus luteum regression: a role for apoptosis. Reprod Biomed Online 11: 93–103.

Ross, M.H. and Pawlina, W. (2008). *Histology*, 5th edn. Philadelphia: Lippincott Williams & Wilkins

Stevens, A. and Lowe, J. (1992). *Histology*. St Louis: Mosby.

Van Wezel, I.L. Dharmarajan, A.M., Lavranos, T.C., et al. (1999). Evidence for alternative pathways of granulosa cell death in healthy and slightly atretic bovine antral follicles. Endocrinology 140: 2602–2612.

5

The Human Spermatozoa

Allan Pacey and Katrina Williams

Introduction

Spermatozoa are haploid cells (Fawcett 1975) evolved for the purpose of delivering the male genome to the oocyte. To achieve this, they have a highly specialized structure, which is created through the complex process of spermatogenesis over about 72 days. Spermatogenesis occurs in the testicles and is responsible for producing millions of fully differentiated sperm every day (Bronson, 2011). The sperm created are specialized for the journey of traversing the female reproductive tract (Suarez and Pacey 2006) and fertilizing an oocyte. This chapter will review the process of spermatogenesis and how the structure of sperm is essential for their function.

Spermatogenesis

Functional mature spermatozoa are made through the process of spermatogenesis, occurring in the seminiferous tubules, situated in the testes (Sutovsky and Manandhar 2006). The first stage of spermatogenesis involves the mitotic division of nonproliferative type A spermatogonia into type B spermatogonia, which are ready to enter meiosis (Phillips et al. 2010). Type A spermatogonia can either commit to differentiate, or self-renew, a step required in order to maintain a population of progenitor cells within the testis. Type B cells then differentiate into primary spermatocytes, which then progress through meiosis I to half their chromosomal complement and form haploid secondary spermatocytes (Figure 5.1). The final step of spermatogenesis involves a meiosis II division forming haploid round spermatids (reviewed in Wistuba et al. 2007).

Round spermatids then go through a series of morphological changes during the second stage of this process, known as spermiogenesis. During this stage, many spermatid organelles are remodelled or degraded by ubiquitin-dependent proteolysis (Bedard et al. 2011) in order to form a functional sperm with the correct accessory structures. The Golgi apparatus is remodelled to form the acrosomal cap (Moreno et al. 2000) and the cytosol becomes the perinuclear theca (Oko 1995). It is during this step of spermatogenesis that the sperm DNA is remodelled into a more condensed structure more suitable to the function of the spermatozoon (Meistrich et al. 2003). Other features of the spermatid are removed, including half of the mitochondrial load and the nuclear pore complexes, involved in mRNA transport (Sutovsky and Manandhar 2006). Once the round spermatid is remodelled into an elongated form, the process of sperm production is concluded by the release of the sperm from the tight associations with Sertoli cells. This last step is known as spermiation. The elongated spermatid is released into the lumen of the seminiferous tubule where the sperm travel to the rete testis and continue their developmental journey through the male reproductive tract (Bronson 2011).

The architecture of the testis is a complex of looped seminiferous tubules, which end in the rete

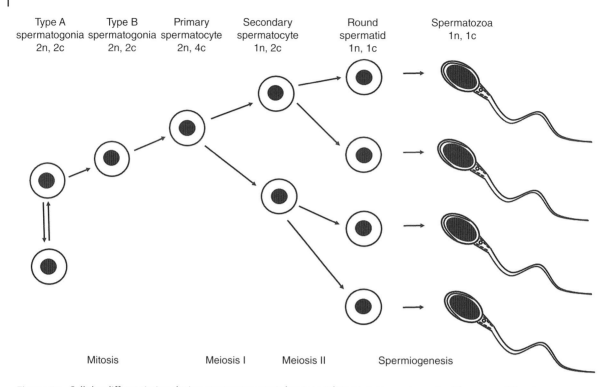

Figure 5.1 Cellular differentiation during spermatogenesis begins with Type A spermatogonia either committing to differentiate into Type B spermatogonia or self-renewal. Type B spermatogonia then further differentiate into primary spermatocytes which are in prophase of meiosis I, consisting of a duplicated complement of DNA, 2n, 4c. In primary spermatocytes, homologous chromosomes line up along the metaphase plate, which allows for homologous recombination, before entering meiosis I and dividing into secondary spermatocytes, which have a haploid complement of chromosomes, with sister chromatids still bound together (1n, 2c). Meiosis I is known as a reductional division as the chromosomal complement has halved to haploid. Secondary spermatocytes then progress through meiosis II to form four round spermatids with one set of chromosomes (1n, 1c). During the final step, spermiogenesis, the round spermatids further differentiate into the specialized form that is required for a functional spermatozoa. Reproduced with permission of Ana-Maria Tomova.

testis. Spermatogenesis occurs in the epithelium of the seminiferous tubules, which is solely populated by spermatogonial and Sertoli cells (Griswold 1995). The Sertoli cells surround the germ cells, providing nutrients and are also involved in the hormonal regulation of spermatogenesis (Griswold 1998). Sertoli cells form tight junctional complexes between each cell, creating a blood–testis barrier, which divides the seminiferous epithelium into two compartments, the basal and adluminal compartments. Spermatogenesis and spermiogenesis occur whilst the spermatogonial cells are in close contact with the Sertoli cells in the basal compartment of the tubule (Griswold 1995). However, the final step of the process, spermiation, involves the release of the differentiated spermatid from the close connections with the Sertoli cells into the immune-privileged lumen of the seminiferous tubule.

The process of spermatogenesis is regulated by a complex endocrine feedback loop (reviewed in Holdcraft and Braun 2004). Gonadotropin-releasing hormones (GnRH) secreted from the hypothalamus act on the pituitary gland. Subsequently, follicle-stimulating hormone (FSH) is released, which acts upon Sertoli cells. The pituitary gland also releases luteinizing hormone (LH), which acts upon Leydig cells. Leydig cells are located in the interstitial space between seminiferous tubules, and upon activation with LH these cells release testosterone. Testosterone then acts upon Sertoli cells, which are involved in the differentiation of spermatogonial stem cells into the spermatozoon.

Epididymal Maturation

After release into the lumen of the seminiferous tubule and passing through the rete testis, sperm enter the epididymis. At this point, they are incapable of fertilizing an oocyte, as they are still biologically immature. Therefore, further maturation occurs during transport through the epididymis where spermatozoa acquire fertilization capability (Moore 1998). Under the influence of epididymal secretory proteins (Brown et al. 1983), spermatozoa acquire the ability to recognize and bind to the oocyte (Hinrichsen and Blaquier 1980). They also acquire progressive motility (Dacheux et al. 1987), through activation of tyrosine phosphorylation signalling pathways (Lin et al. 2006). Upon reaching the tail (cauda) of the epididymis, the final storage place before ejaculation (Robaire and Viger 1995), spermatozoa have acquired the ability to fertilize an egg. This is in comparison to samples taken from the head (caput) of the epididymis, which are still biologically immature (Hinrichsen and Blaquier 1980; Dacheux et al. 1987).

The Structure of Mature Sperm

A spermatozoon consists of two major parts: the sperm head and the tail (Figure 5.2). The major components of the sperm head are the nucleus and the acrosome. The sperm tail can be further divided into four sections, which are connected by the same internal structure: first of all, the connecting piece containing the sperm centriole; the mid piece containing the mitochondria, the source of adenosine triphosphate (ATP) required for sperm motility; the principal piece; and the end piece.

The Sperm Head

The nucleus contains the male DNA in a highly condensed and quiescent form (Brewer et al. 2002; Dadoune, 2003). During spermiogenesis, the histones bound to DNA are replaced by protamines, serving to protect the male genetic information. It is thought that sperm are unable to repair their own DNA (Matsuda et al. 1985), therefore the DNA needs to be protected from any factors, which might

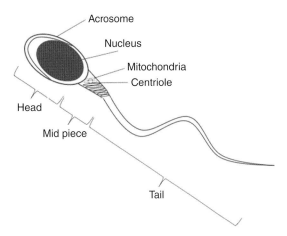

Figure 5.2 The structure of the human spermatozoa. The head contains the acrosome and the condensed male DNA in the nucleus. The head is connected to the tail via the mid (connecting) piece containing the centriole and the mitochondria, wrapped around the axial filament, which runs throughout the entire sperm tail. Reproduced with permission of Ana-Maria Tomova.

compromise its integrity. The condensation of the male DNA is also thought to serve in aiding the transit of sperm through the female reproductive tract and penetration of the oocyte outer layers (Dadoune 2003). The condensed nature of sperm DNA makes it inaccessible to enzymes and therefore it is thought that transcriptional activity and *de novo* gene expression is unlikely to occur. However, evidence pertaining to sperm genomics and proteomics questions this accepted theory, which will be discussed later.

The sperm head also contains the acrosome, a Golgi-derived vesicle, containing hydrolytic enzymes and receptors (Yoshinaga and Toshimori 2003), required for interaction and penetration of the oocyte zona pellucida (ZP) (Osman et al. 1989). Interaction with a ZP glycoprotein, ZP3, initiates an exocytotic reaction, resulting in the release of the acrosomal components and digestion of the ZP, allowing the sperm to penetrate this layer (Brewis et al. 1996). After penetration of the ZP, sperm enter the perivitelline space and are able to bind to the oolemma. After the acrosome reaction occurs, receptors present on the inner acrosomal membrane and at the equatorial segment are unveiled. Receptors located at the equatorial segment, such as fertilin-β were thought to be involved in the fusion with the oolemma (Cho et al. 1998). However, it is now known that a member of a major immunoglobulin family, Izumo1, is the main receptor (Inoue et al. 2005) involved with fusion to the putative egg receptor, Juno (Bianchi et al. 2014).

The remainder of the sperm head is composed of the perinuclear theca (PT), a matrix of structural proteins that provides support and confers head shape. PT proteins located in the posterior part of the sperm head, the postacrosomal segment, are thought to function in signalling during early embryogenesis once the PT is dissolved in the oocyte cytoplasm (Sutovsky et al. 1997).

The Sperm Tail

The sperm tail (or flagellum) provides the motile force for sperm to travel through the female reproductive tract. At the centre of the sperm tail is the microtubule axoneme. This is composed of a nine

plus two arrangement of microtubule doublets, with nine symmetrically arranged outer doublets connected to the two central doublets by radial spokes (Fawcett 1975). The outer doublets are connected by dynein arms, which are the motor proteins responsible for the creation of mechanical energy from ATP (Turner 2003). Coordinated asynchronous movement of dynein arms at each microtubule doublet allows for bending of the axoneme and subsequent flagella movement (Turner 2003). Surrounding the outer doublets are nine outer dense fibres that provide flexibility and support during movement of the flagellum (Figure 5.3).

The sperm tail can be divided into three major sections in addition to the end piece. The connecting piece contains the remaining proximal centriole, leftover from spermatogenesis (Sutovsky and Manandhar 2006). The mid-piece contains approximately 75–100 mitochondria, arranged helically around the central axoneme (Sutovsky and Manandhar 2006). The mitochondria supply ATP

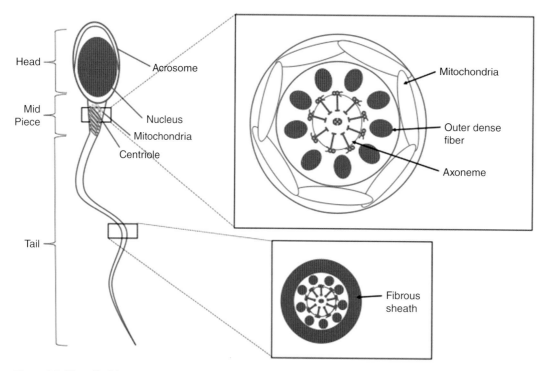

Figure 5.3 The tail of the sperm contains a central skeleton, constructed of 11 microtubules collectively termed the *axoneme*, similar to the structure found in general cilia. Back and forth movement results from a rhythmical longitudinal sliding motion between the anterior and posterior tubules that make up the axoneme. The flagellar (tail) waveform is created by the motor activities of the axonemal dynein arms working against the stable microtubule doublets. This motion propels the sperm and ATP produced by mitochondria supplies energy for this process. Reproduced with permission of Ana-Maria Tomova.

to the axoneme for conversion into mechanical energy, required for the movement of the flagellum (Piomboni et al. 2012). The principal piece has the addition of a fibrous sheath, which is thought to provide support. It is thought that the fibrous sheath is involved in particular steps during capacitation and hyperactivation (Eddy et al. 2003).

The Sperm Transcriptome and Proteome

It was traditionally thought that the spermatozoon only contributed the male DNA to the resulting zygote. However, research into the sperm transcriptome suggests that sperm probably contribute significantly more. It is now known that sperm contain a population of RNAs (Miller et al. 1999), including microRNAs (Ostermeier et al. 2005b). It is thought that the RNA is left over from spermatogenesis. However, there is an apparent selection process regarding which RNAs to keep, as the mature spermatozoon RNA population is significantly different from the testis-specific cell transcripts (Miller et al. 1999). This suggests that the presence of a population of RNA is important to the function of the spermatozoon. One potential function is the *de novo* synthesis of proteins. Despite typically being thought of as a translationally inert cell, there is evidence to suggest that sperm are able to translate these mRNAs into protein using mitochondrial ribosomes (Gur and Breitbart 2006). However, this is also disputed. Other roles for the presence of spermatozoal RNA include a role in early embryonic development (Herrada and Wolgemouth 1997; Ostermeier et al. 2004), epigenetic regulation of genes (Gapp et al. 2014), or a structural role within the sperm itself (Miller and Ostermeier 2006).

The presence of an RNA population within a spermatozoon is also believed to be of importance to male factor infertility. Variation of the RNA present in individual men has been reported (Ostermeier et al. 2002) and is thought to contribute to infertility, as when certain elements are missing, the ability to achieve a natural pregnancy can be compromised (Jodar et al. 2015). Interestingly, when assisted reproductive technology (ART) is used, the absence of certain sperm RNA elements does not affect the outcome of these procedures. This suggests a role for these RNAs in the potential of the spermatozoon to reach and fertilize the egg, rather than an inability to initiate embryonic development. Investigation into whether differences in the RNA carriage of fertile and infertile men can be used as markers for infertility is now being explored (Ostermeier et al. 2005a).

Another interesting observation in relation to the sperm genome is the ability to modify histone-bound DNA. Around 15% of human sperm DNA remains associated with histones, rather than protamines (Tanphaichitr et al. 1978). This histone bound DNA is therefore still vulnerable to modification by enzymes. Studies have shown that sperm are able to digest a portion of their histone bound DNA when challenged with exogenous DNA (Maione et al. 1997; Sotolongo et al. 2003). Also, sperm are able to uptake exogenous DNA into their nucleus (Francolini et al. 1993). It is clear from this evidence that sperm are not as silent and inert as previously thought and are able to respond to environmental triggers.

What is also clear from this evidence is that sperm contain a host of proteins, which regulate these processes. The ability to digest DNA upon exposure to exogenous DNA requires the function of endogenous nucleases, which have been shown to be present in sperm (Maione et al. 1997). In addition, whilst the ability for mature sperm to undergo apoptosis is a controversial point, sperm do possess proteins involved in the apoptotic pathway, including caspase-3 (Weng et al. 2002). In addition to these unexpected proteomic findings, sperm also contain proteins involved in the fundamental processes of sperm hyperactivation and capacitation, such as AKAP4 and the CatSper channels (Miki and Eddy 1998; Ren et al. 2001). Sperm also contain numerous receptors involved in egg recognition and penetration, including Izumo1 (Inoue et al. 2005) and fertilin-β (Cho et al. 1998). Other receptors have shown to be present on the spermatozoon, including epidermal growth factor (EGFR) (Jaldety et al. 2012), fibroblast growth factors (FGFR) (Saucedo et al. 2015), heparin sulphate proteoglycans (Foresta et al. 2011), Toll-like receptor (TLR)-2 (Saeidi et al. 2014), lactoferrin receptor (Wang et al. 2011), as well as receptors for binding progesterone (Tantibhedhyangkul et al. 2014) and oestrogen (Rago et al. 2014). These receptors serve different functions for the spermatozoon, from acquisition of motility, ability to undergo the acrosome reaction and defence to exposure of pathogens. It is clear that we are only just beginning to realize the true complexity of a sperm cell, both inside and out.

Ejaculation and Post-Ejaculatory Changes to Sperm Physiology

At ejaculation, mature spermatozoa are transported through the vas deferens to the urethra, accompanied by secretions from the seminal vesicles and prostate gland, which constitute the seminal fluid (Nojimoto et al. 2009). The accessory proteins present in the seminal fluid contribute to the protection of sperm throughout its transport through the female reproductive tract. An alkaline pH serves to neutralize the acidic pH of vaginal secretions (TeviBenissan et al. 1997) and protection from the female immune system through the presence of immune evasion factors such as TGF-β (Lokeshwar and Block 1992; Robertson et al. 2002).

Capacitation and Hyperactivation

Whilst travelling through the female reproductive tract, sperm undergo two further changes in preparation for fertilization: capacitation and hyperactivation (De Jonge 2005). During this process, sperm undergo multiple membrane changes, such as cholesterol removal (Zarintash and Cross 1996) and binding of a calcium-binding glycoprotein, SABP (Banerjee and Chowdhury 1995), to the sperm head (Banerjee and Chowdhury 1994). These changes constitute the molecular processes of capacitation and cause the sperm head membrane to be more fluid (De Jonge 2005) and more permeable to Ca^{2+} (Banerjee and Chowdhury 1995). During the acrosome reaction, binding to ZP3 induces further calcium influxes within the sperm, resulting in initiation of the acrosome reaction (O'Toole et al. 2000). This process is enabled by the changes to the plasma membrane during capacitation. However, further research has revealed that the acrosome reaction occurs before the sperm reaches the ZP (Jin et al. 2011). Sperm capacitation is also associated with the induction of hyperactivation. This is a change in the

beating of the sperm tail, imparting thrust upon the sperm, necessary for sperm release from storage in the tubual isthmus (Pacey et al. 1995) and penetration of the ZP (Stauss et al. 1995). Hyperactivation occurs as a result of increased intracellular calcium (Suarez et al. 1993) which has been linked (Harayama et al. 2012) to the additional increase in levels of cAMP (Calogero et al. 1998) involved in increased tyrosine phosphorylation, known to be responsible for acquisition of motility (Lin et al. 2006).

Thermotaxis, Chemotaxis, and Rheotaxis

In guiding sperm to the site of fertilization *in vivo*, there are thought to be three complementary mechanisms at work (Perez-Cerezales et al. 2015). The first is a long-range mechanism where capacitated sperm are potentially drawn to the site of fertilization by a temperature difference of up to 2 °C between the (cooler) tubal isthmus close to the uterus and the (warmer) tubal ampulla close to the ovary and where the egg will first appear (Bahat et al. 2003). In combination with this, it has been shown that human sperm are rheotactically responsive (Miki and Clapham 2013). This means they actively orient themselves against a fluid flow and swim towards it. Given that the direction of fluid travel in the Fallopian tube is from ampulla to the isthmus, this will almost certainly mean that the net direction of movement of sperm will be toward the ovary. However, as sperm approach the egg, it has been proposed that a third (short-range) mechanism becomes important, where capacitated sperm chemotactically respond to follicular factor(s), which guide sperm closer to the unfertilized egg (Eisenbach 1999). The molecular mechanism by which chemotaxis is mediated is becoming clearer and has been recently reviewed by Perez-Cerezales et al. (2015).

Conclusion

Spermatozoa are highly specialized cells with specific design features related to their function of navigating the female reproductive tract and fertilizing an oocyte. Clearly, there are many stages of the reproductive process where an individual's sperm function may be inadequate to achieve conception. In this case, *in vitro* fertilization or intracytoplasmic sperm injection will help to simplify the environment in which the sperm have to function and hopefully the embryologist can help the sperm achieve this.

References

Bahat, A., Tur-Kaspa, I., Gakamsky, A. et al. (2003). Thermotaxis of mammalian sperm cells: a potential navigation mechanism in the female genital tract. Nat Med 9: 149–150.

Banerjee, M. and Chowdhury, M. (1994). Purification and characterisation of a sperm-binding glycoprotein from human endometrium. Hum Reprod 9: 1497–1504.

Banerjee, M. and Chowdhury, M. (1995). Induction of capacitation in human spermatozoa in vitro by an endometrial sialic acid-binding protein. Hum Reprod 10: 3147–3153.

Bedard, N., Yang, Y., Gregory, M. et al. (2011). Mice lacking the USP2 deubiquitinating enzyme have severe male subfertility associated with defects in fertilisation and sperm motility. Biol Reprod 85: 594–604.

Bianchi, E., Doe, B., Goulding, D. et al. (2014). Juno is the egg Izumo receptor and is essential for mammalian fertilisation. Nature 508: 483–487.

Brewer, L., Corzett, M. and Balhorn, R. (2002). Condensation of DNA by spermatid basic nuclear proteins. J Biol Chem 277: 38895–38900.

Brewis, I.A., Clayton, R., Barratt, C.L.R. et al. (1996). Recombinant human zona pellucida glycoprotein 3 induces calcium influx and acrosome reaction in human spermatozoa. Mol Hum Reprod 2: 583–589.

Bronson, R. (2011). Biology of the male reproductive tract: its cellular and morphological considerations. Am J Reprod Immunol 65: 212–219.

Brown, C.R., Vonglos, K.I. and Jones, R. (1983). Changes in plasma membrane glycoproteins of rat spermatozoa during maturation in the epididymis. J Cell Biol 96: 256–264.

Calogero, A.E., Fishel, S., Hall, J. et al. (1998). Correlation between intracellular cAMP content, kinematic parameters and hyperactivation of human spermatozoa after incubation with pentoxifylline. Hum Reprod 13: 911–915.

Cho, C., Bunch, D.O., Faure, J-E. et al. (1998). Fertilisation defects in sperm from mice lacking Fertilin β. Science 281: 1857–1859.

Dacheux, J.L., Chevrier, C. and Lanson, Y. (1987). Motility and surface transformations of human spermatozoa during epididymal transit. Ann NY Acad Sci 513: 560–563.

Dadoune, J.P. (2003). Expression of mammalian spermatozoal nucleoproteins. Microsc Res Tech 61: 56–75.

De Jonge, C. (2005). Biological basis for human capacitation. Hum Reprod Update 11: 205–214.

Eddy, E.M., Toshimori, K. and O'Brien, D. (2003). Fibrous sheath of mammalian spermatozoa. Microsc Res Tech 61: 103–115.

Eisenbach, M. (1999). Mammalian sperm chemotaxis and its association with capacitation. Dev Genet 25: 87–94.

Fawcett, D.W. (1975). Mammalian spermatozoon. Dev Biol 44: 394–436.

Foresta, C., Patassini, C., Bertoldo, A. et al. (2011). Mechanism of human papillomavirus binding to human spermatozoa and fertilising ability of infected spermatozoa. PLOS One 6: e15036.

Francolini, M., Lavitrano, M., Lamia, C.L. et al. (1993). Evidence for nuclear internalisation of exogenous DNA into mammalian sperm cells. Mol Reprod Dev 34: 133–139.

Gapp, K., Jawaid, A., Sarkies, P. et al. (2014). Implication of sperm RNAs in transgenerational inheritance of the effects of early trauma in mice. Nature Neurosci 17: 667–669.

Griswold, M.D. (1995). Interactions between germ cells and Sertoli cells in the testis. Biol Reprod 52: 211–216.

Griswold, M.D. (1998). The central role of Sertoli cells in spermatogenesis. Cell Dev Biol 9: 411–416.

Gur, Y. and Breitbart, H. (2006). Mammalian sperm translate nucelar-encoded proteins by mitochondrial-type ribosomes. Genes Dev 20: 411–416.

Harayama, H., Noda, T., Ishikawa, S. et al. (2012). Relationship between cyclic AMP-dependent protein tyrosine phosphorylation and extracellular calcium during hyperactivation of boar spermatozoa. Mol Reprod Dev 79: 727–739.

Herrada, G. and Wolgemouth, D.J. (1997). The mouse transcription factor Stat4 is expressed in haploid male germ cells and is present in the perinuclear theca of spermatozoa. J Cell Sci 110: 1543–1553.

Hinrichsen, M.J. and Blaquier, J.A. (1980). Evidence supporting the existence of sperm maturation in the human epididymis. J Reprod Fertil 60: 291–294.

Holdcraft, R.W. and Braun, R.E. (2004). Hormonal regulation of spermatogenesis. Int J Androl 27: 335–342.

Inoue, N., Ikawa, M., Isotani, A. et al. (2005). The immunoglobulin superfamily protein Izumo is required for sperm to fuse with eggs. Nature 434: 234–238.

Jaldety, Y., Glick, Y., Orr Urtreger, A. et al. (2012). Sperm epidermal growth factor receptor (EGFR) mediates α7 acetylcholine receptor (AChR) activation to promote fertilisation. J Biol Chem 287: 22328–22340.

Jin, M, Fujiwara, E, Kakiuchi, Y, et al. (2011). Most fertilizing mouse spermatozoa begin their acrosome reaction before contact with the zona pellucida during in vitro fertilization. Proc Natl Acad Sci USA 108: 4892–4896

Jodar, M., Sendler, E., Moskovtsev, S.I. et al. (2015). Absence of sperm RNA elements correlates with idiopathic male infertility. Sci Transl Med 7: 295re6.

Lin, M., Lee, Y.H., Xu, W. et al. (2006). Ontogeny of tyrosine phosphorylation-signaling pathways during spermatogenesis and epididymal maturation in the mouse. Biol Reprod 75: 588–597.

Lokeshwar, B.L. and Block, N.L. (1992). Isolation of a prostate carcinoma cell proliferation inhibiting factor from human seminal plasma and its similarity to transforming growth factor beta. Cancer Res 52: 5821–5825.

Maione, B., Pittoggi, C., Achene, L. et al. (1997). Activation of endogenous nucleases in mature sperm cells upon interaction with exogenous DNA. DNA Cell Biol 16: 1087–1097.

Matsuda, Y., Yamada, T. and Tobari, I. (1985). Studies on chromosome aberrations in the eggs of mice fertilised in vitro after irradiation. Mutat Res 148: 113–117.

Meistrich, M.L., Mohapatra, B., Shirley, C.R. et al. (2003). Roles of transition nuclear proteins in speriogenesis. Chromosoma 111: 483–488.

Miki, K, and Clapham, D.E. (2013). Rheotaxis guides mammalian sperm. Curr Biol 23: 443–452.

Miki, K. and Eddy, E.M. (1998). Identification of tethering domains for protein kinase A type Iα regulatory subunits on sperm fibrous sheath protein FSC1. J Biol Chem 273: 34384–34390.

Miller, D., Briggs, D., Snowden, H. et al. (1999). A complex population of RNAs exists in human ejaculate spermatozoa: implications for understanding molecular aspects of spermiogenesis. Gene 237: 385–392.

Miller, D. and Ostermeier, G.C. (2006). Towards a better understanding of RNA carriage by ejaculate spermatozoa. Hum Reprod 12: 757–767.

Moore, H.D.M. (1998). Contribution of epididymal factors to sperm maturation and storage. Andrologia 30: 233–239.

Moreno, R.D., Ramalho-Santos, J., Sutovsky, P. et al. (2000). Vesicular traffic and golgi apparatus dynamics during mammalian spermatogeneis: implications for acrosome architecture. Biol Reprod 63: 89–98.

Nojimoto, F.D., Piffer, R.C., Kiguti, L.R.D. et al. (2009). Multiple effects of sibutramine on ejaculation and on vas deferens and seminal vesicle contractility. Toxicol Appl Pharmacol 239: 233–240.

Oko, R.J. (1995). Developmental expression and possible role of perinuclear theca proteins in mammalian spermatozoa. Reprod Fertil Dev 7: 777–797.

Osman, R.A., Andria, M.L., Jones, A.D. et al. (1989). Steroid induced exocytosis – the human sperm acrosome reaction. Biochem Biophys Res Comm 160: 828–833.

Ostermeier, G.C., Dix, D.J., Miller, D. et al. (2002). Spermatozoal RNA profiles of normal fertile men. Lancet 360: 772–777.

Ostermeier, G.C., Goodrich, R.J., Diamond, M.P. et al. (2005a). Toward using stable spermatozoal RNAs for prognostic assessment of male factor infertility. Fertil Steril 83: 1687–1694.

Ostermeier, G.C., Goodrich, R.J., Moldenhauer, J.S. et al. (2005b). A suite of novel human spermatozoal RNAs. J Androl 26: 70–74.

Ostermeier, G.C., Miller, D., Huntriss, J.D. et al. (2004). Delivering spermatozoan RNA to the oocyte. Nature 429: 154.

O'Toole, C.M.B., Arnoult, C., Darszon, A. et al. (2000). Ca^{2+} entry through store-operated channels in mouse sperm is initiated by egg ZP3 and drives the acrosome reaction. Mol Biol Cell 11: 1571–1584.

Pacey, A.A., Davies, N., Warren, M.A. et al. (1995). Hyperactivation may assist human spermatozoa to detach from intimate association with the endosalpinx. Hum Reprod 10: 2603–2609.

Perez-Cerezales S, Boryshpolets S, Eisenbach M. (2015). Behavioral mechanisms of mammalian sperm guidance. Asian J Androl 17: 628–632.

Phillips, B.T., Gassei, K. and Orwig, K.E. (2010). Spermatogonial stem cell regulation and spermatogenesis. Philos Trans R Soc Biol Sci 365: 1663–1678.

Piomboni, P., Focarelli, R., Stendardi, A. et al. (2012). The role of mitochondria in energy production for human sperm motility. Int J Androl 35: 109–124.

Rago, V., Giordano, F., Brunelli, E. et al. (2014). Identification of G protein-coupled estrogen receptor in human and pig spermatozoa. J Anat 224: 732–736.

Ren, D., Navarro, B., Perez, G. et al. (2001). A sperm ion channel required for sperm motility and male fertility. Nature 413: 603–609.

Robaire, B. and Viger, R.S. (1995). Regulation of epididymal epithelial cell functions. Biol Reprod 52: 226–236.

Robertson, S.A., Ingman, W.V., O'Leary, S., et al. (2002). Transforming growth factor beta – a mediator of immune deviation in seminal plasma. J Reprod Immunol 57: 109–128.

Saeidi, S., Shapouri, F., Amirchaghmaghi, E. et al. (2014). Sperm protection in the male reproductive tract by Toll-like receptors. Andrologia 46: 784–790.

Saucedo, L., Buffa, G.N., Rosso, M. et al. (2015). Fibroblast growth factor receptors (FGFRs) in human sperm: expression, functionality and involvement in motility regulation. PLOS one 10: e0127297.

Sotolongo, B., Lino, E. and Ward, W.S. (2003). Ability of hamster spermatozoa to digest their own DNA. Biol Reprod 69: 2029–2035.

Stauss, C.R., Votta, T.J. and Suarez, S.S. (1995). Sperm motility hyperactivation facilitates penetration of the hamster zona pellucida. Biol Reprod 53: 1280–1285.

Suarez, S.S. and Pacey, A.A. (2006). Sperm transport in the female reproductive tract. Hum Reprod Update 12: 23–37.

Suarez, S.S., Varosi, S.M. and Dai, X. (1993). Intracellular calcium increases with hyperactivation in intact moving hamster sperm and oscillates with the flagellar beat cycle. Proc Natl Acad Sci USA 90: 4660–4664.

Sutovsky, P. and Manandhar, G. (2006). *Mammalian Spermatogenesis and Sperm Structure: The Sperm Cell*, 1st edition. Cambridge: Cambridge University Press. pp. 1–30.

Sutovsky, P., Oko, R., Hewitson, L. et al. (1997). The reomval of the sperm perinuclear theca and its association with the bovine oocyte surface during fertilisation. Dev Biol 188: 75–84.

Tanphaichitr, N., Sobhon, P., Taluppeth, N. et al. (1978). Basic nuclear proteins in testicular cells and ejaculated spermatozoa in man. Exp Cell Res 117: 347–356.

Tantibhedhyangkul, J., Hawkins, K.C., Dai, Q. et al. (2014). Expression of a mitochondrial progesterone receptor in human spermatozoa correlates with a progestin-dependent increase in mitochondrial membrane potential. Andrology 2: 875–883.

TeviBenissan, C., Belec, L., Levy, M. et al. (1997). In vivo semen-associated pH neutralization of cervicovaginal secretions. Clin Diagn Lab Immunol 4: 367–374.

Turner, R.M. (2003). Tales from the tail: what do we really know about sperm motility? J Androl 24: 790–803.

Wang, P., Liu, B., Wang, Z. et al. (2011). Characterisation of lactoferrin receptor on human spermatozoa. Reprod Biomed Online 22: 155–161.

Weng, S-L., Taylor, S.L., Morshedi, M. et al. (2002). Caspase activity and apoptotic markers in ejaculated human sperm. Mol Hum Reprod 8: 984–991.

Wistuba, J., Stukenborg, J.-B. and Luetjens, C.M. (2007). Mammalian spermatogenesis. Funct Dev Embryol 1: 100–117.

Yoshinaga, K. and Toshimori, K. (2003). Organization and modifications of sperm acrosomal molecules during spermatogenesis and epididymal maturation. Microsc Res Tech 61: 39–45.

Zarintash, R.J. and Cross, N.L. (1996). Unesterified cholesterol content of human sperm regulates the response of the acrosome to the agonist, progesterone. Biol Reprod 55: 19–24.

6

The Biology of Fertilization

Michael Carroll

A Brief History

Mankind has pondered the process of fertility and reproduction since the Palaeolithic period, as evidenced by the numerous Venus figurines discovered from that period, which are believed to represent female fecundity (Figure 6.1). However, the mechanism of procreation was attributed at that time to a more mystical modus. The Greek philosopher and 'Father of Medicine', Hippocrates (460–370 BC) approached reproduction rationally and proposed that both males and females produce seeds that combine to give rise to a new human – the 'two seed theory'. Aristotle (384–322 BC) held the view that the unborn child was preformed *in utero*, consisting of female fluids and menstrual blood (catamenia), and awaited the male's semen to elicit its development, bestowing on it form and animation. He considered that the preformed fetus grew like 'the seeds of plants'. His theory of preformation or 'epigenesis' dominated the understanding of reproduction for over 1000 years until the latter part of the European Renaissance.

Renewed interest in reproduction and fertilization ensued; for example, the Italian anatomist Hieronymus Fabricius (1537–1619) and his studies of domestic hens lead him to believe that the semen from the rooster was stored in a little sac near the cloaca where it rendered the whole uterus and eggs fertile. William Harvey (1578–1657), a student of Fabricius and the discoverer of blood circulation, was also interested in reproduction and sought a more active role for semen through dissection of female deer, dogs, rabbits, and chickens. However, he found no 'evidence' of a physical role for semen in reproduction, but ascribed its role as more ethereal, a conclusion more in accord with Aristotle's preformationist idea. Harvey concluded that 'all things come from the egg' (*ex ovo omnia*).

Developments in technology spawn discoveries in science, and the emergence of the microscope is a fine example. The arrival of printed books and manuscripts through mechanical improvements of Gutenberg's printing press during the European Renaissance generated a market for ground lenses as an aid to reading. Around 1600, the Dutch spectacle makers, father and son, Hans and Zacharias Janssen, and Hans Lipperskey are accredited with inventing the first microscope, in which they fashioned two lenses at each end of an adjustable tube. Later the English polymath, Robert Hooke (1635–1703) improved on the design (Figure 6.2) and introduced curious readers to microscopic wonders in his magnificent *Micrographica* (published 1665). This masterpiece contained 38 plates, including a large pullout illustration of a flea, and included the first biological reference to cells.

One likely reader of *Micrographica* was the Dutchman, Antonie van Leeuwenhoek (1632–1723). Leeuwenhoek had no formal university education; he worked as a draper and acted as a minor city official in the Dutch town of Delft. He was a meticulous observer and keen craftsman, designing and making hundreds of microscopes. His unique design was different to the compound double-lens microscopes of Janssen and Hooke. Leeuwenhoek's were mostly small handheld, single-lens microscopes with impressive magnifying and resolving powers (Figure 6.3a) with which he made some remarkable discoveries, notably, the first observations and

Clinical Reproductive Science, First Edition. Edited by Michael Carroll.
© 2019 John Wiley & Sons Ltd. Published 2019 by John Wiley & Sons Ltd.
Companion website: www.wiley.com/go/carroll/clinicalreproductivescience

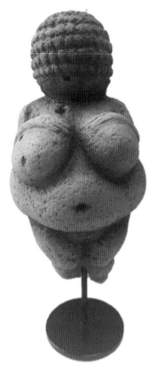

Figure 6.1 The Venus of Willendorf is an 11.1 cm high figurine estimated to have been made between about 28,000 and 25,000 BCE. It was found in 1908 at a palaeolithic site near Willendorf, a village in Lower Austria near the town of Krems.

descriptions of small 'animalcules' – bacteria and protist – in samples of water. He corresponded with the Royal Society in London, whose members (including Hooke) were impressed with his microscopic skills and meticulous descriptions, and made him a foreign member in 1680.

Leeuwenhoek's most famous discovery is that of sperm. He believed that the generation of animals was from these 'animalcules in the male sperm' and noted their presence in abundance in his own semen and that of the dog, rabbit, and cockerel (Figure 6.3b). Leeuwenhoek (Figure 6.3c) ascribed to the preformationist view of generation, stating that he discovered 'the parts and membranes of the fetus', including the head and the shoulders. These animalcules travel to the uterus where they grow and develop – 'the female served only to afford nourishment to the animalcules of the male sperm', akin to a seed planted in nutrient soil (for his letters to the Royal Society see vanleeuwenhoek.com). The younger contemporary of Leeuwenhoek and fellow Dutchman, Nicolas Hartsoeker (1656–1725) predicted that these preformed little men would look like the drawing of the 'homunculi' in these animalcules (Figure 6.3d).

Thus, in the seventeenth and eighteenth century, the concept of reproduction lay in two

(a)

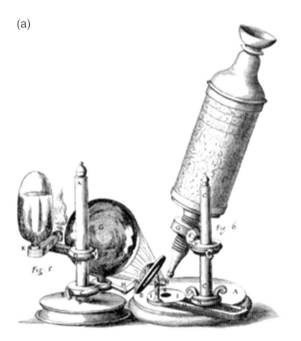

(b)

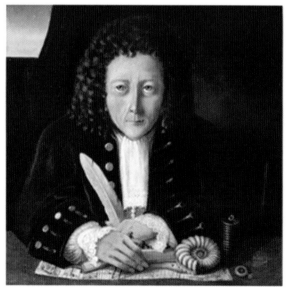

Figure 6.2 (a) Robert Hooke's microscope and (b) Illustration of Robert Hooke. *Source:* https://commons.wikimedia.org.

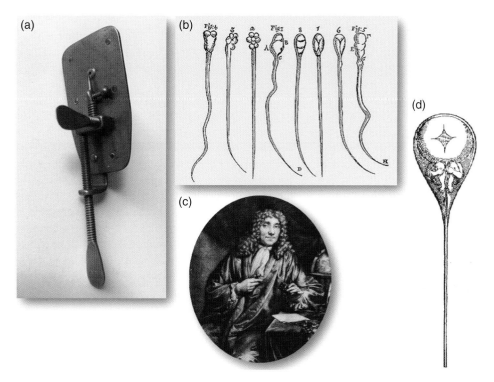

Figure 6.3 (a) Replica of Leeuwenhoek' microscope. *Source:* photo by author. (b) Illustration of sperm as observed by Leeuwenhoek. (c) Leeuwenhoek. (d) The Homunculus as described by Hartsoeker. *Source:* https://commons.wikimedia.org.

preformationist arenas: the ovists, who contended that generation is derived from the preformed residing in the ovum; and the spermists who proposed the idea of the homunculi and the planting of the male seed. It was not until the careful and diligent experimentalist, and Italian Catholic priest, Lazzaro Spallanzani (1729–1799) turned his attention to the question of reproduction that the true role of both ovum and sperm were unraveled.

Spallanzani was a great scientist and thinker – his interests and expertise included physics, chemistry, geology, and biology. He carefully designed controlled experiments, describing the methodology in enough detail for others to repeat his work. In terms of his approach to scientific research, he was ahead of his time. He debunked the theory of spontaneous generation over 100 years before Louis Pasteur's swan-neck flask experiments. He first postulated how bats navigate in the darkness using their ears (echolocation) and observed the regenerative properties of salamander limbs.

However, some of his most ingenious experiments related to fertilization and reproduction. In one experiment, he examined the nature of the sperm's aura spermatica. This was one prevailing theory, which explained the generation of animals and was derived from the ideas of preformationists such as Harvey, proposing that a vapour emanating from semen triggered embryonic development. To investigate this, Spallanzani placed semen from a toad in a watch glass while eggs from the female were placed in the bottom of another watch glass turned upside down. The eggs were separated from the sperm by a few millimetres. After several hours, he noted the eggs were covered 'as if by a dew', from the condensation of the evaporated seminal fluid. However, none of the eggs developed. This refuted the property of the aura spermatica of sperm. In another, rather creative experiment, he prized male frogs from amplexus (the mating position where the males grasps the female with its front legs) and fitted them with tight taffeta britches before replacing them to resume their mating position. In this way, he was able to demonstrate unequivocally, the role of the egg and semen in the generation of animals. Thus, with the taffeta barrier, none of the eggs developed. But when he scraped the semen from the britches and added it to the eggs, they all developed into tadpoles.

This was one of the earliest demonstrations of *in vitro* fertilization (IVF) and the proof that fertilization took place by the physical contact between semen and egg. In an attempt to distinguish which fraction of semen was responsible for fertilization, Spallanzani separated the sperm from the semen by filtration and exposed the eggs to the filtrate upon which they developed. If he had examined these filtrates microscopically, he would have observed swimming little animalcules. However, he did not, and erroneously concluded that semen had the fertilizing property, not the sperm. It would be another 100 years before direct interaction of sperm and eggs could be characterized.

The developments and improvements in optics and microscopic techniques in the mid- to late nineteenth century, together with the elucidation of the cell theory by Virchow, Schwann, and Schleiden paved the pathway for a more accurate explanation and description of the process of fertilization. Two embryologists, Oscar Hertwig (1849–1922) and Hermann Fol (1845–1892) – both students of the great biologist Ernst Haeckel – independently described sperm entry into the egg and the subsequent union of male and female nuclei. To observe fertilization, Hertwig used the sea urchin, while Fol used the starfish – taking advantage of the numerous, large transparent eggs released by both species.

Thus, it was nearly 200 years after Leeuwenhoek's discovery that it was finally recognized that both egg and sperm were intimately involved and the fusion of both gametes was essential for fertilization to take place.

There were many other individuals who played an essential role along this journey; the above mentioned are a few key players. For a more in-depth narrative see: Pinto-Correia (1997), Jardine (1999) and Cobb (2006).

The Journey of the Sperm

Fertilization can be described as a multistep process that results in the restoration of diploidy and the generation of a new organism through the combination of the maternal and paternal (haploid) genomes. To achieve this both gametes must obviously meet. For marine organisms (and other external fertilizers) this can pose a problem, especially when the gametes are spawned in vast volumes of water and their environment is shared with many other species, some possibly close relatives, that may have shed their gametes at the same time, increasing the risk of cross-fertilization.

When the gametes of marine animals are released into the water, in such a dilute concentration, the sperm require some means of attraction to the oocyte of their species. This species-specific sperm attraction is known as sperm chemotaxis and may be defined operationally as a 'modulation of the direction of movement of spermatozoa up a gradient of a chemoattractant' (or down the gradient of a chemorepellent) (Eisenbach 1999). Sperm chemotaxis has been well documented in species such as molluscs, echinoderms (sea urchins and starfish) and ascidians (sea-squirts) (Miller 1985; Yoshida et al. 1993). The precise nature of these sperm attractants varies between species. Most have been identified as sperm-activating peptides or SAPs (Miller 1985). In the sea urchin, the SAP isolated from the egg jelly layer of the sea urchin, *Arbacia punctulata*, is known as 'resact', and is a potent chemoattractant for *A. punctulata* spermatozoa (Ward et al. 1985). In addition, this peptide is specific for *A. punctulata* and stimulates sperm motility by activating the sperm receptor's guanylyl cyclase thus generating cyclic guanosine monophosphate (cGMP) and subsequent influx of Ca^{2+} which controls swimming behaviour during chemotaxis (Cook et al. 1994).

The journey of the sperm is more complicated with internal fertilizers such as mammals where the sperm is placed directly in the female reproductive tract and has to make its way to the region where the oocyte awaits (Figure 6.4).

In humans, the site of sperm deposition is the cranial vagina, at the external os of the cervix (Harper 1994). Soon after ejaculation, human seminal plasma spontaneously coagulates, due to the activity of semenogelin (I–III) proteins expressed exclusively in the seminal vesicles (de Lamirande 2007), which it has been proposed retains the sperm at the cervical external os (Harper 1994), preventing premature capacitation and providing protection from the acidic vaginal environment and from oxidative damage (de Lamirande and Lamothe 2010). This coagulum begins to break down within 30–60 min postejaculation by the proteolytic activity of

Figure 6.4 The journey of sperm in the human female reproductive tract. *Source:* Blausen Medical, https://commons.wikimedia.org.

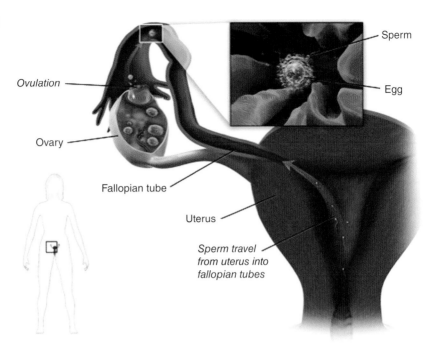

prostate-specific antigen (Mattsson et al. 2014). However, within a few minutes postejaculation, sperm begin to leave the seminal plasma and pass through the cervical canal (Sobrero and McLeod 1962). The cervical mucus provides the first real barrier to sperm movement, and the degree of cervical mucus hydration directly correlates with sperm migration. A mucus sample with the highest percentage of water and lowest protein and glycoprotein concentration has the most positive effect on sperm migration (Morales et al. 1993). Moreover, the percentage hydration can change throughout the ovulatory cycle, (Katz et al. 1997) with maximum mucus hydration levels correlating with increased pregnancy rates (Bigelow et al. 2004).

The cervix is an immunologically competent organ and in humans, coitus and insemination into the vagina stimulate leukocyte (neutrophils and macrophages) migration into the cervix, as well as into the vagina (Pandya and Cohen 1985; Thompson et al. 1992). Neutrophils also migrate readily through midcycle human cervical mucus (Parkhurst and Saltzman 1994). The role of these leukocytes as agents against sperm is uncertain, as their presence does not seem to interfere with fecundity. However, they may be present in response to potential microbial pathogens that can accompany sperm. Another hypothesis proposes that postcapacitated sperm are targeted by leukocytes and phagocytosed, thus removing spent, superfluous sperm (Eisenbach 2003; Oren-Benaroya et al. 2007).

Periovulatory cervical mucus contains IgA, and the vagina and uterus contain elevated levels of IgG. Under normal circumstances, certain immunoglobulins target sperm, and in some women these antisperm antibodies can impair fertility (Jones, 1994; Franklin et al. 1999; Kalaydijev et al. 2002). Furthermore, about one-third of infertile women with a poor post-coital test appear to have anti-sperm antibodies in their cervical mucus (Clarke et al. 1984). However, it seems that sperm have developed methods to evade the immunosurveillance of the female reproductive tract. During maturation in the epididymis, the sperm surface undergoes dramatic changes, acquiring properties that are vital for its survival and performance in the female tract. One such change is the addition to the sperm surface of an atypical β-defensin polypeptide, one of which, the β-defensin DEFB126 becomes adsorbed to the entire sperm surface as it moves through the epididymal duct. Furthermore, it has been proposed that negatively charged glycans on DEFB126 facilitate efficient sperm movement through cervical mucus and cloak sperm from immune surveillance molecules (Yudin et al. 2005; Tollner et al. 2012). Some studies suggest that the cervix also functions as a reservoir, storing sperm in the cervical crypts, since motile sperm have been recovered from the cervix after 5 days of insemination (Gould et al. 1984). These sperm may be protected from the hostile immune environment of the cervix (Tollner et al. 2012), thus providing a source of sperm for a few days after coitus. However, it is unclear if these cervical sperm reach the Fallopian tube.

In 1951, Rubenstein and co-workers removed several motile sperm from the Fallopian tubes of a woman following hysterectomy, 30 min after insemination, and in another study sperm were recovered from the Fallopian tube of women who had a bilateral salpingectomy 5 min after insemination (Settlage et al. 1973). In other words, sperm can traverse the uterus rapidly. However, due to the lack of standardization of the experimental protocols and patient selection more research was warranted. Williams et al. (1993) conducted a more careful study where they inseminated women (attending the clinic for planned hysterectomies) with either their partner's, or donor semen. Approximately 18 h later, both Fallopian tubes were ligatured into ampullary, isthmic, and intramural regions and each region flushed to assess the presence of sperm. Surprisingly, a median of only 251 sperm were recovered with the ovulatory ampulla containing more sperm than the nonovulatory ampulla.

Theoretical calculations on the rate of sperm locomotion and the dimensions of the uterus and tube make it unlikely that the sperm travel through the uterus by intrinsic movement alone. Sperm transport is therefore most probably due to the action of uterine cilia and contractions of the myometrium. It has been reported that uterine smooth muscle contractions increase in intensity during the late follicular phase coinciding with the presence of sperm if sexual intercourse has taken place (Kunz et al. 1996). Furthermore, the role of oxytocin, which is released during intercourse, may further facilitate sperm transport by inducing uterine contractions (Kunz et al. 2007).

The next stage of the sperm's journey is centred on the uterotubal junction, which is filled with mucus and provides a further barrier to sperm such that only those with good motility and morphology are permitted to traverse it. Additionally, the presence of certain sperm surface proteins may play an essential role in the passage (Suarez and Pacey 2006; Suarez 2016).

The Fallopian tube provides a more hospitable milieu than the vagina or cervix, and it has been postulated that the tubal isthmus may function as a sperm reservoir. This is likely for a variety of species (Suarez and Pacey 2006). However, in one study a distinct sperm reservoir was not observed in the human tubes (Williams et al. 1993). Pregnancy can occur as long as 5 days before ovulation (Wilcox et al. 1995) and therefore sperm must be stored at some location(s) along the female reproductive tract. Given that human sperm do attach to endosalpingeal epithelium *in vitro* (Pacey et al. 1995; Vigil et al. 2012) (Figure 6.5), it

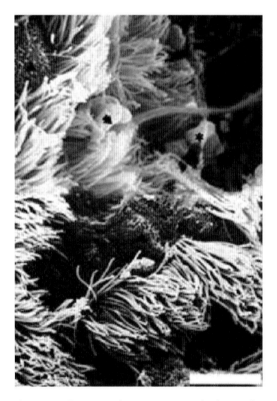

Figure 6.5 Scanning electron micrograph of an explant of human oviduct taken 3 h after insemination with human spermatozoa. Note the spermatozoon (arrow) of normal morphology attached by its acrosomal region to several cilia. Ciliated epithelial cells predominate, but there are also some nonciliated epithelial cells (arrow head) covered by microvilli. Observe the mucous material (asterisk) near the spermatozoon tail. The scale bar represents 10 μm. Reproduced from Vigil et al. (2012) by permission of Oxford University Press.

likely that the human Fallopian tube functions as a sperm reservoir as noted in other mammal species.

Finding the Oocyte

As has been described, of the 200–300 million sperm ejaculated at the cervical external os, only about 200 reach the oocyte. In addition, there are more sperm in the ovulatory ampulla than in the nonovulatory ampulla (Williams et al. 1993). In order for the sperm to reach the site of ovulation there is likely a guidance mechanism involved.

The requirement for a chemoattractant for sperm in mammals was believed to be unnecessary since the sperm were ejaculated directly into the female reproductive tract and a sufficient number of sperm would reach the oocyte. The identity of the mammalian sperm chemoattractant remains unknown. However, the oocyte and cells of the surrounding cumulus oophorus are thought to secrete sperm chemoattractants independently (Sun et al. 2005). Thus, several studies have shown sperm chemotaxis to follicular fluid, and fractions of follicular fluid contain heparin, progesterone, atrial natriuretic peptide, oxytocin, and acetylcholine – all of which demonstrate sperm chemoattractant properties (Eisenbach 1999).

There is growing evidence supporting a role for progesterone as the mammalian sperm chemoattractant (Teves et al. 2006). This hormone is secreted by the cumulus cells (Guidobaldi et al. 2008) and induces sperm hyperactivation by binding to the Ca^{2+} channel CatSper on the sperm membrane (Lishko et al. 2011; Strünker et al. 2011). However, some data suggest that progesterone might be a weak, but not the major chemoattractant derived from follicular fluid. Progesterone may well cause human sperm accumulation mainly by inducing hyperactivation-like motility and, as a consequence, sperm trapping (Jasiwal et al. 1999).

An unexpected group of receptor proteins – members of the odorant receptor (OR) family normally expressed on ciliary membranes of nasal olfactory sensory neurons – have been detected on sperm (Parmentier et al. 1992) where they may play a role in sperm chemotaxis (Spher et al. 2003). OR hOR17 mediates changes in both sperm intracellular Ca^{2+} and swimming behaviour, via a cyclic adenosine monophosphate (cAMP)-regulated pathway (Spehr et al. 2006). The list of potential OR functions in mammals has now been significantly extended to include sperm–oocyte chemical communication (Flegel et al. 2016). Furthermore, studies are now investigating an important role of sperm ORs and idiopathic infertility in men (Ottaviano et al. 2013).

Capacitation, Hyperactivation, and the Acrosome Reaction

Mammalian fertilization does not occur when mature sperm from a fresh ejaculate are placed with oocytes *in vitro*. This observation bewildered researchers until 1951 when Chang and Austin independently reported that mammalian sperm must reside in the female reproductive tract for a predetermined period of time before they gain the ability to fertilize the oocyte. Austin introduced the term 'capacitation' stating 'the sperm must undergo some form of physiologic change or capacitation before it is capable of penetrating the egg' (Chang 1951; Austin 1952).

Capacitation comprises a reversible set of physiological changes that involve the removal of cholesterol by albumin in the female reproductive tract and a prerequisite for hyperactivation (see below), and the acrosome reaction. *In vivo*, it involves the removal of inhibitory factors from seminal plasma and the interaction of the sperm with components in the female reproductive tract (Jaiswal and Eisenbach, 2002). In humans, capacitation most likely begins in the cervix (Overstreet et al. 1991). However, it has been postulated that not all the sperm will capacitate simultaneously and that the process is more a transient event, occurring throughout the female reproductive tract (Eisenbach 1995).

The removal of cholesterol permits the influx of bicarbonate and Ca^{2+} ions, which in turn activate adenylate cyclase, thereby elevating cAMP concentrations. The increased cAMP levels activate protein kinase A, which then phosphorylates several tyrosine kinases, including chaperone proteins. These migrate to the sperm head where they are phosphorylated. One of these chaperone proteins is Izumo – a protein critical for sperm–egg fusion (see below) (Aitken and Nixon 2013).

During capacitation sperm become hyperactivated – that is, they swim with higher velocity and generate greater force and tail movements. Hyperactivation is brought about by the influx of Ca^{2+} through the opening of the membrane Ca^{2+} channel, CatSper, located on the sperm tail (Quill et al. 2003). Furthermore, progesterone has been identified as a regulator of CatSper (Lishko et al. 2011; Strunker et al. 2011). As progesterone is produced from the cumulus cells and has been proposed to be the sperm chemoattractant, the interaction between this steroid hormone and CatSper becomes more evident.

Hyperactivated sperm are released from the oviductal epithelium and migrate up the Fallopian tube towards the oocyte where they engage the cumulus mass. This directed journey is attributed not only to the activity of chemoattractants and CatSper, but the local environment. For example, alterations in pH can influence the activity of CatSper and it has been proposed there is a temperature gradient of 2 °C between the isthmus of the Fallopian tube and the warmer ampullary region (Bahat and Eisenbach 2006).

Sperm reaching the oocyte have to penetrate the cumulus–oocyte complex which, serves as the final sperm filter in that only a few sperm will penetrate this network of cells. The cumulus–oocyte comple is a matrix rich in proteins and carbohydrates including hyaluronan, an unsulfated glycosaminoglycan. The sperm degrades the hyaluronan by the activity of hyaluronidase, thus enabling the sperm to reach the zona pellucida (ZP) on the surface of the oocyte (Kim et al. 2008).

The ZP is a transparent, porous, glycoprotein coat that surrounds mammalian oocytes and contains the species-specific receptors for sperm (Wassarman 1988). It is a component of the sperm selection process and the last hurdle before fertilization. The major components of the ZP are three glycosylated proteins: ZP1, ZP2, and ZP3. The canonical model has been that the capacitated sperm interact with ZP3 and induce the acrosome reaction. However, there is accumulating evidence that the acrosome reaction takes place before the sperm reach the ZP. Jin et al. (2011) demonstrated that mouse sperm had already undergone the acrosome reaction by the time they reached the cumulus. In another study, it was observed that most of mouse sperm did not initiate the acrosome reaction close to or on the ZP. This demonstrated that a significant proportion of sperm initiate the acrosome reaction in the upper segments of the oviductal isthmus (La Spina et al. 2016). It has also been suggested that the interaction of CatSper and progesterone is involved in the onset of the acrosome reaction (Tamburrino et al. 2014). Taken together these data suggest strongly that the sperm–ZP3 interaction is not required to elicit the acrosome reaction.

The acrosome itself is a Golgi-derived exocytotic organelle that covers the tip of the sperm head. An influx of Ca^{2+} is responsible for acrosomal exocytosis and rearrangement of the acrosomal membrane. The outer acrosomal membrane fuses with the overlying oocyte plasma membrane forming hybrid vesicles containing the acrosomal enzymes (Sosa et al. 2015). The hydrolytic and proteolytic enzymes (such as acrosin) released at the site of sperm–zona interaction along with the enhanced thrust of the hyperactivated beat pattern of the bound sperm are important factors in regulating the penetration of the zona-intact oocyte (Abou-Haila and Tulsiani 2000).

The sperm then makes its way in to the perivitelline space where it can make contact with the oocyte plasma membrane.

Sperm Meets Oocyte

Fusion between the gametes is a key event in the fertilization process involving interactions of specific domains of sperm and oocyte plasma membranes. This process occurs through the interactions of complementary molecules localized on specific domains of sperm and oocyte plasma membranes.

There have been several studies over the past three decades investigating the molecular components involved in sperm–oocyte fusion. Members of the ADAM (A Disintegrin and A Metalloprotease domain) protein family (Wolfsberg et al. 1995), in particular fertilin-α, fertilin-β, and cyritestin, have been implicated (Primakoff 1987; Blobel et al. 1992). Both fertilin-α and fertilin-β are synthesized in the testis and are proteolytically processed during sperm development. Fertilin-β was believed to mediate sperm–oocyte binding, while fertilin-α has been proposed to participate in the subsequent sperm–oocyte fusion (Muga et al. 1994). The role of these disintegrins in sperm–oocyte fusion was supported by experiments showing that recombinant forms of the extracellular portion of these proteins are able to bind to oocytes and inhibit sperm–oocyte binding (Evans et al. 1998). In addition, mouse lacking cyritestin and fertilin-β were found to be infertile (Nishimura et al. 2001).

In 1999, Chen et al. demonstrated that the tetraspan superfamily (TM4SF) integral plasma membrane proteins (CD9) in association with the integrin α6/β1 on the plasma membrane of the oocytes bind to fertilin-β and mediate gamete fusion. However, in mouse knockout experiments showed that fertilization occurs with oocytes lacking the integrin α6/β1 (Miller et al. 2000). Oocytes deficient in CD9 did not fertilize, even though sperm bind to the oocytes (Le Naour et al. 2000). These results suggest that the integrin α6/β1 is not essential for sperm–oocyte fusion and that CD9 must interact with other proteins to function in sperm–oocyte fusion. The data also suggest that fertilin-β does not bind to the integrin α6/β1 as previously thought.

In 2005, Inoue et al. showed that the sperm-specific protein Izumo1 is essential in sperm–oocyte fusion. Using gene disruption studies, they reported that females lacking the protein were phenotypically normal and fertile. In contrast, Izumo-deficient males were completely infertile, despite being phenotypically normal and their sperm having normal morphology and motility. Izumo1 (called after the Japanese marriage shrine) was therefore proposed as the sperm component essential for fusion. However, in a later study it was shown that recombinant Izumo1 binds both wild-type and CD9-deficient oocytes, suggesting Izumo1 interacts with an oocyte receptor other than CD9 (Inoue et al. 2013).

The most recent partner for Izumo1 was found to be a Folate receptor-4 (Folr4), later termed Juno (after the Roman goddess of fertility and marriage) (Bianchi et al. 2014). Folr4 is a GPI-anchored protein expressed on the oocyte surface where it interacts with the sperm Izumo1 protein. As with the Izumo1 study, Bianchi et al. used gene disruption studies and demonstrated convincingly that Juno is the essential oocyte component required for gamete fusion.

Future research on the precise mechanism of mammalian sperm–oocyte fusion and the factors involved will no doubt reveal more players (Klinovska et al. 2014).

During sperm–oocyte fusion the entire content of the sperm head is delivered into the oocyte, together with structural and accessory components such as the axoneme, perinuclear matrix, and some mitochondria. These components are normally discarded or degraded soon after fertilization. The sperm also delivers the centrosome, which is essential for embryonic cell division (Sutovsky and Schatten 2000; Krawetz 2005). It is increasingly acknowledged that the paternal contribution at this time has important implications for early embryo developmental processes and ultimately, on the health of a child. This can be achieved through the delivery of methylated sites on specific promoter regions of paternal genes and a host of messenger RNA and microRNAs, which can influence the translation of oocyte and embryo transcripts (Krawetz 2005; Al-Gazi and Carroll 2015; Nevin and Carroll 2015). The oocyte also receives a number of sperm-specific proteins and one of the most essential is that responsible for oocyte activation, the sperm factor (Figure 6.6).

Sparks of Life – Oocyte Activation

Activation of oocyte development in nearly all animals and plants is initiated by the fertilizing sperm triggering an acute rise in cytosolic free Ca^{2+} concentration ($[Ca^{2+}]i$) (Stricker 1999). In mammals, the union of sperm and oocyte leads to a distinctive series of cytosolic Ca^{2+} oscillations that are a prerequisite for normal embryo development (Miyazaki et al. 1993; Stricker 1999). This Ca^{2+} signalling phenomenon arises from increases in inositol 1,4,5-trisphosphate (IP_3) concentrations, which activate IP_3 receptor-mediated Ca^{2+} release from intracellular stores (endoplasmic reticulum, ER) in the oocyte (Miyazaki et al. 1993; Berridge and Boothman 1996). The rise in $[Ca^{2+}]i$ results in the activation of the oocyte and the subsequent release from its state of meiotic arrest. In most mammals, the oocyte is arrested in metaphase II of meiosis (Jones, 1998). The rise in $[Ca^{2+}]i$ is responsible for cortical granule exocytosis, vitelline envelope lift-off and cortical

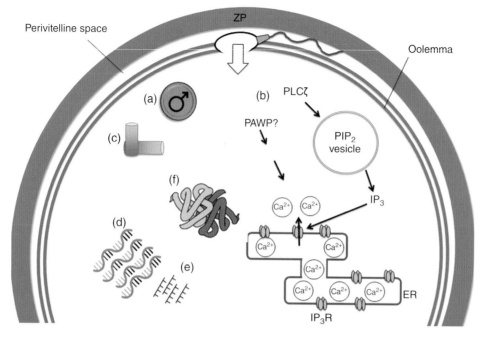

Figure 6.6 The sperm introduces several factors to the oocyte during fertilization. (a) The paternal haploid genome. (b) The sperm factor required for egg activation. (c) The centrioles. (d) Sperm-derived mRNA. (e) Noncoding RNAs. (f) Sperm-specific proteins. ER, endoplasmic reticulum; IP_3R, inositol 1,4,5- trisphosphate receptor; PAWP, postacrosomal WW-domain binding protein; PIP_2, phosphatidylinositol 4,5, bisphosphate; PLCζ, phospholipase C ζ; ZP, zona pellucida.

contraction. The Ca^{2+} oscillations also initiate the ejection of zinc from the oocyte into the extracellular milieu. These 'zinc sparks' decrease the intracellular zinc content permitting cell cycle resumption (Kim et al. 2011).

The IP_3/Ca^{2+} Signalling Cascade: An Overview

Ca^{2+} functions as a key second messenger in many cellular events, ranging from the control of developmental processes, gene transcription, differentiation, muscle contraction, secretion, metabolism, proliferation, cell death (apoptosis), neurotransmitter release and of interest here, oocyte activation at fertilization (Berridge 1997; Berridge 2009).

The production of IP_3 is the primary mechanism for the release of Ca^{2+} from the ER. The membrane phospholipid, phosphatidylinositol 4,5, bisphosphate (PIP_2) is cleaved by the activity of the enzyme phospholipase C (PLC) to yield two compounds – IP_3 and diacylglycerol (DAG). DAG activates members of the protein kinase family, while IP_3 interacts with receptors (IP_3Rs) on the ER to liberate Ca^{2+} from the internal stores (Figure 6.7) (Berridge 2009).

The PLC enzymes are activated by external ligands including hormones and growth factors binding to their respective receptors. Upon binding, a cascade of intracellular events occur involving effectors such as G-coupled proteins and kinase activation, which in turn activate PLCs (Berridge 2009).

The free cytosolic Ca^{2+} can influence the activation or inhibition of a myriad of proteins involved in cellular functions such as proliferation, apoptosis, and gene expression (Berridge 1997; Berridge 2009). Ca^{2+} release from the internal stores can give rise to further localized Ca^{2+} release by sensitizing neighbouring IP_3Rs on the ER. Clusters of Ca^{2+} release channels are then stimulated, eliciting a global Ca^{2+} signal manifested as a propagating Ca^{2+} wave (Bootman and Berridge 1995; Marchant and Parker 2001). Furthermore, cytosolic Ca^{2+} has a biphasic action in both facilitating and inhibiting the opening of the IP_3Rs and as a

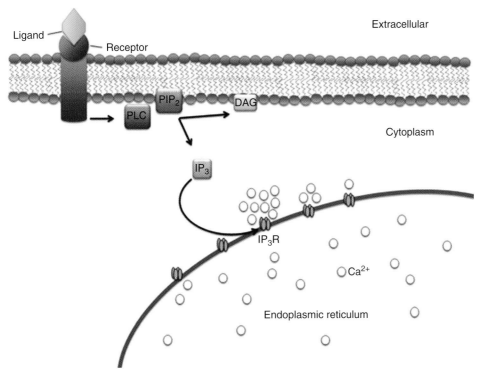

Figure 6.7 The Ca^{2+} signalling pathway and DAG, diacyglycerol; IP_3, inositol 1,4,5- trisphosphate; IP_3R, inositol 1,4,5- trisphosphate receptor; PIP_2, phosphatidylinositol 4,5, bisphosphate; PLC, phospholipase C.

result Ca^{2+} waves are generated in an oscillatory fashion, providing a digital coding system (frequency and amplitude) for signal transduction (Uhlén and Fritz 2010).

The Ca^{2+} transient observed in nearly all species during fertilization occurs as a Ca^{2+} wave. This was first observed by Jaffe and co-workers as a dramatic rise in the free Ca^{2+} concentration occurring within the cytoplasm of an activating medaka fish oocyte during fertilization. This rise in Ca^{2+} was found to be autocatalytic, involving Ca^{2+}-stimulated Ca^{2+} release that propagated across the oocyte in the form of a wave from the point of sperm fusion to its 'antipode' on the opposite side of the cell (Ridgway et al. 1977; Jones 1998; Carroll et al. 2003). Since then, Ca^{2+} signals at fertilization have been observed in numerous species with few exceptions (Stricker, 1999). The subsequent Ca^{2+} oscillations are generated, periodically, from a 'Ca^{2+} wave pacemaker' originating at the cortex of the oocytes (Dumollard et al. 2002; Carroll et al. 2003). In mammalian oocytes these

Ca^{2+} oscillations generally consist of a long-lasting series of approximately 10-fold changes in free Ca^{2+} levels, with each transient lasting about 1 min, and continuing for up to 4 h (Jones 1998).

A Brief History of Oocyte Activation

The idea of oocyte activation by the fertilizing sperm can be dated back to the late nineteenth century when, in 1898, Loeb first proposed that oocyte activation was a biochemical process involving changes in the concentration of ions within the oocyte cytoplasm (Loeb 1899). Loeb's idea was based on experiments he carried out using sea urchin oocytes. He demonstrated that the oocytes could be induced to develop parthenogenetically by altering the proportion of ions in the solution bathing the oocytes. He posited that the sperm initiated such a change in ionic composition within the oocyte cytosol by adding a 'sperm factor' during gamete fusion. This was a concept decades ahead of his time. However, an alternative model of oocyte activation was suggested by Frank Lillie, in 1913, who proposed that the process was triggered by an interaction between a sperm ligand and a receptor on the oocyte membrane – the oolemma (Lillie, 1913). These two hypotheses were to be researched and debated for several years.

It is now widely accepted that IP_3 is responsible for the Ca^{2+} release at fertilization, a phenomenon observed in species as varied as the hamster (Miyazaki et al. 1993) and sea urchin (Swann and Whitaker 1986). Just how PIP_2 is hydrolysed to IP_3 and DAG at fertilization, and the subsequent rise in cytosolic Ca^{2+}, remained unknown until relatively recently. There were three main hypotheses:

1) Building on the concepts proposed by Loeb, Lionel Jaffe (1991) suggested that Ca^{2+} present in the sperm cytoplasm is transported into the fertilizing oocyte where it stimulates the waves of Ca^{2+} seen at fertilization. This idea was later dubbed the calcium bomb (or sperm conduit) hypothesis. However, it is now known that the polyphosphoinositide messenger system is involved in the activation of oocytes via releasing Ca^{2+} from the ER (Swann and Whitaker 1990) such that an increase in the content of polyphosphoinositides are seen following fertilization in the sea urchin oocyte (Turner et al. 1987) and those of Xenopus (Snow et al. 1996).

2) A second hypothesis proposed a role for a G-protein-linked receptor; it was suggested that the sperm acted like a 'big hormone', binding to a membrane-bound receptor on the surface of the oocytes, linked to a guanine nucleotide binding protein or G-protein. Once activated, the αβγ subunits of the G-protein dissociate releasing the α subunit which then activates PLC-β, which in turn catalyses the hydrolysis of PIP_2 into IP_3 and DAG. IP_3 then releases Ca^{2+} from the ER by binding to the IP_3-dependent Ca^{2+}-releasing channels (Jaffe et al. 1988).

3) The third hypothesis involved a sperm-derived oocyte-activating factor (sperm factor) released into the oocyte upon sperm fusion (Dale et al. 1985; Swann 1990). This factor is believed to activate the oocyte by acting on the phosphoinositide cascade, resulting in the rise in $[Ca^{2+}]i$ (Jones 1998; Swann and Yu 2008).

The Sperm Factor

One of the earliest demonstrations of a sperm factor was reported by Dale et al. (1985) who showed that fertilization membranes form around unfertilized sea urchin oocyte after microinjection of soluble sperm fraction, indicating that sperm contain a component that triggers an increase in cytosolic Ca^{2+}. It was also demonstrated that the activating mechanism did not require oocyte membrane receptors. In 1990, Karl Swann showed that injection of hamster sperm extract into an oocyte was capable of inducing Ca^{2+} oscillations similar to those seen at fertilization (Swann 1990) and these results consolidated the sperm factor hypothesis first proposed by Loeb over 100 years ago. The identification of the elusive sperm factor was finally revealed as a novel isozyme of PLC, PLC-zeta (PLCζ), which was found to be specifically expressed in the mouse sperm (Saunders et al. 2002). It was also reported that injection of cRNA encoding PLCζ into mouse eggs could produce fertilization-like Ca^{2+} oscillations and subsequent early embryonic development up to the blastocyst. In addition, it was shown that the expressed level of PLCζ for initiation of Ca^{2+} oscillations was comparable to the amount estimated to be contained in a single mouse spermatozoon. Moreover, the Ca^{2+} oscillation-inducing activity of sperm extract was lost when PLCζ was immunodepleted from the sperm extract (Saunders et al. 2002). A further study used RNA interference to produce mouse sperm partially deficient in PLCζ, which then exhibited deficiencies in their ability to elicit Ca^{2+} oscillations in mouse oocytes, clearly demonstrating the necessity of PLCζ for physiological oocyte activation (Knott et al. 2005). PLCζ is also present in human sperm and was found to be localized to the equatorial region of the sperm head (Grasa et al. 2008). It is likely to play the same role in activating the human oocyte at fertilization as demonstrated in the mouse. Furthermore, human PLCζ can elicit the Ca^{2+} oscillations when injected into mouse oocytes similar to those seen at fertilization. These results are consistent with the proposal that sperm PLCζ is the molecular trigger for oocyte activation during fertilization and that the role and activity of PLCζ is highly conserved across mammalian species (Cox et al. 2002).

The evidence for PLCζ as the sperm-derived activating factor is compelling (Swann and Lai 2016).

However, other candidates are being described. One in particular is the postacrosomal WW-domain binding protein (PAWP), which is a sperm-specific protein found in the postacrosomal region of the perinuclear matrix of the sperm head. PAWP has been reported to be involved in the Ca^{2+} signal transduction events within the fertilized oocyte and compulsory for meiotic resumption and pronuclear development during oocyte activation (Wu et al. 2007). Arabi et al (2014) demonstrated that sperm-borne PAWP acts upstream of Ca^{2+} oscillations and is required for activation of human and mouse oocytes and most likely induces calcium oscillation/release through the WWI domain module. However, Nomikos et al. (2014) compared the ability of mouse PAWP and mouse PLCζ to elicit Ca^{2+} oscillations in mouse oocytes and reported PAWP was unable to increase $[Ca^{2+}]i$ in the oocytes. Further research is required to establish for certain the true nature of the sperm factor – currently PLCζ is the leading contender (Kashir et al. 2015).

Clinical Relevance

Since its inception, intracytoplasmic sperm injection (ICSI) has become a pivotal procedure in assisted reproductive technology (ART). During ICSI, a single sperm is injected directly into the ooplasm, thus circumventing any natural barriers the sperm may encounter during normal fertilization or during *in vitro* insemination (Palermo et al. 1992). ICSI is possible with sperm obtained from ejaculation, microsurgical epididymal sperm aspiration, percutaneous epididymal sperm aspiration, or testicular sperm extraction. Indications for ICSI include idiopathic infertility and repeated conventional IVF failures. The fertilization rate with ICSI is in the region of 60% (Sarkar 2007). However, approximately 3% of ICSI cycles result in complete fertilization failure, where no pronuclei, or only one pronuclei are produced. Most of the oocytes (83%) contain a spermatozoon and, in the majority of these oocytes, the sperm head is partially or completely decondensed. Consequently, failure of oocyte activation is the principal cause of fertilization failure (Flaherty et al. 1998).

In cases of failed ICSI fertilizations, oocytes have been treated with Ca^{2+} ionophores as a clinical treatment in order to overcome activation failure (Eldar-Geva et al. 2003; Nasr-Esfahani et al. 2010). Assisted oocyte activation (AOA) using Ca^{2+} ionophores (such as ionophore A23187, or ionomycin) or strontium aims to mimic the sperm-induced spatiotemporal Ca^{2+} oscillations by increasing $[Ca^{2+}]i$ through the release of Ca^{2+} from cytoplasmic stores; alternative methods such as an electrical stimulus promote influx of Ca^{2+} from the extracellular medium, and some treatments such as ethanol promote both effects (Javed, Esfandiari and Casper, 2010; Nasr-Esfahani et al. 2010). Live births have been achieved using AOA through a combination of ICSI and treatment with strontium (Chen et al. 2010), or through a combination of ICSI with Ca^{2+} ionophores (Eldar-Geva et al. 2003). Strontium and ionophores elicit a Ca^{2+} transient sufficient for oocyte activation. However, the potential cytotoxicity of these compounds has to be investigated in more detail before they are used in routine AOA.

The sperm factor (PLCζ) is presumed to play a role in activating human oocytes after ICSI. During ICSI, the sperm membrane is disrupted prior to injection of the sperm and this is likely to aid the release of factors such as PLCζ. There are some cases of oocyte activation failure after ICSI and it is possible that the sperm may sometimes lack the activating factor (Yoon et al. 2008). It is feasible therefore to consider the use of recombinant human PLCζ as part of AOA treatment in cases of ICSI fertilization failure. The use of PLCζ would result in a more physiological Ca^{2+} transient than produced by chemical Ca^{2+} ionophores. Furthermore, there is increasing evidence suggesting that the physiological significance of oscillatory Ca^{2+} signalling can influence not only the oocyte activation, but peri-implantation gene expression and development (Ozil et al. 2006).

Conclusion

The award, very much belated, of the Nobel Prize for Physiology or Medicine to Robert Edwards for his development of IVF came in 2010 (www.nobelprize.org). Edwards was a reproductive physiologist and his work on *in vitro* culture of early embryo and gamete manipulations bridged the gap between basic research and clinical medicine, when in 1978, he and his collaborator, Patrick Steptoe, successfully produced the first IVF baby. Since the inception of IVF, research has played a pivotal role in the development of this field of medicine and our understanding of the process of fertilization has advanced greatly in the last 150 years. Beginning with the observations of Hertwig and Fol, to the early work by Loeb and Lillie and continuing research into sperm–oocyte interaction, together with other areas of cellular physiology, the gap between basic research and clinical medicine has been bridged through elucidation of the mechanism of oocyte activation and discovery of the mammalian sperm factor (unravelling the mechanism of oocyte activation), and the use of AOA has enabled couples who had failed ICSI fertilization to conceive a child.

The discoveries of the biology of reproduction are as rich in their diversity and complexity as the process they explain. The story and the players involved, from Leeuwenhoek to Edwards, have unravelled the mysteries of reproduction. However, the story is not complete and there are many gaps yet to fill in this narrative.

References

Aarabi, M., Balakier, H., Bashar, S. et al. (2014). Sperm-derived WW domain-binding protein, PAWP, elicits calcium oscillations and oocyte activation in humans and mice. FASEB J 28: 4434–4440.

Abou-Haila, A. and Tulsiani, D.R. (2000). Mammalian sperm acrosome: formation, contents, and function. Arch Biochem Biophys 379: 173–182.

Aitken, R.J. and Nixon, B. (2013). Sperm capacitation: a distant landscape glimpsed but unexplored. Mol Hum Reprod 19: 785–793.

Al-Gazi, M.K. and Carroll, M. (2015). Sperm-specific micrornas – their role and function. J Hum Genet Clin Embryol 1: 003.

Austin, C.R. (1952). The 'capacitation' of mammalian sperm. Nature 170: 327.

Bahat, A. and Eisenbach. M (2006). Sperm thermotaxis. Mol Cell Endocrinol 252: 115–119.

Berridge, M.J. (1997). Annual Review Prize Lecture: Elementary and Global Aspects of Calcium Signalling. J Physiol 499: 291–306.

Berridge, M.J. (2009). Inositol trisphosphate and calcium signalling mechanisms. Biochim Biophys Acta 1793: 933–940.

Berridge, M.J. and Bootman, M.D. (1996). Calcium signaling. In: *Modular texts in Molecular and Cell Biology 1, Signal Transduction* (ed. C.H. Heldin and M. Purton). London: Chapman and Hall.

Bianch, E., Doe, B., Goulding D. et al. (2014). Juno is the egg Izumo receptor and is essential for mammalian fertilisation. Nature 508(7497): 483–487

Bigelow, J.L., Dunson, D.B., Stanford, J.B. et al. (2004). Mucus observations in the fertile window: a better predictor of conception than timing of intercourse. Hum Reprod 19: 889–892.

Bootman, M.D. and Berridge, M.J. (1995). The elementary principles of calcium signaling. Cell 83: 675–678.

Blobel, C.P., Wolfsberg, T.G., Turck, C.W. et al. (1992). A potential fusion peptide and an integrin ligand domain in a protein active in sperm-egg fusion. Nature 356: 248–252.

Carroll, M., Levasseur, M., Wood, C. et al. (2003). Exploring the mechanism of action of the sperm-triggered calcium-wave pacemaker in ascidian zygotes. J Cell Sci 116: 4997–5004.

Chang, M.C. (1951). Fertilizing capacity of spermatozoa deposited into the fallopian tubes. Nature 168: 697–698

Chen, M.S., Coonrod, S.A., Takahashi Y. et al. (1999). Role of the integrin-associated protein CD9 in binding between sperm ADAM 2 and the egg integrin alpha6beta1: implications for murine fertilisation. Natl Acad Sci 96: 11830–11835.

Chen, J., Qian, Y., Tan, Y. et al. (2010). Successful pregnancy following oocyte activation by strontium in normozoospermic patients of unexplained infertility with fertilisation failures during previous intracytoplasmic sperm injection treatment. Reprod Fertil Dev 22: 852–855.

Clarke, G.N., Stojanoff, A., Cauchi, M.N. et al. (1984). Detection of antispermatozoal antibodies of IgA class in cervical mucus. Am J Reprod Immunol 5: 61–65.

Cobb, M. (2006). *The Egg Sperm Race – Seventeenth-Century Scientists Who Unravelled the Secrets of Sex*, Live and Growth. The Free Press.

Cook, S.P., Brokaw, C.H., Muler, C.H. et al. (1994). Sperm chemotaxis: egg peptides control cytosolic calcium to regulate flagellar responses. Developmental Biology 165: 10–19.

Cox, L.J., Larman, M.G., Saunders, C.M. et al. (2002). Sperm phospholipase Czeta from humans and cynomolgus monkeys triggers Ca^{2+} oscillations, activation and development of mouse oocytes. Reproduction 124: 611–623.

Dale, B., DeFelice, L.J. and Ehrenstein, G. (1985). Injection of a soluble sperm fraction into sea urchin eggs triggers the cortical reaction. Experientia 41: 1068–1070.

de Lamirande, E. (2007). Semenogelin, the main protein of the human semen coagulum, regulates sperm function. Semin Thromb Hemost 33: 60–68.

de Lamirande, E. and Lamothe, G. (2010). Levels of semenogelin in human spermatozoa decrease during capacitation: involvement of reactive oxygen species and zinc. Hum Reprod 25: 1619–1630.

Dumollard, R., Carroll, J., Dupont, G. et al. (2002). Calcium wave pacemakers in eggs. J Cell Sci. 115(Pt 18): 3557–64.

Eisenbach, M. (1995). Sperm changes enabling fertilization in mammals. Curr Opin Endocrinol Diabetes 2: 468–475.

Eisenbach, M. (1999). Sperm chemotaxis. Rev Reprod 4: 56–66.

Eisenbach, M. (2003). Why are sperm cells phagocytosed by leukocytes in the female genital tract? Med Hypoth 60: 590–592.

Eldar-Geva, T., Brooks, B., Margalioth, E.J. et al. (2003). Successful pregnancy and delivery after calcium ionophore oocyte activation in a normozoospermic patient with previous repeated failed fertilisation after intracytoplasmic sperm injection. Fertil Steril 79 Suppl 3: 1656–1658.

Evans, J.P., Schultz, R.M., Kopf, G.S. (1998). Roles of the disintegrin domains of mouse fertilins alpha and beta in fertilisation. Biol Reprod 59: 145–152.

Flaherty, S.P., Payne, D. and Matthews, C.D. (1998). Fertilisation failures and abnormal fertilisation after intracytoplasmic sperm injection. Hum Reprod 13 Suppl 1: 155–164.

Flegel, C., Vogel, F., Hofreuter, A. et al. (2016). Characterization of the olfactory receptors expressed in human spermatozoa. Front Mol Biosci 2: 73.

Franklin, R.D. and Kutteh, W.H. (1999). Characterization of immunoglobulins and cytokines in human cervical mucus: influence of exogenous and endogenous hormones. J Reprod Immunol 42: 93–106.

Gould, J.E., Overstreet, J.W. and Hanson, F.W. (1984) Assessment of human sperm function after recovery from the female reproductive tract. Biol Reprod 31: 888–894.

Grasa, P., Coward, K., Young, C. et al. (2008). The pattern of localization of the putative oocyte activation factor, phospholipase C zeta, in uncapacitated, capacitated, and ionophore-treated human spermatozoa. Hum Reprod 23: 2513–2522.

Guidobaldi, H.A., Teves, M.E., Unates, D.R. et al. (2008). Progesterone from the cumulus cells is the sperm chemoattractant secreted by the rabbit oocyte cumulus complex. PLoS ONE 3: e3040.

Harper, M.J.K. (1994). Gamete and zygote transport. In: *The Physiology of Reproduction*, 2nd edition (ed. E. Knobil and J. D. Neill), 123–187. New York: Raven Press.

Inoue, N., Hamada, D., Kamikubo, H. et al. (2013). Molecular dissection of IZUMO1, a sperm protein essential for sperm-egg fusion. Development 140: 3221–3229.

Inoue, N., Ikawa, M., Isotani, A. et al. (2005). The immunoglobulin superfamily protein Izumo is required for sperm to fuse with eggs. Nature 434: 234–223.

Jaffe, L.F. (1991) The path of calcium in cytosolic calcium oscillations. A unifying hypothesis. Proc Natl Acad Sci USA 88: 9883–9887.

Jaffe, L.A., Turner, P.R., Kline, D. et al. (1988). G-proteins and egg activation. Cell Differ Dev 25(Suppl): 15–18.

Jaiswal, B.S. and Eisenbach, M. (2002). Capacitation. In: *Fertilization* (ed. D. Hardy), 57–117. New York: Academic Press.

Jaiswal, B.S., Tur-Kaspa, I., Dor, J. et al. (1999). Human sperm chemotaxis: is progesterone a chemoattractant? Biol Reprod 60: 1314–1319.

Jardine, L (1999). *Ingenious Pursuits, Building the Scientific Revolution*. Boston: Little, Brown and Co.

Javed, M., Esfandiari, N. and Casper, R.F. (2010). Failed fertilisation after clinical intracytoplasmic sperm injection. Reprod Biomed Online 20: 56–67.

Jin, M., Fujiwara, E., Kakiuchi, Y. et al. (2011). Most fertilizing mouse spermatozoa begin their acrosome reaction before contact with the zona pellucida during in vitro fertilization. Proc Natl Acad Sci USA 108: 4892–4896.

Jones, K. (1998). Ca^{2+} oscillations in the activation of the egg and development of the embryo in mammals. Int J Dev Biol 42: 1–10.

Jones, W.R. (1994). Gamete immunology. Hum Reprod 9: 828–841.

Kalaydjiev, S.K., Dimitrova, D.K., Trifonova, N.L. et al. (2002). The age-related changes in the incidence of 'natural' anti-sperm antibodies suggest they are not auto-/isoantibodies. Am J Reprod Immunol 47: 65–71.

Kashir, J., Nomikos, M., Swann, K. et al. (2015). PLCζ or PAWP: revisiting the putative mammalian sperm factor that triggers egg activation and embryogenesis Mol Hum Reprod 21: 383–388.

Katz, D.F., Slade, D.A. and Nakajima, S.T. (1997). Analysis of preovulatory changes in cervical mucus hydration and sperm penetrability. Adv Contracep 13: 143–151.

Kim, A.M., Bernhardt, M.L., Kong, B.Y. et al. (2011). Zinc sparks are triggered by fertilisation and facilitate cell cycle resumption in mammalian eggs. ACS Chem Biol 6: 716–723.

Kim, E., Yamashita, M., Kimura, M. et al. (2008). Sperm penetration through cumulus mass and zona pellucida. Int J Dev Biol 52: 677–682.

Klinovska, K., Sebkova, N. and Dvorakova-Hortova, K. (2014). Sperm-egg fusion: a molecular enigma of mammalian reproduction. Int J Mol Sci 15: 10652–10668.

Knott, J.G., Kurokawa, M., Fissore, R.A. et al. (2005). Transgenic RNA interference reveals role for mouse sperm phospholipase C zeta in triggering Ca^{2+} oscillations during fertilisation. Biol Reprod 72: 992–996.

Krawetz, S.A. (2005). Paternal contribution: new insights and future challenges. Nat Rev Genet 6: 633–642.

Kunz, G., Beil, D., Deininger, H. et al. (1996). The dynamics of rapid sperm transport through the female genital tract: evidence from vaginal sonography of uterine peristalsis and hysterosalpingoscintigraphy. Hum Reprod 11:627–632.

Kunz, G., Beil, D., Huppert, P. et al. (2007). Oxytocin –a stimulator of directed sperm transport in humans. Reprod Biomed Online 14: 32–39.

La Spina, F.A., Puga Molina, L.C., Romarowski, A. et al. (2016). Mouse sperm begin to undergo acrosomal exocytosis in the upper isthmus of the oviduct. Dev Biol 411: 172–182.

Le Naour, F., Rubinstein, E., Jasmin, C. et al. (2000). Severely reduced female fertility in CD9-deficient mice. Science 287: 319–321.

Lillie F.R. (1913). The mechanism of fertilisation. Science 38: 524–528.

Lishko, P.V., Botchkina, I.L. and Kirichok, Y. (2011). Progesterone activates the principal Ca2+ channel of human sperm. Nature 471(7338): 387–391.

Loeb, J. (1899). On the nature of the process of fertilisation and the artificial production of normal larvae (Plutei) from the unfertilized eggs of the sea urchin. Am J Physiol 3: 135–138.

Marchant, J.S. and Parker, I (2001). Role of elementary Ca^{2+} puffs in generating repetitive Ca2+ oscillations. EMBO J 20: 65–76.

Mattsson, J.M., Ravela, S., Hekim, C. et al. (2014). Proteolytic activity of prostate-specific antigen (PSA) towards protein substrates and effect of peptides stimulating PSA activity. PLoS One 19:9.

Miller, B.J., Georges-Labouesse, E., Primakoff, P. et al. (2000). Normal fertilisation occurs with eggs lacking the integrin a6b1 and is CD9-dependent. J Cell Biol 149: 1289–1295.

Miller, R.L. (1985). *Sperm Chemo-Orentiation in the Metazoa*. New York: Academic Press.

Miyazaki, S., Shirakawa, H., Nakada, K. et al. (1993). Essential role of the inositol 1,4,5-trisphosphate/ Ca^{2+} release channel in Ca^{2+} waves and Ca^{2+} oscillations at fertilisation of mammalian eggs. Dev Biol 158: 62.

Morales, P., Roco, M. and Vigil, P. (1993). Human cervical mucus: relationship between biochemical characteristics and ability to allow migration of spermatozoa. Hum Reprod 8:78–83.

Muga, A., Neugebauer, W., Hirama, T. et al. (1994). Membrane interaction and conformational properties of the putative fusion peptide of PH-30, a protein active in sperm-egg fusion. Biochemistry 33:4444–4448.

Nasr-Esfahani, M.H., Deemeh, M.R. and Tavalaee, M. (2010). Artificial oocyte activation and intracytoplasmic sperm injection Fertil Steril 94: 520–526.

Nevin, C. and Carroll, M. (2015). Sperm DNA methylation, infertility and transgenerational epigenetics. J Hum Genet Clin Embryol 1: 004.

Nishimura, H., Cho, C. Branciforte, D.R. et al. (2001). Analysis of loss of adhesive function in sperm lacking cryriestin or fertilin B. Dev Biol 233: 204–213.

Nomikos, M., Sanders, J.R., Theodoridou, M. et al. Sperm specific post acrosomal WW domain binding protein (PAWP) does not cause Ca^{2+} release in mouse oocytes. *Mol Hum Reprod* 2014: 938–947.

Oren-Benaroya, R., Kipnis, J. and Eisenbach, M. (2007). Phagocytosis of human post-capacitated spermatozoa by macrophages. Hum Reprod 22: 2947–2955.

Ottaviano, G., Zuccarello, D., Menegazzo, M. et al. (2013). Human olfactory sensitivity for bourgeonal and male infertility: a preliminary investigation. Eur Arch Otorhinolaryngol 270: 3079–3086.

Overstreet, J.W., Katz, D.F. and Yudin, A.I. (1991). Cervical mucus and sperm transport in reproduction. Semin Perinatol 15: 149–155.

Ozil, J.-P., Banrezes, B., Toth, S. et al. (2006). Ca2+ oscillatory pattern in fertilized mouse eggs affects gene expression and development to term. Dev Biol 300: 534–544.

Pacey, A.A., Hill, C.J., Scudamore, I.W. et al. (1995). The interaction in vitro of human spermatozoa with epithelial cells from the human uterine (fallopian) tube. Hum Reprod 10:360–366.

Palermo, G., Joris, H., Devroey, P. et al. (1992). Pregnancies after intracytoplasmic injection of single spermatozoon into an oocyte. Lancet 340(8810): 17–18.

Pandya, I.J. and Cohen, J. (1985). The leukocytic reaction of the human uterine cervix to spermatozoa. Fertil Steril 43: 417–421.

Parkhurst, M.R. and Saltzman, W.M. (1994). Leukocytes migrate through three dimensional gels of midcycle cervical mucus. Cell Immunol 156: 77–94.

Parmentier, M., Libert, F., Schurmans, S. et al. (1992). Expression of members of the putative olfactory receptor gene family in mammalian germ cells. Nature 355: 453–455.

Pinto-Correia, P (1997). *The Ovary of Eve: Egg and Sperm and Preformation.* Chicago: University of Chicago Press.

Primakoff, P., Hyatt H. and Tredick-Kline, J. (1987). Identification and purification of a sperm surface protein with a potential role in sperm-egg membrane fusion. J Cell Biol 104: 141–149.

Quill, T.A., Sugden, S.A., Rossi, K.L. et al. (2003). Hyperactivated sperm motility driven by CatSper2 is required for fertilization. Proc Natl Acad Sci USA 100: 14869–14874.

Ridgway, E.B., Gilkey, J.C. and Jaffe, L.F. (1977). Free calcium increases explosively in activating medaka eggs. Cell Biology 74: 623–627.

Rubenstein, B.B., Strauss, H., Lazarus, M.L. et al. (1951). Sperm survival in women. Fertil Steril 2:15–19.

Sarkar, N.N. (2007). Intracytoplasmic sperm injection: an assisted reproductive technique and its outcome to overcome infertility. J Obstet Gynaecol 27: 347–353.

Saunders, C.M., Larman, M.G., Parrington, J., et al. (2002). PLC zeta: a sperm-specific trigger of Ca^{2+} oscillations in eggs and embryo development. Development 129: 3533–3544.

Settlage, D.S.F., Motoshima, M. and Tredway, D.R. (1973). Sperm transport from the external cervical os to the fallopian tubes in women: a time and quantitation study. Fertil Steril 24:655–661.

Snow, P., Yim, D L., Leibow, J D., et al. (1996). Fertilisation stimulates an increase in inositol trisphosphate and inositol lipid levels in Xenopus eggs. Dev Biol 180: 108–118.

Sobrero, A.J. and McLeod, J. (1962). The immediate postcoital test. Fertil Steril 13: 184–189.

Sosa, C.M., Pavarotti, M.A., Zanetti, M.N. et al. (2015). Kinetics of human sperm acrosomal exocytosis. Mol Hum Reprod 21: 244–254.

Spehr, M., Gisselmann, G., Poplawski, A. et al. (2003). Identification of a testicular odorant receptor mediating human sperm chemotaxis. Science 299(5615): 2054–2058.

Spehr, M., Schwane, K., Riffell, J.A. et al. (2006). Odorant receptors and olfactory-like signaling mechanisms in mammalian sperm. Mol Cell Endocrinol 250: 128–136.

Stricker, S.A. (1999). Comparative biology of calcium signaling during fertilisation and egg activation in animals. Dev Biol 211: 57–76.

Strünker, T., Goodwin, N., Brenker, C. et al. (2011). The CatSper channel mediates progesterone-induced Ca2+ influx in human sperm. Nature 471(7338): 382–386.

Suarez, S.S. (2016). Mammalian sperm interactions with the female reproductive tract. Cell Tissue Res 363: 185–194.

Suarez, S.S and Pacey, A. (2006). Sperm transport in the female reproductive tract. Hum Reprod Update 12: 23–37.

Sun, F., Bahat, A., Gakamsky, A. et al. (2005). Human sperm chemotaxis: both the oocyte and its surrounding cumulus cells secrete sperm chemoattractants. Hum Reprod 20: 761–767.

Sutovsky, P. and Schatten, G. (2000). Paternal contributions to the mammalian zygote: fertilization after sperm-egg fusion. Int Rev Cytol 195: 1–65.

Swann, K. (1990). A cytosolic sperm factor stimulates repetitive calcium increases and mimics fertilisation in hamster eggs. Development 110: 1295–1302.

Swann, K. and Lai, F.A. (2016). The sperm phospholipase C-ζ and Ca2+ signalling at fertilisation in mammals. Biochem Soc Trans 44: 267–272.

Swann, K. and Yu, Y. (2008). The dynamics of calcium oscillations that activate mammalian eggs. Int J Dev Biol 52: 585–594.

Swann, K. and Whitaker M. (1986). The part played by inositol trisphosphate and calcium in the propagation of the fertilization wave in sea urchin eggs. J Cell Biol 103: 2333–2342.

Swann, K. and Whitaker, M.l. (1990). Second messengers at fertilisation in sea-urchin eggs. J Reprod Fertil 42: 141–153.

Tamburrino, L., Marchiani, S., Minetti, F. et al. (2014). The CatSper calcium channel in human sperm: relation with motility and involvement in progesterone-induced acrosome reaction. Hum Reprod 29: 418–428

Teves, M.E., Barbano, F., Guidobaldi, H.A. et al. (2006). Progesterone at the picomolar range is a chemoattractant for mammalian spermatozoa. Fertil Steril 86: 745–749.

Thompson, L.A., Barratt, C.L., Bolton, A.E. et al. (1992). The leukocytic reaction of the human uterine cervix. Am J Reprod Immunol 28: 85–89.

Tollner, T.L., Bevins, C.L. and Cherr, G.N. (2012). Multifunctional glycoprotein DEFB126–-a curious story of defensin-clad spermatozoa. Nat Rev Urol 9: 365–375.

Turner, P.l.R., Jaffe, L.A. and Fein, A. (1987). Regulation of cortical vesicle exocytosis in sea urchin eggs by inositol 1,4,5-trisphosphate and gtp-binding protein. J Cell Biol 102: 70–76.

Uhlén, P. and Fritz, N. (2010). Biochemistry of calcium oscillations. Biochem Biophys Res Comm 396: 28–32.

Vigil, P., Salgado, A.M. and Cortés, M.E. (2012). Ultrastructural interaction between spermatozoon and human oviductal cells in vitro. J Electron Microsc (Tokyo) 61: 123–126.

Ward, G.E., Brokaw, C.J., Garbers, D.L. et al. (1985). Chemotaxis of Arbacia punctulata spermatozoa to resact, a peptide from the egg jelly layer. J Cell Biol 101: 2324–2329.

Wassarman, P.M. (1988). Zona pellucida glycoproteins. Annu Rev Biochem 57: 415–442.

Wilcox, A.J., Weinberg, C.R. and Baird, D.D. (1995). Timing of sexual intercourse in relation to ovulation. Effects on the probability of conception, survival of the pregnancy, and sex of the baby. N Engl J Med 333: 1517–1521.

Williams, M., Hill, C.J., Scudamore, I. et al. (1993). Sperm numbers and distribution within the human fallopian tube around ovulation. Hum Reprod 8: 2019–2026.

Wolfsberg, T.G., Primakoff, P., Myles, D.G. et al. (1995). ADAM, novel family of membrane proteins containing a disintegrin and metalloprotease domain: multipotential functions in cell-cell and cell–matrix interactions. J Cell Biol 131: 275–278.

Wu, A.T., Sutovsky, P., Manandhar, G. et al. (2007). PAWP, a sperm-specific WW domain-binding protein, promotes meiotic resumption and pronuclear development during fertilization. J Biol Chem 282: 12164–12175.

Yoon, S.Y., Jellerette, T., Salicioni, A.M. et al. (2008). Human sperm devoid of PLC, zeta 1 fail to induce Ca(2+) release and are unable to initiate the first step of embryo development. J Clin Invest 118: 3671–3681.

Yoshida, M., Inaba, K. and Morisawa, M. (1993). Sperm chemotaxis during the process of fertilization in the ascidians Ciona savignyi and Ciona intestinalis. Dev Biol 157: 497–506.

Yudin, A.I., Generao, S.E., Tollner, T.L. et al. (2005). Beta-defensin 126 on the cell surface protects sperm from immunorecognition and binding of anti-sperm antibodies. Biol Reprod. 73: 1243–1252.

7

Human Embryo Development: From Zygote Stage to Peri-Implantation Blastocyst

Stéphane Berneau and Michael Carroll

Human Embryo Cleavage

After the fertilization and the fusion of the sperm and oocyte, resumption of the oocyte metabolism occurs (Kaji and Kudo 2004). Approximately 6–8 h postfertilization, the male and female pronuclei form simultaneously, each containing male and female haploid genomes respectively. The male pronuclei usually form near the site of sperm fusion, while the female pronuclei forms at the site of the meiotic spindle. Both pronuclei migrate towards the centre of the cytoplasm, where they eventually fuse during the process called syngamy (Payne et al. 1997). At this stage, fertilization is complete and a single-cell zygote prepares for the first series of mitotic cell divisions. In humans, the sperm-derived centrosome controls the first mitotic division, which occurs approximately 24 h after fertilization. Each division results in daughter cells called blastomeres. In humans, this process is isolecithal and rotational, producing blastomeres of equal size. The early embryo is encapsulated within the zona pellucida (ZP), which is a protective glycoprotein layer. It plays an essential role for embryo development up to the compaction stage by clustering the embryonic cells (al-Nuaim and Jenkins 2002).

Human embryos produced via *in vitro* fertilization techniques are graded depending on various morphology criteria and development speed (see Chapter 25). It is not uncommon to observe the formation of nucleate cellular debris during embryo cleavage. This phenomenon is the result of successive breakdowns of cell membrane during mitosis and is also found in *in vivo*-developed embryos retrieved from uteri for assessment. If these cytoplasmic fragments appear at an early cleavage stage, the reduction of cell cytoplasm available for nucleate blastomeres division will impair subsequent steps of development such as compaction. Thus, high fragmentation human embryos are less likely to implant (Hardarson et al. 2001; Alikani et al. 1999).

Recently, studies have demonstrated methods to select the best embryo to transfer, based on a mathematical model of cell division and noninvasive observations of embryos using a specific time-lapse incubator (i.e. Embryoscope, Primo Vision or EEVA) (Wong et al. 2010; Kovacs 2014). The speed of embryo growth/division and its viability are correlated: a slow development is linked to a weaker viability (Lee et al. 2012).

The second division of the human embryo occurs approximately 2 days after fertilization. The embryo undergoes a series of mitotic divisions, with no discernible increase in cell size, as it transgresses along the Fallopian tubes (Figure 7.1). Early asynchronous division is often reported *in vitro* via the observation of a temporary three-cell embryo and this difference in blastomeres division timing can be detected up to compaction.

In humans, by the third round of mitotic cell division, eight-cell stage, a major developmental transition occurs – the maternal to zygotic transition (MZT) and subsequent embryonic genome activation (EGA). Here *de novo*-expressed genes replace the developmental programme that was initially directed by maternally inherited transcripts and proteins (Telford et al. 1990). The time of human EGA was first identified by the failure of stopping

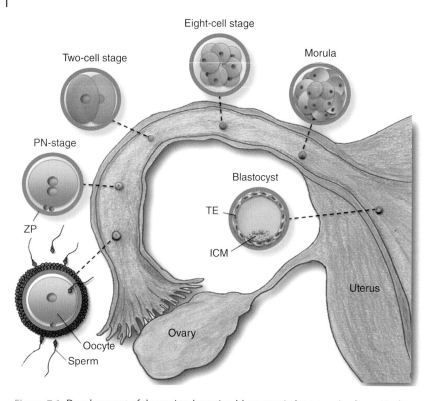

Eight-cell stage

Two-cell stage

Morula

PN-stage

Blastocyst

TE

ICM

ZP

Uterus

Oocyte

Sperm

Ovary

Figure 7.1 Development of the preimplantation blastocyst in humans. A schematic diagram illustrating the temporal and spatial development of a human embryo during the first week from fertilization until the preimplantation phase. Fertilization occurs in the Fallopian tube: a spermatozoa must successfully penetrate the zona pellucida (ZP) of the oocyte and fuse to share the paternal genetic material. From 1 to 3–4 days after fertilization, the embryo cleavage takes place by successive mitotic divisions. Thus, the embryo develops itself through various stages: pronucleus (PN), two-cell, four-cell, eight-cell and morula. After 5–6 days, the embryo becomes a blastocyst. A cavity, called a blastocoele, is formed and filled with fluid. Moreover, at the late blastocyst stage, two distinct cells types are visible: the monolayer of trophectoderm (TE) at the periphery and the inner cell mass (ICM, orange).

the embryo cleavage before the four-cell stage using transcription inhibitors (Tesarík et al. 1987; Braude et al. 1988). MZT is believed to be essential in down-regulating oocyte-specific maternal genes, whilst supporting the developing embryo through upregulating genes responsible for growth and differentiation (Dobson et al. 2004).

The MZT/EGA occurs in waves where degradation of maternal transcripts followed by upregulation of embryonic-specific genes starting at the two-cell stage, with a second wave at the four-cell stage. The genes actively transcribed during these waves represent earlier signs of embryonic genome activity, needed to coordinate the later gene activation. The subsequent waves occur at the 8–10-cell stage and blastocyst (Vassena et al. 2011). During the early stages of cleavage, all the blastomeres are

totipotent (can give rise to all cell types), as indicated by the fact that embryo splitting and birth occur following the transfer of four- to eight-cell embryos with a single viable embryo.

A human embryo reaches the eight-cell stage approximately 72 h after fertilization. In cases of a history of miscarriage, repeated unsuccessful IVF cycles, or risk of known genetic disease, couples can be offered the choice to have a preimplantation genetic diagnosis. The embryo biopsy is performed from the eight-cell stage where one to two cells are collected to be analysed using fluorescence *in-situ* hybridization (FISH) and genomic sequencing (see Chapter 30 for more detail). However, chromosomal mosaicism between blastomeres is detected in pre-implantation embryos and is an issue to predict genetic abnormalities (Harton et al. 2017). At the

8–16-cell stage, the cytoplasmic membrane of blastomeres undergoes changes in structure and composition such as the induction of cytoplasmic polarization and embryonic genome activated-induced expression of intercellular gap and tight junctions. These changes occur when the flattening and compaction of blastomeres begins.

Compaction and Morula

During compaction, a cellular mass is formed with an indistinguishable cell membrane due to newly created intercellular junctions. Compaction is a relatively quick process in embryonic development (occurring around 72 h after fertilization). At this stage, blastomeres become closely apposed forming the morula (meaning 'mulberry'). The blastomeres flatten against neighbours, and the distribution of microvilli and various plasma membrane components become restricted to the free surface. Cell-to-cell adhesion, gap and tight junctions (desmosomes), and cytoplasmic polarization first appear at this stage. Water and salts migrate through the gap junctions forming a fluid-filled cavity – the blastocoel – giving rise to the blastocyst (Nikas et al. 1996)

In mice, the morula is composed of inner apolar and outer polar blastomeres generated from asymmetric divisions, differentiating into trophectoderm (TE) and inner cell mass (ICM) cellular lineages at the blastocyst stage respectively. In humans, it has been suggested that cells lose their totipotency due to their position in the embryo. Cells losing their totipotency are predetermined to follow a certain cell lineage (Condic 2014). However, asymmetric divisions have yet to be demonstrated fully in the human morula. Figure 7.2 demonstrated the morphological changes that occur during early preimplantation development.

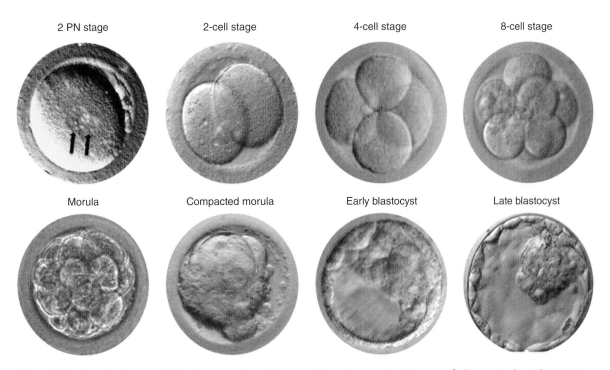

| 2 PN stage | 2-cell stage | 4-cell stage | 8-cell stage |

| Morula | Compacted morula | Early blastocyst | Late blastocyst |

Figure 7.2 *In vitro* development of the human embryo. Representative phase contrast images of a human embryo during its early development. After fertilization, pronuclei are visible: originating from oocyte and spermatozoa they are easily identifiable inside the single cell (arrow). Moreover, at the surrounding of the cell, polar bodies resulting from successful oocyte meiosis are visible until their deterioration (red star). Human embryos are *in-vitro* cultured and observed at each development stage: two-cell (day 2), eight-cell (day 3), morula/compaction (day 3–4), early blastocyst and late blastocyst stage (day 5–6)
Source: Images courtesy of the Association of Clinical Embryologists.

Blastocyst

At the early blastocyst stage, the blastocoel is formed approximately 5 days after fertilization (Dard 2008). This cavity is filled with fluid (water and salts) pumped by TE cells using the recently expressed gap junctions. TE cells will develop into the extraembryonic organs such as the placenta whereas ICM cells will become the fetus. The cell differentiation into each type of embryonic cells is well studied and identifiable using specific transcriptional markers. Early on, transcription markers EOMES, CDX2, and GATA3 are expressed in differentiated TE cells and CDX2 plays a role in the maintenance of TE cells (Sritanaudomchai et al. 2009). Meanwhile, the specification of cells within the ICM is regulated by OCT4, NANOG, and the dysregulation of an activator of CDX2 expression, TEAD4 (Hansis et al. 2000; De Paepe et al. 2013). During embryo cleavage, the embryo travels down the Fallopian tube into the uterine cavity by a secreted fluid and wafting of microvilli and cilia in the tube. After 6 days postfertilization (roughly the 20th day of the menstrual cycle), the blastocyst is in the lumen of the receptive endometrium. Uterine receptivity is hypothetically defined by the presence or upregulation of adhesive proteins at the luminal surface of the endometrium and synchronized secretion of their ligands (Aplin 2006; Aplin and Ruane 2017).

At the late blastocyst stage, the main morphological characteristics are an expanded embryo with thinning of the ZP, a single monolayer of TE, and a distinct and tightly packed ICM. At the late blastocyst stage, differentiation of the ICM into epiblast and primitive endoderm is observed in humans and mice (Piliszek et al. 2016). In culture, the blastocyst is observed to expand and contract, a possible attempt to break free from the ZP or 'hatch' in preparation for implantation.

Implantation

Implantation is a process characterized by sequential steps (Figure 7.3). Implantation is initiated by hatching of the embryo from the surrounding ZP (Hardarson et al. 2012). This first step involves the lysis of the ZP using a trypsin-like proteinase that is expressed by the embryo itself (Yoshinaga 2013). Then, the blastocyst breaks free through the newly-generated hole by repeated expansion and collapsing movements (Kirkegaard et al. 2012).

Initial apposition of the embryo onto receptive endometrial cells is considered to be an unstable attachment phase (Cakmak and Taylor 2011). Using an *in vitro* model, apposition to endometrial epithelial cells induces the activation of the blastocyst for implantation via a change in the transcription of

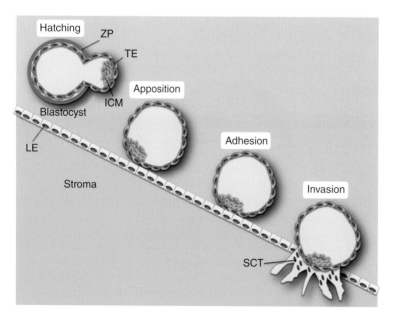

Figure 7.3 Steps of human embryo implantation. A schematic diagram of the implantation process including embryo hatching, apposition, attachment, and invasion into the endometrium. The peri-implantation stage embryo is a blastocyst composed of two differentiated cell types: trophectoderm (TE) and inner cell mass (ICM). Through hatching, the embryo breaks free from its zona pellucida (ZP) in the uterine lumen. The embryo apposes onto luminal epithelial cells (LE). Cell interactions between both epithelia are strengthened: adhesion. Then, the TE cell differentiation into syncytiotrophoblast (SCT) occurs, allowing the embryo to breach the epithelial endometrial monolayer and invade the endometrial stroma.

essential factors such as Cdx2, Hand1 and Gata3 (mouse embryos) (Ruane et al. 2017). TE cells interact more stably with the luminal epithelium as the first cellular contacts are strengthened and this phenomenon is called adhesion. During attachment, the ICM in human embryos is believed to be oriented towards the endometrium. Therefore, at first contact, embryonic adhesion occurs via the polar TE cells (which are adjacent to the ICM).

After attaching, the human blastocyst breaches into the barrier of endometrial epithelial cells to invade the uterine stroma (Armant 2005). In humans, the mechanism of invasion via epithelial cell displacement is unclear. However, Carson et al. (2000) identified various mechanisms using different animal models: (i) TE cells induce apoptosis of endometrial epithelial cells to access the stroma (mice); (ii) TE cells at the operculum of the ZP generate a cone of penetration in the luminal epithelium and therefore invade at the same time as the embryo hatches (guinea pigs); (iii) TE cells form a syncytium and fuse to luminal epithelial (LE) cells prior to penetration (rabbits); (iv) Syncytial trophoblast cells in contact with LE cells adjacent to the ICM penetrate between the LE cells to reach the stroma (primates).

Human trophoblast cells generate a cone of penetration between the lateral membranes of the LE cells (Bentin-Ley et al. 2000), recently called the 'invadopodium', a term borrowed from the mechanism of cancer cell invasion (Alblazi and Siar 2015). Then, a more extensive syncytial layer, named syncytiotrophoblast, is formed (Bentin-Ley et al. 2000). Ultrastructural studies of embryo invasion suggest that the invasion process in nonhuman primates is the most representative of the human situation. The invasion of the human blastocyst into the stroma is the final stage of implantation (Bischof and Campana 1996).

Conclusion

Much has been learnt about human preimplantation embryo development over the past decade, and this has been aided by the use of time-lapse culture of embryos, where human embryos can be monitored undisturbed *in vitro*. Understanding the cellular physiology and biology of human embryology will enhance the selection of viable embryo and pregnancy outcomes in assisted reproductive techniques.

References

Alblazi, K.M. and Siar, C.H. (2015). Cellular protrusions –lamellipodia, filopodia, invadopodia and podosomes –and their roles in progression of orofacial tumours: current understanding. Asian Pac J Cancer Prev 16: 2187–2191.

Alikani, M., Cohen, J., Tomkin, G. et al. (1999). Human embryo fragmentation in vitro and its implication for pregnancy implantation. Fertil Steril 71: 836–842.

al-Nuaim, L.A. and Jenkins, J.M. (2002). Assisted hatching in assisted reproduction. BJOG 109: 856–862.

Aplin, J.D. (2006). Embryo implantation: the molecular mechanism remains elusive. Reprod Biomed Online 13: 833–839.

Aplin, J.D. and Ruane, P.T. (2017). Embryo–epithelium interactions during implantation at a glance. J Cell Sci 130: 15–22.

Armant, D.R. (2005). Blastocysts don't go it alone. Extrinsic signals fine-tune the intrinsic developmental program of trophoblast cells. Dev Biol 280: 260–280.

Bentin-Ley, U., Horn, T., Sjogren, A. et al. (2000). Ultrastructure of human blastocyst-endometrial interactions in vitro. J Reprod Fertil 120: 337–350.

Bischof, P. and Campana, A. (1996). A model for implantation of the human blastocyst and early placentation. Hum Reprod Update 2: 262–270.

Braude, P., Bolton, V. and Moore, S. (1988). Human gene expression first occurs between the four- and eight-cell stages of preimplantation development. Nature 332(6163): 459–461.

Cakmak, H. and Taylor, H.S. (2011). Implantation failure: molecular mechanisms and clinical treatment. Hum Reprod Update 17: 242–253.

Carson, D.D., Bagchi, I., Dey, S.K. et al. (2000). Embryo implantation. Dev Biol 223: 217–237.

Condic, M.L. (2014). Totipotency: what it is and what it is not. Stem Cells Dev 23: 796–812.

Dard, N. (2008). Compaction and lineage divergence during mouse preimplantation embryo development. Gynecol Obstet Fertil 36: 1133–1138.

De Paepe, C., Cauffman, G., Verloes, A. et al. (2013). Human trophectoderm cells are not yet committed. Hum Reprod 28: 740–749.

Dobson, A.T., Raja, R., Abeyta, M.J. et al. (2004). The unique transcriptome through day 3 of human preimplantation development. Hum Mol Genet J 13: 1461–1470.

Hansis, C., Grifo, J.A. and Krey, L.C. (2000). Oct-4 expression in inner cell mass and trophectoderm of human blastocysts. Mol Hum Reprod 6: 999–1004.

Hardarson, T., Van Landuyt, L. and Jones, G. (2012). The blastocyst. Hum Reprod 27(Suppl 1): i72–91.

Hardarson, T., Hanson, C., Sjögren, A. et al. (2001). Human embryos with unevenly sized blastomeres have lower pregnancy and implantation rates: indications for aneuploidy and multinucleation. Hum Reprod 16: 313–318.

Harton, G.L, Cinnioglu, C. and Fiorentino, F. (2017). Current experience concerning mosaic embryos diagnosed during preimplantation genetic screening. Fertil Steril 107:1113–1119.

Kirkegaard, K., Agerholm, I.E. and Ingerslev, H.J. (2012). Time-lapse monitoring as a tool for clinical embryo assessment. Hum Reprod 27: 1277–1285.

Kovacs, P. (2014). Embryo selection: the role of time-lapse monitoring. Reprod Biol Endocrinol 12: 124.

Kaji, K. and Kudo, A. (2004). The mechanism of sperm-oocyte fusion in mammals. Reproduction 127: 423–429.

Lee, M.J., Lee, R.K. Lin, M.H. et al. (2012). Cleavage speed and implantation potential of early-cleavage embryos in IVF or ICSI cycles. J Assist Reprod Genet 29: 745–750

Nikas, G., Ao, A., Winston, R.M. et al. (1996) Compaction and surface polarity in the human embryo in vitro. Biol Reprod 55: 32–37.

Payne, D., Flaherty, S.P., Barry, M.F. et al. (1997). Preliminary observations on polar body extrusion and pronuclear formation in human oocytes using time-lapse video cinematography. Hum Reprod 12:532–541.

Piliszek, A., Grabarek, J.B., Frankenberg, S.R. et al. (2016). Cell fate in animal and human blastocysts and the determination of viability. Mol Hum Reprod 22: 681–690.

Ruane, P., Berneau, S., Koeck, R. et al. (2017). Apposition to endometrial epithelial cells activates mouse blastocysts for implantation. Mol Hum Reprod 23: 617–627.

Sritanaudomchai, H., Sparman, M., Tachibana, M. et al. (2009). CDX2 in the formation of the trophectoderm lineage in primate embryos. Dev Biol 335: 179–187.

Telford, N.A., Watson, A.J. and Schultz, G.A. (1990). Transition from maternal to embryonic control in early mammalian development: a comparison of several species. Mol Reprod Dev 26: 90–100.

Tesarík, J., Kopecný, V., Plachot, M. et al. (1987). Ultrastructural and autoradiographic observations on multinucleated blastomeres of human cleaving embryos obtained by in-vitro fertilization. Hum Reprod 2: 127–136.

Vassena, R., Boué, S., González-Roca, E. et al. (2011). Waves of early transcriptional activation and pluripotency program initiation during human preimplantation development. Development 138: 3699–36709.

Wong, C.C., Loewke, K.E., Bossert, N. et al. (2010). Non-invasive imaging of human embryos before embryonic genome activation predicts development to the blastocyst stage. Nature Biotech 28: 1115–1121.

Yoshinaga, K. (2013). A sequence of events in the uterus prior to implantation in the mouse. J Assist Reprod Genet 30: 1017–1022.

Further Reading

Schoenwolf, G.C., Bleyl, S.B., Brauer, P.R. et al. (2014). *Larsen's Human Embryology, 5e*. Edinburgh: Churchill Livingstone.

Veek, L.L. (1999). *An Atlas of Human Gametes and Conceptuses: An Illustrated Reference for Assisted Reproductive Technology*. Boca Raton: CRC Press.

8

The Female Reproductive Tract and Early Embryo Development: A Question of Supply and Demand

Henry J. Leese and Daniel R. Brison

Introduction

Fertilization and the cleavage stages of preimplantation development occur in the oviduct (termed the 'Fallopian tube' or 'tube' in women). At about the morula stage of development, the embryo is transported into the uterus where blastocyst formation and expansion occur prior to implantation, which in the human begins on day 7 postfertilization and is completed by around day 14. During this time, the embryo has a 'demand' for oxygen, nutrients, and other small and large molecules, which are provided via the environments in the lumen of the oviduct and uterus, i.e., the 'supply' side referred to in the title. This chapter considers each side of the equation in turn before asking how closely 'demand' and 'supply' are matched; a question complicated by the considerable autonomy exhibited by the early embryo. The focus is on events that occur in the oviduct, though the uterine environment is considered where appropriate.

A further complication is that oviduct and uterine fluids contain hundreds of physiologically relevant molecules and to consider them all is obviously beyond the scope of this chapter. Therefore, the molecules in oviduct and uterine fluids which are included in embryo culture media will be the focus. These were documented in a quantitative comparison of the composition of 12 commercially available human embryo culture media (Morbeck et al. 2014a). Thirty-nine compounds were measured, divided into four categories: glucose and organic acids (principally, pyruvate, lactate, and citrate); amino acids; ions (principally Na, K^+, and Cl^-) and elements, such as copper, iron, zinc, and trace elements (which will not be

considered further). Not included in the list but present in virtually all media used to culture human embryos, is human serum albumin (considered in 'Other molecules in embryo culture media' later). The source of human serum albumin may be significant, as Zhu et al. (2014) have shown that even using the same culture medium, albumin from different sources is associated with an effect on birthweight.

The chapter concludes by considering the challenges in devising culture conditions in which the development of the embryo can occur in as physiological manner as possible.

Nutrient Demand: Satisfying the Needs of the Embryo

Nutrients

It might have been imagined that culturing early embryos *in vitro* would require a complex medium such as that used to maintain somatic cells. However, this turned out not to be the case. Thus, Biggers (1998), summarizing the pioneering work of Whitten in the 1970s, stated that 'A surprise from Whitten's work was that the 8-cell mouse embryo would develop into a blastocyst in a very simple solution based on a physiological saline, described earlier by Krebs and Henseleit supplemented only with a carbon source (glucose) and bovine plasma albumin'. Building on this observation, Biggers, Brinster, Wales, Whitten, and Whittingham established the critical role of pyruvate in supporting the first cleavage division, the importance of glucose in the later

Clinical Reproductive Science, First Edition. Edited by Michael Carroll.
© 2019 John Wiley & Sons Ltd. Published 2019 by John Wiley & Sons Ltd.
Companion website: www.wiley.com/go/carroll/clinicalreproductivescience

stages of development, and the large increase in metabolic activity that coincided with blastocyst formation. A good account of the history of these events has been provided by Baltz (2013).

The basic nutrient requirements of preimplantation embryos discovered in the 1970s have not changed fundamentally, such that Leese (2012), almost 40 years later, was able to provide the following, contemporary account:

> The Krebs cycle and oxidative phosphorylation provide the main source of energy throughout the preimplantation period.* Pyruvate is a central energy substrate during the first cleavage in those species in which energy source requirements of the embryo have been examined, although it is not obligatory for all species (e.g. porcine). Other substrates, notably, amino acids, lactate and endogenous fatty acids derived from triglyceride, combine with pyruvate to provide embryos with a range of potential energy sources through to, and including, the blastocyst stage. These nutrients have numerous, overlapping, metabolic roles. Prior to the morula stage, glucose consumption and metabolism is low, although some glucose is necessary for intracellular signalling purposes. With blastocyst formation, large increases in oxygen consumption and the uptake and incorporation of carbon occur and there is a sharp increase in glycolysis, at least *in vitro*. The embryo goes from a relatively inactive metabolic tissue at ovulation to a rapidly metabolizing tissue at implantation.

Until recently, metabolic research on early embryos tended to focus on the utilization of the exogenous substrates mentioned above (pyruvate, lactate, glucose, and amino acids) (e.g. Brison et al. 2004), while the role of endogenous substrates, especially fat, was largely ignored. This was despite the egg being the largest diameter cell in the female mammal, with a high content of triglyceride, at least in large animals such as the cow, pig, rabbit, and sheep as well as the human. The pioneering work on endogenous nutrients was carried out by Kane and Foote, who pointed out in the early 1970s (summarized by Kane 1987) that 'the 1-cell rabbit embryo has sufficient endogenous energy sources to allow up to 3 or more cleavage divisions in culture in the absence of any possible added energy substrate'. This work has been rediscovered in the past few years, with the realization that fatty acid metabolism plays a pivotal role in egg maturation and could potentially sustain the entire energy requirement of the embryo over the preimplantation period (Sturmey et al. 2009; Dunning et al. 2010; Jungheim et al. 2011; McKeegan and Sturmey 2011; Van Hoeck et al. 2011).

The significance of endogenous reserves will be considered further in the context of embryo autonomy and adaptability.

Ions

In comparison with the wealth of data on the uptake and fate of nutrients by mammalian eggs and early embryos, much less is known about the requirement for ions. The major role of ions in somatic cells is in cell volume regulation. The history of this subject in embryos is also described in the account by Baltz (2013) mentioned previously, which considers the control of intracellular pH and the role of organic osmolytes (especially the amino acids glycine and glutamine) in protecting the embryo *in vitro* against the effects of osmotic stress and changes in cell volume. Certain ions have specific functions in gamete and early embryo survival (Chan et al. 2012); thus, the cystic fibrosis transmembrane conductance regulator (CFTR) is involved in the transport of bicarbonate ions necessary for sperm capacitation and embryo development (Chan et al. 2009). The high bicarbonate concentration also contributes to the alkalinity of oviduct fluid. The mechanism of bicarbonate transport is closely linked to the movement of potassium ions, long known to be present at elevated concentrations in oviduct fluid (Keating and Quinlan, 2012). It should also be noted that gametes (at least sperm) and embryos will only be present in the oviduct following mating but that ion and fluid

---

* This account failed to do justice to the remarkable rat preimplantation embryo, which is able to develop from the eight-cell to blastocyst stage in the complete absence of oxygen or the presence of cyanide and other inhibitors of oxidative phosphorylation (Brison and Leese 1994).

secretion will be required at all times, for example, to keep the surface of the oviduct moist and protect it from potential pathogens.

Other Molecules in Embryo Culture Media

There are numerous proteins in oviduct and uterine fluids (for reviews, see Coy et al. 2012, Ghersevich et al. 2015, and Miller 2015 and the section on Proteins later in this review) but the only one added routinely to culture media is albumin (in various forms summarized by Morbeck et al. 2014b), which is required to act as a macromolecular source, with functions as diverse as 'stabilizing' embryo membranes, facilitating handling of embryos *in vitro*, and acting as a source of energy and of 'contaminating' molecules such as fatty acids and growth factors which may act as embryotrophic agents. In clinical in vitro fertilization (IVF), this is added in the form of human serum albumin. Complex protein supplements in human embryo culture media are also considered by Morbeck et al. (2014b). A further protein, granulocyte–macrophage colony-stimulating factor (GM-CSF), present at the time of writing in one embryo culture medium only, is considered later.

Summary of the 'Demand' for Molecules by the Preimplantation Embryo

It is straightforward to list the minimum requirements of the early embryo in *qualitative* terms: the ions (Na^+, K^+, Mg^{++}, Ca^{++}, Cl^-, $PO4^-$, $HCO3^-$ and nutrients); pyruvate, lactate, glucose, amino acids, plus the macromolecule albumin, with a pH buffered to around 7.2 and an osmolarity in the range 250–290 mOsmol (Brinster 1965). However, specifying *quantitative* demands is more difficult.

While ion concentrations tend to reflect those in physiological salts solutions with an increase in K^+ concentration reflecting oviduct fluid, specifying the quantities of nutrients is not straightforward, as discussed by Leese (2003). Although most media are formulated to an osmolarity of 280–290 mOsmol, with a high Na concentration, at least one medium, KSOM (Lawitts and Biggers 1993) was based on empirical observations, with an osmolarity below 260 mOsmol and a correspondingly lower Na concentration.

As another example, one might start by measuring how much of a given nutrient the embryo consumes, but this depends on how much is provided (the higher the concentration the higher the consumption will tend to be) as well as the concentration of other nutrients in the medium. For example, a high lactate concentration will tend to dampen down glucose consumption, and while glutamine as a single amino acid substrate is consumed avidly by early embryos it is only taken up to a minor extent in the presence of all 20 amino acids (these are two of numerous such examples). Adopting an approach to defining quantitative requirements based on the kinetic properties of a given nutrient transport process is similarly flawed (Leese 2003).

In addition, overriding these considerations is the autonomy of the egg and early embryo, first documented by McLaren in 1976, who remarked that: Eggs and embryos are relatively autonomous and have astonishing regulatory powers (McLaren 1976). The most remarkable feature of embryo autonomy is the ability to develop through the whole preimplantation period when removed from the natural environment, while the 'astonishing regulatory powers' were well-illustrated in a review by Lonergan et al. (2001) who summarized the capacity of oviducts from a variety of species to act as surrogate 'hosts' for embryos from different species. Thus, the ligated rabbit oviduct supports the development of sheep, cattle, pig, and horse embryos; excised, intact, mouse oviducts support sheep, cattle, pig, and hamster embryos; and the intact sheep oviduct supports embryos from sheep, cattle, pigs, and horses. The lumen environment will differ in each case, but this is obviously not critical to embryo development.

It is important to note that while the oviduct offers a benign, supportive environment to preimplantation embryos at all stages, this is not the case for the uterine environment, which, with the exception of the human and other primates, is hostile to embryos unless they are at the equivalent developmental stage (Hunter 2002).

These examples of embryo autonomy and adaptability are consistent with the high concentration of endogenous reserves mentioned previously, which will provide a buffer against changes in nutrient availability from the external environment.

Nutrient Supply: The Formation and Composition of the Environments in the Oviduct and Uterus

Until relatively recently, oviduct and uterine fluid formation were neglected topics for research such that a review by Leese et al. (2001) was entitled: 'Formation of Fallopian tubal fluid; role of a neglected epithelium'. Major reasons for this neglect were the difficulty in ensuring that the reproductive tract fluids collected were representative of the physiological environment (Leese et al. 2008), the lack of robust methods to study oviduct and uterine fluid transport *in vitro*, and the success of IVF and other assisted reproductive technologies (ARTs) which led to the impression that the oviduct was dispensable and hence, not a priority for research.

However, evidence had been obtained by the turn of the last century that oviduct function was worthy of study in its own right as well as being related to gamete/early embryo requirements. Some typical research findings from work in the 1980s and 1990s are as follows:

- Rabbit oviduct fluid formation is consistent with the need to sustain the embryo up to day 3 following fertilization, after which time there is a reduction in fluid volume and nutrients as the embryo passes into the uterus (Gott et al. 1988).
- Glucose concentration in pig oviductal fluid falls sharply following ovulation consistent with a strategy of protecting the early embryo from a high glucose concentration (Nichol et al. 1992).
- Oxygen tension values in the oviduct and uterus of the rhesus monkey *in situ* are consistent with aerobic respiration during cleavage and the potential for glycolysis in the blastocyst (Fischer and Bavister 1993).
- Human oviduct and uterine fluid pyruvate, glucose, and lactate concentrations are consistent with the use of pyruvate during early cleavage with an increase in glucose consumption at the blastocyst stage (Gardner et al.1996).
- Oviduct and uterine epithelia transport nutrients selectively; in the case of amino acids 'the free amino acid content is totally original when compared with serum' (Menezo and Guerin 1997).
- The main driving force for human tubal fluid formation is the transepithelial secretion of chloride ions into the oviduct lumen (Dickens et al. 1993; Downing et al. 1997).
- The oviduct epithelium is sensitive to candidate signalling molecules (e.g. adenosine triphophate, platelet activating factor, cyclic adenosine monophosphate) released by sperm and early embryos (Dickens et al. 1996; Downing et al. 1997, 1999).

Although not specifically concerned with oviduct fluid, it has long been known that the oviduct regulates sperm storage and movement; specifically, that sperm became arrested in the isthmus, from where small numbers moved to the site of fertilization in the ampulla. Two of the pioneers who established this 'sperm reservoir' concept in the 1980s were Hunter (1984) and Suarez (1987). For subsequent reviews, see Bosch and Wright (2005), Suarez (2008), and Ghersevich et al. (2015). However, although this information has been well-known for several years, it has not led to changes in human-assisted conception practices; specifically, the composition of embryo culture media.

In light of such evidence, Leese (1995) in considering the role of oviduct secretions, cited the conclusion of Moor et al. (1990) that 'contributions from the oviduct should be seen as important facilitators, rather than obligatory determinants of early development'. In support of this conclusion, Lonergan et al. (2006) reported that when *in vitro*-produced cattle zygotes were cultured in the sheep oviduct, the quality of the blastocysts produced was increased; conversely, *in vivo*-produced bovine embryos cultured *in vitro* gave rise to poor quality blastocysts

A final way of illustrating the contribution of the female tract is provided by the data from Merton et al. (2003), which show that the development of cattle zygotes to blastocysts occurs with greatest success when the entire process is carried within the naturally mated animal. Success then diminishes progressively, with the use of ovarian stimulation to produce a larger number of eggs, and egg maturation, fertilization, and preimplantation development are carried out *in vitro*.

Recent Developments in Oviduct Physiology and Function

While findings such as those by Merton et al. were well-known to those in the animal research community, they had little influence on those who worked in human reproductive medicine where the prevailing view was of the oviduct being 'accommodating' and sometimes, a mere 'conduit' for gamete and embryo development, rather than an active participant. This notion has changed markedly in recent years with the appreciation that there is dynamic interaction between the female tract and the gametes and early embryo, well-summarized by Coy et al. (2012) and Maillo et al. (2015) and that ultimately, this could lead to a reformulation of embryo culture media.

Four examples of this gamete/embryo/maternal dialogue follows.

Cytokines

A number of cytokines are secreted by the oviduct and uterus, which influence embryo survival. Most cytokines found in maternal tract fluid have a dual origin; they are produced both by the embryo and the female tract, while others are unique to the tract. This has important implications for embryo development *in vitro* as the embryo has the ability to provide its own supply of cytokines, provided the volume of medium used is sufficiently low and the time of incubation sufficiently long to allow these to be concentrated to biologically active levels. Thus, there might be a logical argument against supplementing embryo culture media with cytokines of embryonic origin, since the levels of these can be manipulated more easily by simply altering the volume of the medium and the frequency with which it is changed.

Well-characterized cytokines solely of maternal origin are GM-CSF and colony stimulating factor 1 (CSF1). Cytokines exert pro- and antiapoptotic effects and have been referred to as providing 'fine-tuning' of embryo development, possibly by epigenetic remodelling (Robertson et al. 2015). It is worth noting that numerous cytokines are present in the environment of the egg prior to ovulation, i.e. follicular fluid (Field et al. 2014) where their roles involve follicular survival and atresia, and oocyte maturation.

Sperm

Sperm are now known to regulate oviduct gene expression, such that the oviduct may be involved in sperm motility, selection for fertilization, and possibly, the guided movement of sperm towards the egg

(Holt and Fazeli 2010). Constituents in seminal fluid, long thought to be of little biological significance, have also been proposed to influence sperm integrity and protection, and to act as agents which signal the female tract to produce embryotrophic cytokines that may protect embryos from cellular stress (Bromfield et al. 2014). Such molecules clearly do not have an essential role, since ARTs, which eliminate seminal plasma entirely are obviously successful, but nonetheless they may have an important facilitatory role (Bedford 2015).

Proteins

Over 150 proteins have been identified in oviduct fluids; some derived from plasma, others produced and secreted by the epithelial cells. Of the second category, the best characterized is an oestrogen-dependent oviductal glycoprotein (OVGP1) known as 'oviductin' which was discovered in the 1980s and is considered to be conserved across different mammalian species. Oviductin binds to the sperm head plasma membrane and to the zona pellucida of the oocyte. Proposed functions of oviductin include the promotion of sperm capacitation and penetration of the zona, and the induction of transient zona hardening which may limit polyspermy. However, oviductin is thought to have different roles in different species; a topic explored in an excellent review by Aviles et al. (2010). Further proteins that have attracted research interest include: osteopontin, glycodelins, atrial natriuretic peptide, glycosidase enzymes, proteases, sperm adhesion molecule 1 and lactoferrin (Ghersevich et al. 2015), and glycans (Miller 2015).

Ghersovich et al. (2015) provides a contemporary view of the role of the oviduct in reproductive processes and illustrates the way in which this organ is no longer regarded as a passive conduit for the gametes and early embryos (Figure 8.1).

Maternal Diet

While oviduct and uterine fluids provide the local environments of the gametes and embryo, it is now well established that they can be influenced by the mother's diet and lead to changes in the embryo's phenotype, which may have lifelong effects. The person who contributed more than anyone to pioneer this idea, which led to the concept known as the

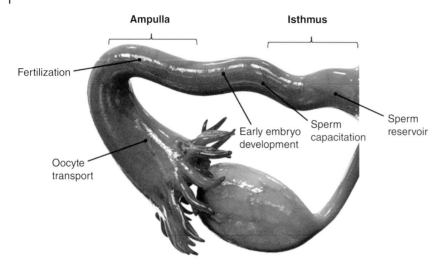

Figure 8.1 Schematic representation of the oviduct and its suggested involvement in the reproductive process. *Source:* Image from shutterstock.com/Magic mine.

'Developmental Origins of Health and Disease' was the late David Barker (1938–2014) (Barker 1989). It is only possible here to give a snapshot of the numerous studies which have provided support for this proposition. For example:

- Administration of a low-protein maternal diet to mice solely over the preimplantation period gives rise to embryos with altered developmental and metabolic characteristics which are associated with altered fetal weight and a variety of adverse changes in the offspring when they became adults; notably, cardiovascular and neurological ('hyperactive') disorders (Eckert et al. 2012).
- Children conceived by IVF have a lower birthweight (Hansen et al. 2002) and exhibit cardiovascular changes in early adulthood, especially an increase in blood pressure (Ceelen et al. 2008).
- Human embryos conceived by IVF from overweight and obese women have an elevated triglyceride content and impaired glucose consumption at the blastocyst stage (Leary et al. 2015)

For recent summaries of this very active field see Lane et al. (2014), Leese (2014), Tarry-Adkins and Ozanne (2014), and Feuer and Rinaudo (2016).

Conclusion

The preimplantation period is uniquely vulnerable to external influences since a number of key developmental events take place at this stage, including reorganization of the embryonic genome to incorporate male and female genetic material, reorganization of the epigenome, and the first cell fate choice in development, to form either inner cell mass (giving rise to the fetus) or trophectoderm (placenta). External influences such as maternal nutrition, low protein content, and infections have been associated with programming of long-term cardiometabolic health in offspring (Figure 8.2). Some of these effects may be mediated by the artificial environment experienced during assisted reproductive technology (ART) procedures, including altered nutrition in different culture media, and a changed material milieu associated with ovarian stimulation regimes. Lane et al. (2014) provides an excellent summary of these effects.

Can Knowledge of the Maternal Environment Help Us Improve Culture Media?

The above discussion provides a number of examples of potentially important maternal tract components which are absent from *in vitro* embryo culture systems. It might therefore seem obvious that adding some of these components to the *in vitro* system would improve embryo development and viability and hence success rates in ART, and more importantly,

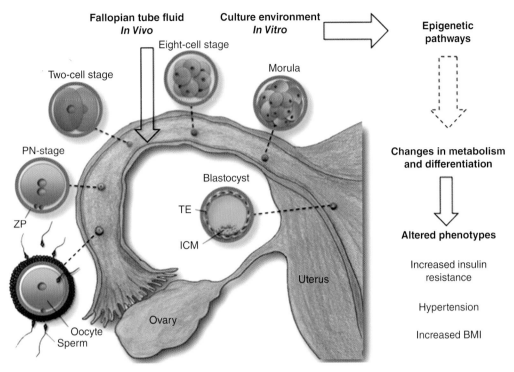

Figure 8.2 Environmental effects on embryogenesis. During progression from conception, through first cleavage to morula and blastocyst stages, a preimplantation embryo is vulnerable to perturbations in its nutritional, biochemical, and physical environment. Influences exerted in the oviduct *in vivo*, or the culture dish *in vitro*, operate via epigenetic pathways to program the embryo developmental trajectory, resulting in an altered adult phenotype. BMI, body mass index; PN, pronucleus; TE, trophoectoderm; ICM, inner cell mass; ZP, zona pellucida.

have a positive impact on the long-term health of ART children. This approach does indeed seem promising when one considers important maternally derived cytokines such as Granulocyte-macrophage colony-stimulating factor (GMCSF) (Robertson 2015) and the plethora of oviductal proteins now identified which might play important roles (Aviles et al. 2010). Having said that, there are at least two important barriers to translation of knowledge of the maternal tract directly into improvements in culture medium.

The first is the sheer complexity of the maternal system. In order to replicate this faithfully *in vitro* one would have to replace a large number of components at their concentrations found in the maternal tract, and additionally, replicate changes in time during development. Furthermore, one would have to replicate the maternal environment in terms of oxygen concentration, the mixing of components by the actions of cilia and muscular activity, and perhaps most difficult, physical interactions between maternal

epithelia and the embryo. In light of these considerations it might seem futile to attempt to replace just one component of the maternal milieu. The second barrier is the emerging awareness of the need for careful testing of new components introduced into IVF (Harper et al. 2012; Brison et al. 2013; Chronopoulou and Harper 2015). Although this has generally not been done through the history of ART, one could argue that we now have sufficient evidence from the cohort of existing ART children to be confident that existing practices are safe, at least in the short term.

However, this obviously does not apply to the assessment of new components, which needs to be rigorous, especially in light of increased scientific knowledge of the impact of epigenetic changes in early embryonic development on long-term health (Brison et al. 2013; Feuer and Rinaudo, 2016). Harper et al. (2012) suggested a framework whereby new development should be tested in animal models, followed by spare human embryos donated to research, before entering into clinical practice in the form of a clinical trial, with consequent follow-up studies of children arising from the new treatment. A recent example of this strategy is afforded by the addition of GMCSF to embryo culture media. This followed more than 10 years of careful work with mouse and human embryos, followed by a large multicentre randomized controlled trial (Ziebe et al. 2013; Robertson 2015). The trial showed that GMCSF did not have a beneficial impact on success rates unless embryos were cultured in suboptimal media, or if the patients had had a previous miscarriage. For the majority of patient cycles using conventional culture media there was no beneficial effect of adding this cytokine (Ziebe et al. 2013).

Although this example illustrates the difficulty in translating basic information on the female tract and early embryo into improvements in ART practice, it should not detract from further efforts of this type based on rigorous research and development. It seems highly likely that increasing consideration of the role of the maternal tract environment will lead to significant improvements in ART conditions and procedures. However, the twin watchwords which should guide efforts to improve assisted conception practices are 'efficacy' and 'safety'. Efficacy should include an understanding of how a new intervention works at as many levels as possible, from the gametes and early embryo, throughout pregnancy and early infancy; safety should also include these areas as well as potential long-term effects. The challenge is to persuade practitioners and regulators to adopt such lifelong thinking since all who work in this area have a responsibility to give ART children 'the best start in life'.

References

Aviles, M., Gutierrez-Adan, A. and Coy, P. (2010). Oviductal secretions: will they be key factors for the future of ARTs? Mol Hum Reprod 16: 896–1206.

Baltz, J.A. (2013). Connections between preimplantation embryo physiology and culture. J Assist Reprod Genet 30: 1001–1007.

Barker, D.J.P. (1989). The foetal and infant origins of inequalities in health in Britain. J Publ Health Med 13: 64–68.

Bedford, J.M. (2015). The functions – or not – of seminal plasma? Biol Reprod 92: 1–3.

Biggers, J.D. (1998). Reflections on the culture of the preimplantation embryo. Int J Dev Biol 42: 879–884.

Bosch, P. and Wright, R.W. Jr. (2005). The oviductal sperm reservoir in domestic mammals. Arch Med Vet 37: 95–104.

Brinster, R.L. (1965). Studies on the development of mouse embryos in vitro. (i) the effect of osmolarity and hydrogen ion concentration. J Exp Zool 158: 49–57.

Brison, D.R., Houghton, F.D., Falconer, D. et al. (2004). Identification of viable embryos in IVF by non-invasive measurement of amino acid turnover. Hum Reprod 19: 2319–2324.

Brison, D.R. and Leese, H.J. (1994). Blastocoel cavity formation by preimplantation rat embryos in the presence of cyanide and other inhibitors of oxidative phosphorylation. J Reprod Fertil 101: 305–309.

Brison, D.R., Roberts, S.A. and Kimber, S.J. (2013). How should we assess the safety of IVF technologies? Reprod Biomed Online 27: 10–21.

Bromfield, J.J., Schkenken, J.E., Chin, P.Y. et al. (2014). Maternal factors contribute to paternal seminal fluid impact on metabolic phenotype in offspring. Proc Natl Acad Sci USA 111: 2200–2205.

Ceelen, M., van Weissenbruch, M.M., Vermeiden, J.P. et al. (2008). Cardiometabolic differences in children born after in vitro fertilization: follow-up study. J Clin Endocrinol Metabol 93: 1682–1688.

Chan, H.C., Chen, H., Ruan, Y. et al. (2012). Physiology and pathophysiology of the epithelial barrier of the female reproductive tract. In: *Biology and Regulation of Blood-Tissue Barriers* (ed C.Y. Cheng). Landes Bioscience and Springer Sciences+Business Media.

Chan, H.C., Ruan, Y.C., He, O. et al. (2009). The cystic fibrosis transmembrane conductance regulator in reproductive health and disease. J Physiol 15: 2187–2195.

Chronopoulou, E. and Harper, J.C. (2015). IVF culture media: past, present and future. Hum Reprod Update 21: 39–55.

Coy, P., Garcia-Vasquez, F.A., Visconti, P.E. et al. (2012). Roles of the oviduct in mammalian fertilization. Reproduction 144: 649–660.

Dickens, C.J., Comer, M., Southgate, J. et al. (1996). Human Fallopian tubal epithelial cells in vitro:

establishment of polarity and potential role of intracellular calcium and ATP in fluid secretion. Hum Reprod 11: 212–217.

Dickens, C.J., Southgate, J. and Leese, H.J. (1993). Use of primary cultures of rabbit oviduct epithelial cells to study the ionic basis of tubal fluid formation. J Reprod Fertil 98: 603–610.

Downing, S.J., Chambers, E.L., Maguiness, S.D. et al. (1999). Effect of inflammatory mediators on the electrophysiology of the human oviduct. Biol Reprod 61: 657–664.

Downing, S.J., Maguiness, S.D., Watson, A. et al. (1997). Electrophysiological basis of human Fallopian tubal fluid formation. J Reprod Fertil 111: 29–34.

Dunning, K.R., Cashman, K., Russell, D.L. et al. (2010). Beta-oxidation is essential for mouse oocyte developmental competence and early embryo development. Biol Reprod 83: 909–918

Eckert, J.J., Porter, R., Watkins, A.J. et al. (2012). Metabolic induction early responses of mouse blastocyst developmental programming following maternal low protein diet affecting life-long health. PLoS ONE 7: e52791.

Feuer, S. and Rinaudo, P. (2016). From embryos to adults: a DOHaD perspective on in vitro fertilization and other assisted reproductive technologies. Healthcare (Basel) 4: pii: E51.

Field, S.L., Dasgupta, T., Cummings, M. et al. (2014). Cytokines in ovarian folliculogenesis, oocyte maturation and luteinisation. Mol Reprod Dev 81: 274–314.

Fischer, B. and Bavister, B.D. (1993). Oxygen tension in the oviduct and uterus of rhesus monkeys, hamsters and rabbits. J Reprod Fertil 99: 673–679.

Gardner, D.K., Lane, M., Calderon, I. et al. (1996). Environment of the preimplantation human embryo in vivo: metabolite analysis of oviduct and uterine fluids and metabolism of cumulus cells. Fertil Steril 65: 349–353.

Ghersevich, S., Massa, E. and Zumoffen, C. (2015). Oviductal secretion and gamete interaction. Reproduction 149: R1–R14.

Gott, A.L., Gray, S.M., James, A.F. et al. (1988). The mechanism and control of rabbit oviduct fluid formation. Biol Reprod 39: 758–763.

Hansen, M., Kurinczuk, J., Bower, C. et al. (2002). The risk of major birth defects after intracytoplasmic sperm injection and in vitro Fertilisation. N Engl J Med 346: 725–30.

Harper, J., Magli, M.C., Lundin, K. et al. (2012). When and how should new technology be introduced into the IVF laboratory? Hum Reprod 27: 303–313.

Holt, W.V. and Fazeli, A. (2010). The oviduct as a complex mediator of mammalian sperm function and selection. Mol Reprod Dev 77: 934–943.

Hunter, R.H.F. (1984). Pre-ovulatory arrest and peri-ovulatory distribution of competent spermatozoa in the isthmus of the pig oviduct. J Reprod Fertil 72: 203–211.

Hunter, R.H. (2002). Tubal ectopic pregnancy: a patho-physiological explanation involving endometriosis. Hum Reprod 17:1688–1691.

Jungheim, E.S., Macones, G.A., Odem, R.R. et al. (2011). Associations between free fatty acids, cumulus oocyte complex morphology and ovarian function during in vitro fertilization. Fertil Steril 95: 1970–1974.

Kane, M.T. (1987). Minimal nutrient requirements for culture of one-cell rabbit embryos. Biol Reprod 37: 775–778.

Keating, N. and Quinlan, L.R. (2012). Small conductance potassium channels drive ATP-activated chloride secretion in the oviduct. Am J Physiol Cell Physiol 302: C100–109.

Lane, M., Robker, R.L. and Robertson, S.A. (2014). Parenting from before conception. Science 345: 756–759.

Lawitts, J.A. and Biggers, J.D. (1993). Culture of preimplantation embryos. Methods Enzymol 225: 153–164.

Leary, C., Leese, H.J. and Sturmey, R.G. (2015). Human embryos from overweight and obese women display phenotypic and metabolic abnormalities. Hum Reprod 30: 122–132.

Leese, H.J. (1995). Metabolic control during preimplantation mammalian development. Hum Reprod Update 1: 63–72.

Leese, H.J. (2003). What does an embryo need? Human Fertility 6: 180–185.

Leese, H.J. (2012). Metabolism of the preimplantation embryo: 40 years on. Reproduction 143: 417–427.

Leese, H.J. (2014). Effective nutrition from conception to adulthood. Hum Fertility, 7: 252–256.

Leese, H.J., Hugentobler, S.A., Gray, S.M. et al. (2008). Female reproductive tract fluids: composition, mechanism of formation and potential role in the developmental origins of health and disease. Reprod Fertil Dev 20: 1–8.

Leese, H.J., Tay, J.I., Reischl, J. et al. (2001). Formation of fallopian tubal fluid: role of a neglected epithelium. Reproduction 121: 339–346.

Lonergan, P., Fair, T., Corcoran, D. et al. (2006). Effect of culture environment on gene expression and developmental characteristics in IVF-derived embryos. Theriogenology 65: 137–152.

Lonergan, P., Rizos, D., Ward, F. et al. (2001). Factors influencing oocyte and embryo quality in cattle. Reprod Nutr Dev 41: 27–437.

Maillo, V., Gaora, P.O., Forde, N. et al. (2015). Oviduct-embryo interactions in cattle: two-way traffic or a one-way street? Biol Reprod 92: 1–8.

McKeegan, P.J. and Sturmey, R.G. (2011). The role of fatty acids in oocyte and early embryo development. Reprod Fertil Dev 24: 59–67.

McLaren, A. (1976). *Mammalian Chimaeras*. Cambridge: Cambridge University Press, Cambridge. p. 22.

Menezo, Y. and Guerin. P. (1997). The mammalian oviduct: biochemistry and physiology. Eur J Obstet Gynecol 73: 99–104.

Merton, J.S., de Roos, A.P.W., Mullaart, E. et al. (2003). Effect on embryo production of the origin of the oocyte and the successive steps of maturation, fertilization and early development performed in vivo and/or in vitro in cattle. Theriogeneology 59: 651–674.

Miller, D.J. (2015). Regulation of sperm function by oviduct fluid and the epithelium: insight into the role of glycans. Reprod Domest Anim 50(Suppl 2): 31–39.

Moor, R.M., Nagai, T. and Gandolfi, F. (1990). Somatic cell interactions in early mammalian development. In: *From Ovulation to Implantation*. VIIth Reinier De Graaf Symposium (ed. J.H.L Evers and M.J. Heineman), 177–191. Amsteram: Excerpta Medica.

Morbeck, D.E., Krisher, R.L., Herrick, J.R. et al. (2014a). Composition of commercial media used for human embryo culture. Fertil Steril 102: 759–766.

Morbeck, D.E., Paczkowski, M., Fredrickson, J.R. et al. (2014b). Composition of protein supplements used for human embryo culture. J Assist Reprod Genet 31: 1703–1711.

Nichol, R., Hunter, R.H.F., Gardner, D.K. et al. (1992). Concentrations of energy substrates in oviductal fluid and blood plasma of pigs during the peri-ovulatory period. J Reprod Fertil 96: 699–707.

Robertson, S.A., Chin, P-Y, Schjenken, J.E. et al. (2015). Female tract cytokines and developmental programming in embryos. In: *Cell Signaling during Mammalian Early Embryo Development* (ed. H.J. Leese and D.R.Brison). New York: Springer Science ۱ Business Media.

Sturmey, R.G., Reiss, A., Leese, H.J. et al. (2009). Role of fatty acids in energy provision during oocyte maturation and early embryo development. Reprod Domest Anim 44(Suppl 3): 50–58.

Suárez, S.S. (1987). Sperm transport and motility in the mouse oviduct: Observations in situ. Biol Reprod 36: 203–221.

Suarez, S.S. (2008). Regulation of sperm storage and movement in the mammalian oviduct. Int J Dev Biol 52: 455–462.

Tarry-Adkins, J. and Ozanne, S.E. (2014). The impact of early nutrition on the ageing trajectory. Proc Nutr Soc 73: 289–301.

Zhu, J., Li, M., Chen, L. et al. (2014). The protein source in embryo culture media influences birthweight: a comparative study between G1 v5 and G1-PLUS v5. Hum Reprod 29: 1387–1392.

Ziebe, S., Loft, A., Povlsen, B.B. et al. (2013). A randomized clinical trial to evaluate the effect of granulocyte-macrophage colony-stimulating factor (GM-CSF) in embryo culture medium for in vitro fertilization. Fertil Steril 99: 1600–1609.

Section Two

Clinical Reproductive Science

Causes of Male and Female Infertility

9

Disorders of Male Reproductive Endocrinology

Michael Carroll

Introduction

Testicular function is regulated by complex positive and negative feedback loops originating from the pulsatile release of gonadotropin-releasing hormone (GnRH) from the hypothalamus, which is followed by secretion of gonadotropins by the anterior pituitary gland. The pituitary gonadotropins – luteinizing hormone (LH) and follicle-stimulating hormone (FSH) – stimulate the Leydig cells and Sertoli cells respectively producing sex steroids and inhibin, which in turn exert a negative feedback on GnRH, LH and FSH secretion (see Chapter 3 for review). In men, the testis has two main functions: synthesis of testosterone and spermatogenesis. The loss of one or both of these functions is termed male hypogonadism. Hypogonadism is classified into primary hypogonadism or secondary hypogonadism:

- In primary hypogonadism, the testes are primarily affected where serum testosterone concentrations are lowered, spermatogenesis is impaired, and concentrations of gonadotropins are raised (also termed hypergonadotropic hypogonadism).
- Secondary hypogonadism is characterized by low serum testosterone concentrations, reduced spermatogenesis and low or abnormal concentrations of gonadotropins (termed hypogonadotropic hypogonadism). Both primary and secondary hypogonadism may arise from several congenital and acquired disorders (Table 9.1).

Diagnosis

In men with low or absent sperm in their ejaculate a complete clinical history and physical examination should be undertaken. Hormonal analysis should include serum testosterone, inhibin, serum FHS, and LH (Figure 9.1). Specific childhood illness such as mumps, orchitis, testicular torsions, and cryptorchidism should be investigated. Physical examination should include hair distribution, body proportions, voice, and development of breast tissue (gynecomastia). Examination of the penis including the location of the urethral meatus, scrotal examination for evidence of varicocele or cryptorchidism, and measurement of testicular volume by Prader orchidometer (Figure 9.2) should also be carried out.

It is important that a clear clinical diagnosis of hypogonadism in men is made early as clinical implications may affect treatment management. The diagnosis of acquired hypogonadism is important, not only in terms of fertility treatment but also for its potential impact on general health. For instance, hypogonadism caused by a pituitary tumour may be associated with symptoms such as tiredness, headaches, and visual problems, which may be related to the tumour. Furthermore, manifestations due to elevated or reduced secretions of other anterior pituitary hormones can present as diabetes insipidus resulting from hypothalamic antidiuretic hormone deficiency. These patients require management of

Clinical Reproductive Science, First Edition. Edited by Michael Carroll.
© 2019 John Wiley & Sons Ltd. Published 2019 by John Wiley & Sons Ltd.
Companion website: www.wiley.com/go/carroll/clinicalreproductivescience

Table 9.1 Causes of hypogonadism in the male.

Primary Hypogonadism	Secondary Hypogonadism
Congenital	**Congenital**
Klinefelter syndrome	Kallmann syndrome (hypogonadotropic hypogonadism)
Y-chromosome microdeletions	Prader–Willi syndrome
Myotonic dystrophy	Laurence–Moon–Bardet–Biedle syndrome
Cryptorchidism	Hereditary haemochromatosis
Noonan's syndrome	**Acquired**
Acquired	Obesity
Orchitis	Smoking
Mumps	Recreational drugs
Varicocele	Anabolic steroid use
Testicular injury/torsion	Increased glucocorticoid levels
Chemotherapy	Increased oestrogen/testosterone levels
Gonadotoxins	Hyperthyroidism/hypothyroidism
	Hyperprolactinaemia

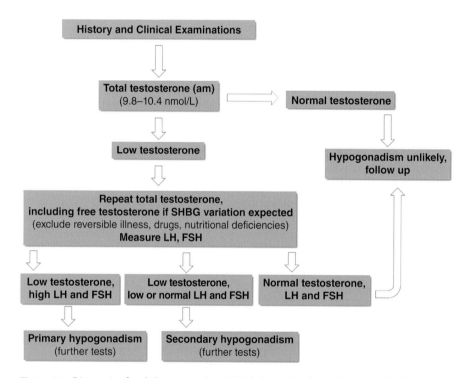

Figure 9.1 Diagnosis of male hypogonadism. FSH, follicle-stimulating hormone; LH, luteinizing hormone; SHBG, sex hormone binding globulin.

the primary disorder (the tumour) in addition to treating their hypogonadism. Secondary hypogonadism resulting from lifestyle factors, disease, or trauma may be reversible by treating the underlying condition (e.g. nutritional deficiency, obesity, infection, or injury) or discontinuation of medicines or gonadotoxic agents. In men with primary hypogonadism, fertility cannot be restored with testosterone replacement treatment; alternative assisted reproductive techniques are suggested.

The causes of male infertility are complex and multifactorial. Recent consensus guidelines have presented

(a)

(b)

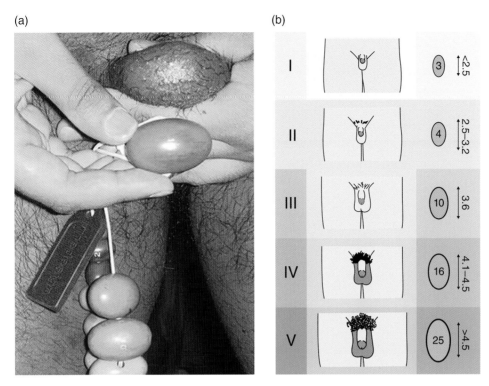

Figure 9.2 Testicular volume measurements by orchidometer. (a) The volume of each testis can be measured by comparing testicular size with those on the orchidometer. (b) Expected testis volume and Tanner scale of testis development. The beads are compared with the testicles of the patient, and the volume is read off the bead that matches most closely in size. *Source:* Astanak, 2011. https://commons.wikimedia.org/wiki/File:Orchidometry.jpg.CC BY-SA 3.0.

an evidence-based approach for the diagnosis of male infertility (Barratt et al. 2017). However, much remains to be done to fully appreciate the status of male reproductive health and infertility diagnosis. This chapter will review the causes of hypogonadism, how it impairs male fertility, and treatment options.

Primary Hypogonadism

Klinefelter syndrome

Harry Klinefelter first described a syndrome in patients with gynecomastia, small testes, sterility, and increased excretion of FSH – later to be named Klinefelter syndrome (Klinefelter et al. 1942). Klinefelter syndrome occurs in approximately 1 in 500 live births and is the most common genetic cause of hypogonadism and male infertility (Lanfranco et al. 2004). This syndrome is caused by congenital aneuploidy of the sex chromosomes, with

the majority (80%) of patients having the 47-XXY karyotype (Figure 9.4), and the remainder having mosaic 47-XXY/46-XY (different chromosome number in different cells), supernumerary X chromosome aneuploidy (48-XXY; 49-XXXXY) or additional Y-chromosomes (48-XXYY). These chromosomal abnormalities are due to chromosomal nondisjunction during maternal and paternal gametogenesis (Tüttelmann and Gromoll 2010).

Clinical presentations of Klinefelter syndrome are small firm testes, low serum testosterone concentrations, and azoospermia. However, some men with mosaicism can have normal testicular size and active spermatogenesis at puberty, but spermatogonial stem cells are progressively lost over time, reducing mature sperm counts dramatically. Patients with Klinefelter syndrome may also display symmetrical gynecomastia and tall stature with long legs and a short trunk. Beard growth and other secondary sexual hair growth are often sparse (see Figure 9.3 for a summary). Diagnosis of Klinefelter syndrome is

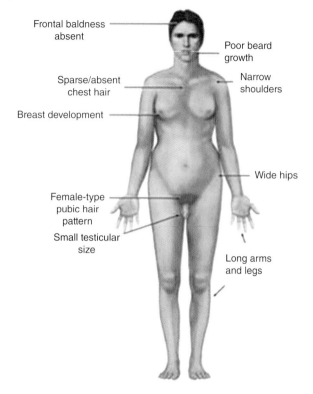

Figure 9.3 Characteristics of Klinefelter syndrome. *Source:* image via Wikimedia.org.

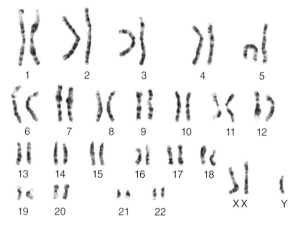

Figure 9.4 Karyotype for Klinefelter syndrome. *Source:* image via Wikimedia.org.

confirmed by karyotyping (Figure 9.4) (Lanfranco et al. 2004; Nieschlag 2013).

Treatment of Klinefelter syndrome involves testosterone replacement therapy, which can attain increased masculinity including increased muscle mass and strength, increased bone density, and thicker secondary hair growth. Increased libido and a decrease in erectile dysfunction and depressive moods and are also achieved (Vignozzi et al. 2010).

Although fertility cannot be restored in men with Klinefelter syndrome, biological fatherhood can be achieved, in some cases, using surgical sperm retrieval and intracytoplasmic sperm injection (ICSI) (Bakircioglu et al. 2011; Greco et al. 2013).

A recent study has demonstrated that during reprogramming to induced pluripotent stem cells (iPSC), fibroblasts from sterile trisomic XXY and XYY mice lose the extra sex chromosome, by a phenomenon termed trisomy-biased chromosome loss. The resulting euploid XY iPSCs can then be differentiated into functional sperm that can be used in ICSI to produce chromosomally normal, fertile offspring. The findings have relevance to overcoming infertility and other trisomic phenotypes, like Klinefelter syndrome (Hirota et al. 2017).

Y-chromosome microdeletions

The Y chromosome is the smallest chromosome containing 60 million base pairs, and is divided into a long arm (Yq) and a short arm (Yp). The genetic information on the Y chromosome contains the *SRY* gene, which is important for male sex determination, and different spermatogenesis loci named azoospermia factors (AZFa, b, and c – see Figure 9.5). Deletions in these regions remove one or more of the candidate genes (*DAZ, RBMY, USP9Y,* and *DBY)* and cause severe testiculopathy leading to male infertility and decreased or absent spermatogenesis (Chandley 1998; Li, Haines and Han 2008; Krausz and Casamonti 2017). A fourth AZF region, between AZFb and AZFc, termed AZFd, has been described and found in patients with mild oligozoospermia or even normal sperm counts and abnormal sperm morphology (Kent-First et al. 1999; Müslümanoglu et al. 2005).

Approximately 7% of men with severe oligospermia and 13% of men with azoospermia have microdeletions of the Y chromosome (Najmabadi et al. 1996). Deletions removing the entire AZFa or AZFb regions (complete deletions) are associated with azoospermia due to Sertoli cell-only syndrome and spermatogenic arrest, respectively. The partial deletions of AZFa and AZFb are associated with residual sperm production. The complete AZFc deletions are associated with a variable semen sperm content

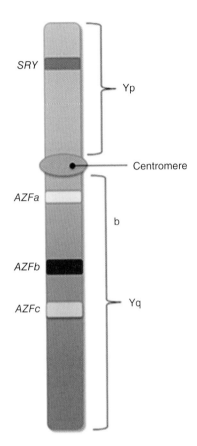

Figure 9.5 Y chromosome showing p and q arms with associated location of *SRY* and *AZF* genes.

achieved in some cases through the use of surgical sperm retrieval and ICSI. However, Y chromosomal microdeletions can be transmitted from a father to a son via ICSI suggesting that the microdeletions may be expanded during such transmission. It is imperative, therefore, that genetic counselling is offered for infertile couples contemplating ICSI in cases where the male carries Y chromosomal microdeletions (Komori et al. 2002).

Noonan Syndrome

Noonan syndrome is a relatively common genetic disorder (1 in 1000 to 1 in 2500) with multiple congenital abnormalities. It is characterized by short stature and broad webbed neck, facial dysmorphia, sternal deformity (pectus carinatum and/or excavatum), and congenital heart disease (Tafazoli et al. 2017). Noonan syndrome is genetically heterogeneous with approximately half the cases caused by activating germline mutations in the *PTPN11* gene, but other cases have since been shown to be because of gain-of-function mutations in *KRAS,6 SOS1,7,8* and *RAF1.9* (Tartaglia et al. 2001).

Cryptorchidism has been reported in 80% of boys with Noonan syndrome. In many cases LH and testosterone levels are essentially normal in men, while FSH levels are raised in the men with cryptorchidism. Although sexual function is not affected in men with Noonan syndrome, the onset of sexual activity can be delayed with late onset of puberty. Bilateral cryptorchidism appears to be the main factor contributing to impairment of fertility in men with Noonan syndrome, which can result in azoospermia or oligozoospermia (Elsawi et al. 1994). However, in other reports, men with normal testicular descent displayed signs of Sertoli cell dysfunction, indicating that bilateral cryptorchidism may not be the main contributing factor to impairment of testicular function in Noonan syndrome (Marcus et al. 2008).

Acquired Primary Hypogonadism

Chemical insult, injury, or infection of the testis can result in testicular dysfunction and impaired spermatogenesis resulting in infertility. See Chapter 13 for more detail on the pathologies of the testis and how this can impact on testicular function. Chapter 14 covers the impact of infection on fertility and Chapter 17 details the impact of environmental

ranging from oligozoospermia (fewer than 2 million sperm/mL) to azoospermia (sperm absent in semen). In hormone analysis, concentrations of testosterone and LH in serum are generally normal, but FSH concentration is raised because of decreased production of inhibin B and loss of negative feedback (Krausz and Casamonti 2017). In some cases of Y chromosome, microdeletions can present with cryptorchidism (Foresta et al. 1999).

The diagnosis of microdeletions is performed by multiplex polymerase chain reaction (PCR) amplification of selected regions of the long arm of the Y chromosome from genomic DNA derived from white blood cells. Lack of PCR amplification suggests the presence of a microdeletion, which should be confirmed by a separate PCR reaction based on different primers (Nakashima et al. 2002; Hopps et al. 2003).

Treatment of men with Y-chromosome microdeletions will depend on the region deleted on the Y chromosome, with successful biological fatherhood exposures on testicular function. The following is a brief description of factors responsible for primary hypogonadism.

Orchitis

Infections and inflammations of the testis (orchitis) are responsible for the most frequent causes of reduced sperm quality. Bacterial infections can result in activation of the immune cells and mediators involved in the inflammatory processes, inducing irreversible damage to seminiferous tubules leading to reduced spermatogenesis and corresponding decline of sperm quality and number (Trojian et al. 2009). Infection of the testis that spreads to the epididymis is referred to as epididymo-orchitis (Kaver et al. 1990). Bacterial testicular infection may result in permanent azoospermia or oligospermia, which can lead to male infertility (Osegbe 1991; Schuppe 2010). In men under 35 years of age, epididymo-orchitis is most commonly caused by sexually transmitted *Neisseria gonorrhoeae* or *Chlamydia trachomatis* infection. In those younger than 14 years or older than 35 years, epididymo-orchitis is generally caused by infection with common urinary tract pathogens, such as *Escherichia coli* (Walker and Challacombe 2013).

The symptoms of orchitis are often difficult to differentiate from those of other acute testicular conditions such as testicular torsion, which is the most important differential diagnosis of acute testicular pain, especially in younger men (Arap et al. 2007). If there is any suspicion of testicular torsion, the patient should be referred to secondary care immediately as surgery is required within 4–6 h. Patients who are in severe pain or systemically unwell should be referred for analgesia, intravenous antibiotics, and hydration (Walker and Challacombe 2013).

Mumps-Related Orchitis

Mumps (epidemic parotiditis) is a highly contagious viral disease caused by a single-stranded RNA virus belonging to the genus Rubulavirus and the family Paramyxoviridae. This virus can spread from human to human by direct contact, airborne droplets, and from fomites contaminated saliva. The clinical presentations of mumps are headache, malaise and low-grade pyrexia, followed by unilateral or bilateral parotid swelling in 60–70% of infections, and in 95% of patients are symptomatic. In prepubertal males the most common symptoms are those associated with infectious parotitis. Since the implementation of widespread vaccinations, the presentation of orchitis related to mumps is seen in pubertal and postpubertal males (Philip et al. 2006; Singh et al. 2006). Orchitis is seen in 15–30% of men with mumps and presents as painful testicular enlargement.

Testicular damage is believed to be a result of parenchymal oedema, which leads to congestion of the seminiferous tubules and perivascular infiltration of lymphocytes. This subsequently results in testicular necrosis fibrosis and atrophy of the testes (Lane and Hines 2006). Additionally, mechanisms linking anti-mumps immune responses and alterations of spermatogenesis-associated antigens have been linked to azoospermia and oligospermia observed in males who have had mumps (Kanduc 2014). Due to the reduction in the uptake of measles–mumps–rubella (MMR) vaccine there has been a recent increase in mumps orchitis among pubertal and postpubertal males. Unvaccinated postpubertal males diagnosed with mumps virus frequently develop mumps orchitis. It is therefore important that diagnosis and treatment is prompt, and investigations of any effect on sperm quality are carried out (Davis et al. 2010).

Testicular Injury and Torsion

Due to their external position, the testes are predisposed to injury and trauma. Blunt trauma can lead to testicular atrophy. Testicular torsion results in interruption of testicular perfusion, leading to hypoxia and tissue death. Surgical correction within 6–8 h can preserve testicular viability. See Chapter 13 for more detail on testicular injury and torsion.

Other Scrotal/Testicular Conditions

Conditions such as varicocele, hydrocele, and carcinoma can have a negative impact on testicular function and sperm production. Chapter 13 covers these conditions in more detail.

Chemical and Radiation-Induced Hypogonadism

Testicular exposure to medications/recreational drugs and environmental chemicals that have gonadal toxicity can result in acquired hypogonadism, reducing testosterone production and spermatogenesis. Chapter 17 covers the impact of environmental chemicals, and medical and recreational drugs on testicular function and their impact on male reproduction.

The use of chemotherapeutic agents and radiotherapy in cancer treatment can affect testicular function by damaging germ cells, Sertoli cells, Leydig cells and/or testicular tissue. The resultant gonadal toxicity can be temporary, long term, or permanent depending on the agents and cumulative dosage used.

In treatment with chemotherapeutic agents that do not kill spermatogonial stem cells, there is usually a return of normal sperm count and potential fertility in many individuals within 12 weeks after the cessation of chemotherapy (Meistrich et al. 1997). Patients with testicular germ cell tumours treated with cycles of bleomycin, etoposide, and cisplatin (BEP) initially all develop azoospermia with recovery of spermatogenesis in 48% after 2 years and in 80% after 5 years (Lampe et al. 1997).

Alkylating agents such as mustine, vincristine procarbazine, and cyclofosfamide, used to treat lymphomas can cause permanent azoospermia in up to 90% of patients.

Chemotherapeutic treatment of Hodgkin lymphoma with a combination of nonalkylating agents such as adriamycin, bleomycin, vinblastine, and dacarbazine (ABVD) results in post-treatment recovery in sperm production in 90% of patients (Fossa and Magelssen 2004). However, treatment of non-Hodgkin lymphoma with cyclophosphamide, doxorubicin, vincristine, and prednisolone (CHOP) results in permanent azoospermia in 30% of patients (Howell and Shalet 2005).

Many combination anticancer regimens include treatment with radiation or chemotherapy drugs (e.g. alkylating agents) that kill spermatogonial stem cells, resulting in azoospermia that lasts much longer than the 12 weeks.

Radiation usually acts by killing cells by inducing apoptosis or by damaging the cell cycle machinery of dividing germ cells. The level and duration of the radiation exposure can impact on the degree of damage. Doses of between 0.35 and 0.5 Gy cause reversible azoospermia (Damewood and Grichow 1986). Radiation noticeably reduces the numbers of spermatocytes up to the leptotene stage at 2 weeks postexposure; a significant depletion of pachytene spermatocytes occurs by 25 days after radiation treatment, and a dramatic decline in ejaculated sperm counts occur at about 10 weeks after radiation. However, the reduction of type A spermatogonia to their lowest levels after single radiation doses between 0.2 and 4 Gy occur progressively over 21 weeks (Paulsen 1973; Rowley et al. 1974; Meistrich 2013).

Due to advancing medical and radiological treatments, cancer patients are experiencing improved outcomes and increased longevity and thus issues such as fertility are discussed, especially in younger patients. Patients with planned cancer treatment that involves chemotherapy and/or radiotherapy fertility preservation (via sperm cryopreservation) can typically be administered quickly and without disruption of the overall treatment plan (Trost and Brannigan 2012).

Secondary Hypogonadism

Congenital Hypogonadotropin Hypogonadism

Kallmann Syndrome

Kallmann syndrome was first identified as a clinical condition in 1944 by the American medical geneticist, F.J. Kallmann, who carried out a study on the occurrence of hypogonadism accompanied by anosmia (lack of smell) in the affected families (Kallmann et al. 1944). The prevalence of Kallmann syndrome is about 1 in 10 000 males and is four times higher than in females (Seminara et al. 1998).

Kallmann syndrome is characterized by a deficiency of hypothalamic GnRH or its function. As a result of GnRH deficiency, the secretion of gonadotropins from the pituitary is impaired, which leads to reduced or absent testosterone production and subsequent azoospermia. Kallmann syndrome may also be accompanied by other dysmorphogenetic symptoms including congenital deafness, harelip, cleft palate, craniofacial asymmetry, renal abnormalities, and red–green colour blindness.

The deficiency in GnRH secretion is due to the lack of GnRH neurons in the hypothalamus. During normal embryonic development, precursors of the

**Genes involved in GnRH neuron development
and migration**

KAL1, FGFR1, FGF8, PROKR2, PROK2, CHD7, NELF

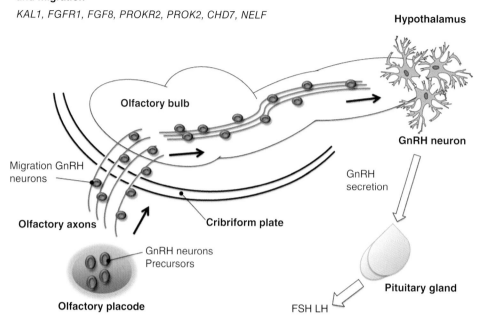

Figure 9.6 Migration of gonadotropin-releasing hormone (GnRH)-releasing neurons along the olfactory bulb towards the hypothalamus during early brain development, and associated genes with Kallmann syndrome. FSH, follicle-stimulating hormone; LH, luteinizing hormone.

GnRH neurons migrate from the nasal olfactory epithelium (olfactory placode) to the basal hypothalamus (Figure 9.6). This neuronal migration is regulated by a number of genes, which are disturbed in patients with Kallmann syndrome. *KAL1* is located on the X chromosome and is mutated or deleted in patients with positive family history and X chromosomal recessive mode of inheritance. The *KAL1* gene product, anosmin 1, is a protein of the extracellular matrix that is localized in the olfactory bulb and involved in the signal transduction of the fibroblast growth factor receptor 1 (FGFR1). Other genes responsible for Kallmann syndrome include prokineticin 2 (*PROK2*) and its receptor (PROK2R) and the *CHD7* gene. Mutations of the *CHD7* gene are usually found in CHARGE syndrome (and acronym for coloboma, heart anomalies, choanal atresia, retardation of growth and/or development, genital and ear anomalies). CHARGE is a multisystem autosomal dominant disorder that includes symptoms such as anosmia and hypogonadism.

CHARGE syndrome has an estimated birth incidence of 1 in 8500–12 000 (Dodé and Hardelin 2009).

Diagnosis and Treatment

Most cases of Kallmann syndrome are diagnosed at the time of puberty due to the lack of sexual development, identified by small testes and absent virilization in males. Diagnosis of Kallmann syndrome is confirmed when low serum gonadotropins and testosterone are coupled with anosmia or hyposmia, and magnetic resonance imaging (MRI) of the forebrain to show the hypoplasia or aplasia of the olfactory bulbs and tracts.

The treatment of hypogonadism in Kallmann syndrome aims to initiate virilization and to develop fertility. Hormone replacement therapy with testosterone is the treatment to stimulate the development of secondary sexual characteristics. To restore fertility, either gonadotropins or pulsatile GnRH can be used to obtain testicular growth and sperm production. Both treatments restore fertility in a vast majority of affected individuals (Buchter et al. 1998; Delemarre-van de Waal 2004).

Prader–Willi Syndrome

Prader–Willi syndrome is a complex syndrome caused by deletions of a gene cluster in the region 15q11–q13 located on the long arm of chromosome 15. It is characterized by severe hypotonia (low muscle tone) and feeding difficulties in infancy. In early childhood, excessive eating can result in the gradual development of morbid obesity. Language development and motor control are delayed and all individuals display some degree of cognitive impairment and behavioural problems. Short stature is common, and characteristic facial features, strabismus, and scoliosis are often present (Butler 2011).

Hypogonadism is present in both males and females and manifests as genital hypoplasia, incomplete or delayed pubertal development, and infertility. Male children typically have a micropenis and uni- or bilateral cryptorchidism. Children with Prader–Willi syndrome display a particular form of combined hypothalamic (low LH) and peripheral (low inhibin B and high FSH) hypogonadism, which indicates a primary defect in Sertoli and/or germ cell maturation or an early germ cell loss (Eiholzer et al. 2006). Furthermore, testicular biopsies show atrophy of the seminiferous tubules and absent spermatogonia. It is therefore likely that all men with Prader–Willi syndrome are infertile (Vogels et al. 2008).

In addition to assessment of physical traits, clinical diagnostic criteria are confirmed by DNA methylation testing to detect abnormal parent-specific imprinting within the Prader–Willi critical region on chromosome 15 (Sanjeeva et al. 2017).

Testosterone or gonadotropin treatment can improve virilization, and growth hormone has shown to be efficacious for improving stature. However, individuals remain infertile.

Hereditary Haemochromatosis

Hereditary haemochromatosis is a common autosomal recessive disorder (one in 200 in white people of northern European descent) and is characterized by abnormally high gastrointestinal iron absorption, resulting in an increased saturation coefficient of transferrin (≥45%), increased concentration of serum ferritin (≥300 μg/L in a human), and parenchymal iron deposition caused by low levels of hepcidin (Janssen and Swinkels 2009). This excessive iron storage causes damage in a number of tissues, in particular the liver, pancreas, heart, joints, skin, gonads, and pituitary gland. Furthermore, iron overload causes endocrine dysfunction, particularly on the pituitary axis, with a potential impact on fertility (Pelusi et al. 2016).

After diabetes, secondary hypogonadism is the most common endocrinopathy associated with hereditary haemochromatosis, which results in androgen deficiency and impairment in sperm production. This is due to iron overload in the pituitary gland and the resultant gonadotropin deficiency. Serum testosterone levels, sperm counts, and LH and FSH levels are low. Iron overload also occurs in the testes and may cause a reduction in testosterone response to gonadotropin stimulation, resulting in combined primary and secondary hypogonadism. However, in most cases, gonadotropin treatment is able to stimulate normal testicular function, including spermatogenesis and fertility (El Osta et al. 2017). Hypogonadism may be reversed with therapeutic phlebotomy, usually early in the course of iron overload (Lufkin et al. 1987).

Acquired Secondary Hypogonadism

Acquired secondary hypogonadism can occur from any disturbance of the hypothalamic–pituitary–gonadal (HPG) axis. A dysfunctional HPG axis can be brought about in men developing hyperprolactinaemia, pituitary damage from tumours, infection (tuberculosis) or infiltrative disease (haemochromatosis, sarcoidosis, or histiocytosis), head trauma (causing stalk injury), or acute systemic illness. Additionally, lifestyle and environmental exposures can affect the HPG axis. These include the use of medications or recreational drugs (cannabinoids, opioids, glucocorticoids, GnRH agonists or antagonists), obesity or diabetes, eating disorders, and excessive exercise. The likely cause of testicular dysfunction in these cases is a dysfunction of hypothalamic GnRH secretion.

Hyperprolactinaemia

Prolactin, produced by the pituitary, is a hormone with roles in reproduction, lactation, and metabolism. Its major role is in stimulating the breast to initiate and maintain lactation. Prolactin secretion from pituitary lactotrophs is predominantly under the negative control of dopamine from the hypothalamic neurons. There are also several prolactin secretion factors that stimulate prolactin release such as as thyrotropin and vasoactive intestinal peptide. The prolactin receptor is expressed mainly in cells of the anterior pituitary, but is also expressed in many other tissues (endometrium, myometrium, brain, mammary gland, lymphocytes, spleen, thymus, prostate, and testis). The role of prolactin on reproduction in men is mostly unknown. However, excess prolactin secretion – hyperprolactinaemia – can induce hypogonadism in men.

Hyperprolactinaemia can impair male infertility on multiple pathways. The clinical manifestations are infertility, hypogonadism, impotence, and galactorrhea. The cause of hyperprolactinaemia in men is multifactorial and can include pituitary adenomas, acromegaly, hypothalamic dysfunction, drug use (cocaine, tricyclic antidepressants, monoamine oxidase inhibitors), liver cirrhosis, renal disease, and stress (Rastrelli et al. 2015).

Prolactin has inhibitory actions of LH on Leydig cells (Odell and Larsen 1984) and the prolactin receptor is found on the seminiferous epithelium, and spermatogenic cells, indicating a direct effect on sperm production (Hondo et al. 1995). Male patients with increased prolactin levels can demonstrate low serum testosterone levels. The diagnosis of hyperprolactinemia should be kept in mind when evaluating subfertile males who demonstrate decreased androgen levels or symptoms associated with pituitary mass. Men with serum prolactin levels greater than $200\,\mu g/L$ is often associated with the presence of an adenoma. It is therefore essential that men presenting with hyperprolactinaemia should be evaluated by MRI to determine the size of the tumour if present.

The goals of treatment are to normalize prolactin levels, restore gonadal function, and reduce the effects of chronic hyperprolactinaemia. Dopamine agonists are the treatment of choice for the majority of patients. Transsphenoidal surgery is reserved for patients who are intolerant of or resistant to dopamine agonists or when hyperprolactinaemia is caused by nonprolactin-secreting tumours compressing the pituitary stalk. The use of cabergoline has shown to be effective in the treatment of hyperprolactinaemia, both reducing tumour size and prolactin levels. In cases of hyperprolactinaemia caused by stress or liver/renal disease, appropriate treatment of the primary cause is required (Verhelst and Abs 2003; Gillam et al. 2006).

Lifestyle and Environmentally Induced Secondary Hypogonadism

Marijuana, cocaine, methamphetamines, opioid narcotics, and anabolic steroids all negatively impact male fertility, and adverse effects have been reported on the hypothalamic–pituitary–testicular axis, sperm function, and testicular structure (Fronczak et al. 2012).

Several *in vivo* and *in vitro* studies have reported the role that marijuana plays in disrupting the HPG axis, spermatogenesis, and sperm function such as motility, capacitation, and the acrosome reaction (Gundersen et al. 2015). When consumed (smoked/ingested), marijuana releases the psychoactive cannabinoid compound called Δ^9-tetrahydrocannabinol (THC), which acts on the cannabinoid receptors, CB1 and CB2. These cannabinoid receptors are present in testicular tissue, including Sertoli and Leydig cells as well as spermatozoa. They are also localized in areas of the hypothalamus responsible for the production of GnRH and can thus exert a role via the HPG axis. THC may negatively affect male reproductive physiology through disruption of the HPG axis, with marijuana users having decreased levels of LH (Vescovi et al. 1992). An early study of chronic marijuana smokers showed users to have significantly lower plasma testosterone compared with age-matched controls who had never used marijuana (Kolodny et al. 1974). However, in a recent population-based study reported, there was no difference in serum testosterone levels among ever users of marijuana compared to never users (Thistle et al. 2017).

In humans, CB1 and CB2 are present on sperm cells and incubation with selective cannabinoid receptor agonists induce a significant reduction in the proportion of rapidly progressive motile spermatozoa, and whereas the CB1 agonist increases the proportion of immobile sperm cells, the CB2 receptor agonist increases the slow/sluggish progressive sperm cell population (Agirregoitia et al. 2010).

Other recreational or illicit drugs such as cocaine, methamphetamines, and opioid narcotics all negatively impact male fertility, and adverse effects have been reported on the HPG axis, testicular function, and sperm function. It is imperative therefore that after ceasing the usage of such drugs, close monitoring of serum testosterone and semen analysis is carried out (Fronczak et al. 2012).

Anabolic-androgenic steroids (AAS) are frequently used in competitive bodybuilding and other sports as an enhancer for muscle building and performance. Supraphysiologic levels of exogenous AAS exert negative feedback on the HPG axis and subsequently reduce FSH, LH, and testosterone concentration. These hormonal changes can lead to azoospermia, oligospermia, testicular atrophy, hypogonadotropic hypogonadism, and an increased percentage of morphologically abnormal sperm with amorphous spermatozoa and defects in the head and center pieces (Bonetti et al. 2008).

Cessation of AAS use may result in spontaneous recovery of normal spermatogenesis if sufficient time is allowed for recovery (McBride and Coward 2016). However, some patients may not recover normal spermatogenesis and exposure time, ethnicity, and age may result in a prolonged recovery time after treatment cessation (Ly et al. 2005). In such cases the available agents to recover HCG activity and spermatogenesis include injectable gonadotropins, selective estrogen receptor modulators, and aromatase inhibitors (Rahnema et al. 2014).

Other lifestyle and environmental influences on male reproductive endocrinology include diet, obesity, diabetes type-2, and exposure to endocrine-disrupting chemicals (EDCs). EDCs are exogenous compounds that can cause disturbances in the HCG axis. Mass industrial production and widespread use of EDCs have resulted in global contamination. Accumulating evidence suggest that human exposure to EDCs is related to the impairment of male reproductive function (Sidorkiewicz et al. 2017) (see Chapter 17 for more details).

Conclusion

Male hypogonadism has a multifactorial aetiology from genetics to acquired hypogonadism. Over the past two decades advances in diagnosis and treatment has improved gonadotropin and testosterone levels, and increased sperm numbers. Moreover, advances in assisted reproductive technology, including surgical sperm retrieval and sperm cryopreservation, has bequeathed biological fatherhood to many men. The use of testosterone replacement therapy has brought great benefit in many cases of hypogonadism. However, patients should be monitored for side effects such as polycythemia, peripheral edema, cardiac, and hepatic dysfunction.

References

Agirregoitia, E., Carracedo, A., Subiran, N. et al. (2010). The CB(2) cannabinoid receptor regulates human sperm cell motility. Fertil Steril 93: 1378–1387.

Arap, M.A., Vicentini, F.C., Cocuzza, M. et al. (2007). Late hormonal levels, semen parameters, and presence of antisperm antibodies in patients treated for testicular torsion. J Androl 28: 528–532.

Bakircioglu, M.E., Ulug, U., Erden, H.F. et al. (2011). Klinefelter syndrome: does it confer a bad prognosis in treatment of nonobstructive azoospermia? Fertil Steril 95: 1696–1699

Barratt, C.L.R., Björndahl, L., De Jonge, C.J. et al. (2017). The diagnosis of male infertility: an analysis of the evidence to support the development of global WHO guidance – challenges and future research opportunities. Hum Reprod Update, pp. 1–21.

Bonetti, A., Tirelli, F., Catapano, A. et al. (2008). Side effects of anabolic androgenic steroids abuse. Int J Sports Med 29: 679–687.

Buchter, D., Behre, H.M., Kliesch, S. et al. (1998). Pulsatile GnRH or human chorionic gonadotropin/human menopausal gonadotropin as effective treatment for men with hypogonadotropic hypogonadism: a review of 42 cases. Eur J Endocrinol 139: 298–303.

Butler, M.G. (2011). Prader-Willi Syndrome: obesity due to genomic imprinting. Curr Genomics 12: 204–215.

Chandley, A.C. (1998). Chromosome anomalies and Y chromosome microdeletions as causal factors in male infertility. Hum Reprod 13: 45–50.

Damewood, M.D. and Grochow, L.B. (1986) Prospects for fertility after chemotherapy or radiation for neoplastic disease. Fertil Steril 1986 45: 443–459.

Davis, N.F, McGuire, B.B., Mahon, J.A. et al. (2010). The increasing incidence of mumps orchitis: a comprehensive review. BJU Int 105: 1060–1065

Delemarre-van de Waal, H.A. (2004). Application of gonadotropin releasing hormone in hypogonadotropic hypogonadism – diagnostic and therapeutic aspects. Eur J Endocrinol 151(Suppl 3): U89–94.

Dodé, C. and Hardelin, J.P. (2009). Kallmann syndrome. Eur J Hum Genet 17: 139–146.

Eiholzer, U., l'Allemand, D., Rousson, V. et al. (2006). Hypothalamic and gonadal components of hypogonadism in boys with Prader-Labhart-Willi syndrome. J Clin Endocrinol Metab 91: 892–898.

El Osta, R., Grandpre, N., Monnin, N. et al. (2017). Hypogonadotropic hypogonadism in men with hereditary hemochromatosis. Basic Clin Androl 827: 13.

Elsawi, M.M., Pryor, J.P., Klufio, G. et al. (1994). Genital tract function in men with Noonan syndrome. J Med Genet 31: 468–470.

Foresta, C., Moro, E., Garolla, A. et al. (1999). Y chromosome microdeletions in cryptorchidism and idiopathic infertility. J Clin Endocrinol Metab 84: 3660–3665.

Fossa, S.D. and Magelssen, H. (2004). Fertility and reproduction after chemotherapy of adult cancer patients: malignant lymphoma and testicular cancer. Ann Oncol 15 (Suppl. 4):iv259–iv265.

Fronczak, C.M., Kim, E.D. and Barqawi, A.B. (2012). The insults of illicit drug use on male fertility. J Androl 33: 515–528.

Gillam, M.P., Molitch, M.E., Lombardi, G. et al. (2006). Advances in the treatment of prolactinomas. Endocr Rev 27: 485–534.

Greco, E., Scarselli, F., Minasi, M.G. et al. (2013). Birth of 16 healthy children after ICSI in cases of nonmosaic Klinefelter syndrome Hum Reprod 28: 1155–1160.

Gundersen, T.D., Jørgensen, N., Andersson, A.M. et al. (2015) Association between use of marijuana and male reproductive hormones and semen quality: a study among 1,215 healthy young men. Am J Epidemiol 182: 473–481.

Hirota, T., Ohta, H., Powell B.E. et al. (2017). Fertile offspring from sterile sex chromosome trisomic mice. Science 357(6354): 932–935.

Hondo, E., Kurohmaru, M., Sakai, S. et al. (1995). Prolactin receptor expression in rat spermatogenic cells. Biol Reprod 52: 1284–1290.

Hopps, C.V., Mielnik, A., Goldstein, M. et al. (2003). Detection of sperm in men with Y chromosome microdeletions of the AZFa, AZFb and AZFc regions. Hum Reprod 18: 1660–1665.

Howell, S.J. and Shalet, S.M. (2005). Spermatogenesis after cancer treatment: damage and recovery. J Natl Cancer Inst Monogr 34: 12–17.

Janssen, M.C.H. and Swinkels, D.W. (2009). Hereditary haemochromatosis. Best Pract Res Clin Gastroenterol 23: 171–183.

Kallmann, F.J., Schoenfeld, W.A. and Barrera, S.E. (1944). The genetic aspects of primary eunuchoidism. Am J Mental Deficiency XLVIII: 203–236.

Kanduc, D. (2014). Describing the potential crossreactome between mumps virus and spermatogenesis-associated proteins. Endocr Metab Immune Disord Drug Targets 14: 218–225.

Kaver, I., Matzkin, H. and Braf, Z.F. (1990). Epididymo-orchitis: a retrospective study of 121 patients. J Fam Pract 30: 548–552.

Kent-First, M., Muallem, A., Shultz, J. et al. (1999). Defining regions of the Y-chromosome responsible for male infertility and identification of a fourth AZF region (AZFd) by Y-chromosome microdeletion detection. Mol Reprod Dev 53: 27–41.

Klinefelter, H.F., Reifenstein, E.C. and Albright, F. (1942). Syndrome characterized by gynecomastia, aspermatogenesis without A-Leydigism, and increased excretion of follicle-stimulating hormone. J Clin Endocrinol II: 615–627.

Kolodny, R.C., Masters, W.H., Kolodner, R.M. et al. (1974) Depression of plasma testosterone levels after chronic intensive marihuana use. N Engl J Med 290: 872–874.

Komori, S., Kato, H., Kobayashi, S. et al. (2002). Transmission of Y chromosomal microdeletions from father to son through intracytoplasmic sperm injection. J Hum Genet 47: 465–468.

Krausz, C. and Casamonti, E. (2017). Spermatogenic failure and the Y chromosome Hum Genet 136: 637–655.

Lampe, H., Horwich, A., Norman, A. et al. (1997). Fertility after chemotherapy for testicular germ cell cancers. J Clin Oncol 15: 239–245.

Lane, T.M. and Hines, J. (2006). The management of mumps orchitis. BJU Int 97: 1–2

Lanfranco, F., Kamischke, A., Zitzmann, M. et al. Klinefelter's syndrome. Lancet 2004 364: 273–283.

Li, Z., Haines, C.J. and Han, Y. (2008). 'Micro-deletions' of the human Y chromosome and their relationship with male infertility. J Genet Genomics 35: 193–199.

Lufkin, E.G., Baldus, W.P., Bergstralh, E.J. et al. (1987). Influence of phlebotomy treatment on abnormal hypothalamic-pituitary function in genetic hemochromatosis. Mayo Clin Proc 62: 473–479.

Ly, L.P., Liu, P.Y. and Handelsman, D.J. (2005). Rates of suppression and recovery of human sperm output in testosterone-based hormonal contraceptive regimens. Hum Reprod 20: 1733–1740.

Marcus, K.A., Sweep, C.G., van der Burgt, I. et al. (2008). Impaired Sertoli cell function in males diagnosed with Noonan syndrome. J Pediatr Endocrinol Metab 21: 1079–1084.

McBride, A.J. and Coward, R.M. (2016). Recovery of spermatogenesis following testosterone replacement therapy or anabolic-androgenic steroid use. Asian J Androl 18: 373–380.

Meistrich, M.L. (2013). Effects of chemotherapy and radiotherapy on spermatogenesis in humans. Fertil Steril 100: 1180–1186.

Meistrich, M.L., Wilson, G., Mathur, K. et al. (1997). Rapid recovery of spermatogenesis after mitoxantrone, vincristine, vinblastine, and prednisone chemotherapy for Hodgkin's disease. J Clin Oncol 15: 3488–3495.

Müslümanoglu, M.H., Turgut, M., Cilingir, O. et al. (2005). Role of the AZFd locus in spermatogenesis. Fertil Steril 84: 519–522.

Najmabadi, H., Huang, V., Yen, P. et al. (1996). Substantial prevalence of microdeletions of the Y-chromosome in infertile men with idiopathic azoospermia and oligozoospermia detected using a sequence-tagged site-based mapping strategy. J Clin Endocrinol Metab 81: 1347–1352.

Nakashima, M., Koh, E., Namiki, M. et al. (2002). Multiplex sequence-tagged site PCR for efficient screening of microdeletions in Y chromosome in infertile males with azoospermia or severe oligozoospermia. Arch Androl 48: 351–358.

Nieschlag, E. (2013). Klinefelter syndrome: the commonest form of hypogonadism, but often overlooked or untreated Dtsch Arztebl Int 110: 347–353.

Odell, W.D. and Larsen, J.L. (1984). In vitro studies of prolactin inhibition of luteinizing hormone action on Leydig cells of rats and mice. Proc Soc Exp Biol Med 177: 459–464

Osegbe, D.N. (1991). Testicular function after unilateral bacterial epididymo-orchitis. Eur Urol 19: 204–208.

Paulsen, C.A. U.S. Department of Energy (1973). The study of radiation effects on the human testis: including histologic, chromosomal and hormonal aspects. Final progress report of AEC contract AT(45–1)-2225, Task Agreement 6. RLO-2225-2. p. 1–36.

Pelusi, C., Gasparini, D.I., Bianchi, N. et al. (2016). Endocrine dysfunction in hereditary hemochromatosis. J Endocrinol Invest 39: 837–847.

Philip, J., Selvan, D. and Desmond, A.D. (2006). Mumps orchitis in the non-immune postpubertal male: a resurgent threat to male fertility? BJU Int 97: 138–141

Rahnema, C.D., Lipshultz, L.I., Crosnoe, L.E. et al. (2014). Anabolic steroid-induced hypogonadism: diagnosis and treatment. Fertil Steril 101: 1271–1279.

Rastrelli, G., Corona, G. and Maggi, M. (2015). The role of prolactin in andrology: what is new? Rev Endocr Metab Disord 16: 233–248.

Rowley, M.J., Leach, D.R., Warner, G.A. et al. (1974). Effect of graded doses of ionizing radiation on the uman testis. Radiat Res 59: 665–678.

Sanjeeva, G.N., Maganthi, M., Kodishala, H. et al. (2017). Clinical and molecular characterization of Prader-Willi Syndrome. Indian J Pediatr 84: 815–821.

Schuppe, H.C., Pilatz, A., Hossain, H. et al. (2010). Orchitis and male infertility. Urologe A 49: 629–635.

Seminara, S.B., Hayes, F.J. and Crowley, W.F. (1998). Gonadotropin-releasing hormone deficiency in the human (idiopathic hypogonadotropic hypogonadism and Kallmann's syndrome): pathophysiological and genetic considerations. Endocr Rev 19: 521–539.

Sidorkiewicz, I., Zaręba, K., Wołczyński, S. et al. (2017). Endocrine-disrupting chemicals-Mechanisms of action on male reproductive system. Toxicol Ind Health 33: 601–609.

Singh, R., Mostafid, H, Hindley RG. (2006). Measles, mumps and rubella—the urologist's perspective. Int J Clin Pract 60: 335–339

Tafazoli, A., Eshraghi, P., Koleti, Z.K. et al. (2017). Noonan syndrome – a new survey. Arch Med Sci 113: 215–222.

Tartaglia, M., Mehler, E.L., Goldberg, R. et al. (2001). Mutations in PTPN11, encoding the protein tyrosine phosphatase SHP-2, cause Noonan syndrome. Nat Genet 29: 465–468.

Thistle, J.E., Graubard, B.I., Braunlin, M. et al. (2017). Marijuana use and serum testosterone concentrations among U.S. males. Andrology 5: 732–738.

Trojian, T.H., Lishnak, T.S. and Heiman, D. (2009). Epididymitis and orchitis: an overview. Am Fam Physician 79: 583–587.

Trost, L.W. and Brannigan, R.E. (2012). Oncofertility and the male cancer patient. Curr Treat Options Oncol 13: 146–160.

Tüttelmann, F., Gromoll, J. (2010). Novel genetic aspects of Klinefelter's syndrome. Mol Hum Reprod 16: 386–395.

Verhelst, J. and Abs, R. (2003). Hyperprolactinemia: pathophysiology and management. Treat Endocrinol 2: 23–32.

Vescovi, P.P., Pedrazzoni, M., Michelini, M. et al. (1992). Chronic effects of marihuana smoking on luteinizing hormone, follicle-stimulating hormone and prolactin levels in human males. Drug Alcohol Depend 30: 59–63.

Vignozzi, L., Corona, G., Forti, G. et al. (2010). Clinical and therapeutic aspects of Klinefelter's syndrome: sexual function. Mol Hum Reprod 16: 418–424.

Vogels, A., Moerman, P., Frijns, J.P. et al. (2008). Testicular histology in boys with Prader-Willi syndrome: fertile or infertile? J Urol 180(4 Suppl): 1800–1804.

Walker, N.A. and Challacombe, B. (2013). Managing epididymo-orchitis in general practice. Practitioner 257: 21–25, 2–3.

10

Disorders of Female Reproductive Endocrinology

Mahshid Nickkho-Amiry and Cheryl T. Fitzgerald

Introduction

Infertility may originate from hormonal causes leading to anovulation or to more subtle cycle disturbances that reflect a poor ovarian reserve, compromised oocyte quality, or poor endometrial response. Treating women with disorders of reproductive endocrinology first requires elucidating its underlying cause, assessing menstrual pattern and ovarian reserve, and performing a physical examination to look for signs of specific hormonal disturbances.

The World Health Organization (WHO) categorized women with anovulatory disorders in three major groups according to the causative factors of the disorders. Hyperprolactinaemia is considered as a separate group (WHO Report 1976). Group I includes women with hypogonadotropic hypogonadal anovulation disorders. In 5–10% of women with anovulation, this is attributed to low gonadotropin and oestradiol levels secondary to reduced pulsatile hypothalamic secretions of gonadotropin-releasing hormone (GnRH). Group II, the largest, includes women with normo-gonadotropic normo-oestrogenemic anovulation disorders. In 75–85% of anovulatory women, follicle-stimulating hormone (FSH) and oestradiol levels are normal whereas luteinizing hormone (LH) levels may be elevated. The most common disorder in this group is polycystic ovary syndrome (PCOS).

Group III includes women with hypergonadotropic anovulation disorders. In 10–20% of women with anovulation, FSH levels are elevated and the functional ovarian reserve is diminished. The most severe disorder in this group is premature ovarian failure (POF), which is associated with a serum FSH concentration higher than 40 IU/L and at least 4 months of amenorrhoea before the age of 40 years (Bukman and Heineman 2001).

Hyperprolactinaemic anovulation occurs in 5–10% women with elevated levels of prolactin. Hyperprolactinaemia may be associated with pituitary dysfunction, pituitary adenoma, dopamine insufficiency, or primary hypothyroidism, or it may be the result of taking certain medications (Yazigi et al. 1997). Pituitary imaging is necessary when secondary causes for hyperprolactinaemia have been excluded. Dopaminergic drugs often restore normal ovulatory cycles and fertility (Turkalj et al. 1982).

In this chapter, the impact of different endocrine disorders on the reproductive female function, potentially leading to female infertility, will be discussed (for an overview on female reproductive endocrine function – see Chapters 3 and 4).

Causes of Hormonal Infertility

Hypogonadotropic Hypogonadal Anovulation

Group I is the smallest and often the most challenging of the WHO groups to treat. Hypothalamic amenorrhoea results from a change in the normal pattern of episodic secretion by the GnRH pulse generator with failure of ovulation and amenorrhoea. The causes are functional hypothalamic amenorrhoea (triggered by excessive exercise, nutritional deficits, or psychological distress), physiological

Clinical Reproductive Science, First Edition. Edited by Michael Carroll.
© 2019 John Wiley & Sons Ltd. Published 2019 by John Wiley & Sons Ltd.
Companion website: www.wiley.com/go/carroll/clinicalreproductivescience

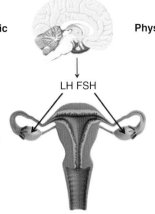

Functional hypothalamic amenorrhoea

Nutritional deficits
Psychological distress
Excessive exercise

LH FSH

Psychiatric disorders
Anorexia
Bulimia

Physiological hypothalamic amenorrhoea

Postpartum
Breast feeding

Figure 10.1 Causes of hypogonadotropic hypogonadal anovulation. FSH, follicle-stimulating hormone; LH, luteinzing hormone. *Source:* https://pixabay.com/en/brain-anatomy-neurology-medical-1132229/. CC0 1.0.

hypothalamic amenorrhoea (postpartum and breast feeding), pharmacological anovulation (opiates) and amenorrhoea associated with psychiatric disorders, such as anorexia–bulimia. Hypothalamic amenorrhoea may also result from organic defects of the hypothalamic–pituitary axis, including congenital GnRH deficiency (idiopathic hypogonadotropic hypogonadism).

Functional hypothalamic amenorrhoea is the absence of menstrual cycles for more than 6 months without evidence of anatomical or organic abnormalities, and thus is a diagnosis of exclusion. Three main types of functional hypothalamic amenorrhoea have been recognized, associated with stress, weight loss, or exercise. Being underweight is not a prerequisite for this diagnosis. Reduced calorific intake appears to be the critical factor in both weight loss and exercise-induced forms of hypothalamic amenorrhoea. Careful history taking will elucidate these factors. Leptin appears to play a critical role in the regulation of hypothalamic dysfunction, and leptin administration has been shown to induce GnRH pulsatility and menstruation. Rare variants in genes associated with idiopathic hypogonadotropic hypogonadism have been identified in women with hypothalamic amenorrhoea. Weight gain, exercise reduction, and appropriate psychological counselling are usually effective in relieving the symptoms of amenorrhoea in young patients (Caronia et al. 2011).

Hypothalamic lesions, although rare, such as infiltrative diseases or tumors, can result in decreased GnRH secretion and amenorrhoea. Idiopathic hypogonadotropic hypogonadism usually can be distinguished from functional amenorrhoea since it presents with primary amenorrhoea and associated symptoms, including anosmia (Figure 10.1).

Normogonadotropic Anovulation

The largest WHO group of women with anovulation, Group II, includes women with normal gonadotropins and oestrogen levels. PCOS is the most frequent endocrine disorder in women of reproductive age. Being a heterogeneous condition, diagnostic criteria may vary but currently the 'Rotterdam criteria' are the most popular for defining this disorder (Rotterdam ESHRE/ASRM 2004). PCOS is diagnosed when at least two of the following three clinical findings are present: oligo- or anovulation, clinical or biochemical signs of hyperandrogenism, and polycystic ovaries on ultrasound or direct inspection (Figure 10.2). The ultrasound criteria to define polycystic ovaries are the presence of 12 or more subcapsular ovarian cysts with a diameter of less than 10 mm or an increase in ovarian volume of more than 10 mL (Balen et al. 2003). Using the newer 'Rotterdam criteria', the prevalence of PCOS may be as high as 18% in a community-based population (March et al. 2010). In women with oligomenorrhoea or hirsutism, the reported prevalence was respectively 85–90% and 70% (Sirmans and Pate 2014).

The aetiology of PCOS has been attributed to three major mechanisms:

1) PCOS has a strong familial occurrence, therefore hereditary factors are very likely.
2) There are indications that an ovarian dysfunction at the level of steroidogenesis may be present because of deficiencies in the cytochrome P450 pathway.

(a)

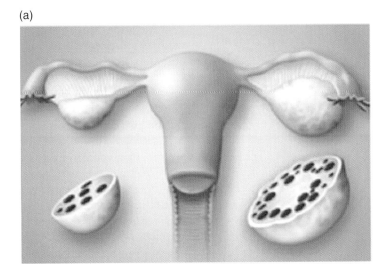

(b) (c)

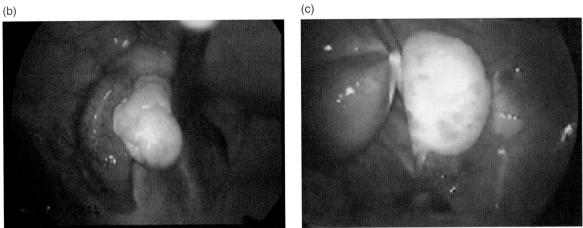

Figure 10.2 (a) Schematic depiction of PCOS. (b) Laparascopic view of a normal ovary. (c) Laparascopic view of a polycystic ovary. Reproduced with permission of Dr Saad Amer (http://www.saadamer.com).

3) Hyperinsulinaemia may interfere with follicular maturation preventing selection of a dominant follicle (Carmina 2013). A decrease in insulin-mediated glucose utilization or 'insulin resistance' is indeed a common finding in women with PCOS and they have a two- to fourfold higher risk for developing diabetes even after adjusting for BMI.

Although women with hirsutism and/or hyperandrogenaemia, and polycystic ovaries on ultrasound, i.e. PCOS according to the 'Rotterdam criteria', can have regular menstrual cycles (Carmina and Lobo 2001) and 60% of PCOS women are reported to be fertile (Brassard et al. 2008), the condition is associated with a higher risk of reproductive failure. This is not only because of oligo- or anovulation but also because they have an increased risk for preterm labour, pre-eclampsia, and gestational diabetes (Legro 2007). The first-line treatment for infertility because of PCOS should focus on weight reduction since 90% of infertile women with PCOS are overweight and obesity independently contributes to infertility. Exercise and diet programmes conceived for PCOS women are highly cost-efficient in overcoming infertility because a weight loss of 5–10% may restore a regular menstrual pattern (Clark et al. 1998).

Hypergonadotropic Anovulation

Included in WHO Group III are young women with hypergonadotropic hypo-oestrogenaemia who were also diagnosed as having POF or, in milder cases, a diminished ovarian reserve. Although ovarian reserve markers are mostly used to assess the prognosis of treatments assisted by reproductive technology, they may also be predictive of the duration of a woman's reproductive life. The combination of low antral follicle count and low serum levels of anti-müllerian hormone, even in relatively young women, is associated not only with a severe decline in ovarian follicle pool and fertility potential, but also with approaching menopause (Hansen et al. 2011).

The strictest definition of POF, a condition affecting approximately 1% of all women, is a secondary amenorrhoea of at least 4 months, along with FSH levels consistently higher than 40 IU/L and decreased E2 concentrations before the age of 40 years (Coulam et al. 1986).

POF may develop from various causes, including gonadotoxic chemotherapeutic agents and radiation as well as extensive abdominal surgery and partial oophorectomy (DeVos et al. 2010). Autoimmunity, in particular against the thyroid, has also been associated with POF, but the mechanisms need further evaluation (Hoek et al. 1997). A high proportion of POF cases derive from numerical or structural chromosomal abnormalities (Mattei et al. 1982). However, for most women with POF no cause can be found.

Regardless of the cause of POF, in all cases they lead to early depletion of functional ovarian follicles (Rebar and Connolly 1990). As a result the menstrual cycle is lost, whether abruptly or gradually, with increasing intervals between menstrual periods. Menopausal symptoms such as hot flushes and night sweats may occur. Although ovarian function may resume temporarily or intermittently, the overall lifetime chance of spontaneous conception remains extremely low at less than 10% (Rebar and Connolly 1990).

Hyperprolactinaemia

Prolactinomas are the most common pituitary tumors. Hyperprolactinaemia, as a result of prolactin-secreting adenoma, is a frequent cause of pathological hyperprolactinaemia. However, serum concentrations of prolactin increase physiologically in pregnancy, during lactation and stress situations. Other pathological situations include pituitary stalk compression, drugs such as dopamine antagonists, hypothyroidism, or renal disorders (Melmed et al. 2011).

Women usually present with menstrual abnormalities, galactorrhoea, and infertility. In addition, women may complain of a decrease in libido and dyspareunia due to oestrogen deficiency. Ovulation can be restored in these women when pulsatile GnRH is given. This confirms the presence of abnormalities in GnRH secretion in these patients (Bergh et al. 1985).

Evaluation of patients includes a full history and a thorough examination. The most useful single investigation is the measurement of serum prolactin in a basal state on two or three independent visits. Repeated measurement obviously is not necessary if the first value is reported to be extremely high (>1000 ng/mL). Endocrine testing of gonadotropin reserve is performed only if indicated. Magnetic resonance imaging is necessary to exclude pituitary adenomas.

Thyroid Disease

Thyroid hormones play an important role in normal reproductive function, directly for their effects on the ovaries and indirectly by interacting with sex hormone binding proteins. Thyroid dysfunction can lead to menstrual irregularities and infertility but it is usually treatable.

The prevalence of hypothyroidism among women between the ages of 20 and 40 years varies between 2 and 4% (Verma and Kaur 2012). In this age group, autoimmune thyroid disease is the most common cause of hypothyroidism. Primary hypothyroidism is commonly associated with ovulatory dysfunction due to the numerous interactions of thyroid hormones with the female reproductive system. Hypothyroidism should be suspected in women with a history of fatigability, lack of energy, weight gain, constipation, intolerance to the cold, and irregular menstrual cycles. Some women may be totally asymptomatic except for anovulation, infertility, or repeated spontaneous abortions. Measuring serum levels of thyroid-stimulating hormone (TSH) and thyroxine (T4) has proven useful in the evaluation and detection of hypothyroidism (Gerhard et al. 1991). Normal TSH levels exclude hypothyroidism and hyperthyroidism. High TSH levels, on the other hand, require measuring free T4 levels; if low, a diagnosis of hypothyroidism will be made.

Hyperthyroidism is five to 10 times more common in women than in men. Its predominant primary cause in premenopausal women is Graves' disease, manifested by the presence of toxic diffuse goiter (Lazarus 1997). Besides the usual symptoms of hyperthyroidism, Graves' disease is often associated with ophthalmopathy and pretibial oedema. It is caused by autoantibodies with TSH properties, which thus activate TSH receptors and stimulate the thyroid gland to secrete large amounts of thyroid hormones. The elevated levels of antibodies to TSH receptors distinguish Graves' disease from other toxic goiters. In women with hyperthyroidism, menstrual activity ranges from normal regular cycles to oligomenorrhoea and amenorrhoea. The classic symptoms of hyperthyroidism are weight loss, restlessness, disturbed sleep, heat intolerance, sweating, palpitations, and diarrhoea.

Thyrotoxicosis results in increased serum levels of the serum sex hormone binding globulins (SHBG) and oestradiol (E2) levels compared with those in euthyroid women. The increase in E2 levels may be due to the increased SHBG levels or to an increased production of E2. Mean plasma levels of testosterone and androstenedione are increased, as well as the conversion ratio of androgens to oestrone and E2.

Adrenal Diseases

Congenital adrenal hyperplasia (CAH) is an autosomal recessive disorder associated with deficiency in any of the several adrenocortical enzymes necessary for cortisol biosynthesis, with the following effects: decrease in cortisol production, compensatory increase in ACTH levels, hyperplasia of the zona reticularis of the adrenal cortex, and accumulation of the substrate for the affected enzyme in the bloodstream. More than 90% of cases of CAH are caused by a 21-hydroxylase (CYP21) deficiency. There are three types of 21-hydroxylase deficiencies. Two are the classic forms, known as the salt-wasting and the simple virilizing types. The third is called the nonclassic type or adult-onset adrenal hyperplasia (AO-CAH), which manifests itself in late childhood or puberty. Its prevalence was reported to be between 1 and 4% of the female population (Speiser and White 2003).

Reduced fertility can also derive from the overproduction of sex steroid precursors that characterizes Cushing syndrome. Affected women may experience hyperandrogenism, with accompanying oligomenorrhoea or amenorrhoea, hirsutism, acne, and baldness, in association with specific clinical signs originating from increased glucocorticoid action. This condition leads to a catabolic state that causes muscle weakness, osteoporosis, atrophy of the skin, reduced immune resistance, as well as glucose intolerance resulting from an antagonism to insulin action and enhanced gluconeogenesis. Women with Cushing syndrome are generally obese and show a characteristic redistribution of fat over the abdomen, clavicles, trunk, and cheeks and around the neck. Menstrual dysfunction and decreased fertility are common findings in this syndrome. Many features of Cushing syndrome are comparable to those observed in PCOS, such as obesity, low SHBG, increased androgens, and hirsutism.

There is uncertainty as to what the underlying mechanisms responsible for chronic anovulation may be, but several theories have been hypothesized. Adrenal androgen excess in Cushing syndrome of all causes together with obesity may cause excessive extraglandular conversion of androgens to oestrogens in fat cells and inappropriate acyclic feedback to the hypothalamic–pituitary axis (Newell-Price et al. 1998). Increased levels of corticotropin-releasing hormone and adrenocorticotropic hormone (ACTH) in Cushing disease may affect the hypothalamic–pituitary secretion of GnRH and LH, as suggested from hypothalamic chronic anovulation.

In Cushing disease there is a marked reduction of primordial follicles, an absence of cortical stromal hyperplasia and luteinization, fibrosis, and size reduction, which point toward a lack in gonadotropins stimulation (Iannaccone et al. 1959). It is therefore suggested that the chronic hypercortisolaemia blocks both the action of the gonadotropins on the gonads and the GnRH secretion from the hypothalamus, resulting in a low level of oestrogens.

Acromegaly

Acromegaly is a hormonal disorder in which the pituitary gland produces excess hormones. Menstrual dysfunction and decreased fertility are present in >50% of women with acromegaly (Kaltsas et al. 1999). Reasons include hypopituitarism and a decreased gonadotropin reserve due to destruction or compression of gonadotroph cells. A multicentre study of 363 patients showed that hypogonadism was present in 57% of the included women. The prevalence of hypogonadism was similar in both macro-and microadenomas (54 and 38% respectively) (Katznelson et al. 2001). Moreover, PCOS is a common finding in women with acromegaly (Kaltsas et al. 2007). It is believed that this is either a direct effect of the excessive growth hormone(GH)/insulin-like growth factor (IgF-I) secretion on the ovaries or secondary to a GH-induced increased insulin resistance.

Treatment Principles

Hypogonadotropic Hypogonadism (WHO Group I)

Treatment for women in Group I should be directed to the cause. Surgery may be indicated in cases of intracranial tumours. Women with anorexia nervosa may benefit from psychotherapy and weight gain after extensive counselling. Ovulation can be induced by pulsatile GnRH administration (for hypothalamic causes) or gonadotropins (containing FSH and LH) if anovulation persists despite optimization of body weight (European Recombinant Human LH Study Group 1998).

Normogonadotropic Anovulation (WHO Group II)

Weight reduction should be the first-line treatment in obese women with PCOS, and this may result in resumption of spontaneous ovulation and also improve their response to ovulation induction if indicated. Ovulation induction can be achieved with clomiphene citrate or aromatase inhibitors. Patients who do not respond to oral treatment may be offered gonadotropins or ovarian drilling.

Other causes of androgen excess should be managed accordingly.

Hypergonadotropic Hypogonadism (WHO Group III)

Women with hypergonadotropic hypogonadism may present with primary or secondary amenorrhoea with elevated FSH and low oestradiol levels. About 50% of young women with ovarian failure may have intermittent and unpredictable ovulation, and spontaneous pregnancies have been reported in about 5–10% of cases subsequent to the diagnosis (van Karsteren and Schoemaker 1999). Any form of ovulation induction treatment, however, is not advisable in these women. The only realistic option is assisted reproduction using donor eggs.

Hyperprolactinaemia

Asymptomatic women with hyperprolactinaemia can be observed without treatment. In anovulatory women with hyperprolactinaemia, a dopamine agonist is the first-line treatment to lower the prolactin level and reduce the prolactinoma if present. Surgical treatment by transphenoidal pituitary adenectomy and rarely radiotherapy may be required if medical treatment fails to shrink a macroadenoma (Casanueva et al. 2006).

Conclusion

The management of female hormonal causes of infertility involves a thorough understanding of all the potential disorders that may interfere with normal ovulatory function. These disorders may involve endocrine organs of the reproductive and nonreproductive systems, nonendocrine organs, metabolic disorders, use of medications, and genetic causes. A systematic evaluation of women with anovulation, consisting of a comprehensive medical and family history, a thorough physical examination, and the use of appropriate laboratory and imaging tests, is therefore necessary. A multidisciplinary approach in aiding the diagnosis of an endocrine disorder is needed, ultimately to assist in the appropriate treatment and outcome of a pregnancy and the birth of a healthy infant.

References

Balen, A.H., Laven, J.S., Tan, S.L. et al. (2003). Ultrasound assessment of the polycystic ovary: international consensus definitions. Hum Reprod Update 9: 505–514.

Bergh, T., Skarin, G., Nillius, S.J. et al. (1985). Pulsatile GnRH therapy: an alternative successful therapy for induction of ovulation in infertile normo- and hyperprolactinaemic amenorrhoeic women with pituitary tumours. Acta Endocrinol 110: 440–444.

Brassard, M., AinMelk, Y. and Baillargeon, J.P. (2008). Basic infertility including polycystic ovary syndrome. Med Clin North Am 92: 1163–1192.

Bukman, A. and Heineman, M.J. (2001). Ovarian reserve testing and the use of prognostic models in patients with subfertility. Hum Reprod Update 7: 581.

Carmina, E. (2013). Obesity, adipokines and metabolic syndrome in polycystic ovary syndrome. Front Horm Res 40: 40–50.

Carmina, E. and Lobo, R.A. (2001). Polycystic ovaries in hirsute women with normal menses. Am J Med 111: 602–606.

Caronia, L.M., Martin, C., Welt, C.K. et al. (2011). A genetic basis for functional hypothalamic amenorrhea. N Engl J Med 364: 215–225.

Casanueva, F.F., Molitch, M.E., Schlechte, J.A. et al. (2006). Guidelines of the Pituitary Society for the diagnosis and management of prolactinomas. Clin Endocrinol 65: 265–273.

Clark, A.M., Thornley, B., Tomlinson, L. et al. (1998). Weight loss in obese infertile women results in improvement in reproductive outcome for all forms of fertility treatment. Hum Reprod 13: 1502–1505.

Coulam, C.B., Adamson, S.C., Annegers, J.F. (1986). Incidence of premature ovarian failure. Obstet Gynecol 67:604–6.

DeVos, M., Devroey, P. and Fauser, B.C.J.M. (2010). Primary ovarian insufficiency. Lancet 376(9744):911–921.

European Recombinant Human LH Study Group (1998). Recombinant human luteinizing hormone (LH) to support recombinant human follicle-stimulating hormone (FSH)-induced follicular development in LH- and FSH-deficient anovulatory women: a dose-finding study. J Clin Endocrinol Metabol 83: 1507–1514.

Gerhard, I., Becker, T., Eggert-Kruse, W. et al. (1991). Thyroid and ovarian function in infertile women. Hum Reprod 6: 338–345.

Hansen, K.R., Hodnett, G.M., Knowlton, N. et al. (2011). Correlation of ovarian reserve tests with histologically determined primordial follicle number. Fertil Steril 95: 170–175.

Hoek, A., Schoemaker, J. and Drexhage, H.A. (1997). Premature ovarian failure and ovarian auto-immunity. Endocr Rev 18: 107–134.

Iannaccone, A., Gabrilove, J.L., Sohval, A.R. et al. (1959). The ovaries in Cushing's syndrome. N Engl J Med 261: 775–780.

Kaltsas, G.A., Androulakis, I., Tziveriotist, K. et al. (2007). Polycystic ovaries and the polycystic ovary syndrome phenotype in women with active acromegaly. Clin Endocrinol 67: 917–922.

Kaltsas, G.A., Mukherjee, J.J., Jenkins, P.J. et al. (1999). Menstrual irregularity in women with acromegaly. J Clin Endocrinol Metabol 84: 2731–2735.

Katznelson, L., Kleinberg, D., Vance, M.L. et al. (2001). Hypogonadism in patients with acromegaly: data from the multi-centre acromegaly registry pilot study. Clin Endocrinol 54: 183–188.

Lazarus, J.H. (1997). Hyperthyroidism. Lancet 349(9048): 339–343.

Legro, R.S. (2007). Pregnancy considerations in women with polycystic ovary syndrome. Clin Obstet Gynecol 50: 295–304.

March, W.A., Moore, V.M., Willson, K.J. et al. (2010). The prevalence of polycystic ovary syndrome in a community sample assessed under contrasting diagnostic criteria. Hum Reprod 25: 544–551.

Mattei, M.G., Mattei, J.F., Ayme, S. et al. (1982). X-autosome translocations: cytogenetic characteristics and their consequences Hum Genet 61: 295–309.

Melmed, S., Casanueva, F., Hoffman, A. et al. (2011). Diagnosis and treatment of hyperprolactinemia: an endocrine society clinical practice guideline. J Clin Endocrinol Metabol 96: 273–288.

Newell-Price, J., Trainer, P., Besser, M. et al. (1998). The diagnosis and differential diagnosis of Cushing's syndrome and pseudo-Cushing's states. Endocr Rev 19: 647–672.

Rebar, R.W. and Connolly, H.V. (1990). Clinical features of young women with hypergonadotropic amenorrhea. Fertil Steril 53:804–810.

Rotterdam ESHRE/ASRM (2004). Revised 2003 consensus on diagnostic criteria and long-term health risks related to polycystic ovary syndrome (PCOS). Rotterdam ESHRE/ASRM-Sponsored PCOS consensus workshop group. Hum Reprod 19: 41–47.

Sirmans, S.M. and Pate, K.A. (2014). Epidemiology, diagnosis, and management of polycystic ovary syndrome. Clin Epidemiol 6: 1–13.

Speiser, P.W. and White, P.C. (2003). Congenital adrenal hyperplasia. N Engl J Med 349: 776–788.

Turkalj, I., Braun, P. and Krupp, P. (1982). Surveillance of bromocriptine in pregnancy. JAMA 247: 1589.

van Karsteren, Y.M. and Schoemaker, J. (1999). Premature ovarian failure: a systematic review on therapeutic interventions to restore ovarian function and achieve pregnancy. Hum Reprod Update 5: 483–492.

Verma, I., Sood, R., Juneja, S. et al. (2012). Prevalence of hypothyroidism in infertile women and evaluation of response of treatment for hypothyroidism on infertility. Int J Appl Basic Med Res 2: 17–19.

World Health Organization Scientific Group (1976). *Agents Stimulating Ovarian Function in The Human*. Geneva: World Health Organization. Report No. 514.

Yazigi, R.A., Quintero, C.H. and Salameh, W.A. (1997). Prolactin disorders. Fertil Steril 67: 215.

11

Oocyte Aneuploidy and the Maternal Age Effect

Mary Herbert

Introduction

Reproductive Consequences of Female Ageing

Errors arising during the meiotic divisions are generally catastrophic as they affect every cell of the embryo. Thus, the majority of meiotic segregation errors involving autosomal chromosomes are not compatible with the establishment of a clinically recognized pregnancy. Rare exceptions include trisomic conceptions involving chromosome 21 (Down syndrome), chromosome 18 (Edwards syndrome), and chromosome 13 (Patau syndrome), which can develop to term. Trisomy 16 is also compatible with implantation, but generally does not develop beyond the first trimester and is the most common chromosomal cause of miscarriage. With the exception of the X chromosome, there are no reports of monosomy in clinically recognized pregnancies.

The incidence of chromosomal abnormalities among live births is estimated to be 0.4%, increasing to 3% and 35% respectively for stillborn babies and spontaneous miscarriages (Hassold and Hunt 2001). Analysis of human embryos indicates that 95% of meiotic errors are of maternal origin and that the incidence increases dramatically as women get older. However, it is important to note that chromosome segregation errors during the early mitotic divisions of human embryos are also common. This gives rise to karyotypic mosaicism in which some cells are aneuploid while others are euploid. Alternatively all cells may be aneuploid, but for different chromosomes. In contrast to meiotic errors, the incidence of

post-zygotic errors does not appear to be related to maternal age (Fragouli et al. 2013).

As a consequence of the high risk of meiotic segregation errors in oocytes from older women, female age is the biggest risk factor for infertility, miscarriage, and trisomy. The complete rescue of these effects by using eggs from younger (<35 years old) donors dispels any doubt that the maternal age effect is due to an oocyte problem. Cytogenetic and molecular genetic analyses of human oocytes show a clear age-related increase in the proportion of oocytes affected. Moreover, oocytes of older women are more likely to be aneuploid for multiple chromosomes (Handyside et al. 2012; Fragouli et al. 2013).

Mechanics and Mechanisms of Female Meiosis

During mitotic cell division, DNA replication gives rise to sister chromatids, which remain tethered until anaphase when the chromatids come apart and segregate to daughter cells. Cohesion between sister chromatids is provided by cohesin, a ring-shaped protein complex thought to entrap newly replicated sister chromatids. Cleavage of cohesin's alpha-kleisin subunit by the protease separase at anaphase onset enables sister chromatids to separate and segregate to daughter cells (Peters et al. 2008; Nasmyth 2011; Haarhuis et al. 2014). Thus, alternating rounds of DNA replication and chromosome segregation enable daughter cells to inherit a maternal and a paternal copy of each chromosome thereby maintaining diploidy. By contrast, meiotic cells transmit a single copy of each chromosome by undergoing two rounds of chromosome segregation following a single round of DNA replication. The first meiotic division (meiosis I) uniquely involves segregation of homologous chromosomes, and the second (meiosis II) involves segregation of chromatids.

Bivalent Chromosomes Are Formed During Meiotic Recombination

In most organisms, accurate segregation of maternal and paternal homologues depends on the formation of bivalent chromosomes. This depends on meiotic recombination, which occurs during prophase of meiosis I after DNA replication (Hunter 2015; Gray and Cohen 2016). Thereafter, paternal and maternal homologues remain physically linked at the sites where they reciprocally exchange DNA to form crossovers. Thus, in addition to providing genetic variation, meiotic recombination provides the physical linkages between parental homologues, which are essential for their accurate segregation during the first meiotic division. In cytological studies, these physical linkages, corresponding to the sites of crossover formation, are referred to as chiasmata (from the Greek for crosspiece of wood).

Accurate segregation of homologous chromosomes requires at least one crossover known as the obligate crossover. The total number of crossovers formed during female meiosis is estimated to exceed that observed in male meiosis by a factor of approximately 1.7 (Broman et al. 1998; Lynn et al. 2004). However, the proportion of chromosomes failing to form a crossover is higher in females than in males (Nagaoka et al. 2012). This paradoxical situation has recently been attributed to defective regulation of 'crossover maturation' in female meiosis (Wang et al. 2017). In addition, the checkpoint mechanisms responsible for monitoring meiotic recombination appear to be less stringent in female meiosis compared with male meiosis (Nagaoka et al. 2012). Thus, differences in the regulation of crossover formation between male and female meiosis constitute an oocyte-intrinsic risk factor, which may contribute to the vastly disproportionate contribution of oocytes to aneuploidy in human embryos.

Bivalent Chromosomes Are Stabilized by Cohesin

Because bivalent chromosomes are formed after premeiotic DNA replication, each consists of four *chromatids* – a pair from each parental homologue.

As in mitotic cells, sister chromatids are linked by cohesin. In meiosis, this depends on cohesin complexes containing Rec8, a highly conserved meiosis-specific alpha-kleisin subunit. In addition to Rec8, mammalian meiocytes contain the meiosis-specific cohesin subunits Smc1β and Stag3, which are both essential for accurate chromosome segregation during the meiotic divisions (McNicoll et al. 2013; Lee 2017). Crucially, the bivalent chromosome structure is stabilized by cohesin rings distal to the site of crossover formation (Figure 11.1).

In female mammals, bivalent chromosomes are established during fetal life when proliferating oogonia enter the meiotic programme to form oocytes. Each oocyte becomes surrounded by a small number of pregranulosa cells to form a primordial follicle. Primordial follicles formed during fetal life constitute the stock from which oocytes are recruited for growth throughout life. Oocytes remain arrested in prophase of meiosis I until shortly before ovulation when homologues disjoin during anaphase I. As discussed above, accurate segregation of homologues during the first meiotic division requires that bivalents remain intact. Thus, bivalent integrity, which depends on cohesin distal to crossovers, must be maintained from fetal life until shortly before ovulation, which corresponds to decades in humans.

The First Meiotic Division: Resolving Bivalents to Dyad Chromosomes

The transition from prophase to M phase of meiosis I is marked by germinal vesicle breakdown (GVBD) and occurs in response to the luteinizing hormone (LH) surge (Eppig et al. 2004; Jaffe and Egbert 2017). Spindle assembly occurs in the absence of a centriole and the mechanism may differ between mouse and human oocytes (Bennabi et al. 2016). Bivalent chromosomes align on the meiosis I spindle by co-orienting sister centromeres, thereby promoting attachment of sister kinetochores to the same spindle pole (Hauf and Watanabe 2004). Thus, in contrast to mitosis and meiosis II, sister kinetochores establish monopolar rather than bipolar attachment. This is essential for cosegregation of sister centromeres and hence for segregation of homologues during the reductional division of meiosis I.

Disjunction of homologues during anaphase I depends on removal of cohesin from chromosome arms, but not from centromeres. This is accomplished by cleavage of the cohesin's alpha-kleisin

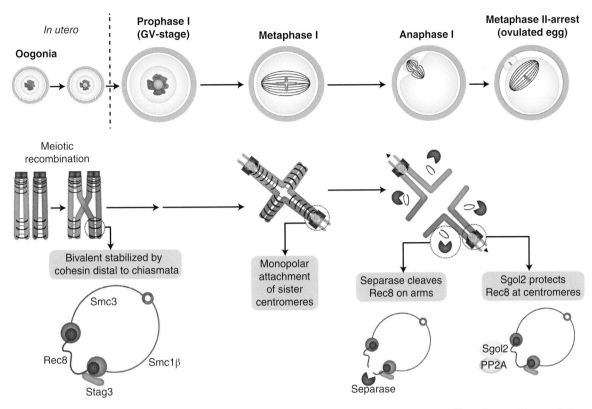

Figure 11.1 Bivalent chromosomes are formed after premeiotic DNA replication. Each consists of four chromatids – a pair from each parental homologue. The bivalent chromosome structure is stabilized by cohesin rings distal to the site of crossover formation. During anaphase I, separase cleaves Rec8 (a subunit of cohesion) on arms but Sgol2 protects Rec8 at centromeres maintaining homologue attachment at the centromeres. *Source:* Illustrated by Mahdi Lamb.

subunit Rec8 by the protease separase. Not surprisingly separase activity is tightly regulated. This is accomplished by degradation of the separase inhibitor securin and cyclin B1 by the anaphase promoting complex (APC/C) under the control of the spindle assembly checkpoint (SAC) (Holt et al. 2013; Herbert et al. 2015). Loss of arm cohesin converts bivalents to two dyad chromosomes, each of which consist of a pair of chromatids linked by cohesin between sister centromeres. Anaphase I occurs at the oocyte cortex and dyads segregating to the outermost spindle pole are lost to first polar body. This enables the oocyte to retain the bulk of the cytoplasm while losing half of its nuclear genome. Dyads remaining in the oocyte align on the meiosis II spindle. In most mammals, including humans, anaphase I occurs before ovulation, and ovulated eggs remain arrested at metaphase of meiosis II until the egg is fertilized.

Protection of Centromeric Cohesion

Work in budding and fission yeast indicates that phosphorylation of Rec8 is essential for its cleavage by separase (Ishiguro et al. 2010; Katis et al. 2010). This property enables protection of centromeric cohesin by recruitment of the phosphatase PP2A by proteins known as Shugoshins (Sgo; Japanese for guardian protector) (Watanabe 2005; Rivera and Losada 2006; Clift and Marston 2011). Protection of centromeric cohesin is essential for accurate segregation of chromatids during meiosis II. In mammalian oocytes, Shugoshin-like 2 (Sgol2) recruits the phosphatase PP2A to protect cohesin at centromeres (Herbert et al. 2015; MacLennan et al. 2015).

The Second Meiotic Division: Resolving Dyads to Single Chromatids

In mammalian oocytes, anaphase II and completion of meiosis is triggered by sperm entry, which activates the APC/C by inactivating cytostatic factor (Schmidt et al. 2006). This leads to a second round of separase activation resulting in cleavage of centromeric cohesin, which resolves dyads to single chromatids (monads) during anaphase II. Cleavage of centromeric cohesin during anaphase II depends on inactivation of the mechanisms responsible for protecting centromeric cohesin during anaphase I (Argüello-Miranda et al. 2017; Jonak et al. 2017). The resulting chromatids segregate equationally (as in mitosis) and are either retained in the oocyte or lost to the second polar body. The maternal and paternal single copy genomes then become separately packaged in pronuclei, where they replicate their DNA in preparation for the first mitotic division (Clift and Schuh 2013). Formation of the pronuclear membrane marks completion of meiosis.

To conclude, in stark contrast to male meiosis, the formation of a single copy maternal genome occurs over a protracted period; decades in humans and months in mice. The process commences during fetal life with the formation of bivalent chromosomes and is not completed until the egg is fertilized. During the intervening period, oocytes remain arrested in prophase of meiosis I, predominantly in the pregrowth stage surrounded by a small number of granulosa cell precursors to form the primordial follicle. Based on findings in mouse oocytes, our current understanding is that bivalent chromosomes are stabilized by cohesin complexes loaded on the DNA early during oogenesis (Chiang et al. 2012; Jessberger 2012), most likely during the premeiotic S phase. This raises the remarkable possibility that cohesin complexes loaded during fetal life in human oocytes maintain cohesion for decades until shortly before the fully grown oocyte is ovulated. As will be discussed later, depletion of cohesin from bivalent chromosomes during prolonged prophase arrest is emerging as a primary culprit in compromising chromosome segregation in oocytes of older women.

Ovarian Ageing Versus Chromosomal Ageing

The idea that females are born with a finite population of oocytes was first proposed in the 1950s. Subsequent claims of *de novo* oogenesis are highly controversial and of questionable physiological significance (Telfer et al. 2005; Handel et al. 2014; Grieve et al. 2015). The number of oocytes present at birth has been estimated to be approximately 1 million, though a recent study involving mathematical modelling reported huge (two orders of magnitude) variation between individuals (Wallace and Kelsey 2010). The pool of primordial follicles becomes depleted throughout life, dwindling to around 1000 by the time of menopause, which generally occurs between 45 and 55 years of age. Only a tiny fraction of oocytes is ovulated, the vast majority being lost due to cell death both before and after birth (Monget et al. 2012; Findlay et al. 2015). Depletion of the ovarian reserve of primordial follicles throughout life culminates in cessation of ovulation at menopause and is generally referred to as 'ovarian ageing'. The circulating level of anti-Müllerian hormone (AMH), which is produced by growing follicles, is considered to be a biomarker of ovarian reserve. Analysis of data from multiple studies indicates that AMH levels peak in the mid-twenties and decline in parallel with the number of primordial follicles (Kelsey et al. 2012). The rate at which a given woman's ovaries age is likely to be a function of the combined effect of the size of the starting pool, the rate or recruitment for growth, and the rate of cell death.

Ovarian ageing occurs in parallel with the age-related increase in oocyte chromosome segregation errors. However, the increase in oocyte aneuploidy precedes menopause by a decade or more. This implies that errors in meiosis are the primary driver of female reproductive ageing. The concept of 'chromosomal ageing' arises from the fact that the lifespan of the bivalent chromosome is approximately equivalent to that of the ovulated egg. A defining feature of oocytes ovulated late in life is that they remain arrested in prophase of meiosis I for an extended period. For example, an oocyte ovulated at the age of 40 faces the biological challenge of maintaining intact bivalents for four decades. A growing body of evidence indicates that ageing is accompanied by deterioration of the bivalent and dyad chromosome architecture required to faithfully transmit a single copy maternal genome (Chiang et al. 2012; Jessberger 2012; Herbert et al. 2015).

In summary, female reproductive ageing is driven by depletion of the ovarian reserve and by deterioration of the chromosome architecture required for accurate segregation during meiosis. The former culminates in the menopause, while the latter results in a decline in fertility due to meiotic segregation errors. In this sense, it could be argued that female reproductive lifespan is curtailed by two biological clocks – the ovarian clock and the chromosomal clock.

Molecular correlates of chromosomal ageing: lessons from mouse oocytes

Contrary to the long-held view that mouse oocytes were immune from the maternal age effect, recent studies showed that oocytes from a range of wild type mouse strains show an increased incidence of prematurely separated chromatids beyond the age of 12 months (Chiang et al. 2010; Lister et al. 2010; Yun et al. 2014). This is the most pervasive defect in oocytes from older women (see later), suggesting that the mouse is an appropriate model for studying the mechanistic basis of the maternal age-effect.

Studies involving oocytes from mice aged >12 months indicate that bivalents lose their structure and that this is correlated with reduced levels of Rec8 (Chiang et al. 2012; Jessberger 2012; Herbert et al. 2015; MacLennan et al. 2015). As discussed previously, Rec8-containing complexes are exclusively responsible for conferring chromosomal cohesion during meiosis (Chiang et al. 2012; McNicoll et al. 2013; MacLennan et al. 2015; Lee 2017). However, because Rec8 is also essential for crossover formation (Yoon et al. 2016), it has been challenging to establish a direct causal relationship between age-related depletion of Rec8 and chromosome missegregation in oocytes.

The first indication that cohesin might be 'the missing link' in female age-related aneuploidy came from studies on oocytes deficient in *Smc1β* which is a meiosis-specific paralogue of Smc1. Crucially, *Smc1β* oocytes showed an age-related deterioration of bivalent structure (Hodges et al. 2005). These findings indicate that Smc1β-containing cohesin complexes are required to stabilize arm and centromeric cohesion during prolonged arrest in prophase of meiosis I. Subsequent studies using oocytes from a variety of wild type mouse strains (Liu and Keefe 2008; Chiang et al. 2010; Lister et al. 2010) indicated that chromosome-associated Rec8 declines markedly during female ageing. This is accompanied by an increase in the prevalence of bivalents in which homologues are linked tenuously and only at telomeres (Chiang et al. 2010; Lister et al. 2010).

Interestingly, the more pervasive effect of female ageing in mouse oocytes is an increase in the distance between sister centromeres (Chiang et al. 2010; Lister et al. 2010). This likely impairs their ability to establish monopolar attachments (Hauf and Watanabe 2004). In addition, recruitment of Sgol2 is reduced in oocytes from older females (Lister et al. 2010). Notably, this was also the case in oocytes from young *Smc1β* females (Lister et al. 2010), indicating that cohesin is either directly or indirectly required for recruitment and/or maintenance of its own protector. This gives ground to the idea that fertility of older females is sabotaged by a two-pronged mechanism, which (i) compromises bivalent architecture by gradual depletion of cohesin during extended arrest in prophase of meiosis I, and (ii) compromises dyad structure by the combined effect of reduced cohesin and reduced recruitment of its protector (Sgol2) to centromeres. This scheme of events is consistent with the age-related increase in premature loss of centromeric cohesin in mouse oocytes (Chiang et al. 2012; Herbert et al. 2015)

High resolution live cell imaging studies of mouse oocytes have provided further insight into the pathways leading to premature resolution of sister centromeres in oocytes from ageing females. During M-phase of meiosis I, a proportion of bivalents in aged oocytes become hyperstretched and undergo premature resolution to dyads. The dyads then congress on the metaphase I plate and undergo a second round of segregation, giving rise to single chromatids during anaphase I (Sakakibara et al. 2015). This indicates that prematurely separated chromatids arise as a consequence of two rounds of chromosome segregation during meiosis I. Evidence from human oocytes suggest that unpaired chromatids in metaphase-II arrested oocytes might arise by a similar pathway (Sakakibara et al. 2015; Zielinska et al. 2015). However, it is worth noting that chromatids may also come apart following completion of anaphase I (Yun et al. 2014).

In summary, the age-related deterioration of bivalent structure in *Smc1β* mouse oocytes together with depletion of chromosomal cohesin in wild-type oocytes gave ground to the 'cohesin deterioration hypothesis'. According to this idea, depletion of cohesin below a threshold level results in destabilization of bivalents and separation of sister centromeres. This in turn compromises monopolar attachment during metaphase I and bipolar attachment during metaphase II. Adding insult to injury, depletion of cohesin is accompanied by reduced recruitment of its own protector Sgol2. These events provide a plausible mechanistic link between female ageing and oocyte aneuploidy.

Are There Other Possible Culprits in the Maternal Age Effect?

While depletion of cohesin and its protector is sufficient to explain the types of aneuploidy observed in oocytes from older mice and women (see later) (Chiang et al. 2012; Herbert et al. 2015), this does not rule out the possibility that other mechanisms may also contribute to age-related oocyte aneuploidy. Indeed, defective regulation of the SAC is frequently invoked as a potential player in the maternal age effect. The canonical function of the SAC is to reduce the risk of aneuploidy by coordinating separase activation with chromosome alignment. This depends on a 'wait anaphase' signal generated from kinetochores that fail to form microtubule attachments (Musacchio and Salmon 2007). While there is a general recognition that the oocyte SAC may not be very sensitive to misaligned chromosomes (Jones and Lane 2013), strong evidence to support an age-related deterioration of SAC function has been lacking. For example, oocytes from young and old mice behave similarly with respect to two hallmarks of SAC function, namely the timing on anaphase onset and the ability to delay anaphase in response to microtubule depolymerization (Chiang et al. 2012; Herbert et al. 2015). However, there may be more subtle effects. For example, it was reported that defective SAC function results in accelerated degradation of the separase inhibitor securin (Ibtissem et al. 2017). This, together with reduced levels of Sgol2, might indeed contribute to premature separation of sister centromeres.

Defects in spindle assembly have also been described in mouse oocytes (Nakagawa and FitzHarris 2017) and in human oocytes (Holubcová et al. 2015; Haverfield et al. 2017). However, it should be noted that the human work is based on oocytes that failed to mature in response to ovarian stimulation (Holubcová et al. 2015) and an earlier report suggests that oocytes

from this source are inherently prone to spindle defects (Coticchio et al. 2013). It will therefore be important to perform experiments using good quality human oocytes.

Maternally Transmitted Aneuploidy in Humans

Insights into the pathways leading to aneuploidy during female meiosis are predominantly based on genetic analysis of trisomy cases (mostly trisomy 21) and human oocytes generated in *in vitro* fertilization (IVF) programmes. Both sources have limitations. In the case of trisomy, analysis is based only on those chromosomes that were retained in the oocyte. In addition, the data are generally based on population studies, which by definition exclude those embryos that fail to implant or miscarry. By contrast, studies on oocytes, particularly when combined with polar body analysis, provide a more comprehensive picture. However, the oocytes available for this type of analysis are generally obtained from women undergoing fertility treatment and may therefore not be representative of the general population.

Evidence from Cases of Trisomy

Typically cases of trisomy are studied by performing genetic mapping studies involving both parents and their trisomic child. These studies yield information on the parental origin of the extra chromosome as well as the number and chromosomal position of crossovers formed during fetal life. Because of mechanisms that supress recombination close to the centromere, polymorphisms in the peri-centromeric region can be used to infer whether the segregation error arose during the first of second meiotic division. Heterozygosity implies a meiosis I error, whereas homozygosity implies a meiosis II error (Lamb et al. 1997).

Failure of crossover formation is a major risk factor for trisomy, accounting for approximately 40% of trisomy 21 cases (Hassold and Hunt 2001; Nagaoka et al. 2012). Absence of crossovers results in two univalent chromosomes (also known as achiasmate homologues), which are expected to segregate independently during anaphase I. Studies in cases of trisomy 21 and 16 indicate that a single crossover positioned close to the telomere (sub-telomeric) is also associated with a high risk of trisomy (Hassold and Hunt 2001). Because bivalents are stabilized by cohesin distal to the site of crossover formation, those with a single sub-telomeric crossover rely on the relatively short stretch of stabilizing arm cohesin. Gradual erosion of this could cause premature resolution of the bivalent to its constituent dyads, even in younger women. In support of this, the incidence of univalent chromosome 16 present in oocytes during M-phase of meiosis I exceeds that detected in fetal ovaries by MLH1 staining, which transiently mark the sites of crossover formation (Garcia-Cruz et al. 2010b).

Crucially, stratification by maternal age indicated that trisomy 21 children born to older women exhibit a similar pattern of crossovers to that observed in euploid offspring (Lamb et al. 2005; Oliver et al. 2008). An implication of this is that all chiasmate configurations become susceptible to missegregation with advancing female age. Interestingly, the presence of a single peri-centromeric crossover, which was not detected in trisomy 21 cases born to younger women, was identified as a risk factor for trisomy 21 in older women and was associated with errors in meiosis II (Oliver et al. 2008). It is tempting to speculate that the age-related errors involving peri-centromeric crossovers may be mechanistically linked to the more general problem of premature separation of sister centromeres in oocytes from older women (see later).

Analysis of trisomic pregnancies is unlikely to provide a comprehensive picture of the whole spectrum of segregation errors in oocytes, or their relationship with crossover formation. More recent developments using next generation sequencing (NGS) to analyse oocytes and polar bodies offers the opportunity to identify the position and number of crossovers by generating genome-wide 'meiomaps' (Hou et al. 2013; Ottolini et al. 2016) for individual oocytes. This approach has the potential to increase our understanding of the relationship between the position and number of crossovers and the risk of chromosome missegregation during the meiotic divisions. However, it will be important to control for technical artifacts such as amplification bias during the whole genome amplification step (Hou et al. 2013).

Evidence from Genetic Analysis of Human Oocytes

Early studies on the chromosomal constitution of human oocytes were largely based on analysis of air-dried chromosome spreads prepared from metaphase II-arrested oocytes that failed to undergo fertilization. This was superseded by fluorescence in-situ hybridization (FISH), which involved the use of fluorescent probes to mark specific chromosomes, generally those such as chromosome 16 and 21, known to be error prone from analysis of trisomic pregnancies. However, detection of multiple chromosomes by FISH is technically challenging and prone to artifact and may have overestimated the extent of oocyte aneuploidy in IVF patients (Pellestor et al. 2006; Nagaoka et al. 2012). The subsequent application of array-based comparative genomic hybridization (aCGH) for analysis of human oocytes and embryos offered the possibility of genome wide detection of numerical abnormalities. This revealed that while no chromosome is immune from missegregation, those detected in trisomic pregnancies were among the most frequent offenders. More recently, the field has been moving towards whole genome amplification (WGA) and NGS, which as discussed previously, has the potential to identify sites of crossover formation as well as numerical and structural abnormalities.

The incidence of aneuploidy reported from studies on human oocytes varies widely. In general, conventional cytogenetic studies of metaphase II-arrested human oocytes obtained from IVF programmes report numerical abnormalities in around 10–17% of oocytes (Pellestor et al. 2006; Nagaoka et al. 2012). By contrast, the larger FISH studies, involving detection of error-prone chromosomes, reported aneuploidy in approximately 45% of oocytes with a range of 20% to >70% (Pellestor et al. 2006; Nagaoka et al. 2012). While technical artifacts may contribute, the generally high incidence of aneuploidy may also reflect the fact that much of the FISH data comes from clinical application in cases thought to be at high risk of aneuploidy. This is also the case for more recent studies involving the use of aCGH. For example, data based on sequential analysis of the first and second polar bodies from 420 eggs from women aged 34–47 years indicates that only 26% underwent normal chromosome segregation in both meiotic divisions (Fragouli et al. 2013). The incidence of aneuploidy was 47% in oocytes obtained from women aged 34–37 years old and this increased to a staggering 78% for those aged 38–47 years (Fragouli et al. 2013). Moreover, the oocytes from older women are frequently aneuploid for more than one chromosome. The evidence indicates an approximately 10-fold increase beyond the age of 40 years (Handyside et al. 2012; Fragouli et al. 2013).

While aneuploidy in metaphase II-arrested oocytes can involve whole chromosomes (dyads) or prematurely separated chromatids, a strikingly consistent finding is that the prevalence of errors involving chromatids increases as a function of female age. This implies that failure to maintain centromeric cohesion until the onset of anaphase II is a predominant cause of age-related aneuploidy in human oocytes. Prematurely separated chromatids exist in several forms in human metaphase II oocytes. A single (unpaired) chromatid can co-exist with an intact dyad resulting in three copies instead of two. Alternatively, three copies are ejected in the first polar body and only one is retained in the oocyte. Finally, two free chromatids from the same chromosome may be retained in the oocyte. In this case the metaphase II oocyte is euploid. However, there is a high risk of missegregation during anaphase II.

Loss or gain of a single chromatid detected in metaphase-II arrested oocytes, which is often referred to as 'unbalanced pre-division', implies a breach of two cardinal rules of meiosis: (i) failure to protect centromeric cohesion and (ii) failure of monopolar attachment, resulting in equational rather than reductional segregation of sister centromeres during anaphase I. 'Balanced pre-division', which refers to the presence of a prematurely separated pair of chromatids could arise by the same pathway, but involving both sets of parental centromeres. In this case, the free chromatids come from different parental homologues (Figure 11.2). An alternative possibility is that both sister centromeres segregate correctly to the same spindle pole, but then lose cohesion either during, or after, anaphase I. In this event, the two free chromatids would be derived from the same dyad and, if retained in the oocyte during anaphase II would give rise to the meiosis II-type errors reported to show an age-related increase in studies of trisomy 21 (Oliver et al. 2008). Consistent with this it has been reported that

balanced pre-division is strongly correlated with female age (Angell 1997; Sandalinas et al. 2002). However, as it does not constitute a numerical abnormality, it cannot be detected by aCGH of metaphase II oocytes and is therefore likely to be under-reported in more recent studies.

Because free chromatids are expected to segregate independently during meiosis II, it is not surprising that studies involving analysis of human zygotes and polar bodies show an increase in the incidence of errors in both meiotic divisions. However, the evidence indicates a disproportionate increase in meiosis II errors during female ageing (Handyside et al. 2012; Fragouli et al. 2013; Herbert et al. 2015) This may be due to an increase in the incidence of oocytes with 'balanced pre-division', which although euploid at metaphase II, have a high risk of error during anaphase II. Furthermore, the relatively low levels of meiosis II errors reported in oocytes from younger women might, in part, be explained by correction of meiosis I errors during anaphase II (Handyside et al. 2012; Fragouli et al. 2013). For example, an extra chromatid present in the metaphase II oocyte may be ejected in the second polar body. However, because oocytes from older women frequently contain multiple free chromatids the chance of becoming euploid by 'correction' during anaphase II is greatly reduced.

In conclusion, genetic studies on human oocytes indicate that the incidence of aneuploidy increases dramatically during female ageing and that this is largely due to premature loss of centromeric cohesion resulting in an increased risk of chromosome missegregation during both meiotic divisions.

What do Genetic Studies on Human Oocytes Reveal About Mechanisms of Aneuploidy?

In mechanistic terms, the evidence from studies on human oocytes indicates that failure to protect centromeric cohesion until anaphase II is a major cause of female age-related meiotic errors. This is consistent with female age-related depletion of Rec8-cohesin and reduced recruitment of Sgol2 reported from studies in mouse oocytes (Chiang et al. 2012; Jessberger 2012; Herbert et al. 2015). Consistent with this, a growing body of evidence indicates that human oocytes exhibit an age-related increase in the

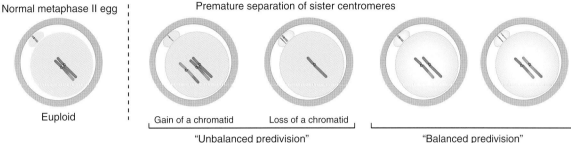

Normal metaphase II egg

Premature separation of sister centromeres

Euploid

Gain of a chromatid

Loss of a chromatid

"Unbalanced predivision"

"Balanced predivision"

Figure 11.2 Premature separation of sister centromeres. Loss or gain of a single chromatid detected in metaphase-II arrested oocytes, which is often referred to as unbalanced predivision, may be due to failure to protect centromeric cohesion and/or failure of monopolar attachment. Balanced predivision, could arise by the same pathways, but involving both sets of parental centromeres. *Source:* Illustrated by Mahdi Lamb.

distance between sister centromeres (Duncan et al. 2012; Zielinska et al. 2015; Patel et al. 2016), which in mouse oocytes is correlated with cohesin depletion (Chiang et al. 2010). However, direct evidence for an age-related decline in cohesin and its protector in human oocytes is scant. While premature loss of Rec8 during anaphase I has been observed in an immunofluorescence study of cohesin in human oocytes (Garcia-Cruz et al. 2010a), the authors did not perform a systematic analysis of the effect of age on oocyte chromosomal cohesin. A subsequent study using human ovarian tissue, indicated a significant reduction in the levels of Rec8 and Smc1β during female ageing (Tsutsumi et al. 2014). Although significant, the magnitude of the effect was modest and was not observed until the age of 49 years (Tsutsumi et al. 2014). This may have been due to the presence of soluble cohesin which, in mouse oocytes, does not decline markedly during female ageing (Chiang et al. 2010). Thus, further work is required to test directly the effect of age on levels of centromeric Rec8 and Sgol2 in human oocytes.

Assisted Reproductive Technologies to Reduce the Risk Of Oocyte Aneuploidy?

Identification of chromosomally normal embryos may help to increase the implantation rate for older women undergoing IVF treatment. However, evidence from aGCH analysis of the first and second polar bodies indicated that 45% of older women (mean age 40 years) produced no euploid zygotes (Geraedts et al. 2011). Some unlikely possibilities have been proposed to help these women. For example, it is difficult to imagine how cytoplasmic donation or 'mitochondrial augmentation' (Chappel 2013) might correct aneuploidies and chromosome defects already present in metaphase II-arrested oocytes. It has also been proposed that the maternal genome contained in the first polar body could be used to rescue age-related infertility (Ma et al. 2017). Again, it is unclear how this might help as the errors in oocytes are inevitably reciprocated in the polar body.

The possibility of using pharmacological agents to activate primordial follicles remaining in the ovary of menopausal women has also been explored (Li et al. 2010). Remarkably, this strategy has been effective in young women affected by premature ovarian failure. However, it was not successful in older women (Kawamura et al. 2013). This is consistent with the idea that 'chromosomal ageing' is a major limiting factor in the reproductive potential of those oocytes remaining in the ovary at the end of a woman's reproductive lifespan.

In conclusion, while genetic testing to identify euploid eggs/embryos may increase the efficiency of IVF treatment for some older women, there are currently no credible options for those who do not produce any euploid eggs. Vitrification and storage of oocytes may offer the possibility of a 'reproductive insurance policy'. However, this would only be effective as an early intervention, before the oocytes succumb to the effects of female age.

Conclusion

While the association between female age, infertility, and oocyte aneuploidy has been known from many generations, the biological basis has been enigmatic. Advances in our understanding of the mechanisms governing chromosome segregation in yeast meiosis paved the way to important mechanistic insights into how mammalian gametes transmit a single copy genome. Moreover, the relatively recent discovery that mouse oocytes exhibit age-related meiotic defects has set the scene for uncovering the molecular basis for the maternal age-effect and considerable progress towards this goal has been made in the past decade. While this research may not lead to a 'cure' for the maternal age effect, an understanding of the difficulties in ameliorating the effects of maternal ageing will, in itself, be of value. In the broader context of reproductive health, the problem of female age-related infertility would benefit from a more prominent position on the public health agenda. In this regard, there is a pressing need to understand better the barriers younger women face in starting a family and their perception of the risks associated with delaying motherhood.

Acknowledgements

Research in the laboratory is supported by the Wellcome Trust and by the EU Horizon 2020 programme. I apologize to authors whose work was not cited due to lack of space. I have tried where possible to reference open-access reviews for further reference.

References

Angell, R. (1997). First-meiotic division non-disjunction in human oocytes. Am J Hum Genet 61: 23–32.

Argüello-Miranda, O., Zagoriy, I., Mengoli, V. et al. (2017). Casein Kinase 1 coordinates cohesin cleavage, gametogenesis, and exit from M phase in meiosis II. Dev Cell 40: 37–52.

Bennabi, I., Terret, M.-E. and Verlhac, M.-H. (2016). Meiotic spindle assembly and chromosome segregation in oocytes. J Cell Biol 215: 611.

Broman, K.W., Murray, J.C., Sheffield, V.C. et al. (1998). Comprehensive Human Genetic Maps: Individual and Sex-Specific Variation in Recombination. The Am J Hum Genet 63: 861–869.

Chappel, S. (2013). The role of mitochondria from mature oocyte to viable blastocyst. Obstet Gynecol Int 2013:183024.

Chiang, T., Duncan, F.E, Schindler K. et al. (2010). Evidence that weakened centromere cohesion is a leading cause of age-related aneuploidy in oocytes. Curr Biol 20: 1522–1528.

Chiang, T., Schultz, R.M. and Lampson, M.A. (2012). Meiotic origins of maternal age-related aneuploidy. Biol Reprod 86: 1–7.

Clift, D. and Marston, A.L. (2011). The role of shugoshin in meiotic chromosome segregation. Cytogen Genome Res 133: 234–242.

Clift, D. and Schuh M. (2013). Restarting life: fertilization and the transition from meiosis to mitosis. Nat Rev Mol Cell Biol 14: 549–562.

Coticchio, G., Guglielmo, M.C., Dal Canto, M. et al. (2013). Mechanistic foundations of the metaphase II spindle of human oocytes matured in vivo and in vitro. Hum Reprod 28: 3271–3282.

Duncan, F.E., Hornick, J.E., Lampson, M.A. et al. (2012). Chromosome cohesion decreases in human eggs with advanced maternal age. Aging Cell 11: 1121–1124.

Eppig, J.J., Viveiros, M.M., Bivens, C.M. et al. (2004). Regulation of mammalian oocyte maturation. In: *The Ovary*, 2nd edn. (ed. EY Adashi and Leung P.C.K.), 113–129. San Diego: Academic Press.

Findlay, J.K., Hutt, K.J., Hickey, M. et al. (2015). How is the number of primordial follicles in the ovarian reserve established? Biol Reprod 93: 111–117.

Fragouli, E., Alfarawati, S., Spath, K. et al. (2013). The origin and impact of embryonic aneuploidy. Hum Genet 132: 1–13.

Garcia-Cruz, R., Brieno, M.A., Roig, I. et al. (2010a). Dynamics of cohesin proteins REC8, STAG3, SMC1 beta and SMC3 are consistent with a role in sister chromatid cohesion during meiosis in human oocytes. Hum Reprod 25: 2316–2327.

Garcia-Cruz, R., Casanovas, A., Brieno-Enriquez, M. et al. (2010b). Cytogenetic analyses of human oocytes provide new data on non-disjunction mechanisms and the origin of trisomy 16. Hum Reprod 25: 179–191.

Geraedts, J., Montag, M., Magli, M.C. et al. (2011). Polar body array CGH for prediction of the status of the corresponding oocyte. Part I: clinical results. Hum Reprod 26: 3173–3180.

Gray, S. and Cohen, P.E. (2016). Control of meiotic crossovers: from double-strand break formation to designation. Ann Rev Genet 50: 175–210.

Grieve, K.M., McLaughlin, M., Dunlop, C.E. et al. (2015). The controversial existence and functional potential of oogonial stem cells. Maturitas 82: 278–281.

Haarhuis, J.H.I., Elbatsh Ahmed M.O. et al. (2014. Cohesin and its regulation: on the logic of X-shaped chromosomes. Dev Cell 31: 7–18.

Handel, M.A., Eppig, J.J. and Schimenti, J.C. (2014). Applying "gold standards" to in-vitro-derived germ cells. Cell 157: 1257–1261.

Handyside, A.H., Montag, M., Magli, M.C. et al. (2012). Multiple meiotic errors caused by predivision of chromatids in women of advanced maternal age undergoing in vitro fertilisation. Eur J Hum Genet 20: 742–747.

Hassold, T.J. and Hunt P. (2001). To err (meiotically) is human: the genesis of human anuploidy. Nat Rev Genet 2: 280 – 291.

Hauf, S. and Watanabe, N. (2004). Kinetochore orientation in mitosis and meiosis. Cell 119: 317–327.

Haverfield, J., Dean, N.L., Nöel, D. et al. (2017). Tri-directional anaphases as a novel chromosome segregation defect in human oocytes. Hum Reprod 32: 1293–1303.

Herbert, M., Kalleas, D., Cooney, D. et al. (2015). Meiosis and Maternal Aging: Insights from Aneuploid Oocytes and Trisomy Births. Cold Spring Harbor Perspectives in Biology 7.

Hodges, C.A., Revenkova, E., Jessberger, R. et al. (2005). SMC1b-deficient female mice provide evidence that cohesins are a missing link in age-related nondisjunction. Nat Genet 37: 1351–1355.

Holt, J.E., Lane, S.I.R. and Jones, K.T. (2013). The control of meiotic maturation in mammalian oocytes. Curr Topics Dev Biol 102: 207–226.

Holubcová, Z., Blayney, M., Elder, K. et al. (2015). Error-prone chromosome-mediated spindle assembly favors chromosome segregation defects in human oocytes. Science 348: 1143.

Hou, Y., Fan, W., Yan, L. et al. (2013). Genome analyses of single human oocytes. Cell 155: 1492–1506.

Hunter, N. (2015). Meiotic Recombination: The Essence of Heredity. Cold Spring Harbor Perspectives in Biology 7.

Ibtissem, N., Grimes, R., Sarna, H. et al. (2017). Maternal age-dependent APC/C-mediated decrease in securin causes premature sister chromatid separation in meiosis II. Nature Communications 8:15346.

Ishiguro, T., Tanaka, K., Sakuno, T. et al. (2010). Shugoshin-PP2A counteracts casein-kinase-1-dependent cleavage of Rec8 by separase. Nat Cell Biology 12: 500–506.

Jaffe, L.A. and Egbert, J.R. (2017). Regulation of mammalian oocyte meiosis by intercellular communication within the ovarian follicle. Ann Rev Physiol 79: 237–260.

Jessberger R. (2012). Age-related aneuploidy through cohesion exhaustion. EMBO reports 13: 539.

Jonak, K., Zagoriy, I., Oz, T. et al. (2017). APC/C-Cdc20 mediates deprotection of centromeric cohesin at meiosis II in yeast. Cell Cycle 16: 1145–1152.

Jones, K.T. and Lane, S.I.R. (2013). Molecular causes of aneuploidy in mammalian eggs. Development 140: 3719–3730.

Katis, V.L., Lipp, J.J., Imre, R. et al. (2010). Rec8 phosphorylation by casein kinase 1 and Cdc7-Dbf4 kinase regulates cohesin cleavage by separase during meiosis. Dev Cell 18: 397–409.

Kawamura, K., Cheng, Y., Suzuki, N. et al. (2013.) Hippo signaling disruption and Akt stimulation of ovarian follicles for infertility treatment. Proc Natl Acad Sci 110: 17474–17479.

Kelsey, T.W., Anderson, R.A., Wright, P. et al. (2012). Data-driven assessment of the human ovarian reserve. MHR: Basic science of reproductive medicine 18: 79–87.

Lamb, N.E., Feingold, E., Savage, A. et al. (1997). Characterization of susceptible chaisma configuration that increases the risk for maternal non-disjunction of chromosome 21. Hum Mol Genet 6: 1391–1399.

Lamb, N.E., Yu, K., Shaffer, J. et al. (2005). Association between maternal age and meiotic recombination for trisomy 21. Am J Hum Genet 76: 91–99.

Lee, J. (2017). The regulation and function of cohesin and condensin in mammalian oocytes and spermatocytes. In: *Oocytes: Maternal Information and Functions* (ed. M. Kloc), 355–372. Cham: Springer International Publishing.

Li, J., Kawamura, K., Cheng, Y. et al. (2010). Activation of dormant ovarian follicles to generate mature eggs. Proc Natl Acad Sci 107: 10280–10284.

Lister, L.M., Kouznetsova, A., Hyslop, L.A. et al. (2010). Age-related meiotic segregation errors in mammalian oocytes are preceded by depletion of cohesin and Sgo2. Curr Biol CB 20: 1511–1521.

Liu, L. and Keefe, D.L. (2008). Defective cohesin is associated with age-dependent misaligned chromosomes in oocytes. Reprod BioMed Online 16: 103–112.

Lynn, A. Ashley, T. and Hassold, T. (2004). Variation in human meiotic recombination. Annual review of genomics and Hum Genet 5: 317–349.

Ma, H., O'Neil, R.C., Marti Gutierrez, N. et al. (2017). Functional human oocytes generated by transfer of polar body genomes. Cell Stem Cell 20: 112–119.

MacLennan, M., Crichton, J.H., Playfoot, C.J. et al. (2015). Oocyte development, meiosis and aneuploidy. Semin Cell Dev Biol 45: 68–76.

McNicoll, F., Stevense, M. and Jessberger, R. (2013). Cohesin in gametogenesis. Curr Top Dev Biol 103: 1–34.

Monget, P., Bobe, J., Gougeon, A. et al. ((2012)The ovarian reserve in mammals: a functional and evolutionary perspective. Mol Cell Endocrinol 356; 2–12.

Musacchio, A. and Salmon, E.D. (2007). The spindle-assembly checkpoint in space and time. Nat Rev Mol Cell Biol 8: 379–393.

Nagaoka, S.I., Hassold, T.J. and Hunt, P.A. (2012). Human aneuploidy: mechanisms and new insights into an age-old problem. Nat Rev Genet 13: 493–504.

Nakagawa, S. and FitzHarris,G. (2017). Intrinsically defective microtubule dynamics contribute to age-related chromosome segregation errors in mouse oocyte meiosis-I. Curr Biol 27: 1040–1047.

Nasmyth, K. (2011). Cohesin: a catenase with separate entry and exit gates? Nat Cell Biol 13: 1170–1177.

Oliver, T.R., Feingold, E., Yu, K. et al. (2008). New Insights into human nondisjunction of chromosome 21 in oocytes. PLoS Genet 4: e1000033.

Ottolini, C.S., Capalbo, A., Newnham, L. et al. (2016). Generation of meiomaps of genome-wide recombination and chromosome segregation in human oocytes. Nat Protocols 11: 1229–1243.

Patel, J., Tan, S.L., Hartshorne, G.M. et al. (2016). Unique geometry of sister kinetochores in human oocytes during meiosis I may explain maternal age-associated increases in chromosomal abnormalities. Biology Open 5: 178.

Pellestor, F., Andreo, B., Anahory, T. et al. (2006). The occurrence of aneuploidy in human: lessons from the cytogenetic studies of human oocytes. Eur J Med Genet 49: 103–116.

Peters, J.M., Tedeschi, A. and Schmitz, J. (2008). The cohesin complex and it roles in chromosome biology. Genes Dev 22: 3089–3114.

Rivera, T and Losada, A. (2006). Shugoshin and PP2A, shared duties at the centromere. BioEssays 28: 775–779.

Sakakibara, Y., Hashimoto, S., Nakaoka, Y. et al. (2015). Bivalent separation into univalents precedes age-related meiosis I errors in oocytes. Nat Commun 6: 7550.

Sandalinas, M., Marquez, C. and Munne, S. (2002). Spectral karyotyping of fresh, non-inseminated oocytes. Mol Hum Reprod 8: 580–585.

Schmidt, A., Rauh, N.R., Nigg, E.A. et al. (2006). Cytostatic factor: an activity that puts the cell cycle on hold. J Cell Sci 119: 1213–1218.

Telfer, E.E., Gosden, R.G., Byskov, A.G. et al. (2005). On regenerating the ovary and generating controversy. Cell 122: 821–822.

Tsutsumi, M. Fujiwara, R., Nishizawa, H. et al. (2014). Age-related decrease of meiotic cohesins in human oocytes. PLoS ONE 9: e96710.

Wallace, W.H.B. and Kelsey, T.W. (2010). Human ovarian reserve from conception to the menopause. PLOS ONE 5: e8772.

Wang, S., Hassold, T., Hunt, P. et al. (2017). Inefficient crossover maturation underlies elevated aneuploidy in human female meiosis. Cell 168: 977–989.

Watanabe, Y. (2005). Shugoshin: guardian spirit at the centromere. Current Opinion in Cell Biology 17: 590–595.

Yoon, S.-W., Lee, M.-S., Xaver, M. et al. (2016). Meiotic prophase roles of Rec8 in crossover recombination and chromosome structure. Nucleic Acids Res 44: 9296–9314.

Yun, Y., Lane, S.I.R. and Jones, K.T. (2014). Premature dyad separation in meiosis II is the major segregation error with maternal age in mouse oocytes. Development 141: 199–208.

Zielinska, A.P., Holubcova, Z., Blayney, M. et al. (2015). Sister kinetochore splitting and precocious disintegration of bivalents could explain the maternal age effect. eLife 4: e11389.

12

Female Reproductive Pathology: Peritoneal, Uterine, and Fallopian Tube Pathologies

Kenneth Ma Kin Yue, Rosa Trigas, and Edmond Edi-Osagie

Introduction

Peritoneal, uterine, and Fallopian tube factors represent a key triad of factors underpinning fertility, the others being ovarian and sperm factors. Pathologies of the peritoneum, uterus, and Fallopian tubes are common amongst women with subfertility and contribute directly or indirectly to more than half of all infertility situations. The most profound peritoneal pathologies impacting on fertility are endometriosis (including adenomyosis) and pelvic adhesive disease, uterine pathologies including uterine fibroids and synechiae, and tubal pathologies including intrinsic and extrinsic tubal blockage.

Endometriosis

Endometriosis is the presence and proliferation of endometrial tissue outside the uterine cavity (Sampson 1927). The ectopic endometrial tissue typically involves various pelvic organs including the ovaries, pelvic peritoneum, uterosacral ligaments, rectovaginal septum, Fallopian tubes, appendix, bladder, and rectum (Figure 12.1). Endometriosis has also been described in distant sites outside the pelvis including upper abdominal organs such as liver and transverse colon, diaphragm, lungs, and central nervous system (brain). The true prevalence of endometriosis is unknown but it is estimated to affect about 10% of women in the general population. Endometriosis is associated with infertility, reportedly affecting about 40% of women with infertility (Ozkan et al. 2008).

Clinical Presentation

Endometriosis is increasingly considered a chronic inflammatory condition and this is reflected in its presentation with pain, infertility, or both. Women with endometriosis typically present with difficulty conceiving (infertility), pain during menstruation (dysmenorrhoea), midcycle (periovulatory) pain, pain during sexual intercourse (dyspareunia), and chronic pelvic pain (Bellelis et al. 2010). Approximately half of these women also demonstrate other comorbidities including chronic fatigue, bowel dysfunction (including bloating, diarrhoea, constipation) and urinary dysfunction (including frequency, urgency, nocturia). Despite these symptoms, the diagnosis of endometriosis is often delayed in the western world with an average delay of 7.5 years from onset of symptoms to diagnosis (Arruda et al. 2003).

Pathophysiology of Endometriosis and Infertility

Neither the cause of endometriosis nor its mechanism for impacting fertility is fully understood. Endometriosis causes inflammation of the pelvic peritoneum with neovascularization (new vessel formation) and adhesion formation which in moderate to severe cases can lead to damage to reproductive organs by way of distortion of pelvic anatomy particularly affecting the Fallopian tubes and ovaries (Figure 12.2).

There appears to be an association between endometriosis and subfertility, but a causal link has not been fully established. The degree of subfertility is

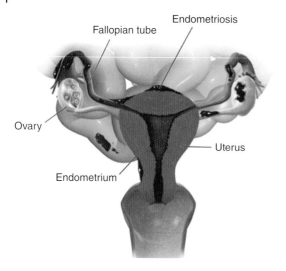

Figure 12.1 Endometriosis explants located on various parts of the female reproductive system. *Source:* Blausen Medical – Wikimedia.

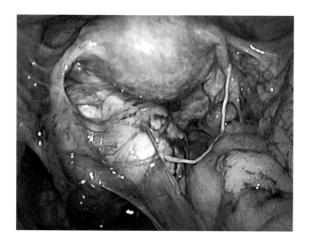

Figure 12.2 Endometriosis with adhesions. *Source:* Wikimedia.

generally related to the severity of endometriosis but not necessarily the intensity of pain as classified by the American Society for Reproductive Medicine (ARSM). This classification utilizes visual assessment at surgery with a score calculated based on the number, size, position, and depth of endometrial lesions and the presence and type of adhesions. The total score is arbitrarily categorized into minimal, mild, moderate, and severe grades of the disease.

The mechanism by which endometriosis impacts fertility in women with minimal or mild endometriosis without adhesion formation or distortion of pelvic organs is poorly understood. A number of mechanisms have been hypothesized including: increased production of prostaglandins, cytokines, and chemokines in the peritoneal fluid interfering with sperm–egg binding and fertilization (Bulun 2009); inhibitory effects of peritoneal fluid on sperm function through the action of macrophages and cytokines (Aeby et al. 1996; Pillai et al. 1998); abnormal cytokine expression and oxidative stress interfering with interaction between sperm and egg (Faber et al. 2001; Baker and Aitken 2004). There is also evidence that endometriosis impacts negatively on oocyte and embryo quality (Al-Azemi et al. 2000; Barcelos et al. 2009). Anti-Müllerian hormone levels in women with endometriosis undergoing *in vitro* fertilization (IVF) has been found to be lower than those in women without endometriosis and this has been correlated to severity of the disease, suggesting endometriosis directly affects ovarian reserve (Shebl et al. 2009).

There is evidence of abnormal endometrial development and function in women with endometriosis with demonstration of abnormal oestradiol production and progesterone resistance with negative effect on implantation (Burney et al. 2007; Dassen et al. 2007). This can be reversed by prolonged ovarian suppression prior to IVF to normalize endometrial development and this has been shown to achieve higher embryo implantation rates (Sallam et al. 2006).

Treatment for Subfertility

The approach to treatment of endometriosis will depend on the symptoms and fertility desire of the patient. Treatment options available aim to reduce or alleviate symptoms of pain and/or improve fertility by reducing or removing ectopic endometrial tissue.

Expectant Treatment

Whilst conception rates of women with endometriosis are reduced compared with women without endometriosis, it is reasonable for the affected couple to continue trying for pregnancy, as long as there are no other factors precluding spontaneous conception. In a prospective study, women with minimal or mild endometriosis treated expectantly achieved conception rates of 21.9% after 9 months of follow-up (Marcoux et al. 1997).

Medical Treatment

Endometriotic glands are hormonally sensitive and so medical treatment for endometriosis aims to block ovarian function. These treatments include hormonal contraceptives, continuous progestogens, GnRH analogues, and Danazol. Hormonal treatments, however, cause anovulation thereby preventing spontaneous conception. Although there is evidence to support their use in reducing symptoms of pain and the risk of recurrence after surgery (De Ziegler et al. 2010; Dunselman et al. 2014), spontaneous conception rate does not improve after cessation of treatment (Hughes et al. 2007). Medical treatment of endometriosis is therefore not recommended for women who also have subfertility.

Surgical Treatment

Surgical treatment of endometriosis aims to remove or destroy peritoneal or deep endometriotic lesions, treat endometriomas, and divide adhesions in order to restore normal pelvic anatomy. Endometriotic deposits are commonly excised or ablated through laparoscopic surgery. Laparoscopic surgery is generally preferred to open surgery because it is associated with better access to the pelvis, less pain, shorter hospital stay, quicker recovery and improved cosmetic outcomes. A variety of techniques have been developed including excision with diathermy scissors or other energy device, or ablation by laser or diathermy. Excision of endometriotic lesions has the advantage of allowing histological examination and diagnosis and ablation is generally not feasible for deep infiltrating lesions (Dunselman et al. 2014).

It has been demonstrated in women with minimal to mild endometriosis that operative laparoscopic treatment is superior to diagnostic laparoscopy alone in improving spontaneous on-going pregnancy rates and symptoms of pain (Jacobson et al. 2010). Although some studies have suggested that CO_2 laser vaporization of endometriosis is associated with higher spontaneous pregnancy rates compared with monopolar electrocoagulation (Chang et al. 1997), there is insufficient evidence to support one technique over the other in achieving on-going pregnancy. For women with endometriosis involving the ovaries (endometrioma), ovarian cystectomy including surgical excision of the endometriotic cyst wall improves symptoms of pain and spontaneous pregnancy rates (Hart et al. 2008). However, reduction of ovarian mass, and in consequence ovarian reserve, is associated with ovarian cystectomy as excision of the endometrioma cyst wall inevitably leads to loss of healthy ovarian tissue (Tsolakidis et al. 2010).

For women with moderate to severe endometriosis, the evidence shows that surgical management is associated with improved quality of life and relief of endometriosis-related pain. However, there is only sparse evidence for increased pregnancy rates compared with expectant management (Dunselman et al. 2014). Surgical management of severe endometriosis is associated with significant complication rates and therefore requires careful prior counselling (Kondo et al. 2011).

Medically Assisted Reproduction

The evidence for surgery improving cumulative spontaneous pregnancy rates is limited in endometriosis patients with compromised tubal function, male factor subfertility, or following other unsuccessful fertility treatments and so these patients are best advised to pursue assisted conception. Intrauterine insemination with controlled ovarian stimulation is a reasonable option in young women since it increases live birth rates (Tummon et al. 1997). If performed within 6 months of surgical treatment, pregnancy rates are similar to those achieved with unexplained subfertility (Werbrouck et al. 2006). A sizeable proportion of women with moderate to severe endometriosis will require assisted conception by way of IVF or intracytoplasmic sperm injection (ICSI). Patients who have had surgical treatment of endometriosis are not at increased risk of recurrence following controlled ovarian stimulation.

There is a specific role for gonadotropin-releasing hormones (GnRH) analogues prior to fertility treatment in patients with endometrioma or adenomyosis who require assisted conception. GnRH analogues for 3–6 months prior to assisted conception have been shown to improve clinical pregnancy rates in such situations (Sallam et al. 2006)

There is doubtful benefit of laparoscopic treatment of stage I/II endometriosis prior to assisted conception. In patients who have endometriomas, there is no evidence that ovarian cystectomy prior to assisted conception improves pregnancy rates (Benschop et al. 2010) and these patients are counselled about the risks of reduced ovarian reserve after surgery. Surgery is, however, recommended in women with endometriosis-associated pain or where access to the ovaries is compromised.

Fallopian Tube Pathology

Fallopian tube pathology is responsible for 25–35% of infertility in women (Schlegel et al. 2013) and tubal pathologies such as peritubal adhesions, proximal and/or distal tubal blockage, hydrosalpinx formation, and endosalpingeal damage all have an adverse impact on fertility (Figure 12.3).

Aetiology

Pelvic inflammatory disease usually resulting from sexually transmitted infections is the commonest cause of tubal damage; 50-70% of tubal factor infertility is the result of *Chlamydia trachomatis*

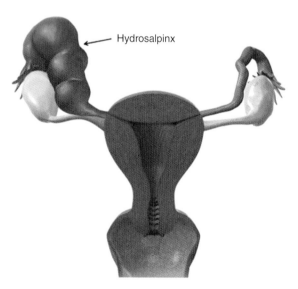

Figure 12.3 Extended Fallopian tube due to hydrosalpinx. *Source:* Bruceblaus, 2016. https://commons.wikimedia.org/wiki/Category:Hydrosalpinx#/media/File:Hydrosalpinx.png. CC BY-SA 4.0.

infection, but other common causative microorganisms include *Neisseria gonorrhoeae*, *Escherichia coli*, and Mycoplasma (Bevan et al. 1995). Infection and inflammation leads to deciliation (loss of tubal cilia) and/or reduced ciliary activity of the Fallopian tubes (Mardh et al. 1979; Cooper et al. 1990). Pelvic inflammatory disease can also result as a complication of miscarriage, termination of pregnancy, puerperal sepsis, and surgical procedures involving the uterine cavity.

In addition to pelvic inflammatory disease, adhesions involving the Fallopian tubes can occur secondary to infection or inflammation associated with surgical procedures (Bhattacharya et al. 2014). The consequences of peritubal adhesions depend on their location, severity, and resultant degree of mechanical distortion of the tubo-ovarian anatomy and distal obstruction of the Fallopian tubes.

Investigations

Investigations for tubal pathology are an essential part of the comprehensive assessment of couples presenting with subfertility. These investigations include hysterosalpingography (HSG) and hysterosalpingo-contrast-sonography (HyCoSy), the standard first-line tests to evaluate tubal patency (NICE, 2013). HSG involves X-ray examination facilitated by injection of contrast material through a cannula inserted into the uterus. HyCoSy involves transvaginal ultrasound scanning whilst injecting contrast into the uterus. Alternative investigations include transvaginal hydrolaparoscopy but this requires expertise that is limited to specialist centres.

Laparoscopic dye test remains the gold standard in evaluating tubal patency (Tsuji et al. 2012) and is recommended as the first-line test for patients who are known to have risk factors for tubal pathology (including history of ectopic pregnancy, pelvic inflammatory disease, endometriosis and prior pelvic surgery). Laparoscopy enables direct visual inspection of the entire external length of the Fallopian tubes and other pelvic organs which improves its diagnostic accuracy and there is the chance of opportunistic treatment of other pathologies (such as endometriosis and periadnexal adhesions) adding a therapeutic benefit (Yalanadu and Narvekar 2014)

Depending on the site of occlusion, tubal pathology can be categorized as proximal or distal tubal disease. Diagnosis of proximal tubal occlusion is usually made at hysterosalpingography and is characterized by failure of contrast medium to advance into the Fallopian tube beyond the intramural–isthmic portion. This is thought to be found in 10–25% of women with tubal pathology (NICE 2013). Occlusion secondary to pelvic inflammatory disease with postinfection fibrosis is thought to be the primary cause, although this may be an artefactual finding or secondary to spasm of the uterine–tubal ostium at hysterosalpingography (Marana et al. 1992).

Distal tubal disease accounts for approximately 85% of tubal infertility (Yalanadu and Narvekar 2014). It is characterized by fimbrial agglutination by adhesions, and phimosis with or without complete occlusion, with hydrosalpinx formation representing the end stage of distal tubal disease. HSG or laparoscopy typically shows tubal fill of contrast media or blue dye but slow or no spillage of the dye into the pelvis.

Treatment of Tubal Disease

Management of tubal pathology depends on the type and severity of tubal damage and presence/absence of other fertility factors. In milder cases surgery can be effective in improving the chances of natural conception but in more severe cases it is generally used to complement assisted conception.

In proximal tubal occlusion, management options include assisted conception or tubal cannulation. Tubal cannulation involves overcoming the proximal tubal occlusion using a guidewire, and this may be achieved hysteroscopically or radiologically. No controlled studies have been performed to evaluate its efficacy but cohort studies report recanalization is successful in approximately 75% of cases with subsequent pregnancy and livebirth rates of 10–20% (Gazzera et al. 1998; Lang and Dunaway 2000).

Prognosis of distal tubal occlusion depends on the severity of damage. Patients with mild adhesions, mildly dilated tubes (<3 cm), and normal endosalpinx with preservation of mucosal folds have better prognosis following surgical treatment (Tulandi et al. 1990). For these patients, surgical correction by laparoscopic neosalpingostomy and fimbrioplasty to open the hydrosalpinx or excise the fimbrial phimosis may be successful in increasing the chances of spontaneous intrauterine pregnancy rates to 58–77%. In comparison, surgical management in patients with severe disease only achieves spontaneous pregnancy rates of 0–22% (Nackley and Muasher 1998).

For patients with extensive peritubal adhesions, massively dilated tubes with thick fibrotic walls, and/or sparse or absent luminal mucosa, salpingectomy may be indicated. Hydrosalpinges have a detrimental effect on IVF success rates with approximately 50% lower rates of pregnancy, implantation, and live birth (Camus et al. 1999). The exact mechanism for this detrimental effect is unclear but may be secondary to mechanical flushing of embryos from the endometrial cavity, decreased endometrial receptivity, or direct toxic effect of the hydrosalpinx fluid on embryos (Mukherjee et al. 1996). In patients with hydrosalpinges, the on-going pregnancy rate with IVF treatment after laparoscopic salpingectomy or tubal occlusion is approximately twofold higher than following IVF in the presence of the hydrosalpinx (Kontoravdis et al. 2006).

Current evidence supports laparoscopic salpingectomy with tubal occlusion as an alternative procedure since there is no significant advantage of either surgical procedure in terms of ongoing pregnancy (Johnson et al. 2010). The evidence base for this is correlated to disease severity and therefore is strongest for ultrasound visible and bilateral disease (Strandell and Lindhard 2000). The presence of bilateral disease, however, raises an ethical dilemma as bilateral salpingectomy renders the woman entirely dependent on IVF for conception. Management of these women is therefore individualized based on age, presence of co-aetiologies and local/personal resources available to fund the treatments.

In younger women, cuff salpingostomy, preferably by laparoscopic approach, may be considered, aiming to create a new ostium of the Fallopian tube with well-everted fimbrial mucosa. The main advantage is that the chance of spontaneous subsequent pregnancy is potentiated while the disadvantage is that reclusion may occur. Further evidence is required to assess the value of ultrasound-guided aspiration of hydrosalpinges.

Uterine Fibroids

Uterine fibroids are benign tumours of the uterine smooth muscle, originating from the myometrium (Islam et al. 2013). They are also known as leiomyomas or myomas and occur in 20–40% of women of reproductive age, with incidence increasing with age (Baird et al. 2003). They are responsive to hormones and oestrogens are known to promote their growth (Marsh and Bulun 2006).

Clinical Presentation

Fibroids are commonly asymptomatic and may be identified incidentally by examination or investigation for other gynaecological problems (such as failure to conceive) or during a routine pregnancy assessment. They can be associated with heavy menstrual bleeding and symptoms related to direct pressure on pelvic organs including bladder and bowel (Donnez and Jadoul 2002).

Mechanism of Infertility

The presence of uterine fibroids is associated with significantly decreased implantation, clinical pregnancy, and ongoing pregnancy/livebirth rates but the magnitude of this impact depends on their size, number, and location (Pritts et al. 2009).

The relationship between fibroids and subfertility is poorly understood and there are a number of hypothesis on how fibroids impact fertility but no studies have shown direct causation. Depending on their size and location, anatomical distortion is thought to have some impact on the transport of sperm, egg, or embryo within the reproductive system. In addition, fibroids are known to influence the contractility of the myometrium and are associated with a chronic inflammatory environment, which may inhibit implantation (Yoshino et al. 2010). The intrauterine cytokine environment important for implantation to occur has also been shown to be different in women with fibroids, with lower levels of IL10 and glycodelin (Ben-Nagi et al. 2010).

Diagnosis

The presence of uterine fibroids is usually suspected on pelvic examination showing an enlarged irregular uterus. Pelvic ultrasound is the imaging study of choice for diagnosing uterine fibroids, having high sensitivity (90–100%) and specificity (87–98%), and appearing to be as efficient as magnetic resonance imaging (MRI) in fibroid detection (Fedele et al.

1991; Becker et al. 2002). MRI is useful if ultrasound findings are inadequate for planning management particularly in cases with more than five lesions, if the diagnosis is uncertain, and to exclude adenomyosis and uterine sarcoma (Dueholm et al. 2002). If there is an intracavitary fibroid (submucosal or intramural that protrudes into the uterine cavity), saline infusion sonography or hysteroscopy is useful to evaluate the uterine cavity.

Classification of Fibroids

Fibroids are classified according to their anatomical location in relation to the endometrium, myometrium, and serosa (Munro et al. 2011) (Figure 12.4). Submucosal fibroids distort the endometrial cavity and are further classified into Type 0, 1, and 2 according to the extent the fibroid protrudes into the cavity. This group of fibroids have the most impact on implantation, clinical pregnancy, ongoing pregnancy and livebirth rates as well as increased risks of spontaneous miscarriage (Pritts et al. 2009). Intramural fibroids lie within the myometrial layer with no extension into the endometrium or serosa. There is evidence to suggest intramural fibroids are

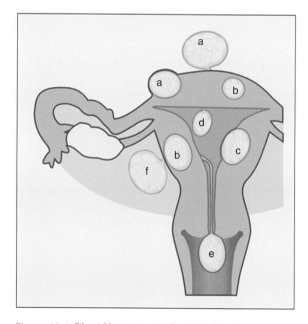

Figure 12.4 Fibroid location. a, Subserosal fibroids; b, intramural fibroids; c, submucosal fibroid;, pedunculated submucosal fibroid; e, fibroid in statu nascendi; f, intraligamental fibroid. *Source:* Wikimedia.

associated with reduction in fertility but their impact, if any, appears to be less significant than submucosal fibroids. Subserosal fibroids lie predominantly under the uterine serosa. Current evidence suggests these fibroids have little impact on fertility or spontaneous miscarriage (Pritts et al. 2009).

Management of Fibroids

Medical Management

No pharmacological agents cure fibroids and so medical management is generally aimed at symptom control by targeting the oestrogen and progesterone pathways. Fibroids are oestrogen-dependent conditions and so it is little surprise that the most commonly used medical strategies target these pathways, including GnRH analogues and selective progesterone receptor modulators, both effective in reducing menstrual blood loss and fibroid volume. They, however, are associated with suppression of ovulation and interfere with the target action of oestrogen and progesterone making them undesirable for the subfertile woman.

Surgical Management

Submucosal fibroids and pedunculated fibroids protruding into the uterine cavity may be removed by hysteroscopic myomectomy. This is minimally invasive and may be carried out as day case surgery. For subfertile women with submucosal fibroids, myomectomy has been shown to increase spontaneous conception and clinical pregnancy rates, but not on-going pregnancy or livebirth rates (Casini et al. 2006; Pritts et al. 2009). Intramural or subserosal fibroids generally require an abdominal approach by open or laparoscopic surgery (Figure 12.5).

Surgical management with the intention of improving pregnancy rates remains controversial for women with intramural fibroids. A few studies have suggested that myomectomy before assisted conception is likely to improve pregnancy outcomes with intramural fibroids >5 cm (Bulletti et al. 2004). However, there is currently no clear evidence to support myomectomy in this situation (Pritts et al. 2009; Metwally et al. 2012). Furthermore, myomectomy is associated with significant morbidity, with risks of intraperitoneal adhesion formation as well as increased risks of uterine rupture and requirement for Caesarean delivery with subsequent pregnancy (Metwally et al. 2012).

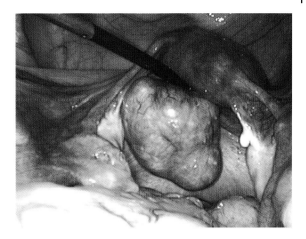

Figure 12.5 Large subserosal leimyoma of the uterus. *Source:* Wikimedia.

Other Interventions

Other interventions less commonly used are uterine artery embolization (UAE) and myolisis (by diathermy, laser, radiofrequency ablation, or MRI-guided focused ultrasound). UAE involves cannulating the femoral artery and identifying the uterine arteries before injecting an embolic agent into them to impair their blood supply. The long-term impact of UAE on fertility remains unknown and so more evidence is needed to establish its role if any in women wishing to retain their fertility (NICE 2013).

Intrauterine Adhesions (Asherman Syndrome)

Intrauterine adhesions, also referred to as intrauterine synechiae, are a consequence of scar tissue developing within the uterine cavity. Intrauterine adhesions accompanied by symptoms (such as subfertility and/or amenorrhoea) is referred to as Asherman syndrome. The true prevalence of intrauterine adhesions is difficult to establish because the condition is rare in the general population and often asymptomatic. Estimates of the prevalence range from 1.5% as an incidental finding at hysterosalpingogram to 21.5% of women with a history of postpartum uterine curettage (Deans and Abbott 2010).

(a) (b)

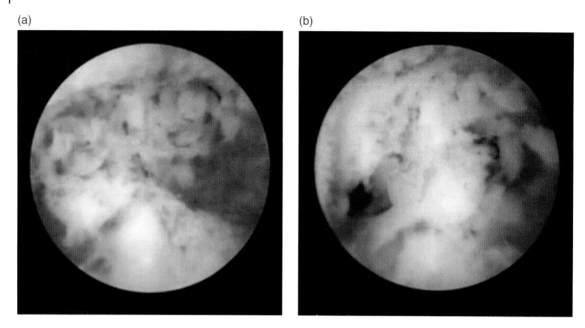

Figure 12.6 Hysteroscopic view of Asherman syndrome. (a) Entrance to the cervix. (b) Adhesions in the uterine cavity. *Source:* https://commons.wikimedia.org/wiki/File:Hysteroscopy_of_Asherman%27s_Syndrome_cropped.jpg?uselang=en-gb. CC BY-SA 2.0.

Aetiology and Risk Factors

Intrauterine adhesions typically result from intrauterine trauma associated with a surgical procedure, although infection may play a minor contributory role. Approximately 90% of cases of severe intrauterine adhesive disease are related to uterine curettage for pregnancy complications, increasing the risk of adhesions if curetting is happening at a later gestational age, 2–4 weeks after delivery, or in cases of repeated curettage following a pregnancy loss (Hooker et al. 2014). Less commonly, it has been associated with uterine compression sutures used to treat severe postpartum haemorrhage (Poujade et al. 2011) and occasionally to intrauterine devices. Adhesions can develop in the nongravid uterus as a result of endometrial injury from procedures such as myomectomy, curettage for indications not related to pregnancy, as a complication of hysteroscopic myomectomy, and after genital tuberculosis. (Al-Inany 2001; Sharma et al. 2008; Mazzon et al. 2014).

Pathogenesis

The basalis layer of the endometrium appears to be more susceptible to damage when curettage is done in the first 4 weeks after delivery or miscarriage, leading to the formation of granular tissue healing on opposing surfaces of the uterus, which eventually fuse and produce tissue bridges. These intrauterine adhesions range from filmy adhesions composed of endometrial tissue to dense adhesions consisting entirely of connective (fibrous) tissue with partial or complete obliteration of the uterine cavity (Figure 12.6). They may impede menstrual flow or interfere with conception or pregnancy. In addition, vascularization may be compromised due to endometrial damage and scarring (Chen et al. 2013).

Clinical Presentation

Intrauterine adhesions may be asymptomatic and found as incidental findings in women undergoing pelvic ultrasound, saline infusion sonohysterography, hysterosalpingography, or hysteroscopy for other indications (such as subfertility or abnormal uterine bleeding). Intrauterine adhesions most commonly present with subfertility or abnormal uterine bleeding patterns (amenorrhoea, hypomenorrhoea) but they can be associated with cyclical pelvic pain and recurrent pregnancy loss. Fertility may be compromised by obstruction of sperm passage into the uterine cavity if the lower uterine segment is occluded or by destruction of the endometrium which will prevent implantation of the embryo. Recurrent pregnancy loss may occur as a result of impaired implantation in areas of denuded endometrium or insufficient vascularization (Deans and Abbott 2010).

Diagnostic Evaluation

The main components of the diagnostic evaluation of intrauterine adhesions are medical history and hysteroscopy. Pelvic imaging may be the initial test that suggests presence of intrauterine adhesions. Other tests such as sonohysterography or hysterosalpingography may detect adhesions but provide less information than hysteroscopy. Hysteroscopy is the gold standard for diagnosis of intrauterine adhesions and can be performed in an office or operating room setting. Hysteroscopy allows diagnosis and treatment in the same procedure and decreases the probability of trauma to the surrounding endometrium compared with blind adhesiolysis (AAGL Practice Report 2010).

Prevention

There are no established approaches to the prevention of intrauterine adhesions but avoidance of vigorous uterine curettage is one potential measure. Medical management of spontaneous miscarriage offers an advantage over surgical management in this regard, as does expectant management. If curettage is performed, it is preferable to avoid delaying the procedure or using metal curettes.

Management

Intrauterine adhesions are treated by hysteroscopic resection of adhesions with the goal of surgery being to restore the size and shape of the uterine cavity, as well as endometrial function and fertility (Yu et al. 2008). Treatment of intrauterine adhesions is indicated only in symptomatic women or those that are planning future childbearing. For asymptomatic women or those who are not actively trying to conceive, treatment of intrauterine adhesions may result in surgical complications in the absence of clinical benefit. A hysterotomy is rarely performed in current practice and is reserved for severe cases where the cavity cannot be entered with the hysteroscope. The recurrence rate following treatment is as high as 33% in women with mild to moderate adhesions and 66% in women with severe adhesions (AAGL Practice Report 2010).

Several treatments have been proposed to prevent recurrence of adhesions after surgery and promote regrowth of the endometrium, including oestrogen therapy, placement of an intrauterine device or bladder catheter immediately after adhesiolysis with removal after 3 months, or use of an intrauterine gel (Orhue et al. 2003). None of these strategies has been demonstrated to be beneficial. Second-look hysteroscopy 2–3 months after adhesiolysis is commonly performed for follow-up assessment, but the use of serial hysteroscopic procedures at shorter time intervals has been described as a further method of preventing adhesion reformation.

Outcome

Data is inconsistent about the efficacy of treatment of intrauterine adhesions in women with subfertility. In a systematic review of 28 studies, pregnancy rates ranged from 40 to 80% with live birth rates of 30–70% (Johary et al. 2014). Women who have hysteroscopic adhesiolysis have a 10% risk of adherent placenta including placenta accreta in subsequent pregnancy (Roy et al. 2010). The likelihood of pregnancy following adhesiolysis appears to vary directly with the severity of the disease. In a retrospective study of 357 women who underwent hysteroscopic adhesion resection and were followed up for a mean of 27 ± 9 months, pregnancy rates after adhesiolysis were 61% for mild disease, 53% for moderate disease, and 25% for severe disease (Chen et al. 2017). The mean time to conception was 9.7 ± 3.7 months, miscarriage rate was 9.4%, and overall live birth rate was 86%.

Conclusion

Uterine and tubal pathologies can account for up to 50% of the causes of female infertility. With careful investigation, a diagnosis can be made, and appropriate treatment options for women with fertility problems can enhance their chances of pregnancy.

References

AAGL Advancing Minimally Invasive Gynecology Worldwide (2010). AAGL practice report: practice guidelines for management of intrauterine synechiae. J Minim Invasive Gynecol 17: 1.

Aeby, T.C., Huang, T. and Nakayama, R.T. (1996). The effect of peritoneal fluid from patients with endometriosis on human sperm function in vitro. Am J Obstet Gynecol 174: 1779–1783.

Al-Azemi, M., Bernal, A.L., Steele, J. et al. (2000). Ovarian response to repeated controlled stimulation in in-vitro fertilization cycles in patients with ovarian endometriosis. Hum Reprod 15: 72–75.

Al-Inany H. (2001). Intrauterine adhesions. An update. Acta Obstet Gynecol Scand 80: 986.

Arruda, M.S., Petta, C.A., Abrão, M.S. et al. (2003). Time elapsed from onset of symptoms to diagnosis of endometriosis in a cohort study of Brazilian women. Hum Reprod 18: 756–759.

Baird, D., Dunson, D.B., Hill, M.C. et al. (2003). High cumulative invidence of uterine leiomyoma in black and white women: ultrasound evidence. Am J Obstet Gynecol 188: 100–107.

Baker, M.A. and Aitken, R.J. (2004). The importance of redox regulated pathways in sperm cell biology. Mol Cell Endocrinol 216: 47–54.

Barcelos, I.D., Vieira, R.C., Ferreira, E.M. et al. (2009). Comparative analysis of the spindle and chromosome configurations of in vitro-matured oocytes from patients with endometriosis and from control subjects: a pilot study. Fertil Steril 92: 1749–1752.

Becker, E., Jr, Lev-Toaff, A.S. and Kaufman, E.P. (2002). The added value of transvaginal sonohysterography over transvaginal sonography alone in women with known or suspected leiomyoma. J. Ultrasound Med 21:237–247.

Bellelis, P., Dias, J.A. Jr., Podgaec, S. et al. (2010). Epidemiological and clinical aspects of pelvic endometriosis-a case series. Rev Assoc Med Bras 56: 467–471.

Ben-Nagi, J., Miell, J., Mavrelos, D. et al. (2010). Endometrial implantation factors in women with submucous uterine fibroids. Reprod Biomed Online 21: 610–615.

Benschop, L., Farquhar, C., van der Poel, N. et al. (2010). Interventions for women with endometrioma prior to assisted reproductive technology. Cochrane Database of Systematic Reviews Issue 11.

Bevan, C.D., Johal, B.J., Mumtaz, G. et al. (1995). Clinical, laparoscopic and microbiological findings in acute salpingitis: report on a United Kingdom cohort. BJOG 102: 407–414

Bhattacharya, S. and Hamilton, M. ed. (2014). *Management of Infertility for the MRCOG and Beyond*, 3rd edn. Cambridge: Cambridge University Press.

Bulletti, C., Ziegler, D., Levi,S.P. et al. (2004). Myomas, pregnancy outcome, and in vitro fertilization. Ann NY Acad Sci 1034: 84–92.

Bulun, S.E. (2009). Endometriosis. N Engl J Med 360:268.

Burney, R.O., Talbi, S., Hamilton, A.E. et al. (2007). Gene expression analysis of endometrium reveals progesterone resistance and candidate susceptibility genes in women with endometriosis. Endocrinology 148: 3814–3826.

Camus, E., Poncelet, C., Goffinet, F. et al. (1999). Pregnancy rates after in-vitro fertilization in cases of tubal infertility with and without hydrosalpinx: a meta-analysis of published comparative studies. Hum Reprod 14: 1243–1249.

Casini, M.L., Rossi, F., Agostini, R. et al. (2006). Effects of position of fibroids on fertility. Gynecol Endocrinol 22: 106–109

Chang, F.H., Chou, H.H., Soong, Y.K. et al. (1997). Efficacy of isotopic 13CO2 laser laparoscopic evaporation in the treatment of infertile patients with minimal and mild endometriosis: a life table cumulative pregnancy rates study. J Am Assoc Gynecol Laparosc 4: 219–223.

Chen, L., Zhang, H., Wang, Q., et al. (2017). Reproductive outcomes in patients with intrauterine adhesions following hysteroscopic adhesiolysis: experience from the largest women's hospital in China. J Minim Invasive Gynecol 24:299.

Chen, Y., Chang, Y. and Yao, S. (2013). Role of angiogenesis in endometrial repair of patients with severe intrauterine adhesion. Int J Clin Exp Pathol 6: 1343–1350.

Cooper, M.D., Rapp, J., Jeffery-Wiseman, C. et al. (1990). Chlamydia trachomatis infection of human fallopian tube organ cultures. J Gen Microbiol 136: 1109–1115.

Dassen, H., Punyadeera, C., Kamps, R. et al. (2007). Estrogen metabolizing enzymes in endometrium and endometriosis. Hum Reprod 22: 3148–3158.

Deans, R. and Abbott, J. (2010). Review of intrauterine adhesions. J Minim Invasive Gynecol 17: 555.

Donnez, J. and Jadoul, P. (2002). What are the implications of myomas on fertility? A need for a debate? Hum Reprod 17: 1424–1430.

Dueholm, M., Lundorf, E., Sørensen, J.S. et al. (2002). Reproducibility of evaluation of the uterus by transvaginal sonography, hysterosonographic examination, hysteroscopy and magnetic resonance imaging. Hum Reprod 17: 195–200.

Dunselman, N., Vermeulen, C., Becker, C. et al. (2014). ESHRE guideline: management of women with endometriosis. Hum Reprod 29: 400–412.

Faber, B.M., Chegini, N., Mahony, M.C. et al. (2001). Macrophage secretory products and sperm zona pellucida binding. Obstet Gynecol 98: 668–673.

Fedele, I., Bianchi, S., Dorta, M. et al. (1991). Transvaginal ultrasonography versus hysteroscopy in the diagnosis of uterine submucous myomas. Obstet Gynecol 77:745–748.

Gazzera, C., Gallo, T., Faissola B. et al. (1998). Tubal catheterisation and selective salpingography. Rays 23: 735–741.

Hart, R.J., Hickey, M., Maouris, P. et al. (2008). Excisional surgery versus ablative surgery for ovarian endometriomata. Cochrane Database Syst Rev 16: CD004992.

Hooker, A.B., Lemmers, M., Thurkow, A.L. et al. (2014). Systematic review and meta-analysis of intrauterine adhesions after miscarriage: prevalence, risk factors and long-term reproductive outcome. Hum Reprod Update 20: 262.

Hughes, E., Brown, J., Collins J.J. et al. (2007). Ovulation suppression for endometriosis. Cochrane Database Syst Rev 3: CD000155.

Islam, M.S., Protic, O., Stortoni, P. et al. (2013). Complex networks of multiple factors in the pathogenesis of uterine leiomyoma. Fertil Steril 100: 178–193.

Jacobson, T.Z., Duffy, J.M., Barlow, D. et al. Laparoscopic surgery for subfertility associated with endometriosis. Cochrane Database Syst Rev 2010: CD001398.

Johary, J., Xue, M., Zhu, X. et al. (2014). Efficacy of estrogen therapy in patients with intrauterine adhesions: systematic review. J Minim Invasive Gynecol 21: 44.

Johnson, N.P., Mak,W. and Sowter, M.C. (2010). Surgical treatment for tubal disease in women due to undergo in vitro fertilisation. Cochrane Database Syst Rev 3: CD002125.

Kondo, W., Bourdel, N., Tamburro, S. et al. (2011). Complications after surgery for deeply infiltrating pelvic endometriosis. BJOG 118: 292–298.

Kontoravdis, A., Makrakis, E., Pantos, K. et al. (2006). Proximal tubal occlusion and salpingectomy result in similar improvements in in vitro fertilisation outcome in patients with hydrosalpinx. Fertil Steril 86: 1642–1649.

Lang, E.K. and Dunaway, H.E. (2000). Efficacy of salpingography and transcervical recanalization in diagnosis, categorisation, and treatment of fallopian tube obstruction. Cardiovasc Int Radiol 23: 427–422.

Marana. R., Muzii, L., Paielli, F.V. et al. (1992). Proximal tubal obstruction: are we over-diagnosing and over-treating? Gynecol Endosc 1: 99–101.

Marcoux, S., Maheux, R., Bérubé, S. and the Canadian Collaborative Group on Endometriosis (1997). Laparoscopic surgery in infertile women with minimal or mild endometriosis. N Engl J Med 337: 217–222.

Mardh, P.A., Baldetorp, B., Hakansson, C.H. et al. (1979). Studies of ciliated epithelia of the human genital tract. 3: mucociliary wave activity in organ cultures of human fallopian tubes challenged with Neisseria gonorrhoeae and gonococcal endotoxin. Br J Vener Dis 55: 256–264.

Marsh, E.E. and Bulun, S.E. (2006). Steroid hormones and leiomyomas. Obstet Gynecol Clin North Am 33: 59–67.

Mazzon, I., Favilli, A., Cocco, P. et al. (2014). Does cold loop hysteroscopic myomectomy reduce intrauterine adhesions? A retrospective study. Fertil Steril 101: 294–298.

Metwally, M., Cheong, Y. and Horne, A. (2012). Surgical management of fibroids for subfertility. Cochrane Database Syst Rev 11: CD003857.

Mukherjee, T., Copperman, A.B., McCaffrey, C. et al. (1996). Hydrosalpinx fluid has embryotoxic effects on murine embrogenesis: a case for prophylactic salpingectomy. Fertil Steril 66: 851–853.

Munro, M.G., Critchley, H.O., Broder, M.S. et al. (2011). FIGO Working Group on Menstrual Disorders. FIGO classification system (PALM-COEIN) for causes of abnormal uterine bleeding in nongravid women of reproductive age. Int J Gynaecol Obstet 113: 1–2.

Nackley, A.C. and Muasher, S.J. (1998). The significance of hydrosalpinx in in vitro fertilization. Fertil Steril 69: 373–384.

National Institute for Clinical Excellence (2013). *Fertility Problems. Assessment and Treatment.* London: RCOG.

Orhue, A.A., Aziken, M.E. and Igbefoh, J.O. (2003). A comparison of two adjunctive treatments for intrauterine adhesions following lysis. Int J Gynaecol Obstet 82:49.

Ozkan, S., Murk, W. and Arici A. (2008). Endometriosis and Infertility. Epidemiology and evidence based treatments. Ann N Y Acad Sci 1127: 92–100.

Pillai, S., Rust, P.F. and Howard L. (1998). Effects of antibodies to transferrin and alpha 2-HS glycoprotein on in vitro sperm motion: implications in infertility associated with endometriosis. Am J Reprod Immunol 39: 235–242.

Poujade, O., Grossetti, A., Mougel, L. et al. (2011). Risk of synechiae following uterine compression sutures in the management of major postpartum haemorrhage. BJOG 118: 433.

Pritts, E.A., Parker, W.H. and Olive, D.L. (2009). Fibroids and infertility: an updated systematic review of the evidence. Fertil Steril 91: 1215–1223.

Roy, K.K., Baruah, J., Sharma, J.B., et al. (2010). Reproductive outcome following hysteroscopic adhesiolysis in patients with infertility due to Asherman's syndrome. Arch Gynecol Obstet 281:355.

Sallam, H.N., Garcia-Velasco, J.A., Dias, S. et al. (2006). Long-term pituitary down-regulation before in vitro fertilization (IVF) for women with endometriosis. Cochrane Database Syst Rev 25: CD004635.

Sampson, J.A. (1927). Peritoneal endometriosis due to premenstrual dissemination of endometrial tissue into the peritoneal cavity. Am J Obstet Gynecol 14: 46.

Shebl, O., Ebner, T., Sommergruber, M. et al. (2009). Anti muellerian hormone serum levels in women with endometriosis: a case-control study. Gynecol Endocrinol 25: 713–716.

Schlegel, P.N., Fauser, B.C., Carrel, D.T. et al. (2013). *Biennial Review of Infertility.* London: Springer.

Sharma, J.B., Roy, K.K., Pushparaj, M. et al. (2008). Genital tuberculosis: an important cause of Asherman's syndrome in India. Arch Gynecol Obstet 277: 37–41.

Strandell, A. and Lindhard, A. (2000). Hydrosalpinx and ART. Salpingectomy prior to IVF can be recommended to a well-defined subgroup of patients. Hum Reprod 15: 2072–2074.

Tsolakidis, D., Pados, G., Vavilis, D. et al. (2010). The impact on ovarian reserve after laparoscopic ovarian cystectomy versus three-stage management in patients with endometriomas: a prospective randomized study. Fertil Steril 94: 71–77.

Tsuji, I., Ami, K., Fujinami, N. et al. (2012). The significance of laparoscopy in determining the optimal management plan for infertile patients with suspected tubal pathology revealed by hysterosalpingography. Tohoku J Exp Med 227: 105–108.

Tulandi, T., Collins, J.A. and Burrows, E. (1990). Treatment-dependent and treatment-independent pregnancy among women with periadnexal adhesions. Am J Obstet Gynecol 162: 354–357.

Tummon, I.S., Asher, L.J., Martin, J.S. et al. (1997). Randomized controlled trial of superovulation and insemination for infertility associated with minimal or mild endometriosis. Fertil Steril 68: 8–12.

Werbrouck, E., Spiessens, C., Meuleman, C. et al. (2006). No difference in cycle pregnancy rate and in cumulative live-birth rate between women with surgically treated minimal to mild endometriosis and women with unexplained infertility after controlled ovarian hyperstimulation and intrauterine insemination. Fertil Steril 86: 566–571.

Yalanadu, N.S. and Narvekar, N.N. (2014). The role of tubal patency tests and tubal surgery in the era of assisted reproductive techniques. TOG 16: 37–45.

Yoshino, O., Hayashi, T., Osuga, Y. et al. (2010). Decreased pregnancy rate is linked to abnormal uterine peristalsis caused by intramural fibroids. Hum Reprod 25: 2475–2479.

Yu, D., Wong, Y.M., Cheong, Y., et al. (2008). Asherman syndrome – one century later. Fertil Steril 89: 759.

de Ziegler, D., Borghese, B. and Chapron, C. (2010). Endometriosis and infertility: pathophysiology and management. Lancet 376: 730–738.

13

Pathologies of the Male Reproductive Tract

Aarush Sajjad, Muhammad A. Akhtar, and Yasmin Sajjad

Introduction

The functional male reproductive tract involves complex processes that includes androgen homeostasis, spermatogenesis, sperm transport and storage, and normal erectile and ejaculatory ability. The control of these functions involves the hypothalamic–pituitary–gonadal axis, central and peripheral nervous systems, and genitalia.

The external male reproductive organs comprise the scrotum, testis, and penis. The testes are responsible for the production of testosterone and spermatozoa. Testosterone and dihydrotestosterone are responsible for the development of male sexual characteristics, which includes the distribution of pubic hair, maturation and enlargement of the penis, and deepening of the voice (by larynx enlargement). During ejaculation, the sperm are transported through the reproductive ducts that include the epididymis, vas deferens, ejaculatory duct, and urethra.

The epididymis is a collection of coiled microscopic tubes that together are almost 6 metres long. Sperm are transported to the epididymis where they remain and mature, gaining functional properties essential for motility. One epididymis lies against each testis. The other ducts include the vas deferens, ejaculatory duct, and urethra. The vas deferens is a firm tube that transports sperm from the epididymis. One such duct travels from each epididymis to the back of the prostate and joins with one of the two seminal vesicles and secretions from bulbourethral glands. These are called the accessory sex glands of the male reproductive system. The reproductive glands produce secretions that become part of semen, which is ejaculated from the urethra; this single duct passes through the penis (Chapter 2 covers the male reproductive anatomy in more detail).

This chapter will discuss only the disorders of the male reproductive tract.

Disorders of the Testes and Epididymis

Cryptorchidism

Testes are not always in the scrotum at birth as they form in the abdomen from the gonadal ridge or indifferent gonad that develops around 3–5 weeks of gestation. At 6 weeks' gestation, primordial germ cell migration occurs leading to testes development. This process is stimulated by the *SRY* gene (sex-determining region on Y chromosome); this gene is the testis-determining factor.

The testes descend prenatally from their initial intra-abdominal location on the urogenital ridge into the low-temperature environment of the scrotum via a complex multistage mechanism (Hutson et al. 1997). Prenatal ultrasonography shows no testicular descent before 28 weeks' gestation, other than transabdominal movement to the internal inguinal ring. Transinguinal migration, thought to be under hormonal control, occurs at 28–40 weeks' gestation, usually resulting in a scrotal testis by the end of a full term of gestation.

Undescended testis, or 'cryptorchidism', is a very common anomaly in male infants and preadolescent

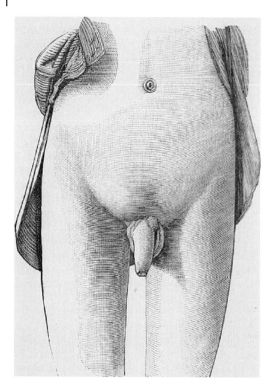

Figure 13.1 Cryptorchidism. The right undescended testis forms a swelling in the inguinal canal in a prepubescent male. Source: https://commons.wikimedia.org.

boys (Figure 13.1), with about one in 20 boys undergoing treatment by the time they reach puberty (Hutson 2013). The incidence of cryptorchidism shows large geographic variation, and in several countries increasing trends have been reported affecting 2–9% of male newborns (Toppari et al. 2010). It could be complete or incomplete failure of intra-abdominal testes to descend into the scrotal sac and is unilateral in most cases.

Factors that predispose or might increase the risk of undescended testes in a newborn include low birth weight and premature birth (Chung and Brock 2011). Exposure to oestrogen *in utero* and prenatal diethylstilbestrol (DES) exposure was associated with an almost twofold risk of cryptorchidism, and a stronger association was observed for exposures starting before the eleventh week of pregnancy (Palmer et al. 2009; Virtanen and Adamsson 2012).

Other factors include family history of undescended testes (Elert et al. 2003), or other problems of genital development, including conditions of the fetus that can restrict growth, such as Down syndrome or an abdominal wall defect (Koivusalo et al. 1998), as well as the mother's exposure to some pesticides (Carbone et al. 2006). These factors may contribute towards failure of the testes to descend into the scrotum at birth.

The mode of treatment for undescended testes has been debated for many years. Recently, a group of specialists in various related disciplines from the Nordic countries summarized the available information from literature, debated the advantages and disadvantages of different treatment modalities, and framed a consensus on the management of undescended testes (Ritzen et al. 2007; Ritzen 2008).

In most cases, the testis will descend without treatment during the child's first year. If this does not occur, treatment may include hormone injections (B-HCG or testosterone) or surgery (orchidopexy) to bring the testis into the scrotum. Orchidopexy is the main treatment for this condition.

Early surgery may prevent damage to the testes that can cause infertility (Ritzen et al. 2007). An undescended testis that is found later in life may need to be removed. Males with undescended testes are 40 times more likely to develop testicular cancer than males without undescended testes (Farrer et al. 1985). Ten percent of testicular cancer cases involve patients with undescended testes (Abratt et al. 1992). There is an increased risk of developing a germ cell tumour, especially seminoma and embryonal carcinoma, in undescended testes. Recent studies have shown that prepubertal orchidopexy reduces this risk (Walsh et al. 2007; Tuazon et al. 2008).

Although successful scrotal repositioning of the testis may reduce the risk, it does not prevent the potential long-term issues of infertility and testis cancer, and appropriate counselling and follow-up of the patient are essential (Kolon et al. 2014).

Testicular Torsion

As discussed previously, the testes develop from condensations of tissue within the urogenital ridge at approximately 6 weeks of gestation. With longitudinal growth of the embryo, and through complex multistage mechanisms under endocrine and paracrine signals, the testes ultimately descend into the scrotum by the third trimester of pregnancy (Hutson et al. 1997). The testes migrate through the inguinal canal and as the testes leave the abdomen it carries the peritoneal lining with it, creating the processus vaginalis. Although the testis is located in the scrotum, it gets its blood supply from an artery that originates in the abdomen, called the spermatic artery. The spermatic arteries and pampiniform venous plexus enter the inguinal canal proximal to the testes, and together with the vas deferens, form the spermatic cord (Barteczko and Jacob 2000). Distally, the testis is attached to the scrotum by the gubernaculum.

It is not clear why testicular torsion happens. Testicular torsion can occur due to testicular injury or congenitally loose attachment of the testis to the scrotum. It often occurs several hours after vigorous activity – a minor injury to the testes can even occur in sleep. Cases of testicular torsion have been documented during periods of cold weather, with an increase in winter (Korkes et al. 2012; Gomes Dde et al. 2015).

It is understood that testicular torsion occurs when the testis rotates, twisting the spermatic cord and its contents (Figure 13.2). It is a surgical emergency, with an annual incidence of 3.8 per 100 000 males younger than 18 years (Zhao et al. 2011). This twisting cuts off the blood supply to the testis, causing the sudden onset of severe pain and swelling.

There is typically a 4–8 h window before significant ischaemic damage occurs, manifested by morphological changes in testicular histopathology and deleterious effects on spermatogenesis (Bartsch et al. 1980). The viability of the testis in cases of torsion is difficult to predict; hence, emergency surgical treatment is indicated despite many patients presenting beyond the 4–8 h time frame (Davenport 1996). If treated quickly, the testis can usually be salvaged. When testicular torsion is not treated for several hours, blocked blood flow can cause permanent damage to the testis. Hence, removal of the testis, called orchidectomy, is performed if the affected testis appears grossly necrotic or nonviable. Torsion accounts for approximately 10–15% of acute scrotal disease in children, resulting in an orchidectomy rate of 42% in boys undergoing surgery for testicular torsion (Barbosa et al. 2013; Liang et al. 2013). Orchidectomy rates vary widely in the literature, typically ranging from 39 to 71% in most series (Jefferson et al. 1997; Kaye et al. 2008; Yang Jr et al. 2011).

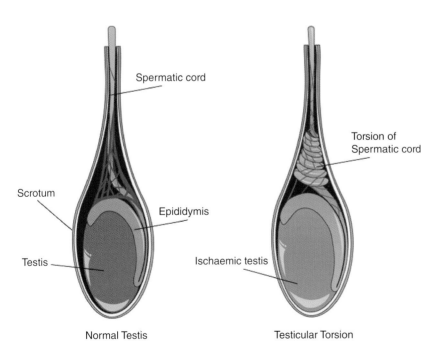

Figure 13.2 Testicular torsion. During testicular torsion a testis rotates, twisting the spermatic cord that supplies blood to the testis. The resultant reduced blood flow causes sudden and often severe pain and swelling. Reproduced with permission of Keith Carroll.

Therefore, prompt restoration of blood flow to the ischaemic testis is critical in cases of testicular torsion (Thomas et al. 1984; Romeo et al. 2010)

If surgery is performed in time and the affected testis is deemed viable, orchidopexy (resolving the torsion) with permanent suture should be performed to permanently fix the testis within the scrotum (Taskinen et al. 2008). It is also recommended that contralateral orchidopexy should be performed regardless of the viability of the affected testis (Bolin et al. 2006). In some cases, damage or loss of a testis affects a male's ability to father children.

Testicular Atrophy

Testicular atrophy is the shrinkage of the testes. There are many causes but it is commonly due to injury to the testes, use of recreational drugs, anabolic steroids and testosterone, cryptorchidism, end stage of inflammatory orchitis, progressive atherosclerotic narrowing of the blood supply in old age, hypopituitarism, generalized malnutrition or cachexia, obstruction to outflow of semen, irradiation, and prolonged administration of hormones. Testicular atrophy can lead to hypogonadism, resulting in reduced testosterone production and poor spermatogenesis, the consequences of which are azoospermia and infertility (Møller et al. 1996).

Testicular Tumours

Testicular tumours are rare (1% of all tumours in men). Each year in the UK around 2300 men are diagnosed with testicular cancer, according to Cancer Research UK. It presents with a painless swelling in the testes with a dull ache or feeling of heaviness in the scrotum.

Risk factors for testicular tumours are:

- Age: common in young and middle-aged men. Men aged 30–34 are more likely to develop testicular cancer and risk reduces after age 49 years.
- Ethnicity: more prevalent in Whites (five times higher) compared with other ethnicities.
- Undescended testes.
- Smoking.
- Subfertility: subfertile men are three times more likely to develop testicular cancer.
- Human immunodeficiency virus.

- Height: taller men (>190 cm tall) are two to three times more likely to develop testicular cancer. The taller you are, the higher the risk. In shorter men (<170 cm) the risk of testicular cancer is reduced by 20%.
- Family history of testicular cancer.

Types of testicular tumours are:

- Germ cell tumours: most common (95% of all cases). Two subtypes, seminoma and nonseminoma, both account for half of all germ cell tumours. They respond well to chemotherapy.
- Leydig cell tumours (1–3% of all cases).
- Sertoli cell tumours (1% of all cases).
- Lymphomas – Hodgkin or non-Hodgkin (4% of all cases).

If a testicular tumour is suspected, it can be investigated either by examination or testicular ultrasound. Refer for an urgent (within 2 weeks) outpatient appointment with a urologist. Measure the tumour markers alpha-fetoprotein (AFP) and human chorionic gonadotrophin (hCG) (NICE 2010; Albers et al. 2015).

Treatment for germ cell tumours is orchidectomy, chemotherapy, radiotherapy, and/or lymph node dissection. Prognosis is excellent following treatment, particularly if the tumour is detected at an early stage. Following treatment, 5-year survival is nearly 100% for nonmetastatic germ cell tumours (Ehrlich et al. 2015). For metastatic disease, 5-year survival is, on average, 85%, but varies from 48 to 92% depending on the stage and type of tumour (NICE 2010; Albers et al. 2015).

Epididymo-Orchitis

Epididymitis refers to inflammation of the epididymis, and may be associated with inflammation extending to the testis itself, in which case the term epididymo-orchitis is used (Tracy et al. 2008). This should be distinguished from isolated orchitis, which is by comparison much less common. Epididymo-orchitis most often presents with acute onset of pain and swelling of the scrotum, which can be a result of bacterial infection, However, this can also be due to non-infectious causes, particularly in children.

In sexually active men under the age of 35 years it is usually caused by a sexually transmitted infection, such as chlamydia or gonorrhoea ascending from the urethra (Zdrodowska-Stefanow et al. 2000). This will be discussed in more detail in Chapter 14.

In older men over the age of 35 years it is usually caused by nonsexually transmitted uropathogens spreading from the urinary tract (Trojian et al. 2009). The majority of cases are bacterial in origin arising from the bladder, prostate, or urethra, which can reflux via ejaculatory ducts into the epididymis. The inflammatory response usually starts in the tail of the epididymis due to the its greatest blood supply before spreading to the body, head, and testis (Mukherjee and Sinclair 2010).

Risk factors include bacterial prostatitis, urinary tract infection, underlying congenital abnormalities (in children), urinary stasis as a result of bladder outlet obstruction, and invasive procedures such as instrumentation/catheterization (Nickel 2007).

Mumps orchitis is a complication of the childhood viral disease. Although less common, incidences of mumps orchitis is increasing, as a result of the decline in vaccinations (Lane and Hines 2006; Phillip et al. 2006). Mumps affect around 20–30% of infected postpubertal males as a result of haematogenous spread, usually 4–11 days after the onset of parotitis (Philip et al. 2006). This viral infection can spread to the epididymis, with bilateral orchitis occurring in 10–30% of cases. Severe infection may result in testicular atrophy and infertility (if mumps orchialgia is bilateral). To reduce the risk of secondary bacterial infection, antibiotic therapy should be given (even with an obvious clinical diagnosis of mumps orchitis) (Lane and Hines 2006).

Less common causes include an operation to the prostrate or urethra. Tuberculous epididymo-orchitis is also considered in patients from high prevalence countries or with a previous history of tuberculosis and particularly in patients with immunodeficiency (Viswaroop et al. 2005). It is usually as a result of disseminated infection and commonly associated with renal TB but can be an isolated finding (Ferrie and Rundle 1983; Viswaroop et al. 2005).

Unilateral and bilateral epididymo-orchitis has also been reported as an adverse effect of amiodarone treatment and will resolve once treatment is ceased (Gasparich et al. 1985). Other rare infective causes include Brucella and fungi such as Candida (Hagely 2003).

Epididymo-orchitis presents characteristically with unilateral scrotal pain and swelling of relatively acute onset. Torsion of the testis is the most important differential diagnosis (Giesler and Krieger 2008). Other symptoms may include pyrexia accompanied by chills, and a sore swelling of the epididymis with hot, reddish scrotal skin. Occasionally, there may be pain in the stomach accompanied by a sick feeling and vomiting.

In sexually transmitted epididymo-orchitis there may be symptoms of urethritis or a urethral discharge; however, the urethritis is often asymptomatic (Hawkins et al. 1986; Mulcahy et al. 1987; Hoosen et al. 1993).

Appropriate rest, analgesia, and scrotal support are recommended. Nonsteroidal anti-inflammatory drugs may be helpful (Walker and Challacombe 2013). Patients should be advised to abstain from sexual intercourse until they and their partner(s) have completed treatment and follow-up in those with confirmed or suspected sexually transmitted epididymo-orchitis (Centre for Disease Control Prevention 2006).

Empirical therapy should be given to all patients with epididymo-orchitis before culture results are available. The antibiotic regimen chosen is determined in light of the immediate tests (urethral or urinalysis) as well as age, sexual history, any recent instrumentation or catheterization, and any known urinary tract abnormalities in the patient.

Antibiotics used for sexually transmitted pathogens may need to be varied according to local knowledge of antibiotic sensitivities. Most commonly a ceftriaxone 500 mg single intramuscular injection is given along with doxycycline 100 mg by mouth twice daily for 10–14 days or ciprofloxacin 500 mg twice daily with a stat dose of azithromycin 1 g (Berger et al. 1979; Hoosen et al. 1993).

Epididymal Cysts

An epididymal cyst is a fluid-filled sac within the epididymis. It is always benign. It can present unilaterally or bilaterally either as single or multiple cysts. It is not associated with any medical conditions or infections. Most epididymal cysts do not require treatment; very rarely, large epididymal cysts require surgical removal. Aspiration of a cyst is not recommended.

Disorders of the Scrotum

Scrotal disorders include inguinal hernias extending to the scrotum, varicocele, hydrocele, scrotal squamous cell carcinoma, cryptorchidism, testicular torsion, and testicular tumours. Some have been described earlier in the chapter.

Inguinal Hernia

Inguinal hernia is protrusion of abdominal contents through the inguinal canal. It presents with a lump in the groin, which can reduce in size with minimal pressure or by lying down. The lump can cause discomfort, which sometimes increases with physical activity. Inguinal hernias are at risk of irreducibility or incarceration, which may result in strangulation and obstruction. However, the risk of strangulation is very low in comparison to femoral hernia (Jenkins and O'Dwyer 2008).

Inguinal hernias can be direct or indirect. Indirect inguinal hernias are more common. Direct inguinal hernia arises from protrusion of abdominal contents through a weakness of the posterior wall of the inguinal canal medial to the inferior epigastric vessels. Indirect inguinal hernias occur due to failure of embryonic closure of the deep (internal) inguinal ring after testicular descent. It is present lateral and superior to the course of the inferior epigastric vessels protruding through the deep inguinal ring into the inguinal canal.

Suspect strangulation if a patient presents with an acutely painful, firm, tender, irreducible inguinal hernia. The risk of strangulation for all inguinal hernias is estimated to be 0.3–3.0% per year (Simons et al. 2009). Suspect obstruction if a patient presents with nausea, vomiting, constipation, absence of flatus, abdominal pain, and distension. In these cases, urgent surgical intervention is required by general surgeons (NICE 2010).

If an inguinal hernia extends into the scrotum, it is almost always indirect (Douglas et al. 2009). It is recommended that any inguinal hernia extending into the scrotum should be repaired (NICE 2010) as the risk of strangulation is 10 times higher for indirect hernias compared with direct inguinal hernias (Simons et al. 2009).

Hydrocele

A hydrocele is defined as presence of a fluid-filled sack along the spermatic cord between the tunica vaginalis and testes within the scrotum (Figure 13.3) (Albino et al. 2010). It can be unilateral or bilateral. The cause can be congenital or acquired. It presents with a painless swollen scrotum (Cimador et al. 2010). A referral to a paediatric surgeon is required if this is present in infancy and young age for any congenital hydrocele. Most hydroceles will resolve spontaneously by the age of two and aspiration is not recommended (NICE 2010). Laparoscopic surgery is offered for treatment of hydrocele in children if needed (Clarke 2010).

Acquired hydroceles may be due to testicular torsion, epididymo-orchitis, testicular cancer, varicocele, inguinal hernia, trauma, or continuous peritoneal ambulatory dialysis, renal or heart failure. Diagnosis is made on examination with transillumination and testicular ultrasound. Approximately 10% of testicular cancers presents with a reactive hydrocele (Albino et al. 2010). Manage according to the cause and if required refer to a urologist. Aspiration of hydrocele is not recommended (NICE 2010).

Varicocele

Varicocele is an enlargement of the scrotal veins due to an abnormally dilated pampiniform venous plexus. It is present in 15% of the normal male population, and present in approximately 40% of infertile males (Nagler et al. 1997). Most cases of varicoceles present as a painless swelling, causing limited or no discomfort (Figure 13.4). Most varicoceles are idiopathic and do not require any intervention. However, in men >40 years old, a newly symptomatic varicocele should be further investigated to rule out a renal tumour. If a varicocele develops only on the right side, vena caval obstruction from a renal carcinoma or any other retroperitoneal tumour should be excluded (NICE 2010).

The cause and pathophysiology of varicoceles is complex and multifactorial. However, there are some indications this condition is age-dependent, as the incidence in prepubertal boys is extremely rare and increases to about 15% in adolescents (Gorelick and Goldstein 1993).

(a)

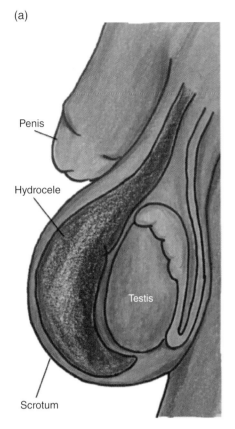

Penis

Hydrocele

Testis

Scrotum

(b)

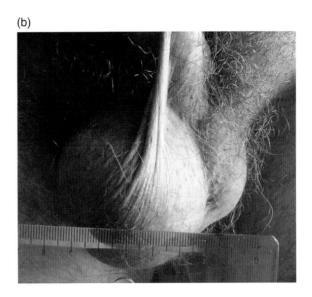

Figure 13.3 Hydrocele. (a) Hydrocele depicted as presence of a fluid-filled sack along the spermatic cord between tunica vaginalis and testes within the scrotum. (b) Presented at a large scrotal swelling. Source: (a) Michael Carroll; (b) https://commons.wikimedia.org).

The relationship between the presence of a varicocele and infertility remains to be firmly established. However, reports have linked varicocele to male factor infertility, testicular hypotrophy, and abnormal semen parameters. There is growing evidence to suggest that oxidative stress is a key element in the pathophysiology of varicocele-related infertility (Cho et al. 2016).

There are various surgical techniques available for varicocele. These include the Palomo technique, microsurgical and laparoscopic varicocelectomy techniques, radiological embolization, and the macroscopic inguinal (Ivanissevich) varicocelectomy technique. A meta-analysis published in 2009 analysing 36 studies reported that the microsurgical varicocelectomy technique has higher spontaneous pregnancy rates and lower postoperative recurrence and hydrocele formation than conventional varicocelectomy techniques in infertile men (Cayan et al. 2009).

It is not recommended that men should be offered surgery for varicoceles as a form of fertility treatment as it does not improve pregnancy rates. The effectiveness of varicocele surgery in men with abnormal semen parameters is uncertain and is not recommended (NICE 2013).

Scrotal Squamous Cell Carcinoma

Scrotal squamous cell carcinoma (SCC) is rare, but it is the most common scrotal malignancy. Other scrotal malignancies are extramammary Paget disease, sarcoma, basal cell carcinoma, melanoma, Bowen disease, and adnexal skin tumours. Median

(a)

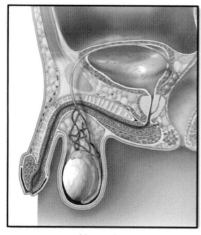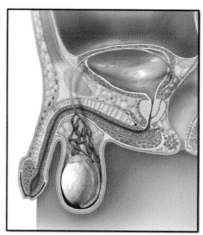

Normal   Varicocele

(b)

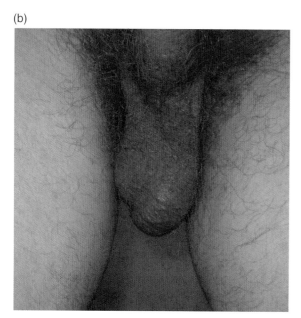

Figure 13.4 Varicocele. (a) Varicocele showing abnormally dilated pampiniform venous plexus dilated and (b) presented as enlargement of the scrotal veins. Source: (a) Blausen Medical, Wikimedia (b) https://commons.wikimedia.org.

age at diagnosis ranges from 52 to 57 years. Most cases occur in White men (Vyas et al. 2014).

The most common presentation of scrotal SCC is of an erythematous scrotal nodule or plaque leading to ulceration and pruritus. It occurs most commonly in the left scrotum, lower and anterior areas. It is commonly related to occupation particularly chimney sweepers, tar and paraffin workers, exposure to mineral and cutting oils, printing, metal working, car and aeroplane manufacture, car mechanics, commercial printing, aluminum workers, shale oil workers, pitch workers, engineering, steel production, and cavalrymen. Immunosuppression and human papillomavirus infection play a role as associating conditions (Vyas et al. 2014).

Treatment is by wide local excision. Inguinal lymphadenectomy, with adjuvant chemotherapy, is considered if inguinal lymphadenopathy persists after antibiotics (often prescribed for 6 weeks) for superimposed local infection (NICE 2010). This should be discussed in the oncology MDT meeting.

Penile Pathologies

The penis is the male copulatory organ, which is a cylindrical pendant organ located anterior to the scrotum and functions to transfer sperm to the vagina.

Penis anatomy is remarkably complex. The internal structure of the penis consists of three columns of erectile tissue that are wrapped in connective tissue and covered with skin. The two dorsal columns are cylinder-shaped vascular tissue bodies called corpora cavernosa and run throughout the penis. The single, midline ventral column surrounds the urethra and is called the corpus spongiosum. Other than that, there is erectile tissue surrounding the urethra, two main arteries, as well as several veins and nerves. The longest part of the penis is the shaft, at the end of which is the head, or glans penis.

The urethra, which extends throughout the length of the corpus spongiosum, opens through the external urethral orifice at the tip of the glans penis. A loose fold of skin, called the prepuce, or foreskin, covers the glans penis.

Some disorders that affect the penis include development abnormalities, such as hypospadias and epispadias, as well as acquired problems like priapism, Peyronie's disease, balanitis, phimosis, paraphimosis, and penile cancer.

Hypospadias

Hypospadias is a congenital abnormality of the penis and is the second most common male genital birth defect with an incidence of one in every 250 male births (Wong and Braga 2015). Hypospadias is the malformation of the urethral groove and urethral canal resulting in an abnormal opening on the ventral surface of the penis (Figure 13.5). These urethral defects can cause urinary tract obstruction and increased risk of infection. Usually the foreskin is lacking in front of the penis. The position of the opening may be only a small distance away from the tip of the penis – this is distal or anterior hypospadias

and is the most commonly encountered variant (Kraft et al. 2010). In more severe cases, it lies away from the tip at the base of the penis, at the scrotum, or even behind the scrotum – this is called proximal or posterior hypospadias (Kraft et al. 2011).

The exact cause of this condition is unknown in most cases. However, some studies have linked the rising rate of hypospadias in boys born prematurely and small for gestational age, boys with low birth weight, and boys born to mothers over 35 years of age (Fisch et al. 2001; Gatti et al. 2001; Fredell et al. 2002). Roberts and Lloyd (1973) noted an 8.5-fold increase in hypospadias in one of monozygotic male twins compared with singleton live male births. It is sometimes present in children with multiple congenital problems. In most cases, it is just a single isolated problem.

A spectrum of abnormalities is commonly associated with hypospadias including a 'hooded' incomplete prepuce, an abortive corpora spongiosum, and in some cases the penis may be bent (chordee) or twisted during erection, or the scrotum may be divided in two halves (Kraft et al. 2011).

Between 8 and 10% of boys with hypospadias have an undescended (cryptorchid) testis, and 9–15% have an associated inguinal hernia (Khuri et al. 1981; Sorber et al. 1997). In boys with more proximal hypospadias, cryptorchidism may occur in as many as 32% (Cerasaro et al. 1986). The incidence of chromosomal anomaly in these groups of patients is much higher (22%) than hypospadias (5–7%) or cryptorchidism (3–6%) occurring alone (Yamaguchi et al. 1991; Moreno-Garcia and Miranda 2002).

Hypospadias and disorders of sex development (DSD) may represent two ends of a spectrum. The more proximal the hypospadias is, the more likely a DSD state exists (Kaefer et al. 1999). Rajfer and Walsh (1976) reported DSD in 27.3% of boys with a normal-sized phallus, cryptorchidism, and hypospadias. Therefore, boys with severe proximal hypospadias and those with hypospadias and cryptorchidism should undergo karyotype analysis and a DSD evaluation as indicated (Kraft et al. 2011).

This condition is treated surgically and the goal is a functional sexual organ that is free of curvature. Equally important is a glanular urethral meatus that allows a boy to void with a laminar flow while standing. The ideal age for genital surgery is between 6 and 12 months of age (Kass et al. 1996).

(a)

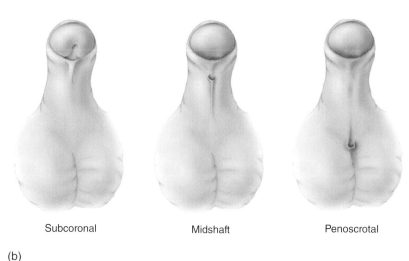

Subcoronal   Midshaft   Penoscrotal

(b)

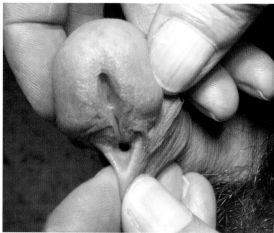

Figure 13.5 Hypospadias. Hypospadias is the malformation of the urethral groove and urethral canal resulting in an abnormal opening on the ventral surface of the penis. (a) Showing locations of hypospadias and (b) example of subcoronal hypospadias. Source: https://commons.wikimedia.org.

Epispadias

Epispadias shares some features with hypospadias. However, in this condition the urethral groove and urethral canal malformation leads to the abnormal opening on the top (dorsal) surface of the penis. Epispadias is a rare occurrence with 1:30 000 live birth incidences (Jeffs 1987). The causes of epispadias are not known. However, it involves abnormal development of the cloaca, the cloacal membrane, the external genitalia, and the pubis (Stephens and Hutson 2005). Epispadias can be associated with bladder extrophy, an uncommon birth defect in which the bladder is inside out, and protrudes through the abdominal wall (Gearhart and Mathews 2007).

Surgical repair of epispadias is recommended in patients with more than a mild case. Surgery generally leads to the ability to control the flow of urine and a good cosmetic outcome. However, some boys with this condition may continue to have urinary incontinence, even after surgery. Ureter and kidney damage and infertility may occur (Elder 2011).

Phimosis

Phimosis is a condition in which the prepuce cannot be retracted over the glans penis, as the orifice of foreskin is too small to permit normal retraction. It could be further defined as physiological, as in infancy and childhood, or pathological. Pathological phimosis can occur from inflammatory or traumatic injury to the prepuce resulting in an acquired inelastic scar that prevents retraction. Physiological phimosis is common in male patients up to 3 years of age, but often extends into older age groups (Gardiner 1949; Oster 1968; Kayaba et al. 1996).

Paraphimosis is a condition where the phimotic foreskin is forcibly retracted over the glans penis resulting in constriction and swelling, where the foreskin cannot be brought back over the glans penis. The glans engorges and the prepuce becomes oedematous because of lymphatic and venous congestion. This could happen because boys have been encouraged to retract the foreskin for physiological phimosis by parents or medical staff (Hayashi et al. 2011). Some authors advise circumcision for paraphimosis because of its tendency to recur, whereas others insist that circumcision is not mandatory because the foreskin will continue to develop normally.

Priapism

Priapism is defined as a painful prolonged and persistent penile erection, unassociated with sexual interest or stimulation, lasting longer than 4 h (Montague et al. 2003). It has further been divided into three main categories: ischaemic, nonischaemic and stuttering priapism, based on the aetiology and pathophysiology of the condition (Montague et al. 2003). Establishing the type of priapism is paramount to safely and effectively treating these episodes.

Ischaemic priapism, formerly known as low-flow priapism, is much more common and is characterized by a veno-occlusive state in which inadequate venous outflow creates an acidotic hypoxic environment leading to a painful prolonged erection (Broderick et al. 2010). Ischaemic priapism is commonly associated with blood dyscrasias (e.g. sickle cell disease, thalassaemia, and leukaemia), advanced pelvic malignancies, and medications such as trazodone (Kulmala and Tamella, 1995; El-Bahnasawy et al. 2002). It is also caused by intracavernous injection of vasoactive drugs used to induce erection in cases of erectile dysfunction (Morales Concepción 1992).

Ischaemic priapism represents a urological emergency and, if not treated in time, can lead to penile fibrosis and erectile dysfunction. Its treatment may involve aspiration/irrigation with sympathomimetic injections, such as phenylephrine at a dosage of 100–250 μg injected into the cavernous body every 2 min until the penis is no longer rigid (Muruve and Hosking 1996). Other treatments involve surgical shunts, and as a last resort, penile prosthesis implantation in cases that are refractory to conservative management (typically those of longer duration) (Brant et al. 2009; Burnett and Pierorazio 2009).

Nonischaemic (formerly known as high-flow) priapism results from continuous flow of arterial blood into the penis most commonly related to perineal or direct penile trauma. Nonischaemic priapism is typically painless and the penis is only semierect (Witt et al. 1990). Patients with arterial priapism typically seek medical attention later than those with ischaemic priapism, due to the fact that nonischaemic priapism causes less pain and discomfort (Montague et al. 2003). This is not an emergency and may be managed conservatively initially, as most of these episodes are self-limiting (Hakim et al. 1996).

Stuttering priapism involves recurrent self-limiting episodes of ischaemic priapism. It is an uncommon form of ischaemic priapism, and its treatment is not yet clearly defined. If left untreated, it may evolve into the classic form of acute ischaemic priapism and lead to erectile dysfunction due to fibrosis of the corpora cavernosa (Migliorini et al. 2016).

The treatment objective for stuttering priapism is to decrease episodes of prolonged erections with systemic treatments, while treating each acute episode as an emergency (Droupy and Giuliano, 2013).

Other causes of priapism include alcohol or drug abuse (especially cocaine), certain medications including some antidepressant and blood pressure medications, spinal cord problems, injury to the genitals and blood diseases, including leukaemia and sickle cell anaemia (Van der Horst et al. 2003).

Peyronie's Disease

Peyronie's disease is a condition, characterized by the presence of localized fibrotic plaques, or a hard lump on the penis. It affects 3.2–8.9% of the adult male population (Mulhall et al. 2004; Taylor and Levine, 2007). The plaque may develop on the upper (more common) or lower side of the penis, in the tunica albuginea, the layers that contain erectile tissue (Taylor and Levine 2007). The plaque often begins as a localized area of irritation, swelling, and inflammation, and can develop into a hardened scar. The scarring reduces the elasticity of the penis in the affected area. It is both a physically and psychologically devastating disorder that causes penile deformity, curvature, hinging, narrowing, and shortening, which may compromise sexual function (Levine and Larsen 2013).

The exact cause of Peyronie's disease is unknown because of incomplete understanding of its aetiopathogenesis and the relative paucity of randomized, placebo-controlled trials. At present, most authorities support the hypothesis that Peyronie's disease generally arises from repetitive microtrauma to the erect penis during sexual activities (Gokce et al. 2013).

However, not all penile trauma leads to the development of Peyronie's disease. Genetically susceptible individuals experience a localized response to endogenous factors such as tumor growth factor-β, which are released in response to microtrauma (Levine and Larsen 2013). Abnormal wound healing appears to be more common in men with Peyronie's disease and there is evidence for a genetic predisposition (De Young and Brock 2011). Furthermore, studies have shown that risk factors for atherosclerosis and endothelial dysfunction such as hypertension, dyslipidemia, diabetes mellitus, and smoking are more common in men with Peyronie's disease (Tefekli et al. 2002; Usta et al. 2004).

Peyronie's disease is generally a progressive disorder that uncommonly resolves completely. It is difficult to predict an individual's prognosis at the initiation of the disease (Gokce et al. 2013). Only penile pain, if present, resolves spontaneously within the first year in the majority of patients (Dorey and James 1990). However, in most circumstances, Peyronie's disease progressively worsens over time (Schiff and Guhring 2006).

Appropriate treatment should be individualized and tailored to the patient's goals and expectations, disease history, physical examination findings, and erectile function. Although a variety of nonsurgical treatments have been suggested, none of these offer a reliable and effective correction of the penile deformity (Larsen and Levine 2012). While medical treatments exist, there is little evidence to support their use (Langston and Carson 3rd 2014). As a result, surgery remains the gold standard treatment option, offering the most rapid and reliable treatment.

Pathologies of the Prostate

The prostate gland is a muscular gland that resides in the true anatomical pelvis and surrounds the first inch of the urethra as it emerges from the bladder. The smooth muscle of the prostate gland contracts during ejaculation to contribute to the expulsion of semen from the urethra. The main role of the prostate as a male reproductive organ is to store and produce a clear and slightly alkaline prostatic fluid constituting up to 30% of semen volume (Frydenberg and Lawrentschuk 2012). The prostatic fluid constituents, and the environment they create, aid sperm motility and nourishment. The seminal vesicle is a convoluted structure attached to the vas deferens near the base of the urinary bladder. About 65–75% of the seminal fluid in humans originates from the seminal vesicles. It contains proteins, enzymes, fructose, mucus, vitamin C, flavins, phosphorylcholine, and prostaglandins. High fructose concentrations provide nutrient energy for the spermatozoa as they travel through the female reproductive system.

Benign Prostatic Hyperplasia

Benign prostatic hyperplasia (BPH) is a benign condition particularly common in men >50 years old. Approximately 40% of men aged >50 years suffer from this condition. It can cause urinary difficulties including frequency, urgency, incomplete voiding, or difficulty voiding. This condition does not increase risk of prostate cancer. In the UK, the International Prostate Symptom Score (IPSS) is completed to assess severity of symptoms. Investigation to aid in diagnosis may include rectal examination, transrectal ultrasound, CT urogram, voiding charts, and uroflowmetry.

Treatment may involve:

- Lifestyle adaptations – reduce caffeine and alcohol intake, bladder retraining.
- Medical – finasteride, alpha blockers.
- Surgical – transurethral resection of the prostate (TURP), transurethral incision of the prostate (TUIP) (Shrivastava and Gupta 2012).

Prostate Cancer

Prostate cancer is the second most common cancer in men in the UK after skin cancer. Approximately 42 000 men are diagnosed each year.

Protective factors:

- Eating food containing lycopene (tomatoes) and selenium (fish, shellfish, eggs, and grains) probably reduce the risk of prostate cancer.
- Being physically active.
- Diabetes.
- Taking aspirin.

Risk factors:

- Age: uncommon <50 years but risk increases with advancing age.
- Family history of cancer.
- Genetics: *BRC2* gene increases the risk of prostate cancer.
- Ethnicity: Afro-Caribbean men are twice as likely to have prostate cancer as White men. Asian men have half the risk of White men.
- History of any other cancer.
- Diet high in calcium.
- Height: taller men at higher risk than short men.
- High BMI.
- Vasectomy: small increase in risk.

Types:

- Acinar adenocarcinoma (most common – 90% of all cases).
- Other types of adenocarcinoma (atrophic, foamy, colloid and signet ring carcinoma).
- Rare types of prostate cancer (10%) could be any of the following:
  – Ductal adenocarcinoma
  – Transitional cell carcinoma
  – Squamous cell carcinoma
  – Carcinoid
  – Small cell carcinoma
  – Sarcomas and sarcomatoid carcinoma.

Diagnosis
Mostly it is asymptomatic. Investigations required for diagnosis are rectal examination, rectal ultrasound, magnetic resonance imaging scan, needle biopsy, and blood test (prostate specific antigen – PSA).

Treatment Options
Appropriate treatment options depend on the stage of the prostate cancer (localized, locally advanced, metastatic, or relapse), the man's prognostic risk, and presence of lower urinary tract symptoms of bladder outlet obstruction, the risk of adverse effects from treatment, his life expectancy, and personal values. This should be discussed in the oncology MDT meeting.

For localized prostate cancer:

- Conservative: surveillance.
- Radical: radical prostatectomy, external beam radiotherapy, brachytherapy.
- Adjuvant therapy: hormonal treatment including androgen blockade and androgen withdrawal – a short course may be given before or during radical radiotherapy.

Treatments for locally advanced prostate cancer, metastatic prostate cancer, or relapse after radical treatment:

- Neoadjuvant and concurrent luteinizing hormone-releasing hormone agonist or antagonist therapy.
- Adjuvant hormonal treatment.
- Radiotherapy: external beam radiotherapy and brachytherapy.
- Prostatectomy: radical prostatectomy, high intensity focused ultrasound, and cryotherapy.
- Chemotherapy.

Prognosis is dependent upon the stage of tumour (NICE 2010; Parker et al. 2015).

Conclusion

Male fecundity is dependent on a healthy reproductive tract. Pathologies of the penis, testis, and accessory glands can impact on the fertility status resulting in decreased sperm production or an inability to transfer sperm sufficiently in the female reproductive tract. Observations of variations and development of the male reproductive anatomy will allow accurate clinical interpretation and subsequent treatment. Urological interventions and treatment is dependent on the cause, where surgery or medical treatment can usually rectify the problem.

References

Abratt, R.P., Reddi, V.B. and Sarembock, L.A. (1992). Testicular cancer and cryptorchidism. Br J Urol 70: 656–659.

Albers, P., Albrecht, W., Algaba, F. et al. (2015). Guidelines on testicular cancer. Eur Urol 68:1054–1068.

Albino, G., Nenna, R., Inchingolo, C.D. et al. (2010). Hydrocele with surprise. Case report and review of literature. Arch Ital Urol Androl 82: 287–290.

Barbosa, J.A., Tiseo, B.C., Barayan, G.A. et al. (2013). Development and initial validation of a scoring system to diagnose testicular torsion in children. J Urol 189: 1859–1864.

Barteczko, K.J. and Jacob M. I. (2000). The testicular descent in humans. Origin, development and fate of the gubernaculum Hunteri, processus vaginalis peritonei, and gonadal ligaments. Adv Anat Embryol Cell Biol 156: 1–98.

Bartsch, G., Frank, S., Marberger, H. et al. (1980). Testicular torsion: late results with special regard to fertility and endocrine function. J Urol 124: 375–378.

Berger, R.E., Alexander, E.R., Harnisch, J.P. et al. (1979). Etiology, manifestations and therapy of acute epididymitis: prospective study of 50 patients. J Urol 121: 750–754.

Bolin, C., Driver, C.P. and Youngson, G.G. (2006). Operative management of testicular torsion: current practice within the UK and Ireland. J Pediatr Urol 2: 190–193.

Brant, W.O., Garcia, M.M., Bella, A.J. et al. (2009). T-shaped shunt and intracavernous tunneling for prolonged ischemic priapism. J Urol 181: 1699–1705.

Broderick, G.A., Kadioglu, A., Bivalacqua, T.J. et al. (2010). Priapism: pathogenesis, epidemiology, and management. J Sex Med 7: 476–500.

Burnett, A.L. and Pierorazio, P.M. (2009). Corporal 'snake' maneuver: corporoglanular shunt surgical modification for ischemic priapism. J Sex Med 6: 1171–1176.

Carbone, P., Giordano, F., Nori, F. et al. (2006). Cryptorchidism and hypospadias in the Sicilian district of Ragusa and the use of pesticides. Reprod Toxicol 22: 8–12.

Cayan, S., Shavakhabov, S. and Kadioğlu, A. (2009). Treatment of palpable varicocele in infertile men: a meta-analysis to define the best technique. J Androl 30: 33–40.

Centre for Disease Control Prevention (2006). Sexually Transmitted Diseases Management Guidelines. MMWR 55, 61–62.

Cerasaro, T.S., Brock, W.A. and Kaplan, G.W. (1986). Upper urinary tract anomalies associated with congenital hypospadias: is screening necessary? J Urol 135: 537–538.

Cho, C.L., Esteves, S.C. and Agarwal, A. (2016). Novel insights into the pathophysiology of varicocele and its association with reactive oxygen species and sperm DNA fragmentation. Asian J Androl 18: 186–193.

Chung, E. and Brock, G.B. (2011). Cryptorchidism and its impact on male fertility: a state of art review of current literature. Can Urol Assoc J 5: 210–4.

Cimador, M., Castagnetti, M. and De Grazia, E. (2010). Management of hydrocele in adolescent patients. Nat Rev Urol 7: 379–385.

Clarke, S. (2010). Pediatric inguinal hernia and hydrocele: an evidence-based review in the era of minimal access surgery. J Laparoendosc Adv Surg Tech A 20: 305–309.

Davenport, M. (1996). ABC of general surgery in children. Acute problems of the scrotum. BMJ 312(7028): 435–437.

De Young, L. and Brock, G.B. (2011). Rat as an animal model for Peyronie's disease research: a review of current methods and the peer-reviewed literature. Int J Impot Res 23: 235–241.

Dorey, F. and James, K. (1990). The natural history of Peyronie's disease. J Urol 144: 1376–1379.

Douglas, G., Nicol, F. and Robertson, C. ed. (2009). *Macleod's Clinical Examination*, 12th edn. Edinburgh: Churchill Livingstone.

Droupy, S. and Giuliano, F. (2013). Priapisms. Prog Urol 23: 638–646.

Ehrlich, Y., Margel, D., Lubin, M.A. et al. (2015). Advances in the treatment of testicular cancer. Transl Androl Urol 4: 381–390.

El-Bahnasawy, M.S., Dawood, A. and Farouk, A. (2002). Low-flow priapism: risk factors for erectile dysfunction. BJU Int 89: 285–290.

Elder, J.S. (2011). Anomalies of the bladder. In: *Nelson Textbook of Pediatrics*, 19th edn. (ed. R.M. Kliegman, R.E. Behrman, H.B. Jenson et al.). Philadelphia: Saunders.

Elert, A., Jahn, K., Heidenreich, A. et al. (2003). The familial undescended testis. Klin Padiatr 215: 40–45.

Farrer, J.H., Walker, A.H. and Rajfer J. (1985). Management of the postpubertal cryptorchid testis: a statistical review. J Urol 134: 1071–1076.

Ferrie, B.G. and Rundle, J.S. (1983). Tuberculous epididymo-orchitis: a review of 20 cases. Br J Urol 55: 437–439.

Fisch, H., Golden, R.J., Libersen, G.L. et al. (2001). Maternal age as a risk factor for hypospadias. J Urol 165: 934–936.

Fredell, L., Kockum, I., Hansson, E. et al. (2002). Heredity of hypospadias and the significance of low birth weight. J Urol 167: 1423–1427.

Frydenberg, M. and Lawrentschuk, N. (2012). Benign prostate disorders. In: *Endotext [Internet]* (ed. L.J. De Groot et al.). South Dartmouth, MA: MDText.com.

Gardiner, D. (1949). The fate of the foreskin: a study of circumcision. Br Med J 2: 1433–1437.

Gasparich, J.P., Mason, J.T., Greene, H.L. et al. (1985). Amiodarone-associated epididymitis: drug-related epididymitis in the absence of infection. J Urol 133: 971–972.

Gatti, J.M., Kirsch, A.J., Troyer, W.A. et al. (2001). Increased incidence of hypospadias in small-for-gestational age infants in a neonatal intensive-care unit. BJU Int 87: 548–550.

Gearhart, J.P. and Mathews, R. (2007). Exstrophy–epispadias complex. In: *Campbell-Walsh Urology*, 9th edn (ed. A.J.Wein), Chapter 119. Philadelphia: Saunders Elsevier.

Geisler, W.M. and Krieger, J.N. (2008). Epididymitis. In: *Sexually Transmitted Diseases, 4*, (ed. K. Holmes et al.). New York: McGraw Hill.

Gokce, A., Wang, J.C., Powers, M.K. et al. (2013). Current and emerging treatment options for Peyronie's disease. Res Rep Urol 5: 17–27.

Gomes Dde, O., Vidal, R.R., Foeppel, B.F. et al. (2015). Cold weather is a predisposing factor for testicular torsion in a tropical country. A retrospective study. Sao Paulo Med J 133: 187–190.

Gorelick, J.I. and Goldstein, M. (1993). Loss of fertility in men with varicocele. Fertil Steril 59: 613–616.

Hagely, M. (2003). Epidiymo-orchitis and epididymitis: a review of causes and management of unusual forms. Int J STD and AIDS 14: 372–378.

Hakim, L.S., Kulaksizoglu, H., Mulligan, R. et al. (1996). Evolving concepts in the diagnosis and treatment of arterial high flow priapism. J Urol 155: 541–548.

Hawkins, D.A., Taylor-Robinson, D., Thomas, B.J. et al. (1986). Microbiological survey of acute epididymitis. Genitourin Med 62: 342–344.

Hayashi, Y., Kojima, Y., Mizuno, K. et al. (2011). Prepuce: phimosis, paraphimosis, and circumcision. Sci World J 11: 289–301.

Hoosen, A.A., O'Farrell, N. and Van den Ende J. (1993). Microbiology of acute epididymitis in a developing country. Genitourin Med 69: 361–363.

Hutson, J.M. (2013). Cryptorchidism and hypospadias. In: *Endotext*. (ed. L.J. De Groot et al.). South Dartmouth, MA: MDText.com.

Hutson, J.M., Hasthorpe, S. and Heyns, C.F. (1997). Anatomical and functional aspects of testicular descent and cryptorchidism. Endocr Rev 18: 259–280.

Jeffs, R.D. (1987). Exstrophy, epispadias, cloacal and urogenital sinus abnormalities. Pediatr Clin North Am 34: 1238–1257.

Jefferson, R.H., Pérez, L.M. and Joseph, D.B. (1997). Critical analysis of the clinical presentation of acute scrotum: a 9-year experience at a single institution. J Urol 158: 1198–1200.

Jenkins, J.T. and O'Dwyer P.J. (2008). Inguinal hernias. BMJ 336(7638): 269–272.

Kaefer, M., Diamond, D., Hendren, W.H. et al. (1999). The incidence of intersexuality in children with cryptorchidism and hypospadias: stratification based on gonadal palpability and meatal position. J Urol 162: 1003–1006; discussion 1006–1007.

Kass, E., Kogan, S.J. and Manley, C. (1996). Timing of elective surgery on the genitalia of male children with particular reference to the risks, benefits, and psychological effects of surgery and anesthesia. Pediatrics 97: 590–594

Kayaba, H., Tamura, H., Kitajima, S. et al. (1996). Analysis of shape and retractability of the prepuce in 603 Japanese boys. J Urol 156: 1813–1815.

Kaye, J.D., Shapiro, E.Y., Levitt, S.B. et al. (2008). Parenchymal echo texture predicts testicular salvage after torsion: potential impact on the need for emergent exploration. J Urol 180(4 suppl): 1733–1736.

Khuri, F.J., Hardy, B.E. and Churchill, B.M. (1981). Urologic anomalies associated with hypospadias. Urol Clin North Am 8: 565–571.

Koivusalo, A., Taskinen, S. and Rintala, R.J. (1998). Cryptorchidism in boys with congenital abdominal wall defects. Pediatr Surg Int 13: 143–145.

Kolon, T.F., Herndon, C.D., Baker, L.A. et al. (2014). American Urological Assocation. Evaluation and treatment of cryptorchidism: AUA guideline. J Urol 192: 337–345.

Korkes, F., Cabral, P.R., Alves, C.D. et al. (2012). Testicular torsion and weather conditions: analysis of 21,289 cases in Brazil. Int Braz J Urol 38: 222–228; discussion 228–229.

Kraft, K.H., Shukla, A.R. and Canning, D.A. (2010). Hypospadias. Urol Clin North Am 37: 167–181.

Kraft, K.H., Shukla, A.R. and Canning, D.A. (2011). Proximal hypospadias. Sci World J 11: 894–906.

Kulmala, R.V. and Tamella, T.L. (1995). Effects of priapism lasting 24 hours or longer caused by intracavernosal injection of vasoactive drugs. Int J Impot Res 7: 131–136.

Lane, T.M. and Hines, J. (2006). The management of mumps orchitis. BJU Int 97: 1–2.

Langston, J.P. and Carson, C.C. 3rd (2014). Peyronie's disease: review and recent advances. Maturitas 78: 341–343.

Larsen, S.M. and Levine, L.A. (2012). Review of non-surgical treatment options for Peyronie's disease. Int J Impot Res 24: 1–10.

Levine, L.A. and Larsen, S.M. (2013). Surgery for Peyronie's disease. Asian J Androl 15: 27–34.

Liang, T., Metcalfe, P., Sevcik, W. et al. (2013). Retrospective review of diagnosis and treatment in children presenting to the pediatric department with acute scrotum. Am J Rentgenol 200: W444–W449.

Migliorini, F., Porcaro, A.B., Baldassarre, R. et al. (2016). Idiopathic stuttering priapism treated with salbutamol orally: a case report. Andrologia 48: 238–240.

Møller, H., Prener, A. and Skakkebaek, N.E. (1996). Testicular cancer, cryptorchidism, inguinal hernia, testicular atrophy, and genital malformations: case-control studies in Denmark. Cancer Causes Control 7: 264–274.

Montague, D.K., Jarow, J., Broderick, G.A. et al. (2003). Members of the Erectile Dysfunction Guideline Update Panel; American Urological Association. American Urological Association Guideline on the Management of Priapism. J Urol 170: 1318–1324.

Morales Concepción, J.C. (1992). Priapism induced by intracavernous injection. Arch Esp Urol 45: 793–795.

Moreno-Garcia, M. and Miranda, E.B. (2002). Chromosomal anomalies in cryptorchidism and hypospadias. J Urol 168; 2170–2172.

Mukherjee, R. and Sinclair, A.M. (2010). Epididymo-orchitis: diagnosis and management. Trends Urol Men's Health 1: 15–18.

Mulcahy, F.M., Bignell, C.J., Rajakumar, R. et al. (1987). Prevalence of chlamydial infection in acute epididymo-orchitis. Genitourin Med 63: 16–18.

Mulhall, J.P., Creech, S.D., Boorjian, S.A. et al. (2004). Subjective and objective analysis of the prevalence of Peyronie's disease in a population of men presenting for prostate cancer screening. J Urol 171: 2350–2353.

Muruve, N. and Hosking, D.H. (1996). Intracorporeal phenylephrine in the treatment of priapism. J Urol 155: 141–143.

Naber, K.G., Bergman, B., Bishop, M.C. et al. (2001). Urinary Tract Infection (UTI) Working Group of the Health Care Office (HCO) of the European Association of Urology (EAU). EAU Guidelines for the Management of Urinary and Male Genital Tract Infections. Eur Urol 40: 576–588.

Nagler, H.M., Luntz, R.K. and Martinis, F.G. (1997). Varicocele. In: *Infertility in the Male* (ed L.I. Lipshultz and S.S. Howards), 336–359. St Louis: Mosby Year Book.

National Institute of Clinical Excellence (2010). Clinical knowledge summaries. http://cks.nice.org.uk/scrotal-swellings

National Institute of Clinical Excellence (2013). Fertility Problems: Assessment and Treatment. NICE guidelines CG156.

Nickel, J. (2007). Inflammatory conditions of the male genitourinary tract: prostatitis and related conditions, orchitis, and epididymitis. In: *Campbell-Walsh Urology*, 9th edn (ed. A.J. Wein), 328–329. Philadelphia: Saunders Elsevier Press.

Oster, J. (1968). Further fate of the foreskin. Incidence of preputial adhesions, phimosis, and smegma among Danish schoolboys. Arch Dis Child 43: 200–203.

Palmer, J.R., Herbst, A.L., Noller, K.L. et al. (2009). Urogenital abnormalities in men exposed to diethylstilbestrol in utero: a cohort study. Environ Health 18: 37.

Parker, C, Gillessen, S., Heidenreich, A. et al. (2015). ESMO Guidelines Committee. Cancer of the prostate: ESMO Clinical Practice Guidelines for diagnosis, treatment and follow-up. Ann Oncol 26(Suppl 5):v69–77.

Philip, J., Selvan, D. and Desmond, A.D. (2006). Mumps orchitis in the non-immune postpubertal male: a resurgent threat to male fertility? BJU Int 97: 138–141.

Rajfer, J. and Walsh, P.C. (1976). The incidence of intersexuality in patients with hypospadias and cryptorchidism. J Urol 116, 769–770.

Ritzen, E.M. (2008). Undescended testes: a consensus on management. Eur J Endocrinol 159: S87–S90.

Ritzén, E.M., Bergh, A., Bjerknes, R. et al. (2007). Nordic consensus on treatment of undescended testes. Acta Paediatr 96: 638–643.

Roberts, C.J. and Lloyd, S. (1973). Observations on the epidemiology of simple hypospadias. Br Med J 1: 768–770.

Romeo, C., Impellizzeri, P., Arrigo, T. et al. (2010). Late hormonal function after testicular torsion. J Pediatr Surg 45: 411–413.

Schiff, J. and Guhring, P. (2006). An analysis of the natural history of Peyronie's disease. J Urol 175: 2115–2118.

Shrivastava, A. and Gupta, V.B. (2012). Various treatment options for benign prostatic hyperplasia: a current update. J Midlife Health 3: 10–19.

Simons, M.P., Aufenacker, T., Bay-Nielsen, M. et al. (2009). European Hernia Society guidelines on the treatment of inguinal hernia in adult patients. Hernia 13: 343–403.

Sorber, M., Feitz, W.F. and de Vries, J.D. (1997). Short- and mid-term outcome of different types of one-stage hypospadias corrections. Eur Urol 32: 475–479.

Stephens, F.D. and Hutson, J.M. (2005). Differences in embryogenesis of epispadias, exstrophy-epispadias complex and hypospadias. J Pediatr Urol 1: 283–288.

Taskinen, S., Taskinen, M. and Rintala R. (2008). Testicular torsion: orchiectomy or orchiopexy? J Pediatr Urol 4: 210–213.

Taylor, F.L. and Levine, L.A. (2007). Peyronie's Disease. Urol Clin North Am 34: 517–534.

Tefekli, A., et al. (2002). A retrospective review of 307 men with Peyronie's disease. J Urol 168; 1075–1079.

Thomas, W.E., Cooper, M.J., Crane, G.A. et al. (1984). Testicular exocrine malfunction after torsion. Lancet 2(8416): 1357–1360.

Toppari, J., Virtanen, H.E., Main, K.M. et al. (2010). Cryptorchidism and hypospadias as a sign of testicular dysgenesis syndrome (TDS): environmental connection. Birth Defects Res A Clin Mol Teratol 88: 910–919.

Tracy, C.R., Steers, W.D. and Costabile, R. (2008). Diagnosis and management of epididymitis. Urol Clin North Am 35: 101–108.

Trojian, T.H., Lishnak, T.S. and Heiman, D. (2009). Epididymitis and orchitis: an overview. Am Fam Physician 79: 583–587.

Tuazon, E., Banks, K., Koh, C.J. et al. (2008). Prepubertalorchiopexy for cryptorchidism may be associated with lower risk of testicular cancer. J Urol 180: 783–784; author reply 784–785.

Usta, M.F., Bivalacqua, T.J., Jabren, G.W. et al. (2004). Relationship between the severity of penile curvature and the presence of comorbidities in men with Peyronie's disease. J Urol 171: 775–779.

Van der Horst, C., Stuebinger, H., Seif, C. et al. (2003). Priapism – etiology, pathophysiology and management. Int Braz J Urol 29: 391–400.

Virtanen, H.E. and Adamsson, A. (2012). Cryptorchidism and endocrine disrupting chemicals. Mol Cell Endocrinol 355: 208–220.

Viswaroop, B.S., Kekre, N. and Goplalkrishnan, G. (2005). Isolated tuberculous epididymitis: a review of 40 cases. J Postgrad Med 51: 109–111.

Vyas, R., Zargar, H., Trolio, R.D. et al. (2014). Squamous cell carcinoma of the scrotum: a look beyond the chimneystacks. World J Clin Cases 2: 654–660.

Walker, N.A. and Challacombe, B. (2013). Managing epididymo-orchitis in general practice. Practitioner 257(1760): 21–25.

Walsh, T.J., Dall'Era, M.A., Croughan, M.S. et al. (2007). Prepubertal orchiopexy for cryptorchidism may be associated with lower risk of testicular cancer. J Urol 178: 1440–1446.

Witt, M.A., Goldstein, I., Saenz de Tejada, I. et al. (1990). Traumatic laceration of intracavernosal arteries: the pathophysiology of nonischemic, high flow, arterial priapism. J Urol 143: 129–132.

Wong, N.C. and Braga, L.H. (2015). The influence of pre-operative hormonal stimulation on hypospadias repair. Front Pediatr 3: 31.

Yamaguchi, T., Kitada, S. and Osada, Y. (1991). Chromosomal anomalies in cryptorchidism and hypospadias. Urol Int 47: 60–63.

Yang, C. Jr, Song, B., Liu, X. et al. (2011). Acute scrotum in children: an 18–year retrospective study. Pediatr Emerg Care 7: 270–274.

Zdrodowska-Stefanow, B., Ostaszewska, I., Darewicz, B. et al. (2000). Role of Chlamydia trachomatis in epididymitis. Part I. Direct and serologic diagnosis. Med Sci Monit 6: 1113–1118.

Zhao, L.C., Lautz, T.B., Meeks, J.J. et al. (2011). Pediatric testicular torsion epidemiology using a national database: incidence, risk of orchiectomy and possible measures toward improving the quality of care. J Urol 186: 2009–2013.

14

The Impact of Infections on Reproduction and Fertility

Val Edwards Jones

Introduction

Men and women are continually exposed to large numbers of microorganisms (bacteria, viruses, fungi, and parasites (predominantly protozoa) and many coexist to form the normal flora in a microbial community or microbiome. The diversity of microbes at each body site under normal environmental conditions is reflective of the age, nutritional status, ecological niche, and immediate partners. Most of these microbes are nonpathogenic but occasionally pathogens can form part of the normal flora and can be problematic for both endogenous and exogenous carriage. As technology improves, so does the information we hold on the interaction of microbes with man and the Human Microbiome Project is using these technologies (16S ribosomal RNA analysis) to determine the diversity of microbial flora at certain body sites and their role in health and disease (metagenomics analysis) (http://hmpdacc.org/micro_analysis/microbiome_analyses.php).

Normal Flora of the Genital Tract

The genital tract has its own microbiome and extensive studies have determined that it plays a mutualistic role in the maintenance of genital health. The common bacteria found colonizing the terminal portion of the urethra of both male and female are *Staphylococcus epidermidis,* diphtheroids, streptococci, lactobacilli, Gram negative bacilli, occasionally yeasts (such as *Candida albicans)* and anaerobic bacteria. These microorganisms can also be found colonizing the foreskin. Internal organs in both male and female are thought to be sterile but recent studies have shown that microorganisms can be found in the uterine cavity (Vertraelen et al. 2016) and placenta postpartum (Aagaard et al. 2014). Implications of these findings have yet to be determined but demonstrate the interaction of microbes and people.

The vaginal microbiome is very complex and diverse and it is known that an imbalance in this microbiome can lead to an unhealthy genital tract and the organisms involved can be sexually transmitted to partners. The microorganisms in the microbiome are attached to their host membranes and exist in a balanced aggregated state encased in mucus, termed a biofilm. The different species of bacteria, occasional fungi, and protozoa present are dependent upon the glycogen content of the vaginal epithelium, which is dependent upon ovarian activity. The predominant bacterium, lactobacillus, breaks down glycogen forming lactic acid, which alters the pH of the vaginal secretions, making it more acidic (Faro 1993). The vaginal microbiome before and after puberty is very similar (being predominantly aerobic bacteria such as staphylococci, enterococci, streptococci, diphtheroids, and coliform bacteria) and differs during parturition (which include predominantly lactobacilli, streptococci, anaerobic bacteria, and some yeasts) (Brotman 2011). The presence of lactobacilli appears to be important in maintaining the equilibrium of normal microflora and preventing overgrowth of potentially pathogenic microorganisms. The most commonly isolated *Lactobacillus* species associated with a healthy vaginal environment are *L. crispatus* and *L. jensenii* (Marrazzo 2011). Production of hydrogen peroxide by lactobacilli is toxic to anaerobic bacteria, which do not produce peroxidase. An imbalance of hormones can impact on the glycogen content and ultimately influence the composition of the vaginal microbiome. The alterations in the dynamics of the microbial community can lead to a shift in hydrogen ion concentration and hydrogen peroxide, allowing an overgrowth of anaerobic bacteria and the subsequent development of vaginitis (Faro 1993). In this instance, the infection is endogenously acquired from the individual's own microflora. Exogenous organisms, which, result in infection, can be acquired during surgery or medical procedures. Occasionally, these microorganisms can be endogenously acquired if part of the microbiome and result from an imbalance in the environment during medical procedures. These infections are usually presented with overt symptoms and if appropriate treatment is administered then there are few sequelae. Genital infections are also acquired through sexual intercourse or other sexual practices and are termed sexually transmitted infection (STI) or sexually transmitted disease (STD). There are over 20 different infections described in man and a number can impact on reproduction: the most commonly described are *Chlamydia trachomatis* and *Neisseria gonorrhoeae*.

Infection and Infertility

Infertility is usually defined as the lack of a conception following at least 1 year of constant, unprotected sexual intercourse. There are a number of reasons for infertility but individuals who do become infertile as a result of infection do so because of the inflammatory response (humoral or cell mediated) in accessory organs and total blockage of Fallopian tubes (Pellati et al. 2008). These infertility problems are considered such an issue that the Centre for Disease Control (CDC) in the USA recommend that all sexually active women under the age of 25 are screened for *C. trachomatis* and *N. gonorrhoeae* as these two common STIs are associated with tubal inflammation and subsequent blockage (CDC 2014).

Female Genital Infections

Vaginitis is an inflammation of the vagina and is associated with an irritation or infection of the vulva. When the inflammation is the result of an infection, it usually has three major causes, namely bacterial (30–35% of cases), candidiasis (20–25%), and trichomoniasis (10–15%) (Faro 1993). It also may be due to a combination of these causes. Symptoms may vary with infection but include vaginal discharge, irritation, inflammation, pain during sexual intercourse, and possibly a foul odour.

Bacterial vaginitis can be caused by a range of bacteria where there is resultant inflammation. Aerobic vaginitis caused by an overgrowth of *Escherichia coli, S. aureus,* Group B streptococci and enterococci (with or without anaerobes) in the absence of lactobacilli (Donders et al. 2005; Tempera and Furneri 2010) and is treated with a combination of antibiotics (often kanamycin or quinolones) and vaginal creams to reduce inflammation. Bacterial vaginosis (BV) is due to an overgrowth of *Gardnerella vaginalis, Mobiluncus* spp., other anaerobic Gram-negative bacilli (e.g. *Prevotella* spp.) and genital mycoplasmas. BV is characterized by an abnormal discharge (often white or yellow) with a fishy odour (due to the production of amines), a vaginal pH >4.5 and the presence of clue cells (vaginal epithelial cells coated with bacteria). Diagnosis is made based on clinical examination and microscopy. It can be asymptomatic and is differentiated from aerobic vaginitis by the absence of succinate, increased sialidase activity, and increased production of cytokines such as interleukin-1, -6 and -8 (Marrazo 2011). Detection of fatty acids (succinic and acetic) in vaginal fluid is indicative of BV, in contrast to lactic acid seen in a healthy vagina (Africa et al. 2014). In women of reproductive age there is an associated risk for adverse pregnancy outcomes such as preterm birth, recurrent abortions, postabortal sepsis, early miscarriages, and still births (Africa et al. 2014).

Fungal vaginitis is caused by a dimorphic fungus *Candida* spp. with *Candida albicans* the most prevalent species (Figure 14.1). Other species such as *C. glabrata* or *C. tropicalis* have also been implicated. These organisms are found on moist skin and mucosal surfaces of the alimentary canal, intestine, and vagina. They can also be found colonizing the foreskin.

(a) (b)

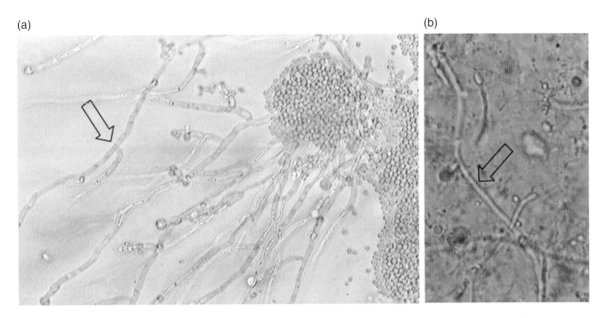

Figure 14.1 (a) *Candidia albicans* in culture on agar showing hyphae (arrow). (b) Vaginal wet mount in candidal vulvovaginitis with hyphae visible (arrow). *Source:* https://commons.wikimedia.org.

Candida spp. can become prevalent as an endogenous infection following antibiotics (which causes an imbalance in bacterial flora allowing it to grow) and its overgrowth can also occur during an imbalance of hormones, either naturally or during treatment, when an individual is stressed or immunosuppressed. *Candida* spp. can be sexually transmitted and colonize the foreskin and glans of the penis. In its invasive form, *C. albicans* will produce hyphae as part of its virulence (Figure 14.1). The resultant inflammation results in itching and oedema and the production of a voluminous soft white cheesy exudate which can form plaques and biofilm on the mucosal surface from the macerated surface. *C. albicans* produce a wide range of virulence factors that are used during the development of genital infections including adhesion, hyphal formation, phenotypic switching, extracellular hydrolytic enzyme production, and biofilm formation (Achkar and Fries 2010).

Trichomoniasis

Trichomonas vaginalis is a sexually transmitted flagellate protozoan causing genital infections in men and women (Figure 14.2). Symptoms develop

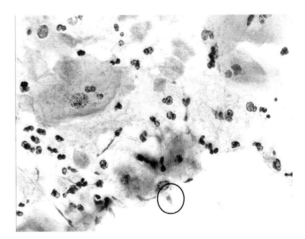

Figure 14.2 Papanicolau stain (×400) showing infestation by *Trichomonas vaginalis* (circle). *Source:* https://commons.wikimedia.org.

within a month of infection, although 50% of infected men and women will be asymptomatic. It causes inflammation, soreness and itching around the vagina, and a green frothy discharge, whereas it manifests in men as urethritis with an associated thin white discharge from the penis, and can also cause prostatitis. *T. vaginalis* is found with increased frequency in infertile women compared with control subjects and is thought to interfere with cervical and tubal factor in female infertility (El-Shazly et al. 2001). It has been shown that secreted factors from *T. vaginalis* interferes with sperm activity, and may contribute to fertility problems (Roh et al. 2015).

Recent molecular studies (using 16s RNA v6 sequencing) comparing healthy women with those with BV and vulvovaginal candidiasis (VVC) showed that the microbiome of normal controls and those with BV had typical patterns. However, a detailed comparison showed that the vaginal microbiota of VVC was complex. The mixed BV and VVC infection group had a unique pattern, with a higher abundance of Lactobacillus than the BV group and a higher abundance of Prevotella, Gardnerella, and Atopobium than the normal control. In contrast, the VVC-only group could not be described by any single profile, ranging from a community structure similar to the normal control (predominated with Lactobacillus) to BV-like community structures (abundant with Gardnerella and Atopobium) (Liu et al. 2013).

Treatment for Vaginitis and Vaginosis

Treatment is varied depending upon the cause but BV and trichomoniasis is commonly treated with metronidazole (with 2% clindamycin cream for BV) and candidiasis with a single oral dose of fluconazole supplemented with a topical clotrimazole or nystatin cream if necessary. Many women have a recurrence of BV within a few months and intravaginal metronidazole gel has been shown to be effective in these cases (Marrazo 2011). Probiotics (either a single strain or a cocktail of lactobacilli) have been used in a number of clinical trials (administered orally or intravaginally) for vaginitis and vaginosis and show some success, but suggest that preparations containing high doses of lactobacilli are required to be effective (Mastromarino et al. 2013).

Unfortunately, some infected women are asymptomatic for vaginitis and vaginosis. If left untreated, pelvic inflammatory disease may develop, which can lead to fertility problems in future years.

Pelvic Inflammatory Disease

Pelvic inflammatory disease (PID) is caused by an ascending infection (which can be endogenous or sexually acquired) of the reproductive organs of women including uterus, Fallopian tubes, and adjacent pelvic structures that are not associated with surgery or pregnancy. The symptoms range from asymptomatic (silent) or subclinical to severe, symptomatic disease. Bilateral lower abdominal pain is the most common symptom but there are others including abnormal vaginal discharge, intermenstrual or postcoital bleeding, menorrhagia, dysuria, fever, and nausea. If left untreated major reproductive health problems can result. However, PID and its sequelae are largely preventable. In the USA it is estimated that there are approximately 780 000 cases annually (Banikarim and Chacko 2005; Paavonen 2005). The most important causative microorganisms are *C. trachomatis*, *N. gonorrhoeae* (which are sexually acquired) and bacteria associated with vaginitis and vaginosis, e.g. *G.vaginalis* and mixed anaerobic organisms. *Ureaplasma urealyticum, Mycoplasma hominis* and *Mycoplasma genitalium* have also been associated with PID (Banikarim and Chacko 2005; Paavonen 2005).

Those at risk for acquiring PID are similar to those for STI. Adolescents who engage in high-risk sexual behaviours, including unprotected sex, and females with multiple partners have an increased risk. There is a slight risk of developing PID following insertion of an intrauterine device if an STI is undiagnosed at the time (Banikarim and Chacko 2005). Risk factors that place an individual at increased risk from STI and PID have been identified: for example, those with cervical eversion (where there are more columnar epithelial cells present) are more at risk of acquiring *N. gonorrhoeae* and *C. trachomatis*; individuals engaging in sexual intercourse close to or during menses can lose the cervical mucus plug and the presence of blood allows growth of endogenous bacteria; and some studies have shown that douching can increase the risk of PID due to a change in environment and alteration of vaginal flora, promoting the development of bacterial vaginosis (Banikarim and Chacko 2005).

Clinical Presentation of PID

The most common symptoms of PID are pain during sexual activity, lower abdominal pain, dysuria, menstrual spotting, and vaginal discharge. The dull abdominal pain can become quite severe and patients may have associated vomiting and fever.

Silent PID, where a patient has mild or no symptoms, can lead to tubal scarring and infertility if left untreated (Paarvonen 2005). Most serological studies undertaken on these individuals show evidence of undiagnosed *C. trachomatis* (WHO 1995). Treatment of PID is with combination therapy using doxycycline plus metronidazole (Paarvonen 2005).

Male Genital Tract Infections

Infections of the male genital tract are a correctable cause of male infertility, causing up to 12% of cases, and include prostatitis, epididymitis, and orchitis (Dohle et al. 2005). Deterioration in spermatogenesis, obstruction of the seminal tract, and defects in spermatozoa function may induced by immunological reactions (humoral and cellular) against microbial agents, as well as by direct influence of some bacterial strains on gametogenic cells (Keck et al. 1998).

Candida Infections and Male Fertility

Candida spp. infections can negatively affect sperm function, as reported in a number of studies. Sperm from healthy volunteers, exposed to *C. albicans,* show decreased sperm motility and increased agglutination (Tuttle et al. 1997). Tian et al. (2007) reported a similar effect on sperm motility with sperm, from healthy donors, exposed to *C. albicans in vitro.* In another *in vitro* study, it was shown that *C. albicans* decreases the functional competence of sperm by reducing motility and membrane mitochondrial potential, which can lead to apoptosis (Burrello et al. 2009).

Prostatitis

There are a number of different categories of prostatitis ranging from asymptomatic presentation through to acute, chronic, and chronic pelvic pain. Symptoms range from acute pain in the genitorectal area and lower urinary tract symptoms including frequency, dysuria, urgency, and obstructive urinary symptoms. Patients may also present with fever, shock, or signs of multiorgan failure (Sharp et al. 2010).

The predominant pathogens isolated in prostatic secretions in up to 80% of prostatitis patients are Gram-negative bacilli, mainly *E. coli,* with Gram-positive enterococci considered the second most common pathogens in prostatitis (Alshahrani et al. 2013). Other pathogens such as *Klebsiella* spp., *Pseudomonas aeruginosa*, *Proteus mirabilis*, and *Enterobacter aerogenes* have been isolated in prostatitis cases. In sexually active men younger than 35 years and older men who engage in high-risk sexual behaviours, *C. trachomatis* and *N. gonorrhoeae* are a frequent cause (Sharp et al. 2010). Mazzoli et al. (2010) also found a high prevalence of *C. trachomatis* in chronic prostatitis (39.1%) but his findings remain controversial. Patients with acquired immune deficiency disease (AIDS) or with human immunodeficiency virus (HIV) infection are susceptible to additional pathogens, such as *Serratia marcescens*, *Salmonella typhi*, *Mycobacterium tuberculosis*, and *Mycobacterium avium*. Nonbacterial organisms (e.g. Candida, Cryptococcus, Histoplasma, and Aspergillus species) should also be considered (Heyns and Fisher 2005; Ludwig et al. 2008).

Penicillin derivatives are used to treat acute bacterial prostatitis with doxycycline, azithromycin, and clarithromycin as second line. However, for chronic prostatitis, fluoroquinolones are recommended as first-line treatment because of better tissue perfusion. Trimethoprim/sulfamethoxazole can be used as an alternative but the tissue penetration may not be as effective (Sharp et al., 2010).

Epididymitis and Orchitis

The symptoms of acute epididymo-orchitis are pain, swelling, and inflammation of the epididymis and testes. It is commonly caused by infections spreading from the urethra or the bladder and more rarely can be the result of structural abnormalities (e.g. a stricture of the urethra allowing a focus of infection to develop). Aetiology varies with age and sexual activity and as such there is a crossover between age groups, and a detailed sexual history is essential for diagnosis (Street et al. 2012). Generally, under 35 years of age it is most often sexually acquired and the common pathogens are *C. trachomatis* and *N. gonorrhoeae* with *U. urealyticum* often reported alongside. *M. genitalium* has also been reported as a potential cause in some cases (Manhart et al. 2011; Lee and Lee 2013). Men who engage in insertive anal intercourse are at risk of epididymitis secondary to sexually transmitted enteric organisms (CDC 2010).

In men over 35 years of age, nonsexually acquired infection is often caused by urinary pathogens with *E. coli* being the most common. Similar bacterial infections may be caused as a complication following catheterization or surgical procedures.

Orchitis is a complication associated with the mumps virus for postpubertal males (especially those born between 1982 and 1986 and not vaccinated) and can occur in up to 40% of patients in comparison with 4.4% in vaccinated males (Yung et al. 2011). Epididymitis can be a complication of mumps and is often misdiagnosed (Wharton et al. 2006). In addition, as a rare complication, tuberculous epididymo-orchitis can occur in patients from countries where there is a high prevalence of tuberculosis (TB), especially disseminated or renal TB and particularly in those with immunodeficiency. These patients also often have signs of systemic TB, occasionally a scrotal sinus, and thickened scrotal sac (Viswaroop et al. 2005).

Clinical Symptoms

Epididymo-orchitis usually presents with acute scrotal pain with an associated urethral discharge. It should not be confused with testicular torsion, which is a medical emergency. Symptoms of mumps typically begin with a headache and fever, parotid swelling (unilateral or bilateral), and unilateral testicular swelling or epididymitis (Wharton et al. 2006) may develop 7–10 days later. Occasionally, testicular involvement following mumps may occur without systemic symptoms (Nickel and Plumb 1986).

In sexually transmitted epididymo-orchitis (irrespective of microbial agent), typical symptoms are urethritis with urethral discharge, dysuria, and penile irritation; however, sometimes urethritis may be asymptomatic (Street et al. 2012).

Sexually Transmitted infections

There are over 20 different STIs described in humans, each with their own specific virulence determinants and disease profiles. However, in the initial infectious stages, some have similar symptoms (such as urethritis, discharge, and inflammation) (e.g. caused by Chlamydia, gonorrhoea, Mycoplasma, Ureaplasma infection) and

laboratory diagnosis is important for administration of correct treatment and epidemiological purposes. Others, such as syphilis and herpes, have very specific symptoms and disease profiles, which makes diagnosis more straightforward. The most common STIs, *C. trachomatis* and gonorrhoea, can have major issues for an individual in terms of infertility and invasive disease as seen in gonorrhoea and syphilis. *C. trachomatis* is also responsible for 25–50% of ectopic pregnancies and 50% of tubular-associated infertility (Paarvonen 2005).

STIs can be broken down into different groups (depending upon the nature of the infecting organism) with bacterial infections being the most common. The most recent STI prevalence report (Public Health England 2016) reported approximately 420 000 cases. The most common was Chlamydia, with 202 546 diagnoses made (49%). Gonorrhoea had increased between 2008 and 2015 from 14 985 to 41 262.

In 2016, gonorrhoea was the most common in men who have sex with men (MSM) with increases of 36%. STIs were most prevalent in young heterosexuals under the age of 25 years and in men MSM (Anon 2014). The report also detailed an increase in STIs in individuals younger than 15 years of age, most likely through unsafe sexual practices (Anon 2014). Statistics on STIs available from the Centre for Disease Control in the USA detail similar findings although there is some variation seen amongst the different age groups. *C. trachomatis* and *N. gonorrhoeae* are still the most prevalent STIs reported with 1 401 906 cases of *C. trachomatis* (representing 446.6 cases per 100 000 population) and 333 004 cases of gonorrhoea (106.1 cases per 100 000 population) (CDC 2013).

Bacterial Sexually Transmitted Infections

Gonorrhoea

Neisseria gonorrhoeae is a Gram-negative intracellular diplococcus and a strict human pathogen. It is sexually transmitted and an essential first step in initiating human infection is colonization of the target mucosal epithelium of the genital tract. Initially Type IV pili attach to the apical surface of epithelial cells at most mucosal surfaces, after which opacity-associated proteins (Opa proteins) drive further adherence and internalization. Organisms devoid of these pili are considered nonpathogenic.

The organisms are detected by immune cells in the epithelium, which may include T helper 17 (TH17) cells, macrophages and dendritic cells via a membrane-associated Toll-like receptor (TLR) and cytoplasmic NOD-like receptor (NLR), and via other pathways promotes local release of interleukin-8 (IL-8), IL-6, tumour necrosis factor, IL-1β and other cytokines, creating a microenvironment that efficiently recruits and activates neutrophils. Following this, symptoms normally follow 2–3 days after infection (Criss and Seifert 2013). *N. gonorrhoeae* modulates phagocytosis by neutrophils and can also survive intracellularly which make them a successful pathogen.

The invasive nature of *N. gonorrhoeae* causes local inflammation in the urethra, vagina, cervix, rectum, and the oropharynx, and manifests with classic overt symptoms of purulent discharge and dysuria. However, up to 35% of women and 5% of men are asymptomatic, which complicates the diagnosis and treatment of gonorrhoea and contributes to its persistence. If left untreated, salpingitis, prostatitis, and epididymitis occur with tubular blockages and obstruction causing the resultant infertility issues (Criss and Seifert 2013). In severe cases, the organism will be transmitted via the bloodstream and lodge in joints causing septic arthritis (often a single joint). Treatment is with penicillins or cephalosporins, with ceftriaxone and cefixime, with or without azithromycin, the most favoured. However, resistance has been reported and these strains (and for persons allergic to the antibiotic) are treated with ciprofloxacin (Bignell et al. 2013). A strain of gonorrhoea resistant to azithromycin was found in the UK and 34 laboratory confirmed cases were reported by Public Health England between November 2014 and April 2016 (Wise 2016).

Chlamydia Trachomatis (D-K serotypes)

Chlamydia trachomatis is an intracellular Gram-negative bacterium that infects the columnar epithelium of the cervix, urethra, and rectum, as well as nongenital sites. There are 18 distinct serotypes identified and D-K causes STIs and neonatal infections.

The cell cycle of Chlamydia is different to other bacteria in that following endocytosis, the bacterium becomes membrane bound and continues to live within the cell in either resting or metabolically inert elementary bodies (EB) or metabolically active replicating bodies (RB) (Paarvonen and Eggert-Kruse 1999). EBs attach to columnar epithelial cells followed by endocytosis and inhibition of lysosomal fusion occurs. These different states (EB and RB) express different antigens during the cell cycle, making antigenically based diagnosis sometimes difficult. Current diagnostic methods are molecularly based looking for specific genes.

Most persons who are infected with *C. trachomatis* are asymptomatic. However, when symptoms of infection are present, in women they most commonly include abnormal vaginal discharge, pelvic pain, vaginal bleeding (including bleeding after intercourse), and dysuria. On physical examination, mucopurulent or purulent discharge from the endocervical canal and cervical friability are common. In men, symptoms may include penile discharge, pruritus, and dysuria. Persons who have receptive anal intercourse can acquire a rectal infection, which can present as pain, discharge, or bleeding (Figure 14.3). Those engaging in oral sex can acquire a pharyngeal infection from an infected partner (Mishori et al. 2012). Chlamydial infections in women are usually asymptomatic and if left untreated have more serious consequences for reproduction. Detailed evidence is lacking but it is suggested that approximately 20% can develop PID, 2–9% ectopic pregnancy, and 4% chronic pelvic pain (Paavonen and Eggert-Kruse 1999) with tubal factor infertility being a major cause (Kavanagh et al. 2013). In addition, pregnant women infected with Chlamydia can pass the infection to their infants during delivery, potentially resulting in neonatal ophthalmia and pneumonia. It is the most frequently reported STI and is the leading cause of infectious blindness in the world (Mishori et al. 2012). In men, Chlamydia infections are implicated in epididymitis, orchitis, and prostatitis. In addition, there is some debate as to whether infection can have an effect on semen quality as well as scarring of the seminal ducts due to chronic inflammation on semen production (Lee and Lee 2013). Furthermore, sperm from infertile men positive for *C. trachomatis* displayed increased sperm-DNA fragmentation compared with uninfected men (Sellami et al. 2014), further implicating *C. trachomatis* infection and decreased sperm quality.

(a)

(b)

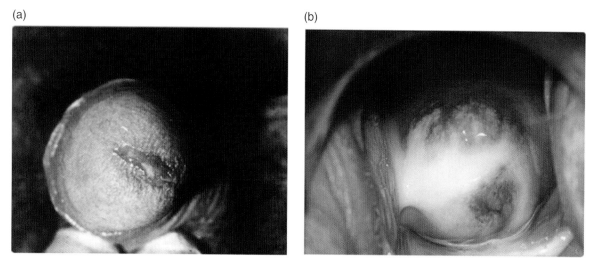

Figure 14.3 (a) *Chlamydia trachomatis* infection in the male, showing penile discharge. (b) Infection in the female displaying purulent discharge from the endocervical canal. *Source:* https://commons.wikimedia.org.

Chlamydia Trachomatis (Lymphogranuloma Venereum) (L1, L2, and L3 Serotypes)

Lymphogranuloma venereum (LGV) is a STI caused by L1, L2, and L3 serovars of *C. trachomatis* that primarily infects the lymphatics and can be transmitted through unprotected vaginal, anal, or oral sexual contact. Three stages of disease have been described:

1) The primary stage (3–30 days) may go undetected when only a painless papule, pustule, or ulceration appears and is diagnosed with serology or more recently, nucleic acid amplification testing.
2) The secondary stage begins within 2–6 weeks after the onset of the primary lesion. Depending on the site of inoculation, LGV can cause inguinal syndrome or anorectal syndrome. Inguinal syndrome presents with painful inflammation of the inguinal (superficial and deep) lymph nodes and occurs mostly in men (Figure 14.4) (occurs in only 20% of women with LGV). It is the most common clinical manifestation of genital LGV among heterosexuals with 66% having unilateral enlargement, inflammation, suppuration, abscesses, and necrosis with lymph nodes developing the classic 'bubo' of LGV.
3) The third stage is seen predominantly in women and is characterized by a chronic inflammatory response and the destruction of tissue, which is followed by the formation of a perirectal abscess,

fistulas, strictures, and stenosis of the rectum causing strictures and fistulas that can cause elephantiasis of the genitals.

LGV is endemic in tropical and subtropical areas of the world (certain areas of Africa, Southeast Asia, India, the Caribbean, and South America). The incidence has been low in the developed world, but in the last 10 years outbreaks have appeared in North America, Europe, and Australia in the form of proctitis among MSM (Ceovic and Gulin 2015).

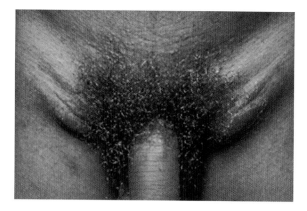

Figure 14.4 Lymphogranuloma venereum is caused by the invasive serovars L1, L2, or L3 of *Chlamydia trachomatis*. Symptoms can include acute onset of tender, enlarged lymph nodes in both groins. *Source:* Herbert. https://commons.wikimedia.org/wiki/File:Lymphogranuloma_venerum_-_lymph_nodes.jpg. CC-BY 2.0.

Syphillis

Treponema pallidum is a spirochaete causing syphilis, which causes reproductive problems and congenital malformations of the fetus if left untreated. Although uncommon in the UK, it is still prevalent in developing countries. The disease profile manifests through three different stages: primary, secondary, and tertiary syphilis. The primary stage involves penetration of mucocutaneous tissues causing a primary painless chancre (ulcer) at the site of entry. During secondary stages (usually several weeks after the chancre has resolved), the spirochaete causes a maculopapular rash, generalized lymphadenopathy, and fever. Other systemic manifestations may occur including meningitis, arthritis, and nephrotic syndrome, to name a few. A latent stage (an asymptomatic stage) between secondary and tertiary stages can persist for several years and causes slow tissue damage in many body organs. The tertiary stage can affect many bodily organs with the underlying gummata (lesions) continuing to degenerate, creating enlargement and ulceration.

Management of syphilis is by administration of antibiotics (penicillin) at all stages to kill the spirochaete and prevent further damage, with clinical support and other medical procedures necessary to rectify resultant tissue damage. Complications of syphilis are related to infection during pregnancy, with early syphilis resulting in abortion and transplacental syphilis resulting in short-term and long-term diseases as a result of malformation to the fetus during its development.

Haemophilus Infection

Haemophilus ducreyi is a Gram-negative coccobacillus that is sexually transmitted. After an incubation period of 2–5 days a chanchroid (a soft ulcer) develops in the genitalia. This ulcer can be mistaken for a primary syphilitic chancre but it is very painful, unlike the painless chancre of syphilis. It is uncommon in the UK but prevalent in the West Indies, south-east USA, the Middle East, China, and North Africa, and is not frequently implicated in infertility issues. Diagnosis is by Gram stain and culture and treatment is with ciprofloxacin or sulphonamides.

Mycoplasma and Ureaplasma

Mycoplasma genitalium and *U. urealyticum* are both mycoplasmas with a role in nonspecific genital infections. These microorganisms do not possess the typical bacterial cell wall, and as such do not respond to antibiotics including cephalosporins or penicillins. Treatment is with erythromycin. Complications of *U. urealyticum* are Reiter's syndrome. *M. genitalium* is associated with acute and chronic urethritis in men and urethritis, cervicitis, pelvic inflammatory disease, and possibly infertility in women. Azithromycin is the drug of choice for treatment and moxifloxacin is used in azithromycin-resistant strains. Persons with persistent PID or clinically significant persistent urethritis or cervicitis should be tested for *M. genitalium.*

Viral Sexually Transmitted Infections

The impact of viral STIs on infertility is suggested but not well understood. Human herpes simplex virus (HSV), HIV, human cytomegalovirus (HCMV), hepatitis B virus, and human papillomavirus (HPV) have all been detected in semen from men attending an infertility clinic.

HPV is a DNA virus establishing infection in the mucous membranes of the genital tract. There are numerous serotypes and type 16 and 18 are associated with cervical cancer and type 6 and 8 with genital warts. HPV infections are often asymptomatic and most of the time, people are infected without being aware. Even if the infection does not necessarily lead to cellular lesions or proliferation, it is unclear whether HPV infections can silently lead to damage that alters reproductive function. A systematic review carried out showed that HPV can be linked to: (i) apoptosis in sperm cells; (ii) alterations of semen quality through cell count decrease, amplitude of lateral head displacement reduction, mobility reduction and increase of antisperm antibodies level; (iii) apoptosis in embryonic cells; (iv) miscarriages or premature rupture of membrane, which ultimately affects infertility (Souhu et al. 2015). Two other viruses, HSV and HCMV, have been implicated in a recent study using DNA detection methods which found a correlation (<5%) between these STIs, leucospermia, and other infertility markers (Bezold et al. 2007).

Fungal and Parasitic Sexually Transmitted Infections

Candida albicans (thrush) and trichomoniasis, previously described, can be sexually acquired if either partner transmits the infectious agent during sexual intercourse; they have been implicated in infertility issues. Other ectoparasites, such as scabies or pubic lice, which are classed as a STIs, have not been implicated in reproductive issues.

Conclusion

Infection and associated infertility is extremely complex and further evidence is required to fully understand the true impact in the long term. Many genital infections, whether endogenous or sexually acquired, are asymptomatic but the resultant immunological damage, whether humoral or cell mediated, can cause long-term tissue damage due to inflammation. Occasionally, some infections can cause problems postconception and can cross the placenta causing fetal damage (Rubella). Infections caught in childhood (such as mumps) can cause long-term effects for the unsuspecting male. Microencephaly and congenital anomalies (referred to as congenital Zika syndrome) have recently been recorded as serious complications of the Zika virus (a member of the genus Flavivirus and family Flaviviridae). This has become a global issue, as it has been determined that this virus can be sexually transmitted as well as transmitted in the usual manner via mosquito bites (WHO 2016).

References

Aagaard, K., Ma, J., Antony, K.M. et al. (2014). The placenta harbours a unique microbiome. Sci Transl Med 6: 237–265.

Achkar, J.M. and Fries, B.C. (2010). Candida infections of the genitourinary tract. Clin Microbiol Rev 23: 253–273.

Africa, C.W.J., Nel, J. and Stemmet, M. (2014). Anaerobes and bacterial vaginosis in pregnancy: virulence factors contributing to vaginal colonisation. Int J Environ Res Public Health 11: 6979–7000.

Alshahrani, S., McGill, J. and Agarwal, A. (2013). Prostatitis and male infertility. J Reprod Immunol 100: 30–36.

Banikarim, C. and Chacko, M.R. (2005). Pelvic inflammatory disease in adolescents. Semin Pediatr Infect Dis 16: 175–180.

Bezold, G., Politch, J.A., Kiviat, N.B. et al. (2007). Prevalence of sexually transmissible pathogens in semen from asymptomatic male infertility patients with and without leukocytospermia. Fertil Steril 87: 1087–1097.

Bignell, C., Unemo, M., Radcliffe, K. et al. (2013). 2012 European guideline on the diagnosis and treatment of gonorrhoea in adults. Int J STD AIDS 24: 85–92.

Brotman, R.M. (2011). Vaginal microbiome and sexually transmitted infections: an epidemiologic perspective. J Clin Invest 121: 4610–4617.

Burrello, N., Salmeri, M., Perdichizzi, A. et al. (2009). Candida albicans experimental infection: effects on human sperm motility, mitochondrial membrane potential and apoptosis. Reprod Biomed Online 18: 496–501.

Centers for Disease Control and Prevention (2010). Sexually transmitted infection guidelines. http://www.cdc.gov/std/treatment/2010/epididymitis.htm.

Centers for Disease Control and Prevention (2013). *Sexually transmitted disease surveillance.* Atlanta: US Department of Health and Human Services, 2014. http://www.cdc.gov/std/stats13/surv2013-print.pdf.

Centers for Disease Control and Prevention (2014). Sexually transmitted disease and infertility. http://www.cdc.gov/std/infertility/default.htm.

Ceovic, R. and Gulin, S.J. (2015). Lymphogranuloma venereum: diagnostic and treatment challenges. Infect Drug Resist 8: 39–47.

Criss, A.K. and Seifert, H.S. (2013). A bacterial siren song: intimate interactions between neutrophils and pathogenic Neisseria. Nat Rev Microbiol 10: 178–190.

Dohle, G.R., Colpi, G.M., Hargreave, T.B. et al. (2005). EAU guidelines on male infertility. Eur Urol 48: 703–711.

Donders, G.G.G., Vereecken, A., Bosmans, E. et al. (2005). Aerobic vaginitis: abnormal vaginal flora entity that is distinct from bacterial vaginosis. Proceedings of the 15th Congress of Gynaecology. Obstet Reprod Med 1279: 118–129.

El-Shazly, A.M., El-Naggar, H.M., Soliman, M. et al. (2001). A study on Trichomoniasis vaginalis and female infertility. J Egypt Soc Parasitol 31: 545–553.

Faro, S. (1993). Infection and infertility. Infect Dis Obstet Gynaecol 1: 51–57.

Heyns, C.F. and Fisher, M. (2005). The urological management of the patient with acquired immunodeficiency syndrome. BJU Int 95: 709–716.

Kavanagh, K., Wallace, L.A., Robertson, C. et al. (2013). Estimation of the risk of tubal factor infertility associated with genital chlamydial infection in women: a statistical modelling study. Int J Epidemiol 42: 493–503.

Keck, C., Gerber-Schafer, C., Clad, A. et al. (1998). Seminal tract infections: impact on male fertility and treatment options. Hum Reprod Update 4: 891–903.

Lee, Y.S. and Lee, K.S. (2013). Chlamydia and male lower urinary tract diseases. Korean J Urol 54: 73–77.

Liu, M.B., Xu, S.R., Hez, Y. et al. (2013). Diverse vaginal microbiomes in reproductive-age women with vulvovaginal candidiasis. PLOS ONE 8: e79812.

Ludwig, M., Velcovsky, H.G. and Weidner, W. (2008). Tuberculous epididymo-orchitis and prostatitis: a case report. Andrologia 40: 81–83.

Manhart, L.E., Broad, J.M. and Golden, M.R. (2011). Mycoplasma genitalium: should we treat and how? Clin Infect Dis 53(S3): S129–142.

Marrazo, J.M. (2011). Interpreting the epidemiology and natural history of bacterial vaginosis: are we still confused? Anaerobe 17: 186–190.

Mastromarino, P., Vitali, B. and Mosca, L. (2013). Bacterial vaginosis: a review on clinical trials with probiotics. New Microbiologica 36: 229–238.

Mazzoli, S., Cai, T., Addonisio, P. et al. (2010). Chlamydia trachomatis infection is related to poor semen quality in young prostatitis patients. Eur Urol 57: 708–714.

Mishori, R., McClaskey, E.L. and Winklerprins, V.J. (2012). Chlamydia trachomatis infections: screening, diagnosis, and management. Am Fam Physician 86: 1127–1132.

Nickel, W.R. and Plumb, R.T. (1986) Mumps orchitis. In: *Campbells Urology*, 5th edn. (ed. J.H. Harrison, R.F. Gittes, A.D. Perlmutter et al.), 977–988. Philadelphia: W.B. Saunders.

Paavonen, J. (2005). Pelvic inflammatory disease. Medicine 33: 41–46.

Paavonen, J. and Eggert-Kruse, W. (1999). Chlamydia trachomatis: impact on human reproduction. Hum Reprod Update 5: 433–437.

Pellati, D., Mylonakis, I., Bertoloni, G. et al. (2008). Genital tract infections and infertility. Eur J Obstet Gynecol Reprod Biol 140: 3–11.

Public Health England (2016). Sexually transmitted infections and chlamydia screening in England, 2016. Health Protection Report, Vol 8, No. 24, 20 June 2014. https://www.gov.uk/government/uploads/system/uploads/attachment_data/file/345181/Volume_8_number_24_hpr2414_AA_stis.pdf accessed 29th April 2015.

Roh, J., Lim, Y.S., Seo, M.Y. et al. (2015). The secretory products of Trichomonas vaginalis decrease fertilizing capacity of mice sperm in vitro. Asian J Androl 17: 319–323.

Sellami, H., Znazen, A., Sellami, A. et al. (2014). Molecular detection of Chlamydia trachomatis and other sexually transmitted bacteria in semen of male partners of infertile couples in Tunisia: the effect on semen parameters and spermatozoa apoptosis markers. PLoS One 9: e98903.

Sharp, V.J., Takacs, E.B. and Powell, C.R. (2010). Prostatitis: diagnosis and treatment. Am Fam Physician 82: 397–406.

Souho, T., Benlemlih, M. and Bennani, B. (2015). Human papillomavirus infection and fertility alteration: a systematic review. PLoS One 10: e0126936.

Street, E.J., Portman, M.D., Kopa, Z. et al. (2012). European guideline on the management of epididymo-orchitis. International Union against Sexually Transmitted Infection (IUSTI) EO Guidelines. http://www.iusti.org/regions/europe/pdf/2013/Epididymo-orchitis-2013IUSTI_WHO.pdf.

Tempera, G. and Furneri, P.M. (2010). Management of aerobic vaginitis. Gynecol Obstet Invest 70: 244–249.

Tian, Y.-H., Xiong, J.W., Hu, L. et al. (2007). Candida albicans and filtrates interfere with human spermatozoal motility and alter the ultrastructure of spermatozoa: an in vitro study. In J Androl 30: 421–429.

Tuttle, J.P. Jr, Bannister, E.R. and Derrick, F.C. (1997). Interference of human spermatozoal motility and spermatozoal agglutination by Candida albicans. J Urol 118: 797–799.

Verstraelen, H., Vilchez-Vargas, R., Desimpel, F. et al. (2016). Characterisation of the human uterine microbiome in non-pregnant women through deep sequencing of the 16S rRNA gene. Peer J 4: e1602.

Viswaroop, B.S., Kekre, N. and Goplalkrishnan, G. (2005). Isolated tuberculous epididymitis: a review of 40 cases (2005). J Postgrad Med 51: 109–111.

Wharton, I.P., Chaudhry, A.H. and French, M.E. (2006). A case of mumps epididymitis. Lancet 367: 9511.

Wise, J. (2016). Antibiotic resistant gonorrhoea increases in England. BMJ 353: i2219.

World Health Organization (1995). World Health Organization Task Force on the Prevention and Management of Infertility. Tubal infertility: serologic relationship to post chlamydial and gonococcal infection. Sex Transm Dis 22: 71–77.

World Health Organization (2016). WHO's response to Zika virus and its associated complications. http://www.who.int/emergencies/zika-virus-tmp/response-zika-2017.pdf?ua=1

Yung, C., Andrews, N., Bukasa, A. et al. (2011). Mumps complications and effects of mumps vaccination, England and Wales, 2002–2006. Emerging Infect Dis 17: 661–667.

15

Nutrition, Fetal Health, and Pregnancy

Emma Derbyshire

Nutritional Demands

During pregnancy the body experiences some of the most physiologically demanding changes ever experienced in human life (Hytten and Chamberlain 1991). Whilst the body adapts to some extent, namely by increasing nutrient absorption via the gut, there are additional dietary requirements for certain nutrients (Table 15.1).

Firstly, energy requirements are mostly unchanged during pregnancy with the exception of the third trimester. The Scientific Advisory Committee on Nutrition reviewed energy requirements for pregnancy, advising that is was not necessary to amend original recommendations of an increment of 0.8 MJ per day (around 200 kcal/day) in the last trimester. It was, however, further noted that women entering pregnancy who are overweight may not need this additional requirement, although data is currently insufficient to formalize this (SACN 2011) (Figure 15.1).

An additional 6 g of protein per day was originally advised by the UK Department of Health. However, Canadian research investigating specific protein requirements during the different stages of pregnancy suggests that protein requirements are higher than original estimations of 0.88 g per kg body weight per day. It is now thought that protein requirements during early and late pregnancy are around 1.22 and 1.52 g per kg body weight per day, respectively (Stephens et al. 2015).

The requirement for the micronutrient folate increases during pregnancy to prevent megaloblastic anaemia and reduce the risk of neural tube defects (NTDs) such as spina bifida (Department of Health 1991). It should be also considered that different modes of food preparation can influence the stability of folate and its bioavailability. This can range from 25 to 50% from foods, 85% from enriched foods, and 100% from supplements (Banjari et al. 2014). In view of this and the tendency towards low habitual intakes of dietary folate the Scientific Advisory Committee on Nutrition advise that women planning a pregnancy should supplement their diet with 400 μg/day of folic acid (5 mg/day for women with a previous pregnancy affected by NTD) prior to conception until the 12th week of pregnancy (SACN 2006).

Vitamin B12 is an essential part of one carbon metabolic pathways and is central to the stability of nucleic acids and methylation of DNA which regulates gene expression. An increasing body of evidence now suggests that low maternal vitamin B12 status (as often seen in vegetarians) may be also be associated with increased NTD risk, alongside low lean fetal mass, excess adiposity, increased insulin resistance, and impaired neurodevelopment in the offspring (Rush et al. 2014). Presently, there is no additional increment for vitamin B12 during pregnancy but women should aim to achieve basic targets of 1.5 μg/day (Table 15.1).

Table 15.1 Increased nutritional demands in pregnancy.

	Non-pregnant women (19–50 years)	Pregnancy increment
Energy (kcal/day)	1940	+200 (third trimester)
Protein (g/day)	45	+6
Thiamin (mg/day)	0.8	+0.1 (third trimester)
Riboflavin (mg/day)	1.1	+0.3
Folate (µg/day)	200	+100
Vitamin B12 (µg/day)	1.5	No Increment
Vitamin C (mg/day)	40	+10
Vitamin A (µg/day)	600	+100
Vitamin D (µg/day)	No reference nutrient intake	+10
Calcium (mg/day)	700	No Increment
Iron (mg/day)	14.8	No Increment
Selenium (µg/day)	60	No Increment
Iodine (µg/day)	140	No Increment

Source: Department of Health (1991).

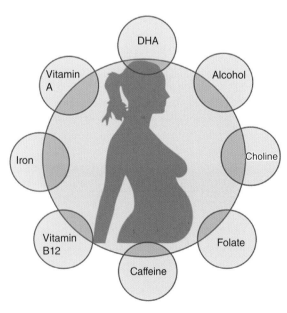

Figure 15.1 The role of nutrition and dietary components during pregnancy. DHA, docosahexaenoic acid.

An increment of 100 µg/day of vitamin A is recommended throughout pregnancy to allow for the rapid growth of the fetus (Department of Health 1991). As well as being important in supporting the development of the fetal eyes it is thought that all-trans retinoic acid (RA) is the form of vitamin A that helps to support embryonic development, which includes the development of the reproductive systems of the fetus *in utero* (Clagett-Dame and Knutson 2011),

In the case of iron, extra maternal and fetal red blood cells are manufactured during pregnancy leading to an increased requirement for iron, yet the UK Reference Nutrient Intake (RNI) for iron does not increase due to enhanced absorption, cessation of menstruation, and mobilization of iron stores. The increased absorption of non-haem iron in pregnancy does, however, increase the vitamin C RNI by 10 mg/day in the last trimester (Department of Health 1991). The risk of pregnancy anaemia, typically defined as blood haemoglobin below 10.5 g/dL can be exacerbated by medical conditions including uterine or placental bleeding, gastrointestinal bleeding, and peripartum blood loss. Subsequently, this can increase the risk of intrauterine growth retardation, prematurity, and peripartum blood transfusion (Breymann 2015).

During pregnancy, calcium is needed to support changes in muscle function, nerve transmission, skeletal development, blood coagulation, and cell membrane function. This demand is mostly met by enhanced absorption and through mobilization of maternal skeleton calcium stores (Hovdenak et al. 2012). Whilst women who begin pregnancy with adequate intake may not need additional calcium, women with suboptimal intakes, defined as <500 mg daily, may need additional amounts to meet both maternal and fetal bone requirements, otherwise the risk of bone loss during pregnancy is likely to be higher (Hacker et al. 2012).

Vitamin D requirements rise to sustain the increase of calcium absorption and utilization during pregnancy and lactation, hence the RNI becomes 10 µg/day (Department of Health, 1991). The Scientific Advisory Committee on Nutrition has proposed that a RNI of 10 µg/day for vitamin D is set for the UK population aged 4 years and over. This is regarded as the amount needed for 97.5% of the population to maintain a serum 25-hydroxyvita-min D concentration of 25 nmol/L when UVB sunshine exposure is minimal (SACN 2015).

Choline

It is well known that folic acid is needed for maternal and fetal health during pregnancy but the role of other nutrients, including choline, is somewhat overlooked. Choline, also a member of the B vitamin family, plays a key role in fetal development, especially of the brain. Human newborns are delivered with blood levels of choline around three times higher than maternal blood concentrations (Caudill 2010).

Choline is found typically in common food sources such as eggs, meat, and dairy products though the trend towards low-fat diets means that there is general tendency for this nutrient to be underconsumed by women of childbearing age. Recently, an assessment of choline intake in European populations identified intakes to be 291–468 mg/day amongst adults (18 to ≤65 years old) (Vennemann et al. 2015). As shown in Table 15.2 pregnancy recommendations are considerably higher than this, demonstrating a gap between habitual intakes and dietary targets.

Table 15.2 Dietary reference intake values for choline.

Adequate intakes	Recommended choline intake (mg/day)
Females 14–18 years	400
Females ≥19 years	425
Pregnancy	450
Lactation	550
Tolerable upper limit (UL)	
Females 14–18 years	3500
Females ≥19 years	3500
Pregnancy	Age-appropriate UL
Lactation	Age-appropriate UL

Source: Institute of Medicine (2006).

Docosahexaenoic Acid

Docosahexaenoic acid (DHA) is an omega-3, essential fatty acid, meaning that it cannot be produced endogenously in amounts needed for optimal health. This is further hampered by the fact that high intakes of omega-6 fatty acids limit the metabolic conversion of alpha-linolenic acid into DHA (Derbyshire 2016). Accumulation of DHA in the fetal brain mainly takes place in the third trimester of pregnancy, with rates of accretion being very high up to the end of the second year of life (Lauritzen et al. 2016).

DHA also accounts for 50% of fatty acids in the retina of the eye (Malcolm et al. 2003). Poor vision has been associated with low DHA status in fetal development (Birch et al. 2005). In particular, DHA is thought to support visual acuity by supporting the normal functioning of photoreceptor cells (Krauss-Etschmann et al. 2008).

The UK recommendation for dietary intake of omega-3 fatty acids is 450 mg per day, which can be achieved by consuming two 140 g portions of fish a week, one of which should be oily (SACN 2004). However, this guideline is aimed at the general population and does not specifically meet the needs of pregnant or lactating women, suggesting that higher omega-3 intakes may be needed for some groups. In Europe, it has been advised that pregnant and lactating women should aim to achieve an average dietary intake of at least 200 mg of DHA per day. Furthermore, intakes of up to 1 g/day of DHA or 2.7 g/day of n-3 long-chain polyunsaturated fatty acids have been used in randomized clinical trials without significant adverse effects (Koletzko et al. 2007).

Alcohol

Alcohol is a well-known teratogen, passing freely across the placenta to the developing child. As amniotic fluid contains less fat than plasma, the concentration of alcohol in amniotic fluid is generally higher than that in the bloodstream which can be potentially toxic to the offspring (Whitehall 2007). The prevalence of birth defects attributed to high rates of alcohol consumption in pregnancy is higher in some regions of the world. A recent meta-analysis identified particularly high rates of fetal alcohol syndrome in South Africa and a high number of alcohol-related birth defects in Australia (Roozen et al. 2016).

If a woman drinks whilst pregnant her baby is at increased risk of being born with fetal alcohol spectrum disorder (FASD). This term is used to categorize a series of structural, behavioural, and neurocognitive impairments that can affect the child. Fetal alcohol syndrome is the most clinically recognizable form of FASD for which three key symptoms must be present: (i) facial malformations; (ii) impaired growth; and (iii) central nervous system dysfunction (Figure 15.2). These children may also experience pre- and postnatal growth restriction leading to poor brain growth and/or development (O'Leary 2004).

In the UK, the Chief Medical Officer's guidelines, published by the Department of Health, advise that if you are pregnant or planning a pregnancy the safest approach is to abstain completely from alcohol consumption. The report emphasizes that drinking in pregnancy can lead to long-term harm to the baby, with the more you drink being proportionately linked to greater risks (Department of Health 2016).

Caffeine

Caffeine is a methylxanthine, a chemical structure that can pass via the placenta to the fetus, potentially leading to poor pregnancy outcomes. Despite considerable research the evidence base from studies is rather mixed. It does, however, seem that the potential adverse effects of caffeine are stronger for the first third of pregnancy when compared with later in pregnancy (Adèn 2011).

Originally, caffeine guidelines were set at ≤300 mg per day. Prospective research in the UK following 2635 women throughout their pregnancies found that higher caffeine intakes were associated with an increased risk of fetal growth restriction (FGR) (CARE 2008). In particular, after adjusting data for several confounders, caffeine consumption was found to increase the risk of FGR by around 50% at intakes of 200–299 mg per day and above.

Subsequently, sensible advice based on findings from the CARE Study Group (2008) is to: monitor caffeine intakes in pregnancy; avoid exceeding Food Standards Agency (2008) guidelines of no more than 200 mg/day; and try to get a feel for 'how much' caffeine is in a mug of tea (about 75 mg), mug of coffee (around 100 mg; instant coffee), and a bar of chocolate (about 25 mg in a 50 g bar of milk chocolate).

Conclusion

In summary, a balanced diet containing adequate amounts of nutrients central to maternal and fetal health is essential during pregnancy. As a general model, the UK Eatwell Guide (Public Health England 2016) is a good basis for a healthy and balanced diet. However, given the limited bioavailability of certain

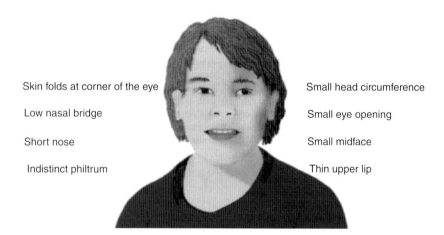

Skin folds at corner of the eye

Low nasal bridge

Short nose

Indistinct philtrum

Small head circumference

Small eye opening

Small midface

Thin upper lip

Figure 15.2 The features and symptoms of fetal alcohol spectrum disorder. *Source:* www.wikicommons.org.

nutrients coupled with the tendency towards low habitual intakes, folic acid, vitamin D, iron, and choline, in particular, may need to be obtained from fortified or supplement sources. Alcohol and caffeine intake should also be considered during this physiologically sensitive time.

References

Adėn, U. (2011). Methylxanthines during pregnancy and early postnatal life. Handb Exp Pharmacol 200: 373–389.

Banjari, I., Matoković, V. and Škoro, V. (2014). The question is whether intake of folic acid from diet alone during pregnancy is sufficient. Med Pregl 67: 313–321.

Birch, E.E., Castenda, Y.S., Wheat, D.H. et al. (2005). Visual maturation of term infants fed long-chain polyunsaturated fatty acid-supplemented or control formula for 12 mo. Am J Clin Nutri 81: 871–879.

Breymann, C. (2015). Iron deficiency anemia in pregnancy. Semin Hematol 52: 339–347.

CARE Study Group (2008). Maternal caffeine intake during pregnancy and risk of fetal growth restriction: a large prospective observational study. BMJ 337: 23–32.

Caudill, M.A. (2010). Pre- and postnatal health: evidence of increased choline needs. J Am Diet Assoc 110: 1198–1206.

Clagett-Dame M. and Knutson D. (2011). Vitamin A in reproduction and development. Nutrients 3: 385–428.

Department of Health (1991). Report on Health and Social Subjects. *Dietary Reference Values for Food Energy and for Nutrients for the United Kingdom*. London: HMSO.

Department of Health (2016). UK Chief Medical Officers' Alcohol Guidelines Review Summary of the proposed new guidelines. Available at: https://www.gov.uk/government/uploads/system/uploads/attachment_data/file/489795/summary.pdf (accessed 8 February 2018).

Derbyshire, E.J. (2016). Docosahexaenoic acid and its principal roles during pregnancy. NHD Mag 111: 16–21.

Food Standards Agency (2008). Food Standards Agency publishes new caffeine advice for pregnant women. Available at: http://www.food.gov.uk/news/pressreleases/2008/nov/caffeineadvice (accessed 8 February 2018).

Hacker, A.N., Fung, E.B. and King, J.C. (2012). Role of calcium during pregnancy: maternal and fetal needs. Nutr Rev 70: 397–409.

Hovdenak, N., Haram, K., Hovdenak, N. et al. (2012). Influence of mineral and vitamin supplements on pregnancy outcome. Eur J Obstet Gynecol Reprod Biol 164: 127–132.

Hytten, F.E. and Chamberlain, G. (1991). *Clinical Physiology in Obstetrics*. Oxford: Blackwell Scientific Publications.

Institute of Medicine (2006). *Dietary Reference Intakes: The Essential Guide to Nutrient Requirements*. Washington, DC: The National Academies Press.

Koletzko, B., Cetin, I., Brenna, JT, Perinatal Lipid Intake Working Group; Child Health Foundation et al. (2007). Dietary fat intakes for pregnant and lactating women. Br J Nutr 98: 873–877.

Krauss-Etschmann, S., Hartl, D., Rzehak, P. et al. (2008). Decreased cord blood OL-4, OL-13, and CCR4 and increased TGF-β levels after fish oil supplementation of pregnant women. J Allergy Clin Immunol 121: 464–470.

Lauritzen, L., Brambilla, P., Mazzocchi, A. et al. (2016). DHA effects in brain development and function. Nutrients 8: pii: E6.

Malcolm, C.A., Hamilton, R., McCulloch, D.L. et al. (2003). Scotopic electroretinogram in term infants born of mothers supplemented with docosahexaenoic acid during pregnancy. Invest Ophthalmol Vis Sci 44: 3685–3691.

O'Leary, C.M. (2004). Fetal alcohol syndrome: diagnosis, epidemiology, and developmental outcomes. J Paediatr Child Health 40: 2–7.

Public Health England (2016). The Eatwell Guide. Available at: https://www.gov.uk/government/publications/the-eatwell-guide (accessed 8 February 2018).

Roozen, S., Peters, G.J., Kok, G. et al. (2016). Worldwide prevalence of fetal alcohol spectrum disorders: a systematic literature review including meta-analysis. Alcohol Clin Exp Res 40:18–32.

Rush, E.C., Katre, P. and Yajnik, C.S. (2014). Vitamin B12: one carbon metabolism, fetal growth and programming for chronic disease. Eur J Clin Nutr 68: 2–7.

Scientific Advisory Committee on Nutrition and Committee on Toxicity (2004). *Advice on Fish Consumption, Benefits and Risks*. London: HMSO.

Scientific Advisory Committee on Nutrition (2006). *Folate and Disease Prevention*. London: TSO.

Scientific Advisory Committee on Nutrition (2011). *Dietary Reference Values for Energy*. London: TSO.

Scientific Advisory Committee on Nutrition (2015). Draft Vitamin D and Health report. Available at: https://www.gov.uk/government/consultations/consultation-on-draft-sacn-vitamin-d-and-health-report (accessed 8 February 2018).

Stephens, T.V., Payne, M., Ball, R.O. et al. (2015). Protein requirements of healthy pregnant women during early and late gestation are higher than current recommendations. J Nutr 145: 73–78.

Vennemann, F.B., Ioannidou, S., Valsta, L.M. et al. (2015). Dietary intake and food sources of choline in European populations. Br J Nutr 114: 2046–2055.

Whitehall, J.S. (2007). National guidelines on alcohol use during pregnancy: a dissenting option. Med J Austr 186: 35–37.

16

The Embryonic Environment and Developmental Origins of Health

Tom P. Fleming and Congshan Sun

Introduction

During the first 5–7 days of life, the early embryo undertakes a complex, challenging developmental programme, set within a tight deadline and comprising a daunting 'tick list' of activities which have been well studied mainly across animal models, with more limited data on the human. The embryo programme of activities can be briefly summarized as:

- Fertilization: with the objectives to complete oocyte meiosis, re-establish diploidy, activate cortical granule exocytosis to block polyspermy, initiate sperm-mediated signalling within the egg necessary for resumption of mitotic cell cycling, and engage with the new development programme (Nomikos et al. 2013; Anifandis et al. 2014).
- Embryonic genome activation: to ensure degradation of maternally encoded transcripts and their attendant biosynthetic profile followed by *de novo* construction and expression from the new integrated paternal and maternal genome belonging to the embryo (Li et al. 2013).
- Cleavage and the onset of early differentiation: including a coordinated pattern of cellular inheritance of zygotic cytoplasm into early blastomeres and their expression of embryonic genome proteins to initiate cellular differentiation, and notably, activation of cell–cell adhesion and embryo compaction together with the onset of cell polarity (Eckert and Fleming 2008; Eckert et al. 2015).
- Generation of embryonic and extra-embryonic cell lineages: to construct an outer epithelium, the trophectoderm (TE) and progenitor of the chorio-allantoic placenta, and an inner cell cluster, the inner cell mass (ICM), which subsequently segregates into epiblast, the pluripotent stem cell pool for gastrulation and formation of the embryonic germ cell lineages, and the primitive endoderm which gives rise to the parietal and visceral yolk sac endoderm extraembryonic lineages (Bedzhov et al. 2014; Sozen et al. 2014; Eckert et al. 2015).
- Morphogenesis: to activate polarized, regulated TE epithelial transport to facilitate blastocyst formation and the expansion of the blastocoelic cavity resulting in a three-dimensional cyst-like organization necessary for implantation (Eckert and Fleming 2008; Chen et al. 2010).
- Metabolism: to provide and maintain an energy budget and homeostasis for the demands of biosynthesis, morphogenesis, and growth (Leese 2012; Gardner and Harvey 2015).
- Epigenetic reorganization of the embryonic genome: to facilitate global active and passive demethylation of paternal and maternal alleles respectively, ensure protection from demethylation of imprinted genes, and initiate the gradual remethylation of genes in a lineage-specific manner from the blastocyst stage onwards to underlie cell-type specific patterns of gene expression (Chen et al. 2010; Rivera and Ross 2013; Zhou and Dean 2015).
- Hatching and implantation: to ensure emergence of the expanded blastocyst from the zona pellucida glycoprotein coat, the gradual apposition and adhesion of the TE with the uterine endometrial epithelium, followed by TE outgrowth and invasion accompanied by endometrial decidualization and embryo implantation (Seshagiri et al. 2009; Cha et al. 2012).

Clinical Reproductive Science, First Edition. Edited by Michael Carroll.
© 2019 John Wiley & Sons Ltd. Published 2019 by John Wiley & Sons Ltd.
Companion website: www.wiley.com/go/carroll/clinicalreproductivescience

The embryo is involved in more than this busy series of classical, inward-looking developmental transitions. Recent research indicates a second more outward-looking programme running in parallel where the embryo interfaces with its environment. This second series of events confers plasticity of the emerging phenotype to promote an optimal growth trajectory and metabolic status best suited to the actual conditions the embryo is experiencing. We believe external conditions such as maternal nutrition, physiology, and health status can be 'sensed' by early embryos resulting in adaptations that support survival and competitiveness of the offspring. These *in vivo* interactions and modifications can also occur *in vitro*, and so are relevant within the clinical setting of assisted reproductive technology (ART) (Figure 16.1). Such sensing and response mechanisms can be considered as embryos making 'decisions' on their future or may reflect perturbations in the inherent programme caused by external factors (Fleming et al. 2015) and stress conditions (Puscheck et al. 2015). This second, extrinsic, programme is the subject of this chapter. Embryo environmental programming has profound consequences with a legacy that persists into late adult life and may associate with increased disease risk, notably cardiometabolic and behavioural. It is clear that the combination of inward- and outward-looking developmental programmes conducted by the early embryo represents a critical phase in the life course and that it is essential to explore further.

In Vivo Environmental Condition and Embryo Plasticity

Overnutrition Models

Maternal physiology and dietary nutrients, both over- and undernutrition, affect follicular and maturing oocytes and early embryos in ways that can permanently affect developmental potential (Sinclair and Watkins 2013). Maternal obesity is well recognized to reduce fertility, increase early pregnancy loss, and promote the risk of congenital abnormalities (Grindler and Moley 2013). Maternal circulating lipids can influence the accumulation of lipid metabolites in follicular fluid and the oocyte. For example, it has been shown that follicular fluid

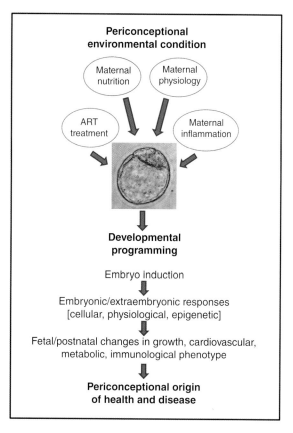

Figure 16.1 Summary of periconceptional developmental programming mediated through maternal and *in vitro* environmental cues that are sensed by embryos resulting in induction of programming and a series of responses or adaptations in embryonic and extra-embryonic cell lineages. Collectively, through cellular, physiological and epigenetic mechanisms, the developmental programme is altered, leading to fetal and postnatal changes in growth and phenotype and ultimately, the origin of health and disease in offspring.

triglyceride concentrations are positively correlated with maternal body mass index (Robker et al. 2009). There is also substantial evidence from small and large animal models that fatty maternal diets lead to increased follicular and oocyte lipid levels with detrimental consequences for oocyte and embryo potential (Dunning et al. 2014). Thus, maternal high fat diet in mice may increase follicular and oocyte lipid content leading to impaired fertilization and poorer embryo quality (Wakefield et al. 2008; Wu et al. 2010) and later fetal abnormalities (Luzzo et al. 2012). Data consistent with these conclusions has been obtained by Leary et al (2015), who related maternal body mass index to the triglyceride content of single blastocysts conceived via *in vitro* fertilization (IVF).

The major cellular defect in oocyte and embryo potential mediated through high fat diet and obesity relates to mitochondrial function, which becomes compromised and associated with increased oxidative and endoplasmic reticulum stress (Igosheva et al. 2010; Wu et al. 2012). These adverse effects on mitochondria following an over-rich diet also include impaired morphology and biogenesis (Igosheva et al. 2010; Luzzo et al. 2012). The longer-term outcomes of maternal obesity and high fat nutrition across animal models have demonstrated that adverse periconceptional programming leads to cardiovascular and metabolic disease in the offspring (Samuelsson et al. 2008; Picone et al. 2011; Torrens et al. 2012) as well as compromising ovarian morphology and function (Cheong et al. 2014) and perpetuating the condition across generations.

Maternal Undernutrition Models

With others, we have focused on the mechanistic basis of maternal undernutrition effects on embryo potential; it is useful to break these down into long-term consequences, early causes, and potential epigenetic regulation.

Consequences

Maternal undernutrition during the periconceptional period has been extensively studied using the mouse isocaloric low protein diet (LPD) model, including maternal protein restriction exclusively during the period of oocyte maturation (Egg-LPD) or preimplantation development (Emb-LPD) and with normal nutrition at all other times and postnatally (Watkins et al. 2008a; Watkins et al. 2008b). As has been discussed for maternal overnutrition, these dietary treatments lead to increased risk of cardiometabolic disease in the adult offspring, notably hypertension, endothelial vascular impairment, nephron deficit, and increased angiotensin-converting enzyme (ACE) activity, in a gender-specific manner (Watkins et al. 2008a; Watkins et al. 2008b; Watkins et al. 2010; Watkins et al. 2011). The Emb-LPD offspring, especially females, also exhibit impaired energy metabolism with excess adiposity and a gene expression profile that indicates a storage,

anabolic metabolism (Watkins et al. 2011). A similar cardiometabolic phenotype occurs in Emb-LPD rat offspring (Kwong et al. 2000). Moreover, Emb-LPD and Egg-LPD adult offspring display a disturbed behavioural phenotype that influences the level of locomotory activity (Watkins et al. 2008a; Watkins et al. 2008b). These diverse adult abnormalities appear to derive from an altered growth trajectory during gestation since the perinatal weight of offspring is positively associated with adult weight and cardiovascular and behavioural conditions (Watkins et al. 2008a).

The sensitivity of periconceptional maternal undernutrition to adult health has also been explored in sheep and similar adverse cardiovascular, metabolic, and behavioural outcomes have been identified (Gardner et al. 2004; Hernandez et al. 2009; Todd et al. 2009; Torrens et al. 2009). Most critically, in limited human maternal nutritional datasets, there is further evidence that periconceptional or early gestational exposure to famine leads to a cardiometabolic and neurological phenotype in adult offspring, which is more severe than exposure during later stages of pregnancy (Roseboom et al. 2011).

Causes

The apparent consistency in embryo vulnerability to poor maternal nutrition across mammalian species has led to more detailed studies on mechanisms, using the mouse Emb-LPD model. These studies have shown that programming of the embryo to maternal Emb-LPD has occurred by the blastocyst stage. This has been demonstrated by transferring blastocyst stage embryos to control-diet foster mothers, which does not prevent the persistence of programming consequences (Watkins et al. 2008a). Analysis of maternal serum and uterine fluid composition has indicated that Emb-LPD reduces insulin and amino acid levels during the period of preimplantation development which may be influential in the induction of embryo programming (Kwong et al. 2000; Eckert et al. 2012). Individual analysis of amino acids has shown specifically that the concentrations of branched-chain amino acids (BCAAs), leucine, isoleucine and valine, are up to 30% reduced in Emb-LPD uterine fluid at the time of blastocyst morphogenesis (Eckert et al. 2012). These metabolites are known mediators of cellular growth and protein translation through the mTORC pathway (Wang and Proud 2009).

Indeed, blastocysts collected from Emb-LPD mothers exhibit both significantly altered pools of free amino acids and reduced mTORC signalling compared with control blastocysts from mothers fed a normal diet, strongly implicating this nutrient pathway in embryo 'sensing' of maternal dietary status (Eckert et al. 2012). The role of insulin and BCAAs in the induction of abnormal fetal growth and onset of cardiovascular disease has been further demonstrated in an *in vitro* model, which mimics the Emb-LPD *in vivo* environment (Velazquez 2014).

Following induction of embryo programming mediated through maternal Emb-LPD, the embryo activates a series of compensatory responses within the extra-embryonic lineages, first evident within the expanding blastocyst, to promote nutrient delivery to the conceptus despite the deficit in maternal nutrient quality. These responses appear critical in promoting survival and competitive fitness of the offspring and affect both (i) trophectoderm – chorio-allantoic placenta and (ii) primitive endoderm – visceral yolk sac cell lineages. Within the trophectoderm, formed on the outer surface of the blastocyst and facing the uterine lumen, there is an increase in the proliferation rate (Eckert et al. 2012) as well as an increase in fluid-phase and receptor-mediated endocytosis and cytoplasmic vesicular organization for enhancing degradation of externally-derived nutrients (Sun et al. 2014). This endocytosis response to Emb-LPD includes upregulation of expression of the megalin endocytic receptor, increased presence of endocytosed vesicles and lysosomes and is regulated by Rho-A GTPase acting on the actin cytoskeleton via mTORC2 signalling (Figure 16.2). Interestingly, we find that the inductive mechanism of adverse developmental programming by Emb-LPD maternal diet mediated through low BCAAs (see above) is responsible for endocytic activation since this phenotype can be generated *in vitro* in control embryos through culture in medium containing low BCAAs to mimic the uterine fluid environment (Sun et al. 2014). Another important functional aspect of this cellular response identified *in vitro* is that whilst a richer nutrient environment will suppress the enhanced endocytic response, only brief exposure (~1 h) of blastocysts to depleted nutrient levels is sufficient to induce the response which, once activated, becomes stabilized and apparently irreversible even if nutrient levels are subsequently increased (Sun et al. 2014). A further

compensatory response by trophectoderm to Emb-LPD maternal diet is to enhance the motility of trophoblast cells during their invasive phase at the time of implantation (Eckert et al. 2012). This response is likely to facilitate early placentation and, following a sustained maternal LPD environment through to E8.5, secondary trophoblast migration from the ectoplacental cone is also enhanced, further facilitating placentation (Watkins et al. 2015). The longer-term consequences of these trophectoderm adaptations to maternal protein restriction is an increased placental efficiency in late gestation (Watkins et al. 2015) coupled with increased placental transport capacity (Coan et al. 2011).

The primitive endoderm (PE) – visceral yolk sac extra-embryonic lineage also responds to maternal Emb-LPD by stimulating endocytosis similar to the TE, first apparent in the early differentiated PE-like outer epithelium formed on embryoid bodies derived from embryonic stem cell lines generated from Emb-LPD blastocysts (Sun et al. 2014). These Emb-LPD embryoid bodies also show increased cell proliferation compared with controls (Sun et al. 2015). The enhanced endocytic phenotype is maintained through to the mature visceral yolk sac epithelium in late gestation (Watkins et al. 2008a) where the yolk sac forms an outer cellular layer to the conceptus, active in endocytic uptake of maternal uterine lumen proteins and their cytoplasmic breakdown and release of amino acids into the fetal circulation (Beckman et al. 1997). Collectively, these extra-embryonic adaptations to maternal protein restriction support the growth trajectory of the fetus despite maternal protein restriction, representing a physiological adaptation to nutrient scarcity underpinned by epigenetic restructuring.

Epigenetics

The maternal protein restriction model comprises an alteration in physiological and metabolic characteristics of the adult phenotype (see Consequences previously). The storage metabolism and high adiposity induced by maternal LPD in rat offspring coincide with altered epigenetic regulation of key transcription factors within liver and heart. Thus, LPD offspring in the rat model exhibit reduced expression and increased promoter DNA methylation of glucocorticoid receptor and peroxisomal proliferator-activated receptor (*PPAR*) genes (Lillycrop et al. 2005; Slater-Jefferies et al. 2011). A similar epigenetic

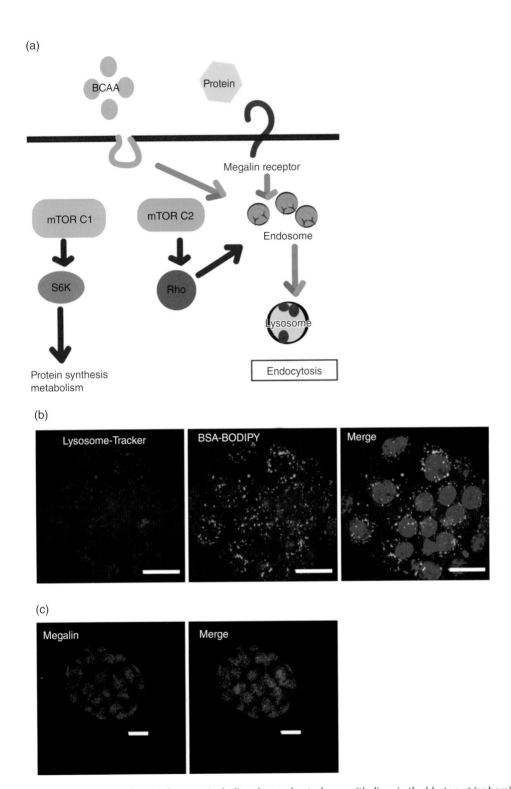

Figure 16.2 Extra-embryonic lineages including the trophectoderm epithelium in the blastocyst (as here) respond to Emb-LPD maternal nutrition by upregulation of cellular endocytosis. (a) Diagram showing both exogenous protein and branched-chain amino acid (BCAA) levels may affect embryonic cell protein synthesis via mTORC1 signalling and endocytosis via mTORC2 signalling (see text for details). (b) Representative images of E3.5 blastocysts labelled to show trophectoderm endocytosis using LysoTracker (red, for lysosomes) and BSA-BODIPY (green, for endocytosed ligand); blue = nuclei. (c) Blastocyst immunostained to show distribution of megalin endocytic receptor in trophectoderm; blue = nuclei. Scale bar = 20 μm.

basis has been identified using the Emb-LPD model in mice, coinciding with the extra-embryonic PE compensatory response of increased proliferation and endocytic activity. Using Emb-LPD embryoid bodies, the expression of Gata6, a key transcription factor regulating PE differentiation, is suppressed; a process mediated through hypoacetylation of the *Gata6* promoter domain (Sun et al. 2015).

Maternal Sickness Model

In vivo developmental programming of the early embryo is not restricted to maternal nutritional signalling but can include other conditions such as maternal health and immune responsiveness. Here, maternal inflammatory sickness, mediated through systemic bacterial endotoxin exposure at the time of conception, is sufficient to activate a proinflammatory cytokine response within mouse dams which, through signalling into the maternal tract, leads to changes in blastocyst morphogenesis (Williams et al. 2011). The consequences of the maternal inflammatory response lead to altered programming of the embryo but, unlike nutritional programming, have minimal or no effect on offspring growth or adult cardiometabolic phenotype but rather alter the innate immune system such that immune responsiveness to endotoxin is suppressed (Williams et al. 2011). The sensing mechanism active in inducing altered immune programming in the embryo has not been defined but may occur via Toll-like receptors and NFkB signalling, known to be present at the maternal–embryonic interface at the time of implantation (Koga et al. 2014). Thus, different periconceptional environments appear to alter embryo developmental potential in different ways, suggesting that plasticity may be 'selective' upon conditions experienced and, in the case of increased periconceptional maternal sickness, acting to protect offspring from autoimmune disorders in a perceived pathogen-rich postnatal world (Williams et al. 2011; Fleming et al. 2015).

In vitro Environmental Condition and Embryo Plasticity

The clinical success of ART to overcome infertility has been clear with over five million children born worldwide and an increasing proportion of ART births occurring in developed countries, some 2–3% in the UK (Brison et al. 2013). Following quite extensive epidemiological investigations, ART children and growing adolescents are generally healthy despite their periconceptional *in vitro* experience (Hart and Norman, 2013b; Hart and Norman, 2013a; Hyrapetian et al. 2014). However, increased incidence relative to natural conception has been recorded for perinatal complications and low birth weight, abnormal placental growth, fetal congenital malformations and imprinting disorders (Haavaldsen et al. 2012; Hart and Norman 2013a, b; Bloise et al. 2014; Hyrapetian et al. 2014). Moreover, although more epidemiological studies are required to confirm these findings, there is increased risk of cardiometabolic disease in ART children and adolescents, notably increased incidence of high blood pressure, adiposity, and glucose intolerance (Ceelen et al. 2008; Hart and Norman 2013b). It has also been proposed that ART offspring may have a small increase in the incidence of neurodevelopmental delay and risk of clinical depression (Hart and Norman 2013a).

Whilst the direct cause of any adversity in ART children, whether related to clinical and/or embryological treatment or the parental reproductive capacity, is unclear, caution in the use of such technologies should be exercised and further use of animal models should be made to understand direct relationships independent of parental fertility. Such an approach is further supported by the existence of complexities such as the relative influence of different ART treatments (superovulation, IVF, embryo culture duration, cryopreservation, embryo transfer, etc.) and how their use may have changed over time as practice has changed. It is interesting that the potential increase in systolic blood pressure in ART-conceived children is related to early childhood growth (Ceelen et al. 2009); a factor also found in the animal Emb-LPD model linking growth rate to later blood pressure (Watkins et al. 2008a). Moreover, human embryo culture medium composition has been shown to relate to subsequent birth weight and early infant weight in some but not all studies and recently further demonstrated in a randomized controlled trial (Kleijkers et al. 2014, 2016; Zandstra et al. 2015). These close relationships between the periconceptional environment and fetal growth trajectory resemble further the Emb-LPD mouse model.

As indicated previously, use of animal models to mimic ART treatments where parental infertility is absent, has tended to reveal the longer-term outcomes identified in human ART offspring, implicating the treatment rather than infertility per se adversely affects outcomes. Thus, combined super-ovulation and embryo culture and transfer have been shown to increase systolic blood pressure and perturb different markers of cardiometabolic health in adult mouse offspring (Watkins et al. 2007). Mouse embryo culture also adversely affects offspring behaviour and memory (Ecker et al. 2004). IVF and embryo culture/transfer can further cause abnormal mouse placental development and organization (de Waal et al. 2015). Mouse IVF has been further shown to modify metabolic activity in adult offspring including fasting glucose level (Chen et al. 2014), adult fat and liver metabolism (Feuer et al. 2014), and the glucocorticoid pathway expression profile that regulates diverse metabolic performance (Simbulan et al. 2016). Clearly, an objective to enhance the safety of ART techniques is still paramount (Brison et al. 2013; Sunde et al. 2016), taking into account the lessons learned from animal models and the specific treatment combinations causing the greatest health risk to offspring.

Conclusion

In this chapter, we have reviewed the evidence indicating that the embryonic period is sensitive to environmental conditions and that this interaction can influence long-term physiology and health status. Different forms of early environment promote different responses suggesting the periconceptional period may in part act to optimize the developmental programme to match prevailing conditions. This is illustrated by programming responses to maternal undernutrition and sickness, which differentially affect extra-embryonic and embryonic/fetal lineages. The embryo environment is altered significantly during human ART treatment to alleviate infertility, and long-term outcomes tend to match those identified using animal models. A safe, healthy maternal and *in vitro* environment around the time of conception is a priority to protect the health of offspring and needs to remain a focus for research in the future.

Acknowledgements

This work was supported through awards from the Biotechnology and Biological Sciences Research Council (BB/I001840/1; BB/F007450/1), The Medical Research Council (G9800781), the NICHD National Cooperative Program (U01 HD044635) and the EU-FP7 EpiHealth and EpiHealthNet programmes to T.P.F. C.S. was in receipt of a University of Southampton postgraduate scholarship bursary.

References

Anifandis, G., Messini, C., Dafopoulos, K. et al. (2014). Molecular and cellular mechanisms of sperm-oocyte interactions opinions relative to in vitro fertilization (IVF). Int J Mol Sci 15: 12972–12997.

Beckman, D.A., Lloyd, J.B. and Brent, R.L. (1997). Investigations into mechanisms of amino acid supply to the rat embryo using whole-embryo culture. Int J Dev Biol 41: 315–318.

Bedzhov, I., Graham, S.J., Leung, C. Y. et al. (2014). Developmental plasticity, cell fate specification and morphogenesis in the early mouse embryo, Philos Trans R Soc Lond B Biol Sci 369(1657).

Bloise, E., Feuer, S.K. and Rinaudo, P.F. (2014). Comparative intrauterine development and placental function of ART conception: implications for human reproductive medicine and animal breeding. Hum Reprod Update 20: 822–839.

Brison, D.R., Roberts, S.A. and Kimber, S.J. (2013). How should we assess the safety of IVF technologies? Reprod Biomed Online 27: 710–721.

Ceelen, M., van Weissenbruch, M.M., Prein, J. et al. (2009). Growth during infancy and early childhood in relation to blood pressure and body fat measures at age 8–18 years of IVF children and spontaneously conceived controls born to subfertile parents. Hum Reprod 24: 2788–2795.

Ceelen, M., van Weissenbruch, M.M., Vermeiden, J.P. et al. (2008). Cardiometabolic differences in children born after in vitro fertilization: follow-up study. J Clin Endocrinol Metab 93: 1682–1688.

Cha, J., Sun, X. and Dey, S.K. (2012). Mechanisms of implantation: strategies for successful pregnancy. Nat Med 18: 1754–1767.

Chen, L., Wang, D., Wu, Z. et al. (2010). Molecular basis of the first cell fate determination in mouse embryogenesis. Cell Res 20: 982–993.

Chen, M., Wu, L., Zhao, J. et al. (2014). Altered glucose metabolism in mouse and humans conceived by IVF. Diabetes 63: 3189–3198.

Cheong, Y., Sadek, K.H., Bruce, K.D. et al. (2014). Diet-induced maternal obesity alters ovarian morphology and gene expression in the adult mouse offspring. Fertil Steril 102: 899–907.

Coan, P.M., Vaughan, O.R., McCarthy, J. et al. (2011). Dietary composition programmes placental phenotype in mice. J Physiol 589: 3659– 3670.

de Waal, E., Vrooman, L.A., Fischer, E. et al. (2015). The cumulative effect of assisted reproduction procedures on placental development and epigenetic perturbations in a mouse model. Hum Mol Genet 24: 6975–6985.

Dunning, K.R., Russell, D.L. and Robker, R.L. (2014). Lipids and oocyte developmental competence: the role of fatty acids and beta-oxidation. Reproduction 148: R15–27.

Ecker, D.J., Stein, P., Xu, Z. et al. (2004). Long-term effects of culture of preimplantation mouse embryos on behavior. Proc Natl Acad Sci USA 101: 1595–1600.

Eckert, J.J. and Fleming, T.P. (2008). Tight junction biogenesis during early development. Biochim Biophys Acta 1778: 717–728.

Eckert, J.J., Porter, R., Watkins, A.J. et al. (2012). Metabolic induction and early responses of mouse blastocyst developmental programming following maternal low protein diet affecting life-long health. PLoS One 7: e52791.

Eckert, J.J., Velazquez, M.A. and Fleming, T.P. (2015). Cell signalling during blastocyst morphogenesis. Adv Exp Med Biol 843: 1–21.

Feuer, S.K., Donjacour, A., Simbulan, R.K. et al. (2014). Sexually dimorphic effect of in vitro fertilization (IVF). on adult mouse fat and liver metabolomes. Endocrinology 155: 4554–4567.

Fleming, T.P., Watkins, A.J., Sun, C. et al. (2015). Do little embryos make big decisions? How maternal dietary protein restriction can permanently change an embryo. Reprod Fertil Dev 27: 684–692.

Gardner, D.K. and Harvey, A.J. (2015). Blastocyst metabolism. Reprod Fertil Dev 27: 638–654.

Gardner, D.S., Pearce, S., Dandrea, J. et al. (2004). Peri-implantation undernutrition programs blunted angiotensin II evoked baroreflex responses in young adult sheep. Hypertension 43: 1290–1296.

Grindler, N.M. and Moley, K.H. (2013). Maternal obesity, infertility and mitochondrial dysfunction: potential mechanisms emerging from mouse model systems. Mol Hum Reprod 19: 486–494.

Haavaldsen, C., Tanbo, T. and Eskild, A. (2012). Placental weight in singleton pregnancies with and without assisted reproductive technology: a population study of 536,567 pregnancies. Hum Reprod 27: 576–582.

Hart, R. and Norman, R.J. (2013a). The longer-term health outcomes for children born as a result of IVF treatment. Part II – Mental health and development outcomes. Hum Reprod Update 19: 244–250.

Hart, R. and Norman, R. J. (2013b). The longer-term health outcomes for children born as a result of IVF treatment: Part I – General health outcomes. Hum Reprod Update 19: 232–243.

Hernandez, C.E., Harding, J.E., Oliver, M.H. et al. (2009). Effects of litter size, sex and periconceptional ewe nutrition on side preference and cognitive flexibility in the offspring. Behav Brain Res 204: 82–87.

Hyrapetian, M., Loucaides, E.M. and Sutcliffe, A.G. (2014). Health and disease in children born after assistive reproductive therapies (ART). J Reprod Immunol 106: 21–26.

Igosheva, N., Abramov, A.Y., Poston, L. et al. (2010). Maternal diet-induced obesity alters mitochondrial activity and redox status in mouse oocytes and zygotes. PLoS One 5: e10074.

Kleijkers, S.H., van Montfoort, A.P., Smits, L. J. et al. (2014). IVF culture medium affects post-natal weight in humans during the first 2 years of life. Hum Reprod 29: 661–669.

Kleijkers, S.H., Mantikou, E., Slappendel, E. et al. (2016). Influence of embryo culture medium

(G5 and HTF) on pregnancy and perinatal outcome after IVF: a multicenter RCT. Hum Reprod 31: 2219–2230.

Koga, K., Izumi, G., Mor, G. et al. (2014). Toll-like receptors at the maternal-fetal interface in normal pregnancy and pregnancy complications. Am J Reprod Immunol 72: 192–205.

Kwong, W.Y., Wild, A.E., Roberts, P. et al. (2000). Maternal undernutrition during the preimplantation period of rat development causes blastocyst abnormalities and programming of postnatal hypertension. Development 127: 4195–4202.

Leary, C., Leese, H.J. and Sturmey, R.G. (2015). Human embryos from overweight and obese women display phenotypic and metabolic abnormalities. Hum Reprod 30: 122–132.

Leese, H.J. (2012). Metabolism of the preimplantation embryo: 40 years on. Reproduction 143: 417–427.

Li, L., Lu, X. and Dean, J. (2013). The maternal to zygotic transition in mammals. Mol Aspects Med 34: 919–938.

Lillycrop, K.A., Phillips, E.S., Jackson, A.A. et al. (2005). Dietary protein restriction of pregnant rats induces and folic acid supplementation prevents epigenetic modification of hepatic gene expression in the offspring. J Nutr 135: 1382–1386.

Luzzo, K.M., Wang, Q., Purcell, S.H. et al. (2012). High fat diet induced developmental defects in the mouse: oocyte meiotic aneuploidy and fetal growth retardation/brain defects. PLoS One 7: e49217.

Nomikos, M., Kashir, J., Swann, K. et al. (2013). Sperm PLCzeta: from structure to Ca2+ oscillations, egg activation and therapeutic potential. FEBS Lett 587: 3609–3616.

Picone, O., Laigre, P., Fortun-Lamothe, L. et al. (2011). Hyperlipidic hypercholesterolemic diet in prepubertal rabbits affects gene expression in the embryo, restricts fetal growth and increases offspring susceptibility to obesity. Theriogenology 75: 287–299.

Puscheck, E.E., Awonuga, A.O., Yang, Y. et al. (2015). Molecular biology of the stress response in the early embryo and its stem cells. Adv Exp Med Biol 843: 77–128.

Rivera, R.M. and Ross, J.W. (2013). Epigenetics in fertilization and preimplantation embryo development. Prog Biophys Mol Biol 113: 423–432.

Robker, R.L., Akison, L.K., Bennett, B.D. et al. (2009). Obese women exhibit differences in ovarian metabolites, hormones, and gene expression compared with moderate-weight women. J Clin Endocrinol Metab 94: 1533–1540.

Roseboom, T.J., Painter, R.C., van Abeelen, A.F. et al. (2011). Hungry in the womb: what are the consequences? Lessons from the Dutch famine. Maturitas 70: 141–145.

Samuelsson, A.M., Matthews, P.A., Argenton, M. et al. (2008). Diet-induced obesity in female mice leads to offspring hyperphagia, adiposity, hypertension, and insulin resistance: a novel murine model of developmental programming. Hypertension 51: 383–392.

Seshagiri, P.B., Sen Roy, S., Sireesha, G. et al. (2009). Cellular and molecular regulation of mammalian blastocyst hatching. J Reprod Immunol 83: 79–84.

Simbulan, R.K., Liu, X., Feuer, S.K. et al. (2016). Adult male mice conceived by in vitro fertilization exhibit increased glucocorticoid receptor expression in fat tissue. J Dev Orig Health Dis 7: 73–82.

Sinclair, K.D. and Watkins, A.J. (2013). Parental diet, pregnancy outcomes and offspring health: metabolic determinants in developing oocytes and embryos. Reprod Fertil Dev 26: 99–114.

Slater-Jefferies, J.L., Lillycrop, K.A., Townsend, P.A. et al. (2011). Feeding a protein-restricted diet during pregnancy induces altered epigenetic regulation of peroxisomal proliferator-activated receptor-alpha in the heart of the offspring. J Dev Orig Health Dis 2: 250–255.

Sozen, B., Can, A. and Demir, N. (2014). Cell fate regulation during preimplantation development: a view of adhesion-linked molecular interactions. Dev Biol 395: 73–83.

Sun, C., Denisenko, O., Sheth, B. et al. (2015). Epigenetic regulation of histone modifications and Gata6 gene expression induced by maternal diet in mouse embryoid bodies in a model of developmental programming. BMC Dev Biol 15: 3.

Sun, C., Velazquez, M.A., Marfy-Smith, S. et al. (2014). Mouse early extra-embryonic lineages activate compensatory endocytosis in response to poor maternal nutrition. Development 141: 1140–1150.

Sunde, A., Brison, D., Dumoulin, J. et al. (2016). Time to take human embryo culture seriously. Hum Reprod 31: 2174–2182.

Todd, S.E., Oliver, M.H., Jaquiery, A.L. et al. (2009). Periconceptional undernutrition of ewes impairs glucose tolerance in their adult offspring. Pediatr Res 65: 409–413.

Torrens, C., Ethirajan, P., Bruce, K.D. et al. (2012). Interaction between maternal and offspring diet to impair vascular function and oxidative balance in high fat fed male mice. PLoS One 7: e50671.

Torrens, C., Snelling, T.H., Chau, R. et al. (2009). Effects of pre- and periconceptional undernutrition on arterial function in adult female sheep are vascular bed dependent. Exp Physiol 94: 1024–1033.

Velazquez, M.A., Sheth, B., Marfy-Smith, S. et al. (2014). Insulin and branched-chain amino acid depletion during mouse in vitro preimplantation embryo development alters postnatal growth and cardiovascular physiology. Reproduction Abstracts 1 (World Congress of Animal Reproduction 2014, Edinburgh UK): P096.

Wakefield, S.L., Lane, M., Schulz, S.J. et al. (2008). Maternal supply of omega-3 polyunsaturated fatty acids alter mechanisms involved in oocyte and early embryo development in the mouse. Am J Physiol Endocrinol Metab 294: E425–434.

Wang, X. and Proud, C.G. (2009). Nutrient control of TORC1, a cell-cycle regulator. Trends Cell Biol 19: 260–267.

Watkins, A.J., Lucas, E.S., Marfy-Smith, S. et al. (2015). Maternal nutrition modifies trophoblast giant cell phenotype and fetal growth in mice. Reproduction 149: 563–575.

Watkins, A.J., Lucas, E.S., Torrens, C. et al. (2010). Maternal low-protein diet during mouse pre-implantation development induces vascular dysfunction and altered renin-angiotensin-system homeostasis in the offspring. Br J Nutr 103: 1762–1770.

Watkins, A.J., Lucas, E.S., Wilkins, A. et al. (2011). Maternal periconceptional and gestational low protein diet affects mouse offspring growth, cardiovascular and adipose phenotype at 1 year of age. PLoS One 6: e28745.

Watkins, A.J., Platt, D., Papenbrock, T. et al. (2007). Mouse embryo culture induces changes in postnatal phenotype including raised systolic blood pressure. Proc Natl Acad Sci USA 104: 5449–5454.

Watkins, A.J., Ursell, E., Panton, R. et al. (2008a). Adaptive responses by mouse early embryos to maternal diet protect fetal growth but predispose to adult onset disease. Biol Reprod 78: 299–306.

Watkins, A.J., Wilkins, A., Cunningham, C. et al. (2008b). Low protein diet fed exclusively during mouse oocyte maturation leads to behavioural and cardiovascular abnormalities in offspring. J Physiol 586: 2231–2244.

Williams, C.L., Teeling, J.L., Perry, V.H. et al. (2011). Mouse maternal systemic inflammation at the zygote stage causes blunted cytokine responsiveness in lipopolysaccharide – challenged adult offspring. BMC Biol 9: 49.

Wu, L.L., Dunning, K.R., Yang, X. et al. (2010). High-fat diet causes lipotoxicity responses in cumulus-oocyte complexes and decreased fertilization rates. Endocrinology 151: 5438–5445.

Wu, L.L., Russell, D.L., Norman, R.J. et al. (2012). Endoplasmic reticulum (ER). stress in cumulus-oocyte complexes impairs pentraxin-3 secretion, mitochondrial membrane potential (DeltaPsi m), and embryo development. Mol Endocrinol 26: 562–573.

Zandstra, H., Van Montfoort, A.P. and Dumoulin, J.C. (2015). Does the type of culture medium used influence birthweight of children born after IVF? Hum Reprod 30: 530–542.

Zhou, L.Q. and Dean, J. (2015). Reprogramming the genome to totipotency in mouse embryos. Trends Cell Biol 25: 82–91.

17

Lifestyle and Environmental Impacts on Fertility

Ana-Maria Tomova and Michael Carroll

Introduction

Both male and female reproductive health is dependent on a functioning endocrine system, reproductive organs, and gametes. Environmental and occupational exposures, lifestyle habits and infectious disease are increasingly considered important modifiable risk factors for infertility (Table 17.1). Lifestyle habits such as smoking tobacco, drinking alcohol and caffeine, and taking recreational drugs are associated with poor sperm quality in men and poor follicular function in women. Environmental contaminants, including endocrine-disrupting chemicals and air pollution, can be deleterious to human reproductive health. Many potentially toxic chemicals can also be found in commonly used products such as linings of food and drink containers, personal care products, textiles, and pesticides.

Damage to reproductive health can be incurred by exposures *in utero*, in neonatal or adolescent stages, or in adulthood. Moreover, several studies have noted increased global incidences of male reproductive problems, such as poor spermatogenesis, testicular cancer, hypospadias, and cryptorchidism. It has been proposed that these disorders have a common origin during fetal development; all represent different symptoms of the same underlying entity known as the testicular dysgenesis syndrome (Skakkebaek et al. 2001; Virtanen et al. 2005).

This chapter will review the effects environmental and lifestyle exposures have on reproductive health.

Reproductive Toxicology: Environmental and Occupational Exposures

Reproductive toxicology is the study of the incidence of adverse effects on the male or female reproductive system resulting from exposure to chemical or physical agents. People are exposed to potentially hazardous chemical compounds during their daily life. These chemical compounds can be derived from both natural sources (toxins) and anthropogenic or synthetic sources (toxicants). Chemical contaminants can occur in the ambient environment such as the air, soil, and water, and in the indoor environment, e.g. in the workplace, school, and home. Exposure, contact, and absorption of the hazardous chemical compounds into the body are necessary to exert any toxic effect.

Route and Site of Exposure

Hazardous chemical compounds can gain access to the body via the major routes of ingestion (gastrointestinal tract), inhalation (lungs), and skin contact (topical, percutaneous, or dermal exposure). Toxic compounds can produce the greatest and most rapid effect when access is directly into the bloodstream through an intravenous route. In addition, the route of exposure can influence the toxicity of the chemical compounds. For example, a compound that is detoxified in the liver would be less toxic when ingested than through inhalation.

Table 17.1 Lifestyle and environmental exposures factors affecting the fertility of men and women.

Modifiable Lifestyle Risks	Environmental Risks
Diet	Occupation
Stress	Environmental toxic chemicals
Infections	Radiation
Recreational drugs	Water (pollutants)
Alcohol consumption	Air (pollution)
Cigarette smoking	

To exert any toxic effect on testicular tissue or sperm cells, the compound or its metabolite would have to breach the blood testis barrier. In women, the uterus, ovary, and follicles can be exposed to compounds ingested, inhaled, or absorbed through the skin. However, the oocyte may have some protection by the surrounding granulosa cells providing a barrier similar to the blood–testis barrier.

Occupational exposure to toxic agents results mostly from breathing contaminated air and/or direct and prolonged contact of the skin with the substance, whereas accidental poisoning occurs most often by ingestion. Factors that can increase toxic effects by any route of exposure are the concentration of the compound, and the duration and rate of exposure. One principle of toxicology is that any compound can exert a toxic effect. The Swiss physician and scientist Paracelsus (1493–1541), is famed for the phrase: '*What is there that is not poison? All things are poison and nothing is without poison. Solely the dose determines that a thing is not a poison*' – or simply put – 'it is the dose that makes the poison'.

Compounds regarded as highly toxic will exert a toxic effect at very low concentrations. An example is botulinum toxin, which is produced by *Clostridium botulinum* bacteria and can be lethal in the ng/kg range. Other well-known toxic compounds such as arsenic or strychnine can be lethal in the mg/kg range.

The exposure to potentially toxic substances can be acute, subacute, subchronic, and chronic. Acute exposure is exposure to a hazardous chemical or agent for fewer than 24 hours. Repeated exposure can be subacute, subchronic, and chronic. Subacute exposure refers to repeated exposure to a hazardous chemical or agent for 1 month or less, subchronic for 1–3 months, and chronic for more than 3 months.

Mechanism of Toxicity

The degree of toxicity depends on the route of exposure, concentration of the hazardous chemical or agent, and duration of exposure. Cellular damage occurs when the toxin/toxicant results in perturbations in cell function and/or structure beyond any repair capacity. Some chemicals can alter the biological microenvironment (Figure 17.1). Heavy metals like cadmium can alter actin filament function, thus disrupting cell structure and tight junctions between cells. A number of agents such as strong acids and bases, nicotine, aminoglycosides, ethylene oxide, heavy-metal ions, hydrogen cyanide, and

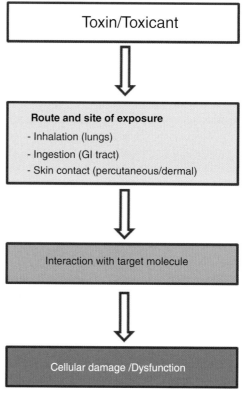

Figure 17.1 Mechanism of toxicity. To exert its toxic effect a chemical compound must reach the target cell/molecule. Cellular damage occurs when the toxin/toxicant results in perturbations in cell function and/or structure beyond any repair capacity. GI, gastrointestinal.

carbon monoxide are directly toxic, whereas the toxicity of other agents can be due to the action of their metabolites. Many chemicals can be genotoxic or mutagenic, damaging DNA, while others can interfere with cellular functions such as metabolism, cell division, and cell membrane integrity. Some chemicals can activate protein target molecules, mimicking endogenous ligands, which can interfere with normal cellular signalling activity. An important class of such chemicals are the endocrine-disrupting chemicals, which interfere with the production, binding, or action of physiological hormones.

Environmental and Occupational Toxicants

Many reproductive health problems are caused by exposure to toxicants in the environment and workplace. These problems include infertility, abnormal fetal development, miscarriage, and poor pregnancy outcomes. Environmental toxicants include: pesticides and herbicides; volatile organic compounds such as benzene and toluene; heavy metals such as lead, mercury, and cadmium; and persistent organic pollutants such as dichlorodiphenyltrichloroethane (DDT) and polychlorinated biphenyls (PCB). Endocrine-disrupting chemicals such as bisphenol-A, phthalates, and certain pesticides (dicofol, atrazine) can alter male and female reproductive hormones in both humans and other vertebrates.

Heavy Metals

Mercury, cadmium, and lead are toxic to humans. There have been associations between welding and reduced sperm motility and concentration.

Lead exposure (primarily from paint) has been concomitant with negative effects on male fertility, with poor sperm motility, lower sperm concentration, and abnormal morphology. Lead exposure has also been implicated as a factor for poor fertilization rates in *in vitro* fertilization (IVF) (Benoff et al. 2003). Lead may affect pituitary function therefore disrupting the hypothalamic–pituitary gonadal axis, leading to hypogonadism. Lead is also known to affect fetal development with long-term effects on cognitive abilities (Schnaas et al. 2006).

Cadmium (a known carcinogen) exposure, usually from food sources such as shellfish, even at low levels has been implicated in poor sperm parameters and altered levels of reproductive hormones, increasing time to pregnancy. Cadmium is associated with human prostate cancer and in animal studies has shown to induce benign Leydig cell tumours, likely due to testicular necrosis and atrophy resulting in overstimulation from luteinizing hormones (LH) (Waalkes 2003). Cadmium's effect on Sertoli cell tight junctions may be due to its actions on the actin filaments associated with these junctions, which results in loss of tight junctional barriers leading to oedema, increased fluid pressure, ischaemia, and tissue necrosis (Li and Heindel 1998). Cadmium-induced capillary toxicity can also affect the pampiniform plexus leading to testicular necrosis and ischaemia.

Mercury exposure can result in abnormal sperm morphology and poor motility, and in women is associated with a doubled risk of miscarriage (Cordier et al. 1991). Methylmercury (exposure typically through a fish-rich diet) can cross the placenta and concentrates 5–7-fold more in the fetal brain than in the mother's blood. High concentration causes widespread damage to the fetal brain, although for low levels of methylmercury exposure the results are inconsistent (Counter and Buchanan 2004).

Endocrine-Disrupting Chemicals

Endocrine-disrupting chemicals can be described as chemicals that can interfere with the endocrine systems. The chemicals usually mimic endogenous hormones either structurally or functionally and can cause a range of disorders: cancerous tumours, metabolism disruption, neurological function disruption, developmental disorders, and congenital defects. Endocrine disruptors affect normal endocrine function and some have severe impacts on the hypothalamic–pituitary gonadal axis, causing infertility. The route of exposure is variable and includes: industrial products, personal care goods, water, air, and food. Endocrine disruptors can also accumulate in the food chain, and although some substances such as DDT and PCBs were banned more than 30 years ago, they are still detected in human bodily fluids due to the lack of biodegradability of these chemicals and their lipophilicity. Chronic exposure to endocrine-disrupting chemicals can occur via inhalation and skin contact. However, the primary source of these chemicals is through food and water. The use of xenoestrogens in the food industry has resulted in amplified levels of sex steroid hormones in processed foods (milk, meat).

Bisphenol A (BPA) is a synthetic compound that is commonly used to make plastics and resins. It has been shown to leach from plastics under normal use. BPA is classed as a xenoestrogen (oestrogen mimicker)/endocrine disrupter. It has never been used as a drug, however; BPA is structurally similar to diethylstilboestrol which was used as a synthetic oestrogen in women and animals until its ban in the 1970s due to its carcinogenicity. When BPA was tested for use as a synthetic oestrogen it was found to be 1000–2000-fold less effective than oestradiol (other studies have shown up to 100 000- fold lowered affinity for oestrogen receptors) but the oestrogen mimicking effects of BPA are due to the similarity of the phenol groups in oestradiol and BPA. In high concentrations BPA binds to the androgen receptor and acts as an antagonist (Kwon et al. 2007; Vandenberg et al. 2007; Vogel, 2009). Unconjugated BPA has repeatedly been measured in human serum, plasma, placenta, amniotic fluid, and breast milk (low ng/mL range) and BPA conjugates are detected in human urine in over 90% of multiple populations in different continents (low ng/mL range) (Vandenberg et al. 2007). BPA has been implicated in many human health issues including cardiovascular disease, diabetes, liver enzyme abnormalities, and obesity. The more significant effects are usually seen when exposed from fetal stage to early childhood leading to secondary sexual development changes, immune disorders, and neurobehavioral changes; therefore pregnant women, infants, and young children are the most at risk groups (Erler and Novak 2010). Other studies have also shown BPA exposure with meiotic spindle disruption in oocytes, reduced ovarian response and poor IVF outcomes, reduced fertilization and poor embryo quality, poor implantation rates, increased risk of miscarriage, premature birth, altered sex hormone concentrations, altered thyroid hormone concentration, and poor sperm quality (Rochester 2013).

PCBs were primarily used as dielectric or coolant fluids in electronic equipment. In the 1960s PCBs were shown to accumulate in the environment,

acting as a persistent organic pollutant, which may be a major source for human exposure. PCBs have been classified as definite human carcinogens, and are known endocrine disruptors. PCBs can produce either oestrogenic or antioestrogenic effects, which can lead to developmental issues for both male and females, poor sexual development, skeletal problems, mental development issues. In males, PCBs negatively correlate with testosterone. In adults, high levels of PCBs have shown to reduce levels of thyroid hormones, which can impact on many other physiological process in humans (growth, metabolism, temperature, and heart rate) (Hagmar et al. 2001; Schell et al. 2014).

Organic Solvents

Organic solvents can have a negative effect on male and female fertility. Aromatic solvent exposure (i.e. toluene, xylene, benzene) is linked to abnormal sperm parameters, and paternal exposure have been associated with spontaneous abortion, congenital malformation, and low birth weight or pre-term birth (Lindbohm, 1995) and increased risk for neural tube defects (Logman et al. 2005). It is postulated that exposure may affect the hypothalamic–pituitary gonadal axis, or by directly affecting spermatogenesis. Maternal occupational exposure to organic solvents is associated with an increased risk for spontaneous abortion and major malformations.

Radiation and Chemotherapy

Radiation and chemitherpy are routinley used in cancer treatment. Both radiation and chemotherapy are cytotoxic, and affect fertility by damaging gonads and gametes. Radiation therapy is typically more damaging to fertility when directed below the diaphragm, reducing fertility by approximately 25% in both males and females. In males, chemotherapy with alkylating agents, regardless of whether combined with radiation below the diaphragm, is associated with approximately 60% inhibited fertility, while the use of chemotherapy with alkylating agents in females seems to have no effect on fertility. However, fertility after radiation and chemotherapy treatment heavily depends on the site of radiation, intensity, and duration/doses of both radiation and chemotherapy (Byrne et al. 1987). Fractioned radiation aimed at the testes is more harmful than an acute large dose up to 600 rad. Fractioned radiation doses larger than 35 rad cause azoospermia and the time taken to recover is increased with each dose; after 200 rad azoospermia can be permanent. In females, age also influences recovery post radiation; 400 rad in young women causes approximately 30% sterility, whereas in women over 40 years of age this becomes 100% sterility (Ash 1980).

Impact of Lifestyle and Reproduction

Lifestyle can affect all aspects of health. Diet, cigarette smoking, alcohol consumption, recreational/ pharmaceutical drugs, mood disorders, and stress have all been shown to affect fertility.

Smoking

Cigarette smoking is well known for its negative effects on health – the evidence supporting this is indisputable. There is no safe level of exposure to second-hand smoke as it causes severe illness in both adults and children (World Health Organization 2007). It is well documented that both male and female fertility is negatively impacted by smoking and exposure to second-hand smoke, not only impacting the gametes, conception, and successful pregnancy, but also the health and fertility of the offspring. In males, smoking is significantly detrimental to sperm parameters (motility, concentration, and morphology) and causes DNA damage in sperm which predisposes the offspring to an increased risk of cancer, genetic diseases, and malformations (Evans et al. 1981; Potts et al. 1999; Vine et al. 1996). In females, smoking is associated with earlier menopause and reduced fertility and fecundity. Smoking may impair oocyte function and viability; in women undergoing IVF, smokers had significantly higher rates of tubal factor infertility, reduced retrieval of oocytes, and also had a significantly higher rate of diploid oocytes and triploid zygotes (Oyesanya et al. 1995; Wilks and Hay 2004). For both men and women, smoking negatively affects (typically delaying) spontaneous conception and IVF/intracytoplasmic sperm injection

rates, reduces oocyte pick up rates (due to potassium cyanide), doubles the rate of ectopic pregnancy, increases the rate of miscarriage by 80%, as well as being associated with previous recurrent miscarriage (Kline et al. 1977; Knoll and Talbot 1998; Saraiya et al. 1998; Suonio et al. 1990; Wallach et al. 1996). *In utero* exposure predisposes offspring to clinically diagnosed asthma as well as a higher risk of childhood cancer (Gilliland et al. 2001; Zenzes 2000). There is evidence to suggest smoking also affects the hypothalamic–pituitary axis, stimulating growth hormone, cortisol, vasopressin, and oxytocin, which then inhibit LH and prolactin, negatively impacting fertility (Mattison 1982; Weisberg 1985). However, the effects of cigarette smoking on fertility may be transient. Smokers who quit have an increased pregnancy rate than active smokers (Watson 2015).

Alcohol Consumption

Alcohol consumption is associated with adverse effects on fertility, severe pregnancy complications, poor fetal development, and fetal alcohol syndrome, which causes developmental problems in the child. Alcohol consumption increases infertility in females due to ovulatory factors or endometriosis by 50% (Grodstein et al. 1994a). Alcohol intake around the time of conception is associated with early pregnancy loss: female alcohol intake is associated with a two to three times increased risk and male intake with a two to five times increased risk (adjusted for confounding factors) of miscarriage (Henriksen et al. 2004). Chronic alcohol consumption in males has been show to increase follicle stimulating hormone (FSH), LH and E2, decrease testosterone and progesterone, and significantly decrease semen volume, sperm count, morphologically normal sperm, and sperm motility (Muthusami and Chinnaswamy 2005). It is postulated that the reproductive toxicity of alcohol is due to an impairment of hypothalamic–pituitary–testicular signalling in males, which is expressed as poor semen quality, and in females it is decreased secretion of LH and reduced ovulation (Sadeu et al. 2010).

Caffeine

There is a lack of consensus regarding caffeine consumption and its effects on fertility. Most studies investigating caffeine and infertility have other confounding factors such as smoking or alcohol intake (Watson 2015). A caffeine intake of no more than 300 mg per day is unlikely to have any effects on both male or female fertility. Women are advised to limit their caffeine intake to 200 mg per day when pregnant or trying to conceive (Anderson *et al.* 2010). However, a very high caffeine intake (>500 mg a day) has been associated with a longer time to pregnancy, miscarriage, and stillbirth (>800 mg a day) (Watson 2015). A recent meta-analysis reported that over four caffeinated drinks per day were likely to negatively impact on male fecundity but three or fewer per day had no effect (Ricci et al. 2017).

Drugs

The illicit drugs that are known to have a negative effect on male fertility are: cannabis, cocaine, methamphetamines, opioids, ecstasy, and anabolic steroids. Cannabis is the most frequently used illicit drug in males of reproductive age. It releases cannabinoids that can act systemically to inhibit the reproductive process. The cannabinoid receptors are found throughout both male and female reproductive tracts, and also on the sperm itself. Cannabis use lowers motility, inhibits acrosome reaction, mitochondrial function, and also inhibits the hypothalamic–pituitary gonadal axis reducing testosterone. In females, regular users have higher rates of primary infertility, reduced fertilization, and poor placental and fetal development. *In utero* exposure is associated with congenital defects and stillbirth.

Prescription opioids suppress the hypothalamic–pituitary gonadal axis by inhibiting gonadotropin-releasing hormone (GnRH) and suppressing LH, with the end result of lowered testosterone levels and lowered spermatogenesis. The same is documented in heroin users. In chronic users of prescription opioids nearly all males showed symptoms of hypogonadism with lack of libido, impotency, and low LH and testosterone. In women, cocaine has teratogenic effects on the fetus during pregnancy. For men the studies have confounding factors with other illicit drug use. However, men with a sperm count of under 20 million/mL were twice as likely to have used cocaine in the past 2 years and men with a history of using cocaine for 5 years or more were twice as likely to have poor sperm motility. There are few studies exploring the effects of methamphetamines and ecstasy on fertility; most have been animal studies. These drugs work by acting on the dopaminergic and serotoninergic systems and have an effect on the secretion of GnRH. *In vivo* and *in vitro* rat studies showed amphetamine injections to decrease the levels of testosterone in the plasma in a dose dependent manner. In mouse studies, injections of methamphetamine induced apoptosis in the seminiferous tubules. Other animal studies indicated that methamphetamine suppressed GnRH and testosterone levels in the serum. Damage to sperm DNA was also found, but sperm motility and morphology remained unaffected (Fronczak et al. 2012).

Anabolic steroids are typically taken by men to aid muscle performance and strength. Anabolic steroids inhibit the hypothalamic–pituitary gonadal axis, causing hypogonadotropic hypogonadism and inhibition of testosterone production; this negatively affects spermatogenesis and causes erectile dysfunction. Anabolic steroids are associated with reduced sperm motility, lower sperm concentration, and increased abnormal morphology. However, these effects are reversible on discontinuation of use (recovery is 4 months to a year).

Other prescription medication such as antibiotics and antidepressants also negatively impact sperm parameters. Nitrofurantoin (used to treat urinary tract infections) causes maturation arrest in the testes in high doses. Minocycline (a broad-spectrum antibiotic) is toxic to sperm in all concentrations. Erythromycin (commonly used to treat respiratory tract infections) may negatively impact sperm motility and concentration. Aminoglycoside antibiotics (often used against Gram-negative bacteria) may inhibit spermatogenesis.

Selective serotonin reuptake inhibitors and tricyclic antidepressants may decrease libido and induce difficulty in reaching climax for both men and women. They may also cause hyperprolactinaemia, which suppresses spermatogenesis, although this is reversible upon discontinuation (Watson 2015).

Diet

Metabolic Syndrome/Obesity

Obesity (defined as having a body mass index (BMI) of 30 and over) is a global health issue, contributing to a wide range of related diseases (heart disease, stroke, diabetes type 2, and some types of cancer) with a high level of morbidity and mortality. Obesity is associated with hypogonadism as well as further disruptions to the endocrine system, which affect fertility in both males and females (Brewer and Balen 2010; Phillips and Tanphaichitr 2010; Reece 2008). Obese women respond poorly to ovarian stimulation protocols during assisted reproductive technology procedures, which can lead to poor fertilization rates and fewer live births. Obese women also have an increased rate of pregnancy complications: increased miscarriage, gestational diabetes, high blood pressure, large fetuses, and therefore delivery complications (Homan *et al.* 2007; Pandey et al. 2010). In men, a high BMI is related to reduced testosterone and poor semen parameters (reduced concentration, poor motility, and abnormal morphology) (Cabler et al. 2010; Eisenberg et al. 2014; MacDonald et al. 2009).

Increased aromatase activity in obese men can lead to hypothalamic–pituitary gonadal axis dysfunction, resulting in hypogonadotropic hyperoestrogenic hypogonadism. Furthermore, adipose tissue-derived factors, such as leptin and adipokines, regulate testosterone production and inflammation, respectively. Increased systemic inflammation results in increased reactive oxygen species and sperm DNA fragmentation. Inactivity, increased midsection, and inner-thigh adiposity can lead to increased scrotal temperature and impairment of spermatogenesis (Kahn and Brannigan 2017).

Underweight

Women who have a very low BMI (<18.5) and low body fat percentage are at higher risk of ovarian disorders and infertility. It is suggested that this infertility in underweight women is due to increased FSH levels, a shortened luteal phase, and secondary amenorrhoea (Cramer et al. 1994; Frisch, 1987; Grodstein et al. 1994b). Underweight women also have lower rates of clinical pregnancy, higher rates of miscarriage when comparing with women of a normal weight (11% in underweight women compared with 0.5% for normal weight women), as well as an increased risk for premature labour and birth of low weight infants (Davies 2006; Han et al. 2010). Amenorrhoea in women who are underweight is associated with a low leptin secretion, suggesting that leptin affects the female hypothalamic–pituitary gonadal axis. It has been suggested that in underweight males, lower levels of leptin are associated with lower levels of LH, FSH, and testosterone. When these males increased their weight, levels of leptin increased and correlated with increased levels of LH, FSH, and testosterone (Wabitsch *et al.* 2001).

Sexually Transmitted Infections

Sexually transmitted infections (STIs) are caused by viruses, bacteria, fungi, and protozoa. STIs are usually due to high risk sexual behaviour (many sexual partners, changing sexual partners often, and not using condoms) and are more commonly seen in sexually active adolescents and young adults (under 25) (Satterwhite et al. 2013; Watson 2015). Many of the reported studies regarding STIs and infertility are related to bacterial infections (Chlamydia and gonorrhoea). When these infections are left untreated, either due to lack of symptoms or repeated infections, this increases the incidence of pelvic inflammatory disease (PID) in females which causes inflammatory obstruction of the reproductive tract. PID can also cause scarring of the Fallopian tubes, increasing the risk of ectopic pregnancy and is a major aspect in tubal factor female infertility (Paavonen and Eggert-Kruse 1999; Lareau and Beigi 2008; Bachir and Jarvi 2014). However, the impact of bacterial STIs on male fertility is less well known. Chlamydial infections in the male have shown to lower semen quality and cause DNA damage in sperm although there is no clear consensus on whether this significantly affects male fertility (Ochsendorf 2008; Pacey 2010). See Chapter 14 for more details on the impact of infection on reproduction.

Conclusion

In order to optimize fertility, it is vital for both men and women to adjust their lifestyles by maintaining a healthy body weight, abstaining from cigarette smoking, alcohol and drugs, minimizing their exposure to STIs, and tackling stress and anxiety. Reducing or eliminating exposure to hazardous compounds in the workplace and environment is important to improve fertility rates.

References

Anderson, K., Nisenblat, V. and Norman, R. (2010). Lifestyle factors in people seeking infertility treatment – a review. Aust NZ J Obstet Gynaecol 50: 8–20.

Ash, P. (1980). The influence of radiation on fertility in man. Br J Radiol 53: 271–278.

Bachir, B.G. and Jarvi, K. (2014). Infectious, inflammatory, and immunologic conditions resulting in male infertility. Curr Manag Male Infertil 41: 67–81.

Benoff, S., Centola, G.M., Millan, C. et al. (2003). Increased seminal plasma lead levels adversely affect the fertility potential of sperm in IVF. Hum Reprod 18: 374–383.

Brewer, C.J. and Balen, A.H. (2010). The adverse effects of obesity on conception and implantation. Reproduction 140: 347–364.

Byrne, J., Mulvihill, J.J., Myers, M.H. et al. (1987). Effects of treatment on fertility in long-term survivors of childhood or adolescent cancer. N Engl J Med 317: 1315–1321.

Cabler, S., Agarwal, A., Flint, M. et al. (2010). Obesity: modern man's fertility nemesis. Asian J Androl 12: 480.

Cordier, S., Deplan, F., Mandereau, L. et al. (1991). Paternal exposure to mercury and spontaneous abortions. Occup Environ Med 48: 375–381.

Counter, S.A. and Buchanan, L.H. (2004). Mercury exposure in children: a review. Toxicol Appl Pharmacol 198: 209–230.

Cramer, D.W., Barbieri, R.L., Xu, H. et al. (1994). Determinants of basal follicle-stimulating hormone levels in premenopausal women. J Clin Endocrinol Metab 79: 1105–1109.

Davies, M.J. (2006). Evidence for effects of weight on reproduction in women. Reprod Biomed Online 12: 552–561.

Eisenberg, M.L., Li, S., Behr, B. et al. (2014). Semen quality, infertility and mortality in the USA. Hum Reprod 29: 1567–1574.

Erler, C. and Novak, J. (2010). Bisphenol A exposure: human risk and health policy. J Pediatr Nurs 25: 400–407.

Evans, H., Fletcher, J., Torrance, M. et al. (1981). Sperm abnormalities and cigarette smoking. The Lancet 317: 627–629.

Frisch, R.E. (1987). Body fat, menarche, fitness and fertility. Hum Reprod 2: 521–533.

Fronczak, C.M., Kim, E.D., Barqawi, A.B. (2012). The insults of illicit drug use on male fertility. J Androl 33: 515–528.

Gilliland, F.D., Li, Y.-F. and Peters, J.M. (2001). Effects of maternal smoking during pregnancy and environmental tobacco smoke on asthma and wheezing in children. Am J Respir Crit Care Med 163: 429–436.

Grodstein, F., Goldman, M.B. and Cramer, D.W. (1994a). Infertility in women and moderate alcohol use. Am J Public Health 84: 1429–1432.

Grodstein, F., Goldman, M.B. and Cramer, D.W. (1994b). Body mass index and ovulatory infertility. Epidemiology 5: 247–250.

Hagmar, L., Rylander, L., Dyremark, E. et al. (2001). Plasma concentrations of persistent organochlorines in relation to thyrotropin and thyroid hormone levels in women. Int Arch Occup Environ Health 74: 184–188.

Han, Z., Mulla, S., Beyene, J. et al. (2010). Maternal underweight and the risk of preterm birth and low birth weight: a systematic review and meta-analyses. Int J Epidemiol 40: 65–101.

Henriksen, T.B., Hjollund, N.H., Jensen, T.K. et al. (2004). Alcohol consumption at the time of conception and spontaneous abortion. Am J Epidemiol 160: 661–667.

Homan, G., Davies, M. and Norman, R. (2007). The impact of lifestyle factors on reproductive performance in the general population and those undergoing infertility treatment: a review. Hum Reprod Update 13: 209–223.

Kahn B.E. and Brannigan, R.E. (2017). Obesity and male infertility. Curr Opin Urol 27: 441–445

Kline, J., Stein, Z.A., Susser, M. et al. (1977). Smoking: a risk factor for spontaneous abortion. N Engl J Med 297: 793–796.

Knoll, M. and Talbot, P. (1998). Cigarette smoke inhibits oocyte cumulus complex pick-up by the oviduct *in vitro* independent of ciliary beat frequency. Reprod Toxicol 12: 57–68.

Kwon, J.-H., Katz, L.E. and Liljestrand, H.M. (2007). Modeling binding equilibrium in a competitive estrogen receptor binding assay. Chemosphere 69: 1025–1031.

Lareau, S.M. and Beigi, R.H. (2008). Pelvic inflammatory disease and tubo-ovarian abscess. Infect Dis Clin North Am 22: 693–708.

Li, L.H. and Heindel, J.J. (1998). Sertoli cell toxicants. In: *Reproduction and Developmental Toxicology* (ed. K.S. Korach), 655–691. New York: Marcel Dekker.

Lindbohm, M.L. (1995). Effects of parental exposure to solvents on pregnancy outcome. J Occup Environ Med 37(8): 908–14.

MacDonald, A., Herbison, G., Showell, M. et al. (2009). The impact of body mass index on semen parameters and reproductive hormones in human males: a systematic review with meta-analysis. Hum Reprod Update 16: 293–311.

Mattison, D.R. (1982). The effects of smoking on fertility from gametogenesis to implantation. Environ Res 28: 410–433.

Muthusami, K. and Chinnaswamy, P. (2005). Effect of chronic alcoholism on male fertility hormones and semen quality. Fertil Steril 84: 919–924.

Ochsendorf, F. (2008). Sexually transmitted infections: impact on male fertility. Andrologia 40: 72–75.

Oyesanya, O.A., Zenzes, M.T., Wang, P. et al. (1995). Cigarette smoking may affect meiotic maturation of human oocytes. Hum Reprod 10: 3213–3217.

Paavonen, J. and Eggert-Kruse, W. (1999). Chlamydia trachomatis: impact on human reproduction. Hum Reprod Update 5: 433–447.

Pacey, A. (2010). Environmental and lifestyle factors associated with sperm DNA damage. Hum Fertil 13: 189–193.

Pandey, S., Maheshwari, A. and Bhattacharya, S. (2010). Should access to fertility treatment be determined by female body mass index? Hum Reprod 25: 815–820.

Phillips, K.P. and Tanphaichitr, N. (2010). Mechanisms of obesity-induced male infertility. Expert Rev Endocrinol Metab 5: 229–251.

Potts, R., Newbury, C., Smith, G. et al. (1999). Sperm chromatin damage associated with male smoking. Mutat Res Mol Mech Mutagen 423: 103–111.

Reece, E.A. (2008). Perspectives on obesity, pregnancy and birth outcomes in the United States: the scope of the problem. Am J Obstet Gynecol 198: 23–27.

Ricci, E., Viganò, P., Cipriani, S. et al. (2017). Coffee and caffeine intake and male infertility: a systematic review. Nutr J 16: 37.

Rochester, J.R. (2013). Bisphenol A and human health: a review of the literature. Reprod Toxicol 42: 132–155.

Sadeu, J., Hughes, C.L., Agarwal, S. et al. (2010). Alcohol, drugs, caffeine, tobacco, and environmental contaminant exposure: reproductive health consequences and clinical implications. Crit Rev Toxicol 40: 633–652.

Saraiya, M., Berg, C.J., Kendrick, J.S. et al. (1998). Cigarette smoking as a risk factor for ectopic pregnancy. Am J Obstet Gynecol 178: 493–498.

Satterwhite, C.L., Torrone, E., Meites, E. et al. (2013). Sexually transmitted infections among US women and men: prevalence and incidence estimates (2008). Sex Transm Dis 40: 187–193.

Savitz, D.A., Sonnenfeld, N.L. and Olshan, A.F. (1994). Review of epidemiologic studies of paternal occupational exposure and spontaneous abortion. American journal of industrial medicine 25(3): 361–383.

Schell, L.M., Gallo, M.V., Deane, G.D. et al. and Task Force on the Environment (2014). Relationships of polychlorinated biphenyls and dichlorodiphenyldichloroethylene (p, p'-DDE) with testosterone levels in adolescent males. Environ Health Perspect 122: 304.

Schnaas, L., Rothenberg, S.J., Flores, M.-F. et al. (2006). Reduced intellectual development in children with prenatal lead exposure. Environ Health Perspect 114: 791.

Skakkebaek, N.E., Rajpert-De Meyts, E. and Main, K.M. (2001).Testicular dysgenesis syndrome: an increasingly common developmental disorder with environmental aspects. Hum Reprod 16: 972–978.

Suonio, S., Saarikoski, S., Kauhanen, O. et al. (1990). Smoking does affect fecundity. Eur J Obstet Gynecol Reprod Biol 34: 89–95.

Vandenberg, L.N., Hauser, R., Marcus, M. et al. (2007). Human exposure to bisphenol A (BPA). Reprod Toxicol 24: 139–177.

Vine, M.F., Chiu-Kit, J.T., Hu, P.-C. et al. (1996). Cigarette smoking and semen quality. Fertil Steril 65: 835–842.

Virtanen, H.E., Rajpert-De Meyts, E., Main, K.M. et al. (2005). Testicular dysgenesis syndrome and the development and occurrence of male reproductive disorders. Toxicol Appl Pharmacol 207(2 Suppl): 501–505.

Vogel, S.A. (2009). The politics of plastics: the making and unmaking of bisphenol a "safety." Am J Public Health 99: S559–S566.

Waalkes, M.P. (2003). Cadmium carcinogenesis. Mutat Res Mol Mech Mutagen 533: 107–120.

Wabitsch, M., Ballauff, A., Holl, R. et al. (2001). Serum leptin, gonadotropin, and testosterone concentrations in male patients with anorexia nervosa during weight gain. J Clin Endocrinol Metab 86: 2982–2988.

Wallach, E.E., Hughes, E.G. and Brennan, B.G. (1996). Does cigarette smoking impair natural or assisted fecundity? Fertil Steril 66: 679–689.

Watson, R.R. (2015). *Handbook of Fertility: Nutrition, Diet, Lifestyle and Reproductive Health*. Cambridge, MA: Academic Press.

Weisberg, E. (1985). Smoking and reproductive health. Clin Reprod Fertil 3: 175–186.

Wilks, D.J. and Hay, A.W. (2004). Smoking and female fecundity: the effect and importance of study design. Eur J Obstet Gynecol Reprod Biol 112: 127–135.

Woodruff, T.J., Janssen, S.J., Guillette Jr, L.J. and Giudice, L.C. eds. (2010). Environmental impacts on reproductive health and fertility. Cambridge University Press.

World Health Organization (2007). *Tobacco Free Initiative. Protection from exposure to second-hand tobacco smoke: policy recommendations*. Geneva: World Health Organization.

Zenzes, M.T. (2000). Smoking and reproduction: gene damage to human gametes and embryos. Hum Reprod Update 6: 122–131.

Section Three

Clinical Reproductive Science In Practice

IVF and Assisted Reproductive Technologies

18

Assessing the Infertile Couple

Narmada Katakam, Ruth Arnesen, Caroline Watkins, Bert Stewart, and Luciano G. Nardo

Introduction

Definitions

1) Infertility is defined as the inability to conceive after regular unprotected sexual intercourse for 12 consecutive months, in the absence of any known cause (NICE 2013).
2) Subfertility is defined as the inability to conceive due to reduced fertility. Clear understanding of the definitions of sub- and infertility is very important for the appropriate management of infertility (Gnoth et al. 2005).
3) Primary infertility is when someone has never conceived in the past and has difficulty conceiving now.
4) Secondary infertility is when someone has had one or more pregnancies in the past and has difficulty conceiving now.

Epidemiology of Infertility

More than 80% of couples conceive in the first year and circa 90% in the second year, with some age dependent differences (Dunson et al. 2004). The remaining couples may require some kind of fertility treatment to achieve a successful pregnancy (te Velde et al. 2000; Taylor 2003a).

Since 1991, 170 000 babies have been born as a result of *in vitro* fertilization (IVF) treatment in the UK, constituting almost 2% of all the newborns in the country (Human Fertilisation and Embryology Authority 2011). Infertility affects one in seven heterosexual couples in the UK, which equates to approximately 3.5 million people (Human Fertilisation and Embryology Authority 2010). These patients should be offered further clinical assessment and tailored investigations. However, earlier referral should be offered when the woman is aged 35 or over and there is a known cause or predisposing factor increasing the risk of infertility. Main reasons for infertility in the UK include male factors (30%), ovulation disorders (25%), unexplained (25%), tubal damage (20%), uterine or peritoneal factors (10%), and both male and female factors (40%). Some couples may have more than one cause (NICE 2013). Other reasons include uterine abnormality, endometrial factors, gamete or embryo defects, and pelvic conditions such as endometriosis, fibroids, and adhesions. Fertility assessments fail to identify an abnormality in up to 25% of infertile couples (Gelbaya et al. 2014).

The number of couples seeking help for fertility is constantly rising. Women delaying starting a family until their late 30s or even early 40s is a significant contributing factor to the changing face of fertility performance in developing countries.

The rate of spontaneous pregnancy amongst subfertile couples is less than the fertile population. Heterosexual couples should be seen together as the process affects both partners. Assessment should take individual needs, underlying medical problems, and treatment preferences into account. The patients should be given adequate information to be able to make well-informed decisions about their management. Thorough assessment is recommended, to include history, clinical examination, and investigations (Kamel 2010) as outlined in Figure 18.1 and 18.2.

Clinical Reproductive Science, First Edition. Edited by Michael Carroll.
© 2019 John Wiley & Sons Ltd. Published 2019 by John Wiley & Sons Ltd.
Companion website: www.wiley.com/go/carroll/clinicalreproductivescience

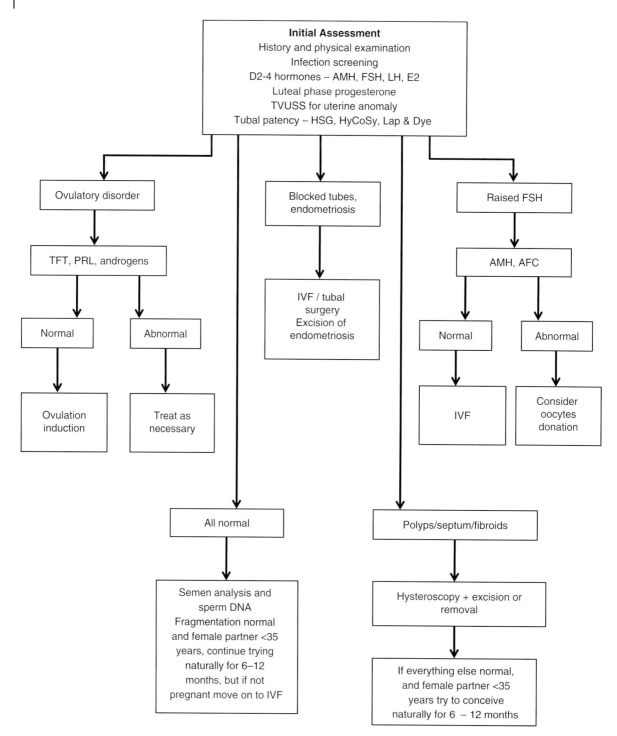

Figure 18.1 Flow diagram outlining initial assessment of the female patient including clinical history, physical examination, and screening. AFC, antral follicle count; AMH, anti-Müllerian hormone; FSH, follicle-stimulating hormone; HSG, hysterosalpingogram; HyCoSy, hysterosalpingo-contrast-sonography; IVF, *in vitro* fertilization; Lap & Dye, laparoscopy and dye test; LH, luteinizing hormone; PRL, prolactin level; TFT, thyroid function test; TVUSS, transvaginal ultrasound scan.

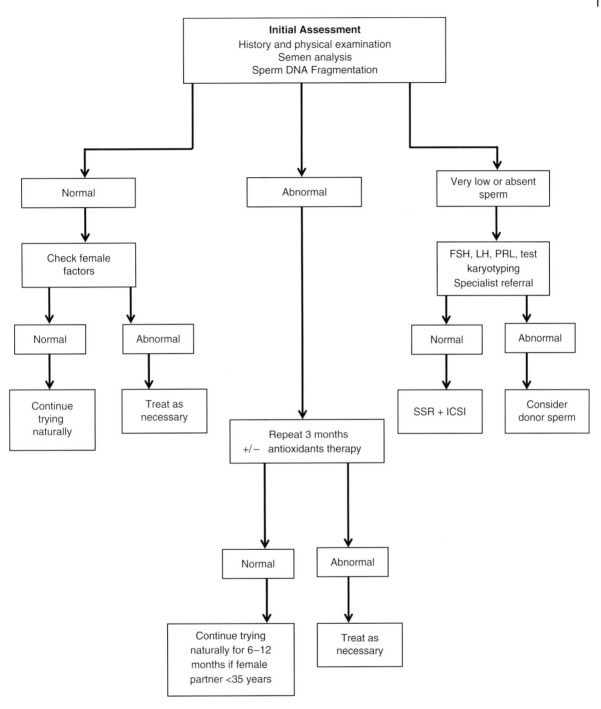

Figure 18.2 Flow diagram outlining initial assessment of the male patient including semen analysis. FSH, follicle-stimulating hormone; ICSI, intracytoplasmic sperm injection; LH, luteinizing hormone; PRL, prolactin level; SSR, surgical sperm retrieval.

Counseling is also an important part of the fertility assessment and should be offered to all patients seeking fertility treatment.

History Taking: Female Partner

General factors that reduce fertility in a couple include (Taylor 2003b):

- Woman aged over 35 years
- No previous pregnancy
- Trying to conceive for >3 years
- Infrequent sexual intercourse
- Woman's body mass index (BMI) <20 or >30
- Regular use of recreational drugs
- Sexually transmitted infections
- Lifestyle factors including smoking in one or both partners, caffeine intake >2 cups of coffee per day.

As shown in Table 18.1, the causes of female infertility can be mainly subdivided into ovulatory disorders, tubal and peritoneal factors, cervical factors, and unexplained causes (Sanders and Debuse 2003). Detailed history from both partners usually indicates the underlying reproductive problem (Forti and Krausz 1998; Whitman-Elia and Baxley 2001; Case 2003; Taylor 2003b). History taking should include details of age, duration of infertility, cervical smears, breast changes and milk-like discharge

Table 18.1 Causes of and influences on female subfertility (Saunders and Debuse 2003).

Causes of Female Subfertlity	Influenced Or Caused By
Ovulatory factors	- Weight loss - Polycystic ovarian syndrome (PCOS) - Premature ovarian failure - Hypothalamicamenorrhoea - Hyperprolactinaemia
Tubal and peritoneal factors	- Pelvic adhesions - Pelvic inflammatory disease (PID) - Endometriosis - H/O ectopic pregnancy - Pelvic surgery
Cervical factors	- Cervical stenosis - Abnormal cervical mucus-hostile to sperm

(galactorrhoea), excessive hair growth with or without acne, hot flushes, recent weight loss or weight gain, and previous fertility treatment.

1) *Menstrual history:* age of menarche, cycle characteristics – frequency, duration, dysmenorrhoea, intermenstrual or postcoital bleeding. Review for any history of primary or secondary amenorrhoea. Women with regular menstrual cycles are very likely to be ovulating and should be reassured.
2) *Obstetric history:* previous pregnancies, if any, and its outcome, recurrent pregnancy loss, terminations, infection or puerperal sepsis.
3) *Contraceptive history:* previous use of contraceptives, any associated problems including lost coil, latest contraceptive methods and when last used. This is particularly relevant for medroxyprogesterone injections and combined pills as the return of fertility can be longer –up to 1 year in some cases.
4) *Sexual history:* frequency of intercourse, timing in relation to the cycle, use of vaginal lubricants, douching after sexual intercourse, dyspareunia, loss of libido, and history of any sexually transmitted infections
5) *Medical history:* diabetes, hypertension, thyroid disorder, cystic fibrosis, sickle cell disease, tuberculosis, and history of ovarian cysts. Enquire about rubella status.
6) *Surgical history:* appendicectomy, tubal surgery, pelvic surgery, laparotomy and bowel surgery, Caesarean sections, and cervical loop excision or conization.
7) *Family history:* consanguinity, diabetes mellitus, hypertension, and cancer.
8) *Social history:* occupation, diet, drug history including recreational drugs such as marijuana and cocaine, smoking, alcohol and caffeine consumption.

Ovulation Disorders

Reducing the body weight in women with a BMI of >30 kg/m^2 may restore ovulation spontaneously, improve response to ovulation induction agents, and have a positive impact on pregnancy outcome. Using drugs such as clomifene citrate or metformin, or a combination of the above, can induce ovulation (see Table 18.2).

Table 18.2 Ovulatory Disorders (WHO 1973).

Group	Cause/Presentation	Hormones
WHO Group 1	Hypothalamic–pituitary failure	No oestrogen No/low FSH or LH
Amenorrhoea	• Severe weight loss • Anxiety • Genetic (Kallman ssyndrome)	Normal prolactin <1% infertility patients
WHO Group 2	Hypothalamic–pituitary dysfunction	Oestrogen present FSH and LH levels – variable from cycle to cycle
Amenorrhoea/ oligomenorrhoea	• Polycystic ovary syndrome (PCOS)	Normal prolactin Mostly PCOS Elevated LH levels in PCOS
WHO Group 3	Ovarianfailure	No oestrogen Raised LH and FSH
Amenorrhoea	• Resistant ovary • Premature ovarianfailure	

FSH, follicle-stimulating hormone; LH, luteinizing hormone.

Polycystic ovary syndrome (PCOS) is one of the most common hormonal disorders affecting women of reproductive age. It is an inherited condition with a prevalence of around 10%. Polycystic ovaries are seen on the scan in 20% of women investigated for infertility (Elsheikh and Murphy 2008). PCOS accounts for approximately 75% of women who suffer from infertility due to anovulation. The precise cause of PCOS remains unknown, but it is thought to be a thecal cell defect in androgen biosynthesis (Johnson 2007).

In PCOS, luteinizing hormone (LH) is raised and follicle-stimulating hormone (FSH) may be normal. This differentiates PCOS from secondary ovarian failure and early menopausal onset where both LH and FSH are raised. Women with PCOS have two to three times the normal number of preantral follicles, which arrest at the early antral stage. There is no dominant follicle. Other aetiologies should be excluded (congenital adrenal hyperplasia, androgen-secreting tumours, Cushing's syndrome). The 2003 Rotterdam Consensus Workshop revised the diagnostic criteria for PCOS to include two out of three of the following (Rotterdam Consensus 2004):

1) Oligo- and/or anovulation.
2) Clinical and/or biochemical signs of hyperandrogenism (hirsutism, weight gain, acne).
3) Polycystic ovaries.

Premature ovarian failure (POF) is amenorrhoea before the age of 40 without obvious cause. POF is characterized by amenorrhoea, hypo-oestrogenism, and elevated gonadotropins. The incidence is 1% (Coulam *et al.* 1986; Shelling 2010).

Causes of premature ovarian failure include:

• Iatrogenic – chemotherapy, radiotherapy
• Surgical removal of the ovaries or repeated cystectomies
• Autoimmune disease (myasthenia gravis or hypothyroidism)
• Genetic abnormalities – mosaic Turner syndrome.

In POF, there is loss of fertility either due to the absence of follicles or lack of response to ovarian stimulation. There is sporadic ovulation and successful pregnancy in 5–10% of patients; however, this response cannot be reliably predicted.

History Taking: Male Partner

1) *Present history:* age, duration of infertility, previous seminal analysis findings, breast changes such as enlargement, previous fertility treatment.
2) *Sexual history:* frequency of intercourse, loss of libido, erectile dysfunction or ejaculatory problems, history of sexually transmitted infections.

3) *Contraceptive history:* previous contraceptives and vasectomy.
4) *Surgical history:* hydrocele, varicocele, undescended testis, inguinal hernia repair, prostate operations.
5) *Medical history:* diabetes, hypertension, and history of mumps.
6) *Family history:* any similar problems amongst the male members, consanguinity, diabetes mellitus, hypertension, and cancer.
7) *Social history:* occupation, diet, drug history including recreational drugs such as marijuana and cocaine, smoking, alcohol and caffeine consumption.

Clinical Examination

Clinical examination of both partners is essential. In some cases, a provisional diagnosis is usually possible by the end of the examination. Investigations are then performed to confirm the clinical diagnosis and exclude any abnormalities (ESHRE Capri Workshop Group 2004; Jose-Miller *et al.* 2007; Macaluso *et al.* 2010).

Clinical Examination: Female Partner

1) *General examination:* vital signs (especially blood pressure), BMI, secondary sexual characteristics, excessive hairs/acne on face or chest, thyroid gland examination, inspection of skin for any abnormal pigmentation such as vitiligo or eczema.
2) *Breast examination:* look for occult galactorrhoea.
3) *Abdominal examination:* abdominal mass, organomegaly, abdominal wall and neck striae, surgical scars.
4) *Genital examination:* vaginal introitus for any vaginismus, vaginal discharge; cervical appearance, size, consistency; mobility and direction of the uterus; adnexal masses and tenderness; check for thickening of the uterosacral ligament and nodules in the cul-de-sac suggestive of endometriosis.

Clinical Examination: Male Partner

1) *General examination:* vital signs (especially blood pressure), BMI, secondary sexual characteristics, thyroid gland examination.
2) *Breast examination:* look for gynaecomastia.

3) *Abdominal examination:* abdominal mass, undescended testis, inguinal hernia, organomegaly, or ascites.
4) *Genital examination:* shape and size of penis, prepuce, position of external urethral meatus; testicular examination to assess volume using a Prader orchidometer to exclude varicocele or hydrocele, palpation of epididymis and vas deferens; perineal sensation, anal sphincter tone, and prostate enlargement by rectal examination (only if indicated by underlying medical conditions and symptoms).

Investigations of an Infertile Couple

It is not always possible to assess the cause of infertility from history taking and clinical examination alone. No treatment should be commenced until basic investigations are performed and results reviewed. Investigations should be arranged after 12 months of trying to conceive. However, in women over 35 years old or in the presence of obvious identifiable reproductive problems, investigations should be arranged without delay.

Common causes of infertility are sperm abnormalities, ovarian disorders, and Fallopian tube obstruction. Therefore, the focus of preliminary investigations for the infertile couple should be semen analysis, detection of ovarian function by hormonal assay (early follicular phase AMH, FSH, LH, E2 levels), and evaluation of pelvic organs and tubal patency by ultrasound scan and hysterosalpingo-contrast-sonography (HyCoSy). Any previous fertility assessment tests should be reviewed. Further investigations should be requested according to the clinical presentation and the results of the preliminary investigations.

Female Partner: Basic Investigations

1) *General:* cervical smear, if it is due.
2) *Basal body temperature recording:* basal body temperature rises by 0.5–1 °C following ovulation and remains elevated for the rest of the luteal phase. Temperature falls just before menstruation.
3) *Infection screening:* viral screening for human immunodeficiency virus (HIV), hepatitis B, and

hepatitis C are performed, not necessarily for assessment of infertility but for further management in the case of specialist referral for assisted conception treatment. All women are screened for Rubella: vaccination is offered to those who are susceptible to prevent Rubella in pregnancy and avoid associated fetal abnormalities. Contraception is advised for at least a month after the vaccination. Vaginal swabs are taken to exclude bacterial vaginosis. Sexually transmitted infection screening for *Chlamydia trachomatis* is performed. Positive cases are treated and screening is advised for the partner.

4) *Hormonal assay:* to assess ovarian reserve – FSH, LH, E2 (day 2–4 of the menstrual cycle). In some cases of irregular periods, serial testing of serum progesterone should be performed to confirm ovulation. In women with longer cycles, this test should be done weekly from 7 days before the next expected menstrual cycle (Table 18.3).

Table 18.3 Hormone Assays.

Progesterone	If low, suggests anovulation or ovulatory dysfunction Rise in mid-luteal phase (>30 nmol/L) suggests ovulation
FSH	Day 2–4 Assesses ovarian reserve Raised level suggests ovarian failure
LH	Day 2–4 Raised-Level (with normal FSH) suggests PCOS
Oestradiol	Day 2–4 Normal – low FSH and lowoestradio on day 3
Sex hormone binding globulin	Low level suggests PCOS or Androgen Excess
Thyroid stimulating hormone	Raised level suggests hypothyroidism
Testosterone	Moderately raised level suggests PCOS
Prolactin	Marginally raised with regular cycles in PCOS Raised with amenorrhoea in case of prolactinoma
AMH	Low levels suggest poor ovarian reserves High levels suggest PCOS

FSH, follicle-stimulating hormone; LH, luteinizing hormone; PCOS, polycystic ovary syndrome.

5) *Ovarian reserve tests:* a woman's chronological age is a very strong predictor of her overall chance of success. Fertility remains relatively stable in the early 30s, at more than 400 pregnancies per 1000 exposed women per year. It begins to decrease significantly thereafter dropping to 100 pregnancies per 1000 exposed women per year by the age of 45 (Heffner 2004). Checking one or more of the following markers can assess ovarian reserve (NICE 2013):

- Total antral follicle count (AFC), defined as the total numbers of follicles measuring between 2 and 6 mm detected by transvaginal ultrasound scan on day 2–4 of the menstrual cycle. An AFC of >16 is prognostic for a high response whereas if <4 it is prognostic for a low response.
- Anti-Müllerian hormone (AMH) is a direct serum marker of the functional ovarian reserve (the number of growing follicles that can be recruited by exogenous FSH stimulation). Granulosa cells of preantral and small antral follicles primarily secrete AMH. Serum AMH levels correlate with the number of primordial follicles in the ovary (Hansen et al. 2011; Dewaily et al. 2014). Serum AMH levels remain relatively stable throughout the menstrual cycle and therefore can be measured on any day of the cycle (van Disseldorp 2010). Age-related serum AMH reference intervals assessed by the Roche automated assay include 13.1–53.8 pmol/L (20–29 years), 6.8–47.8 pmol/L (30–34 years), 5.5–37.4 pmol/L (35–39 years), 0.7–21.2 pmol/L (40–44 years) and 0.3–14.7 pmol/L (45–49 years) (Elecsys AMH Factsheet 2014). Circulating AMH levels can predict excessive and poor ovarian response to exogenous gonadotropin stimulation (Nardo et al. 2009).

AMH and AFC are comparable predictors for ovarian performance. Ovarian volume, ovarian blood flow, and inhibin B are not very accurate and reliable predictors of outcome of fertility treatment.

6) *Transvaginal ultrasound scan (TVUSS):* to detect congenital uterine anomalies including bicornuate or septate uterus, assess the endometrium for polyps, distortion by fibroids, presence of adhesions, to rule out ovarian abnormality including ovarian cysts and polycystic ovaries,

and to exclude the presence of tubal pathologies such as hydrosalpinx and paratubal cysts. Ultrasound scan is also employed to measure the follicular development from day 6 to 7 of the cycle in women undergoing controlled ovarian stimulation and in those having ovulation induction. Sliding sign is assessed to confirm mobility of the ovary and tenderness is assessed in suspected cases of endometriosis.

7) *Hysterosalpingogram (HSG) or HyCoSy:* investigations to assess tubal and uterine dysfunction. These are offered to low risk women to evaluate the uterine cavity and confirm patency of the Fallopian tubes. Tubal patency is different from tubal function; tubal patency can be assessed by these tests but not the function.

HSG is a reliable test to assess tubal patency in women who are not known to have comorbidities (such as pelvic inflammatory disease, previous ectopic pregnancy, or endometriosis). It is less invasive and avoids anaesthesia, hospital stay, and complications of laparoscopy.

HyCoSy is an effective alternative to HSG with equally good results and should be considered where facilities are available. It has the additional advantage of being more dynamic than the HSG and allows the assessment of uterus and the ovaries at the same time. Both HSG and HyCoSy should be performed between day 5 and 10 of the menstrual cycle. Swabs for vaginal infections and Chlamydia should be taken, and if necessary treatment should be prescribed before performing any tubal patency tests.

Female Partner: Additional Investigations

These are offered to women if indicated during history and clinical examination.

1) *Hormonal assay:* prolactin should be checked in women with ovulatory dysfunction, galactorrhoea, visual disturbance, and pituitary tumours. Thyroid function tests should be checked in women with symptoms of thyroid disease, hair loss, lethargy and tiredness; androstenedione, testosterone, sex hormone binding globulin (SHBG), dehydroepiandrosterone (DHEA), and dehydroepiandrosterone sulphate (DHEAS) should be checked in women with irregular cycles, raised BMI, polycystic appearance of the

ovary on scanning, and signs of hyperandrogenism, to confirm PCOS and to exclude other causes of androgen excess.

2) *Laparoscopy and dye test:* the procedure of choice in women with comorbidities, i.e. suspected cases of associated pelvic pathology or adhesions where patency could not be confirmed by HSG or HyCoSy, history of pelvic inflammatory disease, or endometriosis. This not only assesses tubal patency but also other pelvic pathology can be evaluated and in some cases treated at the same time.

3) *Hysteroscopy:* offered when uterine pathology is suspected at TVUSS, HSG, or HyCoSy. These include partial or complete septum, adhesions, or endometrial polyps and fibroids distorting the endometrial cavity. Both laparoscopy and hysteroscopy should be performed in the follicular phase of the cycle (day 5–10).

4) *Karyotyping:* to exclude underlying genetic disorders such as mosaic Turner syndrome, single gene disorders, aneuploidy, and translocations, in the presence of a normal phenotype.

Male Partner: Basic Investigations

1) *General:* viral screening for HIV, hepatitis B, and hepatitis C.

2) *Semen analysis:* it should be an integral part of the initial assessment. The results should be compared to the World Health Organization reference values (Table 18.4). If the results from the first semen analysis are abnormal, the test should be repeated to confirm the findings. This should ideally be undertaken within 3 months after the initial analysis. If the results are grossly abnormal (e.g. azoospermia or severe oligozoospermia) (Table 18.5), the test should be repeated as soon as possible and appropriate referral instigated.

Male Partner: Additional Investigations

1) *Hormonal assay:* FSH, LH, prolactin, and testosterone are performed in cases with abnormal semen analysis and suspected endocrine disorders.

2) *Testicular biopsy:* a fine-needle aspiration biopsy differentiates between obstructive and nonobstructive azoospermia by the presence

of sperm in the sample. This is not only diagnostic but also allows sperm freezing at the same time.

3) *Sperm DNA Fragmentation:* conventional semen analysis continues to be the only routine test to diagnose male factor infertility. However, the quality of the DNA in the sperm head is of paramount importance for normal embryo development. Damage to sperm DNA can be associated with impaired fertilization, disrupted preimplantation embryo development, and higher rates of spontaneous miscarriage (Lewis and Aitken 2005; Bungum et al. 2007; Simon et al. 2010, 2011; Zini 2011; Simon et al. 2013; Lewis et al. 2013). There are two major causes of

DNA damage: (i) oxidative stress via reactive oxygen species (ROS), and (ii) the action of nucleases. It has long been established that sperm need to be protected from oxidative stress; indeed, the seminal plasma is a suspension full of antioxidants helping to prevent free radical attack from ROS (Aitken and Clarkson 1988). It is suggested that sperm cells that have experienced defective chromatin remodelling during spermatogenesis are more prone to DNA damage from ROS (Aitken et al. 2010). The ROS themselves may evolve from immune system cells, which are present in the testis as a result of injury and/or inflammation. Another potential source of damage comes from varicocoele. It is known that men with varicocoele have increased levels of ROS, thus leading to sperm DNA damage (Zini and Dohle 2011).

There are several tests available in the laboratory that have been used extensively to analyse sperm chromatin integrity: sperm COMET assay (Simon et al. 2011), sperm chromatin structure assay (Giwercman et al. 2010), and Halo and TUNEL assays (Sharma et al. 2010). However, there are differences between these tests in how DNA damage is assessed. The studies in the literature have shown a strong correlation between sperm DNA fragmentation and fertility status of men. Using the Comet test, 95% of fertile donors had DNA fragmentation below 25% whereas 98% of infertile men had DNA fragmentation above

Table 18.4 Semen Analysis (WHO 2010).

Semen volume	1.5 mL or more
pH	7.2 or more
Sperm concentration	15 million spermatozoa per mL or more
Total sperm number	39 million spermatozoa per ejaculate
Total motiliy (% of progressive motility and nonprogressive motility)	40% or more motile or 32% or more with progressive motility
Vitality	58% or more live spermatozoa
Sperm morphology (% of normal forms)	4% or more

Table 18.5 Abnormalities in sperm Production.

Azoospermia	Semen contains no sperm Causes: Primary testicular failure, Klinefelter tubal obstruction, vasectomy, chromosomal abnormalities, such as Klinefelter syndrome, in which the body's cells all carry an extra X chromosome, Y chromosome deletion; absence of both vas deferens (an inherited condition known as CBAVD - congenital bilateral absence of the vas deferens)
Oligozoospermia	Reduced sperm, commonly known as a low sperm count Causes: Testosterone deficiency and hyperprolactinaemia
Asthenozoospermia	Decreased sperm quality due to reduced motility or abnormal sperm shape Causes: Antisperm antibodies, infections, raised scrotal temperature
Anospermia	Complete lack of semen Causes: Retrograde ejaculation, ejaculatory duct obstruction
Teratozoospermia	Abnormally-shaped sperm may have reduced motility and be unable to adhere to the oocyte Causes: Hodgkin Crohn disease, coeliac disease, Crohn's disease, etc.
Oligoasthenoteratozoospermia (OATS)	Reduced sperm with reduced motility and morphology

25% (Simon et al. 2011). The latest study using the Comet assay showed that couples with low levels of sperm DNA fragmentation (<25%) had a live birth rate of 33% following IVF treatment. Couples with high levels (>50%) had a much lower live birth rate of 13% following IVF treatment (Simon et al. 2013). There is growing evidence that embryos generated from cycles with high levels of sperm DNA damage have an increased chance of pregnancy loss and this is regardless of the fertilization method used (Robinson et al. 2012).

The main limitation of testing for sperm DNA damage is that each assay renders the tested sperm unsuitable for clinical purpose. Noninvasive tests that have been developed include birefringence, intracytoplasmic morphologically selected sperm injection (IMSI), and hyaluronic acid selection of spermatozoa for intracytoplasmic sperm injection (ICSI) (Sakkas 2013). However, the clinical evidence that associates these methods with detecting sperm with reduced DNA damage is not very robust (McDowell et al. 2014). A study is currently taking place in the UK to try and answer some of these questions.

The current recommendations are that patients who are tested positive for sperm DNA damage should be treated with one or more antioxidants for the duration of spermatogenesis (90 days). This approach will lead to improvement of the patient's sperm DNA quality prior to undertaking any fertility treatment (Gharagozloo and Aitken 2011).

4) *Sperm Aneuploidy:* most human aneuploidy originates in the germ cell line arising from meiotic and mitotic errors in both male and female germinal cells (Bourrouillou et al. 1985; Bond 1987; Van Assche et al. 1996). An increase in the production of aneuploid sperm cells may be as a result of an abnormal somatic cell karyotype, which can be established through a blood test. However, men with a normal somatic cell karyotype, alongside decreased semen parameters, can also produce cytogenetically abnormal spermatozoa (Shi and Martin 2001). Alteration of the intratesticular microenvironment can impair spermatogenesis and also disturb the mechanisms that regulate chromosomal segregation during mitosis and meiosis (Mroz et al. 1999).

Aneuploidy can be either the gain or loss of an entire chromosome or it can be structural involving a gain (trisomy) or loss (monosomy) of a segment of a chromosome. Numerical chromosomal aneuploidy usually consists of a trisomic state in chromosomes 13, 18, 21, X and Y. To date sperm aneuploidy levels have been assessed using fluorescence *in-situ* hybridization (Shi and Martin 2000, 2001; Tempest and Griffin 2004).

It is evident that all men have aneuploid sperm with levels of 3–5% reported amongst the fertile population. Investigation of infertile men, however, has demonstrated a significant increase in aneuploidy levels (Shi and Martin 2000, 2001; Tempest and Griffin 2004), with the highest levels in oligoasthenoteratozoospermia and in testicular biopsies from nonobstructive azoospermia. These higher levels of sperm aneuploidy are associated with recurrent ICSI failure (Petit et al. 2005; Nicopoullos et al. 2008), increased chromosomal abnormalities in embryos (Gianaroli et al. 2005), and lower pregnancy and live birth rates (Nagvenkar et al. 2005). Therefore, it is recommended that patients with very poor semen parameters should be investigated for aneuploidy levels prior to embarking on an IVF programme. However, it is not yet established whether increased levels of sperm aneuploidy actually translate to an increased risk of producing aneuploid conceptions. The approximate threefold increase in sperm aneuploidy observed in infertile populations is apparently reflected in a threefold increase in *de novo* chromosomal abnormalities in children born after ICSI (Aboulghar et al. 2001; Bonduelle et al. 2002; Van Steirteghem et al. 2002; Devroey and Van Steirteghem 2004). Given that we are unable to test individual sperm before it is used, it is not yet clear how aneuploidy assessments can or should be used to counsel patients (Carrell 2008; Tempest and Martin 2009; Hann, Lau and Tempest 2011; Tempest 2011).

5) *Karyotyping:* to confirm a normal genetic make up. Chromosome abnormalities are nearly 10 times more common in infertile males (5.3%) than in the general population (0.6%) (Egozcue 1989). Karyotyping must be performed in men with azoospermia and severe oligozoospermia before undergoing IVF with ICSI. The most frequent

abnormalities are sex chromosome aneuploidies such as the 47,XXY and the 47,XYY karyotypes, autosomal Robertsonian translocations, and Y chromosome microdeletions.

Conclusion

Management of infertility is a challenging task with clearly identifiable outcomes of success, i.e. achievement of pregnancy. Couples should be informed that the chances of live birth are higher in females aged between 23 and 39 years, with a BMI between 19 and 25, and in women who have previously been pregnant.

Initial assessment of a couple seeking pregnancy can be effortlessly and effectively carried out in primary care setting. In 70–85% of cases, the cause of infertility can be identified by detailed history, thorough clinical examination and basic investigations to assess ovulation, tubal function, and semen quality. Investigations play an important role in the initial assessment of the infertile couple. Appropriate tests should be performed at the appropriate time, and the results must be interpreted judiciously and explained to the couple.

Infertility is not a life-threatening situation but can have devastating psychosocial implications (Chen et al. 2004). Unrealistic expectations of pregnancy should not be fostered, and honest and evidence-based information should be given regarding treatment options and success rates (Cahill and Wardle 2002).

References

Aboulghar, H., Aboulghar, M., Mansour, R. et al. (2001). A prospective controlled study of karyotyping for 430 consecutive babies conceived through intracytoplasmic sperm injection. Fertil Steril 76: 249–253.

Aitken, R.J. and Clarkson, J.S. (1988). Significance of reactive oxygen species and antioxidants in defining the efficacy of sperm preparation techniques. J Androl 9: 367–376.

Aitken, R.J., De Iuliis, G.N., Finnie, J.M. et al. (2010). Analysis of the relationships between oxidative stress, DNA damage and sperm vitality in a patient population: development of diagnostic criteria. Hum Reprod 25: 2415–1426.

Bond, D.J. (1987). Mechanisms of aneuploid induction. Mutat Res 181: 257–266.

Bonduelle, M., Van Assche, E., Joris, H. et al. (2002). Prenatal testing in ICSI pregnancies: incidence of chromosomal anomalies in 1586 karyotypes and relation to sperm parameters. Hum Reprod 17: 2600–2614.

Bourrouillou, G., Dastugue, N. and Colombies P. (1985). Chromosome studies in 952 infertile males with a sperm count below 10 million/ml. Hum Genet 71: 366–367.

Bungum, M., Humaidan, P., Axmon, A. et al. (2007). Sperm DNA integrity assessment in prediction of assisted reproduction technology outcome. Hum Reprod 22: 174–179.

Cahill, D.J. and Wardle, P.G. (2002). Management of infertility: clinical review. BMJ 325: 28–32.

Carrell, D.T. (2008). The clinical implementation of sperm chromosome aneuploidy testing: pitfalls and promises. J Androl 29: 124–133.

Case, A.M. (2003). Infertility evaluation and management: strategies for family physicians. Can Family Phys 49: 1465–1472.

Chen, T.H., Chang, S.P., Tsai, C.F. et al. (2004). Prevalence of depressive and anxiety disorders in an assisted reproductive technique clinic. Hum Reprod 19: 2313–2318.

Coulam, C.B., Adamson, S.C. and Annegers, J.F. (1986). Incidence of premature ovarian failure. Obstet Gynecol 67: 604–606.

Devroey, P. and Van Steirteghem, A. (2004). A review of ten years experience of ICSI. Hum Reprod Update 10: 19–28.

Dewailly, D., Andersen, C.Y., Balen, A. et al. (2014). The physiology and clinical utility of anti-Müllerian hormone in women. Hum Reprod Update 20: 370–385.

Dunson, D.B., Baird, D.D. and Colombo, B. (2004). Increased infertility with age in men and women. Obstet Gynecol 103: 51–56.

Egozcue, J. (1989). Chromosomal aspects of male infertility. In *Perspectives in Andrology* (ed. M. Serio), 341–346. New York: Serono Symposia Publications.

Elecsys® AMH Fact Sheet (2014). Electrochemi-luminescence immunoassay (ECLIA). for the in vitro quantitative determination of anti-Mullerian Hormone in human serum and plasma.

Elsheikh, M. and Murphy, C. (2008). *Polycystic Ovary Syndrome (PCOS) - The Facts.* Oxford: Oxford University Press.

ESHRE Capri Workshop Group (2004). Diagnosis and management of the infertile couple: missing information. Hum Reprod Update 10: 295–307.

Forti, G. and Krausz, C. (1998). Evaluation and treatment of the infertile couple. J Clin Endocrinol Metabol 83: 4177–4188.

Gelbaya, T.A., Potdar, N., Jeve, Y.B., et al. (2014). Definition and epidemiology of unexplained infertility. Obstet Gynecol Surv 69: 109–115.

Gharagozloo, P. and Aitken, R.J. (2011). The role of sperm oxidative stress in male infertility and the significance of oral antioxidant therapy. Hum Reprod 26: 1628–1640.

Gianaroli, L., Magli, M.C. and Ferraretti, A.P. (2005). Sperm and blastomere aneuploidy detection in reproductive genetics and medicine. J Histochem Cytochem 53: 261–267.

Giwercman, A., Lindstedt, L., Larsson, M. et al. (2010). Sperm chromatin structure assay as an independent predictor of fertility in vivo: a case-control study. Int J Androl 33: 221–227.

Gnoth, C., Godehardt, E., Frank-Herrmann, P. et al. (2005). Definition and prevalence of subfertility and infertility. Hum Reprod 20: 1144–1147.

Hann, M.C., Lau, P.E. and Tempest, H.G. (2011). Meiotic recombination and male infertility: from basic science to clinical reality? Asian J Androl 13: 212–218.

Hansen, K.R., Hodnett, G.M., Knowlton, N. et al. (2011). Correlation of ovarian reserve tests with histologically determined primordial follicle number. Fertil Steril 95:170–175.

Heffner, L.J. (2004). Advanced maternal age – how old is too old? N Engl J Med 351: 1927–1929.

Human Fertilisation and Embryology Authority (2010). *Fertility Facts and Figures 2008.* London: Human Fertilisation and Embryology Authority.

Human Fertilisation and Embryology Authority (2011). Fertility Treatment in 2010 Trends and Figures. London: Human Fertilisation and Embryology Authority.

Johnson, M.H. (2007). *Essential Reproduction*, 6th edn. Oxford: Blackwell Publishing.

Jose-Miller, A.B., Boyden, J.W. and Frey, K.A. (2007). Infertility. Am Fam Phys 75: 849–856.

Kamel, R.M. (2010). Management of the infertile couple: an evidence-based protocol. Reprod Biol Endocrinol 8: 21.

Lewis, S.E. and Aitken, R.J. (2005). DNA damage to spermatozoa has impacts on fertilization and pregnancy. Cell Tissue Res 322: 33–41.

Lewis, S.E., Aitken, R.J., Conner, S.J. et al. (2013). The impact of sperm DNA damage in assisted conception and beyond: recent advances in diagnosis and treatment. Reprod Biomed Online 27: 325–337.

Macaluso, M., Wright-Schnapp, T.J., Chandra, A. et al. (2010). A public health focus on infertility prevention, detection, and management. Fert Steril 93: 16e1–16e10.

Mroz, K., Hassold, T.J. and Hunt, P.A. (1999). Meiotic aneuploidy in the XXY mouse: evidence that a compromised testicular environment increases the incidence of meiotic errors. Hum Reprod 14: 1151–1156.

McDowell, S., Kroon, B., Ford, E. et al. (2014). Advanced sperm selection techniques for assisted reproduction. Cochrane Database Syst Rev 10:CD010461.

Nardo, L.G., Gelbaya, T.A., Wilkinson, H. et al. (2009). Circulating basal anti-Müllerian hormone levels as predictor of ovarian response in women undergoing ovarian stimulation for in vitro fertilization. Fertil Steril 92: 1586–1593.

Nagvenkar, P., Zaveri, K. and Hinduja, I. (2005). Comparison of the sperm aneuploidy rate in severe oligozoospermic and oligozoospermic men and its relation to intracytoplasmic sperm injection outcome. Fertil Steril 84: 925–931.

National Institute for Health and Care Excellence (NICE) (2013). Fertility. Assessment and treatment for people with fertility problems. Clinical Guideline 156. London: NICE.

Nicopoullos, J.D., Gilling-Smith, C., Almeida, P.A. et al. (2008). The role of sperm aneuploidy as a predictor of the success of intracytoplasmic sperm injection? Hum Reprod 23: 240–250.

Petit, F.M., Frydman, N., Benkhalifa, M. et al. (2005). Could sperm aneuploidy rate determination be used as a predictive test before intracytoplasmic sperm injection? J Androl 26: 235–241.

Practice Committee of the American Society for Reproductive Medicine (2008). Vaccination guidelines for female infertility patients. Fertil Steril 90: S169–S171.

Robinson, L., Gallos, I.D., Conner, S.J. et al. (2012). The effect of sperm DNA fragmentation on miscarriage rates: a systematic review and meta-analysis. Hum Reprod 27: 2908–2917.

Rotterdam ESHRE/ASRM-Sponsored PCOS Consensus Workshop Group (2004). Revised 2003 consensus on diagnostic criteria and long-term health risks related to polycystic ovary syndrome (PCOS). Hum Reprod 19: 41–47.

Sakkas, D. (2013). Novel technologies for selecting the best sperm for in vitro fertilization and intracytoplasmic sperm injection. Fertil Steril 99: 1023–1029.

Sanders, S. and Debuse, M. (2003). *Endocrine and Reproductive Systems*, 2nd edn. Edinburgh: Mosby.

Sharma, R.K., Sabanegh, E. Mahfouz, R. et al. (2010). TUNEL as a test for sperm DNA damage in the evaluation of male infertility. Urology 76: 1380–1386.

Shelling, A.N. (2010). Premature ovarian failure. Reproduction 140: 633–641.

Shi, Q. and Martin, R.H. (2000). Aneuploidy in human sperm: a review of the frequency and distribution of aneuploidy, effects of donor age and lifestyle factors. Cytogenet Cell Genet 90: 219–226.

Shi, Q. and Martin, R.H. (2001). Aneuploidy in human spermatozoa: FISH analysis in men with constitutional chromosomal abnormalities, and in infertile men. Reproduction 121: 655–666.

Simon, L., Brunborg, G., Stevenson, M. et al. (2010). Clinical significance of sperm DNA damage in assisted reproduction outcome. Hum Reprod 25: 1594–1608.

Simon, L., Lutton, D., McManus, J. et al. (2011). Sperm DNA damage measured by the alkaline Comet assay as an independent predictor of male infertility and in vitro fertilization success. Fertil Steril 95: 652–657.

Simon, L., Proutski, I., Stevenson, M. et al. (2013). Sperm DNA damage has a negative association with live-birth rates after IVF. Reprod Biomed Online 26: 68–78.

Taylor, A. (2003a). ABC of subfertility: extent of the problem. BMJ 327: 434–436.

Taylor, A. (2003b). ABC of subfertility: making a diagnosis. BMJ 327: 494–497.

te Velde, E.R., Eijkemans, R. and Habbema, H.D. (2000). Variation in couple fecundity and time to pregnancy, an essential concept in human reproduction. Lancet 355: 1928–1929.

Tempest, H.G. (2011). Meiotic recombination errors, the origin of sperm aneuploidy and clinical recommendations. Syst Biol Reprod Med 57: 93–101.

Tempest, H.G. and Griffin, D.K. (2004). The relationship between male infertility and increased levels of sperm disomy. Cytogenet Genome Res 107: 83–94.

Tempest, H.G. and Martin, R.H. (2009). Cytogenetic risks in chromosomally normal infertile men. Curr Opin Obstet Gynecol 21: 223–227.

Van Assche, E., Bonduelle, M., Tournaye, H. et al. (1996). Cytogenetics of infertile men. Hum Reprod 11(Suppl 4):1–24.

van Disseldorp, J., Lambalk, C.B., Kwee, J. et al. (2010). Comparison of inter- and intra-cycle variability of anti-Mullerian hormone and antral follicle counts. Hum Reprod 25: 221–227.

Van Steirteghem, A., Bonduelle, M., Devroey, P. et al. (2002). Follow-up of children born after ICSI. Hum Reprod Update 8: 111–116.

Whitman-Elia, G.F. and Baxley, E.G. (2001). A primary care approach to the infertile couple: clinical review. J Am Board Fam Pract 14: 33–45.

World Health Organization (1973). Advances in methods of fertility regulation: report of a WHO scientific group. World Health Organization Technical Report Series 527: 1–42.

World Health Organization (2010). *WHO Laboratory Manual for the Examination and Processing Of Human Semen*, 5th edn. Geneva: WHO.

Zini, A. (2011). Are sperm chromatin and DNA defects relevant in the clinic? Syst Biol Reprod Med 57: 78–85.

Zini, A. and Dohle, G. (2011). Are varicoceles associated with increased deoxyribonucleic acid fragmentation? Fertil Steril 96: 1283–1287.

19

Ovarian Stimulation Protocols

Nikolaos Tsampras and Cheryl T. Fitzgerald

Introduction

The introduction of controlled ovarian stimulation (COS) for multiple follicular development significantly increased pregnancy rates (Trounson et al. 1981). Such stimulation protocols have now been developed and refined for more than 25 years in an attempt to prevent premature luteinizing hormone (LH) surge, allow oocyte maturation, and obtain an optimal number of oocytes from each treatment cycle, in order to maximize pregnancy rates per fresh embryo transfer, whilst reducing the risk of over response (Pacchiarotti et al. 2016). The good response to COS is important, as the number of oocytes obtained following stimulation correlates positively with live birth rate (Sunkara et al. 2011).

Prevention of Premature LH Surge

The most commonly used COS protocols are summarized in Figure 19.1.

The classical COS protocols use gonadotropin-releasing hormone (GnRH) agonists or antagonists to prevent premature LH surge through pituitary suppression. Without suppression, high oestrogen levels during *in vitro* fertilization (IVF) cycles can result in an LH surge, with consequent lower number of oocytes retrieved and a reduced pregnancy rate (Toner 2002). Spontaneous ovulation has been reported in 16% of unsuppressed cycles (Kadoch et al. 2008).

GnRH analogues are decapeptides similar to human GnRH in order to interact with GnRH receptors. These analogues have certain amino acid substitutions in the gonadotropin amino acid sequence that increases the half-lives and the receptor-binding affinities of analogues compared with endogenous hormones (Daya 2000; Ortmann et al. 2002). Prolonged activation of GnRH receptors by GnRH agonists leads to desensitization and consequently to suppressed gonadotropin secretion, while GnRH antagonists act as mediators of chemical hypophysectomy (van Loenen et al. 2002; Ortmann et al. 2002). Several agonistic analogues (triptorelin, leuprorelin, deslorelin, goserelin, and nafarelin) and a few antagonistic analogues (cetrorelix and ganirelix) have been introduced into clinical practice (van Loenen et al. 2002).

GnRH Agonist Protocols

The GnRH long agonist protocol starts with administration of the GnRH agonist in the midluteal phase of the cycle immediately preceding stimulation. This diminishes the GnRH agonist's flare effect and suppresses endogenous follicle-stimulating hormone (FSH) production and dominant follicle selection, aiming to promote synchronous follicular growth. After 10–14 days of agonist administration, an ultrasound scan and serum oestradiol level is used to confirm suppression, and gonadotropin stimulation begins (Pacchiarotti et al. 2016). The ovarian response is monitored with frequent transvaginal ultrasound scans and serum oestrogen levels (O'Shea et al. 1988). The adjustment of

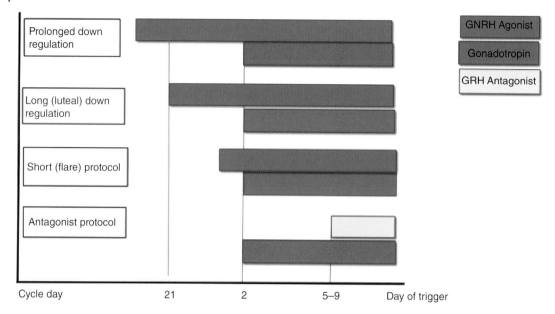

Figure 19.1 Controlled ovarian stimulation (COS) protocols.

gonadotropin dose is based on follicular development. Administration of the GnRH agonist and gonadotropin continues until follicles reach 16–18 mm in size (Pacchiarotti et al. 2016). The oocytes final maturation is triggered by administration of 5000–1000 IU of human chorionic gonadotropin (hCG) (Chen et al. 2014). At 34–36 h after triggering, the oocytes are retrieved transvaginally under ultrasound guidance.

A variation of the long GnRH agonist protocol is the administration of GnRH agonists for a few months prior to COS. It has been suggested that this pretreatment increases the pregnancy rate when endometriosis is present (Sallam et al. 2006).

Short GnRH agonist flare protocols have been advocated for poor responders, attempting to increase oocyte yield. These protocols involve administration of the GnRH agonist in the early follicular phase, aiming to take advantage of the agonist flare effect and increase follicular recruitment (Bstandig et al. 2000). Gonadotropin stimulation begins 1–2 days later while continuing the agonist administration (Pacchiarotti et al. 2016).

GnRH Antagonist Protocols

GnRH antagonists were developed by modifying the GnRH decapeptide at six positions. They compete with GnRH for binding of pituitary receptors. As they have no agonistic activity, they lead to almost immediate endogenous gonadotropin and hence ovarian suppression (Ortmann et al. 2002). Several GnRH antagonist protocols have been developed for assisted reproduction technology (ART). Usually the administration of the antagonist starts on day 3–7 of stimulation and is continuous until the hCG triggering (de Jong et al. 2001; Devroey et al. 2009). Latterly, flexible antagonist protocols have been developed, where the initiation of the antagonist depends on follicular growth (Tarlatzis et al. 2006). The antagonist administration continues, along with gonadotropin stimulation, until follicles reach 16–18 mm. In an antagonist protocol, final oocyte maturation can be achieved either with hCG or alternatively with an agonist trigger. As the duration of the LH surge with the GnRH agonist trigger is short (approximately 34 h), compared with the one provoked by hCG (>6 days), it has been shown to be beneficial for the prevention of ovarian hyperstimulation syndrome (OHSS) (Casper 2015).

Comparison of Stimulation Protocols

The effectiveness of different GnRH agonist protocols as adjuncts to COS was extensively assessed in a recent Cochrane review. Thirty-eight randomized controlled trials (RCT) were included and nine different comparisons between protocols were performed. Several protocols were evaluated regarding administration of the agonist during the follicular or luteal phase, for 2 versus 3 weeks before stimulation, the dose of agonist, and time of discontinuation. The authors concluded that there was no evidence that the GnRH agonist long protocol was associated with an increase in live birth and ongoing clinical pregnancy rates in comparison with the GnRH agonist short protocol, although there was moderate evidence of an increase in clinical pregnancy rates. None of the other comparisons showed any difference in live birth or pregnancy rates between the protocols compared. There was insufficient evidence to make any conclusions regarding adverse effects (Siristatidis et al. 2015).

There is very limited evidence comparing the fixed and the flexible GnRH antagonist protocols. So far, antagonist administration from day 3 onward does not appear to reduce the incidence of an LH rise compared with fixed antagonist administration on day 6 of stimulation (Kolibianakis et al. 2011) and the treatment outcome is not compromised (Tannus et al. 2013).

A comprehensive review by the Cochrane Collaboration compared the GnRH agonist and antagonist protocols in 2011. The study included 47 RCTs and 7511 patients undergoing ART. The authors concluded that there was no evidence of a difference in live birth rates. However, the use of antagonist compared with long GnRH agonist protocols was associated with a large reduction in OHSS (Al-Inany et al. 2011). In addition, antagonist protocols allow the use of a GnRH agonist trigger, for oocyte final maturation, reducing further the risk of OHSS in potentially high responders (Youssef et al. 2014). Therefore, GnRH antagonist protocol is preferable for patients with polycystic ovarian syndrome (PCOS) (Pundir et al. 2012; Nardo et al. 2013; Mathur and Tan, 2014; Tannus et al. 2015).

The GnRH antagonist protocol is recommended for patients diagnosed with a malignancy, undergoing COS before chemotherapy/radiotherapy for oocyte storage for future use. In such an emergency setting, delay of COS may result in a significant delay in cancer treatment that may lead to patients forgoing fertility preservation. Use of an antagonist allows random-start ovarian stimulation, decreasing total time for the COS cycle, without compromising oocyte yield and maturity (Cakmak and Rosen 2015).

Literature suggests that fertilization, implantation, and pregnancy rates with ART are lower in patients with endometriosis compared with patients with tubal factor infertility, possibly as result of poorer oocyte quality (Barnhart et al. 2002). A meta-analysis of three small randomized studies (Sallam et al. 2006) in which prolonged, 3–6 months pretreatment with a GnRH agonist was compared with controls, showed a significant improvement of clinical pregnancy rates. Therefore, the GnRH agonist protocol, with prolonged ovarian suppression prior to COS might be preferable for patients with endometriosis (Nardo et al. 2013)

Follicular Growth in Controlled Ovarian Stimulation: Gonadotropins

The goal of gonadotropin stimulation in ART is the synchronous growth of multiple dominant follicles. FSH is the key hormone in this regard. Therefore, gonadotropin administration is an integral part of stimulation protocols (Practice Committee of the American Society for Reproductive Medicine 2008). Gonadotropin preparations can be classified, based on the source, into urine-derived and those produced using recombinant techniques.

Human menopausal gonadotropins (hMG) are derived from the pooled urine of menopausal women and contain both LH and FSH activity. The LH activity may derive from hCG, which can be preferentially concentrated during the purification process or sometimes added to the preparation (Requena et al. 2014). Initial preparations of hMG were only 5% pure. Further improvement of urine-derived gonadotropins led to the production of purified urinary FSH (urofollitropin, FSH-P), a product with little LH activity (<1 unit per vial as opposed to 75 IU per vial of hMG), but significant nongonadotropin protein content. Continuous attempts to purify the FSH activity further using monoclonal antibodies directed against FSH, resulted in highly purified urinary FSH (FSH-HP). This product has less than 0.1 IU LH activity and 75 IU FSH activity per vial, and less than 5% unidentified urinary protein, making it suitable for subcutaneous use. At the same time, the specific activity of FSH in highly purified preparations was significantly higher, and batch-to batch variability lower, than the previous generation of products (Practice Committee of the American Society for Reproductive Medicine 2008).

Advances in recombinant technology techniques allowed the production of gonadotropin in cell lines that have been transfected with plasmids containing the cloned gene for producing gonadotropin subunits. A major advantage of recombinant products is their high batch-to-batch consistency (Levi Setti 2006). In addition, the activity of the gonadotropin can be assessed by protein content, rather than by biological assays as in the case of urine-derived products (Bassett and Driebergen 2005). This allows superior quality control in recombinant preparations. FSH, LH, and hCG preparations have been produced with recombinant technology. There are two variants of recombinant FSH (r-FSH) available today: (1) follitropin-alpha (α) and (2) follitropin-beta (β). Both variants have the same α- and β-chains as native FSH, but differ in their sialic acid residues as a result of different purification processes. It is not considered that these differences have any clinical implications (Practice Committee of the American Society for Reproductive Medicine 2008).

Modification of the FSH β-subunit using recombinant techniques has led to the production of a new molecule, consisting of the α-subunit of human FSH and a hybrid subunit composed of the C-terminal peptide of the β-subunit of hCG coupled with the FSH β-subunit. This molecule is a long-acting FSH, named corifollitropin alfa (Elonva) or FSH-CTP (carboxy terminal peptide) (Corifollitropin Alfa Dose-finding Study Group 2008; Fauser et al. 2009).

Choice of Gonadotropins

With such an array of available preparations, the clinician should consider efficacy, safety, consistency, ease of administration, and cost, in order to choose the most suitable for each patient.

Efficacy

Van Wely et al. published the landmark Cochrane review, including 42 trials with a total of 9606 cycles, in 2012. Comparison of r-FSH to all other gonadotropins combined did not result in any evidence of a statistically significant difference in live birth rate (28 trials, 7339 couples). When different urinary gonadotropins were considered separately, there were significantly fewer live births after r-FSH than hMG (11 trials, $n = 3197$), although differences were small and considered unlikely to be clinically significant. There was no evidence of a difference in live births when r-FSH was compared with FSH-P (five trials, n = 1430) or when r-FSH was compared with FSH-HP (13 trials, n = 2712 (van Wely et al. 2012). The efficacy of corifollitropin-α was confirmed by a Cochrane review including 2335 patients (Pouwer et al. 2015).

Safety

Ovarian stimulation carries the risk of excessive response and OHSS. The risk of OHSS relates primarily to patient factors, such as polycystic ovaries. The choice of gonadotropin does not appear to influence the risk (Mathur and Tan 2014). In the past, use of human pituitary-derived gonadotropin was associated with the occurrence of Creutzfeldt–Jakob disease (Cochius et al. 1990). It has been reported that prion proteins can be found in the urine of human sufferers of prion disease. However, there is no evidence that any cases of sporadic human prion disease have been associated with the clinical use of urine-derived gonadotropins.

Consistency

It is generally agreed that recombinant preparations have excellent batch-to-batch consistency, although they have not been demonstrated to perform better than urine-derived products in a clinical setting (van Wely et al. 2012).

Ease of Administration

Most preparations are now injectable subcutaneously, using a pen-shaped device (Figure 19.2), or a syringe and needle (Figure 19.3). Very little evidence exists evaluating the ease of administration and patient's experience, using different gonadotropin preparations. Poor quality studies suggest that patients using a prefilled pen system find it less stressful, easier to use, and more convenient than a conventional syringe (Somkuti et al. 2006; Welcker et al. 2010; Schertz et al. 2011).

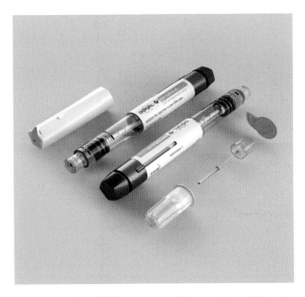

Figure 19.2 Gonal-F. Reproduced with permission of Merck Serono.

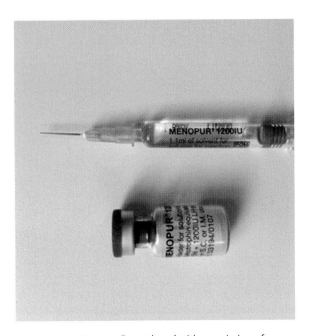

Figure 19.3 Menopur. Reproduced with permission of Ferring.

Cost

Cost should be considered not just on a per unit basis, but over the entire treatment cycle. Different preparations may also have different potential for wastage, depending on the dose contained in each vial or pen, and the dosage regime followed by the clinic. Although per unit based evaluation reveals the higher cost of r-FSH, per treatment cost is not clear. Small studies suggest the higher unit cost of r-FSH may be offset by a lower required dosage compared with hMG (Trew et al. 2010). As the total treatment cost is implicated by multiple factors (length of stimulation, dosage, live birth rate), comparison between different gonadotropins needs further research.

Role of LH Supplementation

Luteinizing hormone activity in gonadotropin preparations can be obtained by LH itself or added hCG. When urinary gonadotropins are used, hCG is added to urinary hMG to replace LH lost during the purification process and to standardize the therapy. The hCG LH-like activity varies compared with LH in its effectiveness and duration of action. A potential advantage of hCG over recombinant LH (r-LH) is the longer half-life of hCG and its greater stimulation of the LH receptor. However, some concerns have been expressed that the pharmacological dose of hCG in hMG may lead to disproportionate LH activity causing premature luteinization, reduced fertilization rates, and down regulation of the LH/hCG receptor expression in the follicular compartment. This concern has not been clinically observed (Trew et al. 2010). The most advanced hMG available contains a combination of FSH, LH and hCG with up to 30% impurities, including growth factors and binding proteins. In contrast, r-LH is relatively free from contaminants and 99% pure. It has been suggested that due to the hCG content, hMG produces fewer, but better quality, oocytes than those stimulated with r-FSH (Hu et al. 2014). Smitz et al. (2007) demonstrated a relation between D6 hCG levels and the frequency of top quality embryos, ongoing pregnancy, and live birth rates. However, the clinical significance of this is unclear. Morphological embryo quality assessment is subjective and not directly related to clinical outcome. Acevedo et al. (2004) reported higher clinical pregnancy rates in donor-recipient cycles administering r-LH, although this difference was not statistically significant. Subsequent studies supported the hypothesis of improved clinical outcome with r-LH supplementation (Franco et al. 2009). A review of the literature by

Hill et al. (2012a,b) highlighted the limited evidence to support the general use of r-LH, but suggested potential benefit for poor responders and older patients. A recent meta-analysis by Lehert et al. (2014) included 40 RCTs (6443 patients). The authors identified a relative increase of 9% in the clinical pregnancy rate for the general population, when additional r-LH was used. The difference was more profound in women with poor ovarian response, reaching 30%. However, there was significant variation between included trials in the r-FSH and r-LH doses used and even in the definition of poor ovarian response. In an extensive literature review, Ezcurra and Humaidan (2014) concluded that current evidence supports r-LH administration to patients with hypogonadotropic hypogonadism, patients who have profound LH suppression in a long GnRH agonist protocol, patients with a suboptimal response to FSH alone, and some patients older than 35 years.

Hypogonadotropic hypogonadism is defined as a medical condition with low or undetectable gonadotropin secretion, associated with a complete arrest of follicular growth and very low oestradiol. Although the role of LH in stimulation of follicles, optimal dosage of LH in stimulation, and its importance in unselected patients remains controversial, the administration of exogenous LH with FSH is obligatory for COS in patients with hypogonadotropic hypogonadism (Krause et al. 2009).

Further research is needed to confirm whether there is an advantage of r-LH supplementation and to develop treatment regimes.

Gonadotropin Regime

The selection of the appropriate and individualized gonadotropin dose is of paramount importance for effective COS and subsequent IVF outcomes. The starting dose of FSH for controlled ovarian hyperstimulation COS should take into account factors that may increase the risk of evoking an excessive or a poor ovarian response. The presence or absence of polycystic ovaries, previous history of OHSS or poor response to COS, young or older age, body mass index, antral follicle count, anti-Müllerian hormone (AMH) levels, and day-2 FSH have been introduced as predictive factors of the response to COS (La Marca and Sunkara 2014). AMH is the best single current available measure of ovarian reserve

for different clinical conditions (Broer et al. 2014) and AMH-guided COS protocols significantly improve positive clinical outcomes (Yates et al. 2011). At present, there are no randomized trials examining a lower starting dose of FSH for patients with risk factors for excessive ovarian response undergoing IVF (van Tilborg et al. 2012). Furthermore, evidence suggests no benefit for any patient exceeding a total dose of 450 IU daily (Devroey et al. 2009). Despite the lack of evidence, an initial dose of 150–225 IU is commonly used as a default with the dose readjusted for potentially high or poor responders (Devroey et al. 2009).

Oocyte Maturation

Since spontaneous LH surges are suppressed in ART cycles, hCG has been used for oocyte maturation. Homology between hCG and LH (identical α subunits) allows for crossreactivity with the LH receptors and induction of final oocyte maturation (Pacchiarotti et al. 2016). When there is concern for OHSS, the GnRH agonist can be substituted for hCG to trigger oocyte maturation, in antagonist protocols. However, this practice has been associated with reduced pregnancy rates in nondonor cycles (Youssef et al. 2015).

hCG Preparations

Recombinant technology has allowed the production of recombinant hCG. Youssef et al. compared the urine-derived and recombinant hCG preparations in a Cochrane review, including 14 RCTs and 2306 patients. The authors concluded that there is no difference in reproductive outcomes between the different forms of hCG used. Continuation of use of urine-derived hCG for final oocyte maturation was recommended, because of the lower cost and increased availability (Youssef et al. 2011).

Luteal Phase Support

The luteal phase during a natural cycle is characterized by progesterone secretion by the corpus luteum, and appropriate endometrial secretory transformation, allowing embryonic implantation and supporting the pregnancy for the first 7–8 weeks

(Palomba et al. 2015). ART treatment might induce iatrogenic luteal phase deficiency via disruption of granulosa cells from follicular aspiration and suppression of endogenous LH secretion through supraphysiological oestrogen levels or GnRH agonist/antagonist administration (Bukulmez and Arici 2004; Jones 2008).

It has been well demonstrated that supplementation of the luteal phase with either exogenous progesterone or hCG is crucial to optimize IVF cycle outcomes (Yanushpolsky 2015). A recent comprehensive Cochrane review evaluated the different forms of luteal support in ART. The authors concluded that both progesterone and hCG during the luteal phase are associated with higher rates of live birth and ongoing pregnancy than placebo. As hCG is associated with higher risk of OHSS, progesterone only has been recommended. The route of administration of progesterone was not found to affect treatment outcomes (van der Linden et al. 2015).

Agonist-triggered cycles frequently result in cryopreservation of the entire embryo cohort (Engmann et al. 2016). However, if a fresh embryo transfer is used after an agonist trigger, LH activity will be further compromised due to the shorter duration of the endogenous induced LH surge and a potential weaker activation of the LH/hCG receptor (Leth-Moller et al. 2014). The result of this is a significant reduction in LH activity throughout the early/mid luteal phase leading to premature luteolysis and implantation failure. After the initial disappointing clinical results, several subsequent studies implemented a modified luteal support with LH activity (Shapiro and Andersen 2015). Using modified luteal phase support, the reproductive outcome increased remarkably and is now comparable to that seen after hCG triggering (Humaidan et al. 2015; Liang et al. 2015; Orvieto, 2015; Engmann et al. 2016). The most optimal luteal phase support after agonist triggering still has to be investigated (Leth-Moller et al. 2014).

Conclusion

Current controlled ovarian stimulation for ART pursues three main objectives: pituitary suppression, multiple follicular growth, and oocyte maturation. The remarkable progress in developing ovarian stimulation protocols over the last three decades has resulted in a multitude of stimulation protocols being available to clinicians. There are many factors to consider in deciding upon the optimal protocol for an individual patient. Further research is essential to continue to enhance the chance of pregnancy whilst limiting risk both to the woman undergoing treatment and future offspring.

References

Acevedo, B., Sanchez, M., Gomez, J.L. et al. (2004). Luteinizing hormone supplementation increases pregnancy rates in gonadotropin-releasing hormone antagonist donor cycles. Fertil Steril 82: 343–347.

Al-Inany, H.G., Youssef, M.A., Aboulghar, M. et al. (2011). Gonadotrophin-releasing hormone antagonists for assisted reproductive technology. Cochrane Database Syst Rev CD001750.

Barnhart, K., Dunsmoor-Su, R. and Coutifaris, C. (2002). Effect of endometriosis on in vitro fertilization. Fertil Steril 77: 1148–1155.

Bassett, R.M. and Driebergen, R. (2005). Continued improvements in the quality and consistency of follitropin alfa, recombinant human FSH. Reprod Biomed Online 10: 169–177.

Broer, S.L., Broekmans, F.J., Laven, J.S. et al. (2014). Anti-Mullerian hormone: ovarian reserve testing and its potential clinical implications. Hum Reprod Update 20: 688–701.

Bstandig, B., Cedrin-Durnerin, I. and Hugues, J.N. (2000). Effectiveness of low dose of gonadotropin releasing hormone agonist on hormonal flare-up. J Assist Reprod Genet 17: 113–117.

Bukulmez, O. and Arici, A. (2004). Luteal phase defect: myth or reality. Obstet Gynecol Clin North Am 31: 727–744.

Cakmak, H. and Rosen, M.P. (2015). Random-start ovarian stimulation in patients with cancer. Curr Opin Obstet Gynecol 27: 215–221.

Casper, R.F. (2015). Basic understanding of gonadotropin-releasing hormone-agonist triggering. Fertil Steril 103: 867–869.

Chen, Y., Zhang, Y., Hu, M. et al. (2014). Timing of human chorionic gonadotropin (hCG) hormone administration in IVF/ICSI protocols using GnRH agonist or antagonists: a systematic review and meta-analysis. Gynecol Endocrinol 30: 431–437.

Cochius, J.I., Burns, R.J., Blumbergs, P.C. et al. (1990). Creutzfeldt-Jakob disease in a recipient of human pituitary-derived gonadotrophin. Aust NZ J Med 20: 592–593.

Corifollitropin Alfa Dose-finding Study Group (2008). A randomized dose-response trial of a single injection of corifollitropin alfa to sustain multifollicular growth during controlled ovarian stimulation. Hum Reprod 23: 2484–2492.

Daya, S. (2000). Gonadotropin releasing hormone agonist protocols for pituitary desensitization in in vitro fertilization and gamete intrafallopian transfer cycles. Cochrane Database Syst Rev CD001299.

De Jong, D., Macklon, N.S., Eijkemans, M.J. et al. (2001). Dynamics of the development of multiple follicles during ovarian stimulation for in vitro fertilization using recombinant follicle-stimulating hormone (Puregon) and various doses of the gonadotropin-releasing hormone antagonist ganirelix (Orgalutran/Antagon). Fertil Steril 75: 688–693.

Devroey, P., Aboulghar, M., Garcia-Velasco, J. et al. (2009). Improving the patient's experience of IVF/ICSI: a proposal for an ovarian stimulation protocol with GnRH antagonist co-treatment. Hum Reprod 24: 764–774.

Engmann, L., Benadiva, C. and Humaidan, P. (2016). GnRH agonist trigger for the induction of oocyte maturation in GnRH antagonist IVF cycles: a SWOT analysis. Reprod Biomed Online 32: 274–285.

Ezcurra, D. and Humaidan, P. (2014). A review of luteinising hormone and human chorionic gonadotropin when used in assisted reproductive technology. Reprod Biol Endocrinol 12: 95.

Fauser, B.C., Mannaerts, B.M., Devroey, P. et al. (2009). Advances in recombinant DNA technology: corifollitropin alfa, a hybrid molecule with sustained follicle-stimulating activity and reduced injection frequency. Hum Reprod Update 15: 309–321.

Franco, J.G., Jr, Baruffi, R.L., Oliveira, J.B. et al. (2009). Effects of recombinant LH supplementation to recombinant FSH during induced ovarian stimulation in the GnRH-agonist protocol: a matched case-control study. Reprod Biol Endocrinol 7: 58.

Hill, M.J., Levens, E.D., Levy, G. et al. (2012a). The use of recombinant luteinizing hormone in patients undergoing assisted reproductive techniques with advanced reproductive age: a systematic review and meta-analysis. Fertil Steril 97: 1108–1114.

Hill, M.J., Levy, G. and Levens, E.D. (2012b). Does exogenous LH in ovarian stimulation improve assisted reproduction success? An appraisal of the literature. Reprod Biomed Online 24: 261–271.

Hu, L., Bu, Z., Wang, K. and Sun, Y. (2014). Recombinant luteinizing hormone priming in early follicular phase for women undergoing in vitro fertilization: systematic review and meta-analysis. J Int Med Res 42: 261–269.

Humaidan, P., Engmann, L. and Benadiva, C. (2015). Luteal phase supplementation after gonadotropin-releasing hormone agonist trigger in fresh embryo transfer: the American versus European approaches. Fertil Steril 103: 879–885.

Jones, H.W., Jr (2008). Luteal-phase defect: the role of Georgeanna Seegar Jones. Fertil Steril 90: e5–7.

Kadoch, I.J., Al-Khaduri, M., Phillips, S.J. et al. (2008). Spontaneous ovulation rate before oocyte retrieval in modified natural cycle IVF with and without indomethacin. Reprod Biomed Online 16: 245–249.

Kolibianakis, E.M., Venetis, C.A., Kalogeropoulou, L. et al. (2011). Fixed versus flexible gonadotropin-releasing hormone antagonist administration in in vitro fertilization: a randomized controlled trial. Fertil Steril 95: 558–562.

Krause, B.T., Ohlinger, R. and Haase, A. (2009). Lutropin alpha, recombinant human luteinizing hormone, for the stimulation of follicular development in profoundly LH-deficient hypogonadotropic hypogonadal women: a review. Biologics 3: 337–347.

La Marca, A. and Sunkara, S.K. (2014). Individualization of controlled ovarian stimulation in IVF using ovarian reserve markers: from theory to practice. Hum Reprod Update 20: 124–140.

Lehert, P., Kolibianakis, E.M., Venetis, C.A. et al. (2014). Recombinant human follicle-stimulating hormone (r-hFSH) plus recombinant luteinizing hormone versus r-hFSH alone for ovarian stimulation during assisted reproductive technology: systematic review and meta-analysis. Reprod Biol Endocrinol 12: 17.

Leth-Moller, K., Hammer Jagd, S. and Humaidan, P. (2014). the luteal phase after GnRHa trigger – understanding an enigma. Int J Fertil Steril 8: 227–234.

Levi Setti, P.E. (2006). The importance of consistent FSH delivery in infertility treatment. Reprod Biomed Online 12: 493–499.

Liang, I.T., Huang, H.Y., Wu, H.M. et al. (2015). A gonadotropin releasing hormone agonist trigger of ovulation with aggressive luteal phase support for patients at risk of ovarian hyperstimulation syndrome undergoing controlled ovarian hyperstimulation. Taiwan J Obstet Gynecol 54: 583–587.

Mathur, R.S. and Tan, B.K. (2014). British Fertility Society Policy and Practice Committee: prevention of ovarian hyperstimulation syndrome. Hum Fertil (Camb) 17: 257–268.

Nardo, L.G., Bosch, E., Lambalk, C.B. et al. (2013). Controlled ovarian hyperstimulation regimens: a review of the available evidence for clinical practice. Produced on behalf of the BFS Policy and Practice Committee. Hum Fertil (Camb) 16: 144–150.

O'Shea, R.T., Forbes, K.L., Scopacasa, L. et al. (1988). Comparison of transabdominal and transvaginal pelvic ultrasonography for ovarian follicle assessment in in vitro fertilisation. Gynecol Obstet Invest 26: 52–55.

Ortmann, O., Weiss, J.M. and Diedrich, K. (2002). Gonadotrophin-releasing hormone (GnRH) and GnRH agonists: mechanisms of action. Reprod Biomed Online 5(Suppl 1): 1–7.

Orvieto, R. (2015). Triggering final follicular maturation – hCG, GnRH-agonist or both, when and to whom? J Ovarian Res 8: 60.

Pacchiarotti, A., Selman, H., Valeri, C. et al. (2016). Ovarian stimulation protocol in IVF: an up-to-date review of the literature. Curr Pharm Biotechnol 17: 303–315.

Palomba, S., Santagni, S. and La Sala, G.B. (2015). Progesterone administration for luteal phase deficiency in human reproduction: an old or new issue? J Ovarian Res 8: 77.

Pouwer, A.W., Farquhar, C. and Kremer, J.A. (2015). Long-acting FSH versus daily FSH for women undergoing assisted reproduction. Cochrane Database Syst Rev 7: CD009577.

Practice Committee of the American Society for Reproductive Medicine (2008). Gonadotropin preparations: past, present, and future perspectives. Fertil Steril 90: S13–20.

Pundir, J., Sunkara, S.K., El-Toukhy, T. et al. (2012). Meta-analysis of GnRH antagonist protocols: do they reduce the risk of OHSS in PCOS? Reprod Biomed Online 24: 6–22.

Requena, A., Cruz, M., Ruiz, F.J. et al. (2014). Endocrine profile following stimulation with recombinant follicle stimulating hormone and luteinizing hormone versus highly purified human menopausal gonadotropin. Reprod Biol Endocrinol 12: 10.

Sallam, H.N., Garcia-Velasco, J.A., Dias, S. et al. (2006). Long-term pituitary down-regulation before in vitro fertilization (IVF) for women with endometriosis. Cochrane Database Syst Rev CD004635.

Schertz, J.C., Saunders, H., Hecker, C. et al. (2011). The redesigned follitropin alfa pen injector: results of the patient and nurse human factors usability testing. Expert Opin Drug Deliv 8: 1111–1120.

Shapiro, B.S. and Andersen, C.Y. (2015). Major drawbacks and additional benefits of agonist trigger–not ovarian hyperstimulation syndrome related. Fertil Steril 103: 874–878.

Siristatidis, C.S., Gibreel, A., Basios, G. et al. (2015). Gonadotrophin-releasing hormone agonist protocols for pituitary suppression in assisted reproduction. Cochrane Database Syst Rev 11: CD006919.

Smitz, J., Andersen, A.N., Devroey, P. et al. (2007). Endocrine profile in serum and follicular fluid differs after ovarian stimulation with HP-hMG or recombinant FSH in IVF patients. Hum Reprod 22: 676–687.

Somkuti, S.G., Schertz, J.C., Moore, M. et al. (2006). Patient experience with follitropin alfa prefilled pen versus previously used injectable gonadotropins for ovulation induction in oligoanovulatory women. Curr Med Res Opin 22: 1981–1996.

Sunkara, S.K., Rittenberg, V., Raine-Fenning, N. et al. (2011). Association between the number of eggs and live birth in IVF treatment: an analysis of 400 135 treatment cycles. Hum Reprod 26: 1768–1774.

Tannus, S., Burke, Y.Z. and Kol, S. (2015). Treatment strategies for the infertile polycystic ovary syndrome patient. Womens Health (Lond Engl) 11: 901–912.

Tannus, S., Weissman, A., Boaz, M. et al. (2013). The effect of delayed initiation of gonadotropin-releasing hormone antagonist in a flexible protocol on in vitro fertilization outcome. Fertil Steril 99: 725–730.

Tarlatzis, B.C., Fauser, B.C., Kolibianakis, E.M. et al. (2006). GnRH antagonists in ovarian stimulation for IVF. Hum Reprod Update 12: 333–340.

Toner, J.P. (2002). Progress we can be proud of: U.S. trends in assisted reproduction over the first 20 years. Fertil Steril 78: 943–950.

Trew, G.H., Brown, A.P., Gillard, S. et al. (2010). In vitro fertilisation with recombinant follicle stimulating hormone requires less IU usage compared with highly purified human menopausal gonadotrophin: results from a European retrospective observational chart review. Reprod Biol Endocrinol 8: 137.

Trounson, A.O., Leeton, J.F., Wood, C. et al. (1981). Pregnancies in humans by fertilization in vitro and embryo transfer in the controlled ovulatory cycle. Science 212: 681–682.

Van Der Linden, M., Buckingham, K., Farquhar, C. et al. (2015). Luteal phase support for assisted reproduction cycles. Cochrane Database Syst Rev 7: CD009154.

Van Loenen, A.C., Huirne, J.A., Schats, R. et al. (2002). GnRH agonists, antagonists, and assisted conception. Semin Reprod Med 20: 349–364.

Van Tilborg, T.C., Eijkemans, M.J., Laven, J.S. et al. (2012). The OPTIMIST study: optimisation of cost effectiveness through individualised FSH stimulation dosages for IVF treatment. A randomised controlled trial. BMC Womens Health 12: 29.

Van Wely, M., Kwan, I., Burt, A. L. et al. (2012). Recombinant versus urinary gonadotrophin for ovarian stimulation in assisted reproductive technology cycles. A Cochrane review. Hum Reprod Update 18: 111.

Welcker, J.T., Nawroth, F. and Bilger, W. (2010). Patient evaluation of the use of follitropin alfa in a prefilled ready-to-use injection pen in assisted reproductive technology: an observational study. Reprod Biol Endocrinol 8: 111.

Yanushpolsky, E.H. (2015). Luteal phase support in in vitro fertilization. Semin Reprod Med 33: 118–127.

Yates, A.P., Rustamov, O., Roberts, S.A. et al. (2011). Anti-Mullerian hormone-tailored stimulation protocols improve outcomes whilst reducing adverse effects and costs of IVF. Hum Reprod 26: 2353–2362.

Youssef, M.A., Abdelmoty, H.I., Ahmed, M.A. et al. (2015). GnRH agonist for final oocyte maturation in GnRH antagonist co-treated IVF/ICSI treatment cycles: systematic review and meta-analysis. J Adv Res 6: 341–349.

Youssef, M.A., Al-Inany, H.G., Aboulghar, M. et al. (2011). Recombinant versus urinary human chorionic gonadotrophin for final oocyte maturation triggering in IVF and ICSI cycles. Cochrane Database Syst Rev CD003719.

Youssef, M.A., Van Der Veen, F., Al-Inany, H.G. et al. (2014). Gonadotropin-releasing hormone agonist versus HCG for oocyte triggering in antagonist-assisted reproductive technology. Cochrane Database Syst Rev 10: CD008046.

20

Oocyte Retrieval Techniques and Culture of Oocytes

Dawn Yell

History of Human Oocyte Retrieval

During the late 1960s the innovative partnership that was Robert Edwards and Patrick Steptoe made huge advances in the recovery of preovulatory oocytes for the purpose of *in vitro* fertilization (IVF). Compared with laparotomy, the laparoscopic method developed by Edwards and Steptoe was a smaller scale procedure that placed fewer demands on the patient, allowed for a short recovery period (approximately 36 h in hospital) and could be repeated on the same individual (Steptoe and Edwards 1970). Their refining of this technique, which recovered oocytes from approximately one-third of follicles, led to its adoption worldwide and the development of the first aspiration needle. In 1978, following laparoscopic oocyte retrieval, IVF, and subsequent embryo transfer, the pioneering work of Edwards and Steptoe led to the birth of Louise Brown, the first successful live birth in the history of IVF. In the early 1980s ultrasound-guided oocyte retrieval techniques emerged with Lenz and Lauritsen first describing the transabdominal transvesical ultrasonically guided approach (Dellenbach et al. 1985). Just a couple of years later, in 1984, Pierre Dellenbach and his team developed the transvaginal oocyte retrieval (TVOR) method (Dellenbach et al. 1985). Such developments coincided with the increasing sophistication of equipment designed for oocyte recovery. Echogenic, Teflon-coated needles, pedal driven vacuum pumps and silicon tubing all led to the 90% recovery rate that we can expect today.

Timing of Oocyte Retrieval

As with many aspects of an IVF cycle, the correct timing of oocyte retrieval, post trigger injection, is crucial. The previous chapter described the oocyte maturational role of the trigger injection by inducing the resumption of meiosis. It is essential that enough time is given so that the oocytes reach nuclear and cytoplasmic maturity, but not so much that they are lost through ovulation or aged *in vivo*. Most clinic protocols aim to perform oocyte retrieval 35–37 h post maturational trigger injection.

Planning Theatre

Careful consideration must be given to the availability of theatre and staff on the planned day of oocyte retrieval. Reasonable time should be allowed for each case (30–45 min in most clinics) and there must be minimal risk of delay. Due to the consequences of a woman undergoing ovulation or retrieving postmature oocytes if the oocyte retrieval is delayed, these cases must have priority. Once appropriate theatre times have been allocated, the patient undergoing oocyte retrieval must be contacted and given clear instructions about the precise timing of her trigger injection. When the patient is admitted to the clinic on the day of oocyte retrieval, it is wise to confirm, as a routine, the date and time she administered the final injection.

Preparation for Oocyte Retrieval

Before oocyte retrieval can take place, significant preparation is required in both theatre and the embryology laboratory to ensure that oocytes are collected under optimal conditions. It is important to understand that oocytes are extremely sensitive to environmental changes and suboptimal retrieval conditions can lead to disruption of homeostasis and have detrimental effects within the oocytes. The successful outcome of an IVF cycle can hinge on the environmental conditions the oocytes encounter at the time of retrieval.

Temperature

The temperature can fluctuate at several points during the oocyte collection process, having a possible impact on the chromosomal integrity of those oocytes. It is widely accepted that at lower temperatures the meiotic spindle of an oocyte is disrupted, leading to chromosomal misalignment on the metaphase plate and abnormal distribution during meiosis (Pickering et al. 1990). Such aberrations result in aneuploidy. At temperatures of 33 °C and below, the meiotic spindle depolymerizes; the speed at which this occurs increases with decreasing temperatures (Wang et al. 2001). Rewarming to 37 °C can induce repolymerization although in many oocytes the process is incomplete (depending on the length of time spent below 33 °C) and those allowed to cool to room temperature never recover (Wang et al. 2001). Similarly, the same has been shown to be true if oocytes experience temperatures of 39 °C and above. Overheating can induce disassembly of the spindle microtubules and even relocation of the spindle in the cytoplasm. If the temperature returns to 37 °C, the microtubules of the spindle may repolymerise but the process is often incomplete and can still lead to aneuploidy via inappropriate chromosome segregation (Sun et al. 2004).

pH

The intracellular pH (pHi) of an oocyte has been shown to be approximately 7.1. In order to offset the acidification that occurs during culture due to intracellular metabolic processes, extracellular pH should be higher (Swain 2010). For this reason, most media suites recommend a pH ranging between 7.2 and 7.4. The most commonly used buffer in IVF culture media is sodium bicarbonate, the pH of which is regulated by the production of carbonic acid and is relative to the amount of CO_2 in the atmosphere immediately surrounding the culture dish. To reach and maintain a desirable pH of 7.2–7.4, such media must be equilibrated in a humidified incubator under specified gaseous conditions (most commonly 6% CO_2, 5% O_2, and 89% N_2) at 37 °C. Raising CO_2 lowers media pH, while lowering CO_2 raises the pH (Swain 2010). Whilst some laboratories continue to make their media in house, most now use commercially available media due to the benefits of quality control and assurance. Many of these media suites offer a handling medium for gametes, which allows the user to work in ambient conditions, on a heated stage, without the risk of gaseous exchange causing an unwanted rise in pH. Zwitterionic buffers such as MOPS and HEPES are used to regulate the pH in ambient conditions (Will et al. 2011). Media of this kind is particularly useful for oocyte retrieval as the collection part of the procedure can vary in length (depending on several factors including follicle number and ease of access to the ovaries); repeated opening of the incubators could lead to detrimental pH fluctuations in other gametes or embryos being cultured and slow the collection process further.

Osmolality

The osmolality of a medium is determined by the amount of solute particles dissolved in the solution and, for IVF culture, should be between 255 and 295 mOsm/kg (Swain et al. 2012). Whilst the manufacturer predetermines this, manipulation of the media in the laboratory can have an effect on its value. Altering the osmolality of the culture media can place osmotic stress on oocytes and disrupt homeostasis. For this reason, laboratories must take great care when preparing cultures dishes, as evaporation will lead to detrimental changes in the osmolality of culture media. Things to be considered during culture dish preparation include temperature of the work surface, airflow within the safety cabinet, the size and number of media drops per dish and the time allowed before adding the oil overlay.

The IVF Laboratory

In addition to the clinical practice described here, performing the optimal oocyte retrieval also depends on many other factors. Laboratory design, culture systems, and incubator choice all have an impact and are discussed in more detail within other chapters.

Preparation for oocyte retrieval usually begins in the IVF laboratory on the afternoon prior to the procedure. As detailed above, media containing bicarbonate buffer requires equilibration in a humidified incubator, a process that can take up to several hours. Volume of media, surface area, use of oil overlay, and even the type of lid/dishware can influence this (Swain 2010). Consequently, each laboratory should validate this equilibration process for its own culture conditions, ensuring optimal pH and temperature are reached and maintained. Each laboratory has its own standard operating procedures around the type and configuration of dish used and thus, consideration must be given to the number of follicles a female has in order that the appropriate number of culture dishes are made for the expected number of oocytes. All dishes and vessels destined to contain gametes or embryos should be appropriately labelled with patient details: name, date of birth, and unique hospital/patient number.

As the handling media described previously does not require equilibration to ensure optimal pH, it can be prepared and warmed, using a warming block or oven, either the day prior to or on the morning of oocyte retrieval. Most media suites also offer a flushing medium which is used to check the retrieval needle is clear of blockages and can be used to irrigate follicles in the cases of poor ovarian response to stimulation (see later). This media does not require equilibration for pH but should be prewarmed to 37 °C before use.

On the day of TVOR, laboratory staff should carry out routine checks to ensure all equipment required for both the procedure and for the warming and equilibration of media is functioning normally. It is also prudent to check that the warming blocks in which tubes containing follicular fluid will be placed are empty before the patient is brought into the procedure room (repeat this step between every patient). Immediately prior to the procedure, the embryologist should prepare the safety cabinet for oocyte collection with the consumables required. Once the patient's identity has been confirmed, the appropriately labelled dishes should then be filled using the prewarmed handling media and placed on a heated surface.

Theatre

Preparation in theatre is usually carried out immediately prior to oocyte retrieval. Once it has been confirmed that the warming blocks do not contain tubes from a previous procedure, they are filled with an appropriate number (related to the number of follicles present) of empty tubes. This is done in order to bring the tubes up to temperature, ready for the collection of follicular fluid.

Aspiration Equipment

Oocytes are collected using a needle, guided by a transvaginal ultrasound probe. Various needles are commercially available for this specific procedure but they can be split into two main categories: single lumen and double lumen. Single lumen needles contain just one channel used for draining follicular fluid in routine TVOR (Figure 20.1a). Double lumen needles, as the name suggests, have two channels. One is used for draining follicular fluid whilst the second is used to expel flushing media into the collapsed follicle (Figure 20.1b).

In keeping with the NICE guidelines regarding flushing, flushing with a double lumen needle is usually employed in females who have had a reduced response to stimulation, having produced fewer than three follicles. In such cases the clinician will first drain the follicle and repeatedly flush and drain to maximize the chance of collecting the oocyte from within. At the time of writing the current NICE guidelines make the following recommendation: 'Women who have developed at least three follicles before oocyte retrieval should not be offered follicle flushing because this procedure does not increase the numbers of oocytes retrieved or pregnancy rates, and it increases the duration of oocyte retrieval and associated pain' (National Institute for Health and Care Excellence 2013). Another feature of the oocyte retrieval needle is the length of the tubing from the needle itself to the collection tube. This is usually kept to a minimum to avoid increased

(a)

(b)

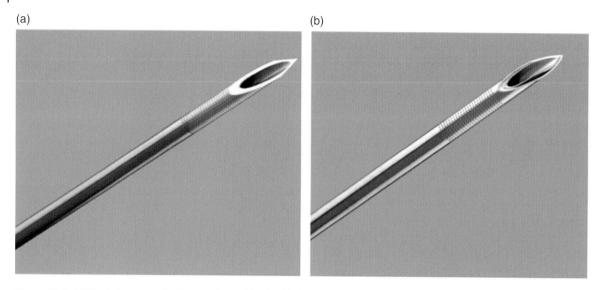

Figure 20.1 (a) Single lumen aspiration needle and (b) double lumen aspiration needle. Reproduced with permission of Cook Medical, Bloomington, Indiana, USA.

exposure of the follicular fluid, and oocytes contained within, to the reduced ambient temperature.

A final consideration should be the pressure on the vacuum pump. This should be high enough to ensure follicular fluid is drained quickly into the warmed collection tubes, but not so high that there is a risk of mechanical damage to the oocytes through sheering.

Transvaginal Oocyte Retrieval

When the patient enters the theatre, an identification check must take place (usually between the clinician and embryologist). It is considered good practice to check three points of identification. Prior to the administration of anaesthetic, the patient should be asked to state her name, date of birth and, for example, the unique patient/hospital number on her wristband. These details should be crossreferenced with the patient notes.

Each clinic has their own anaesthetic/analgesia regime that is the preferred method of the treating clinician and/or anaesthetist. During the early days of laparoscopic oocyte retrieval, general anaesthetic had to be administered. More recently, with the advent of TVOR, there has been a trend towards conscious sedation as it has the benefits of needing

less specialized equipment, causes fewer complications, and is usually well tolerated by the patients (National Institute for Health and Care Excellence 2013). General anaesthetic is most commonly used only in those patients with difficult ovarian access or other medical complications.

Once the patient is sedated, the clinician begins by observing the follicles using the transvaginal probe, and briefly compares this with what was seen on the last scan during follicular tracking. When satisfied that ovulation has not taken place, and there are no unexpected anomalies, the needle and guide are fitted to the probe and TVOR begins. The clinician pushes the needle through the vaginal wall and into the first ovary, puncturing a single follicle at a time (Figure 20.2). Repeated puncture of the vaginal wall and ovaries should be avoided to minimize bleeding, trauma to the ovaries, and postoperative pain. Once in a follicle, the fluid within is drained into the warmed collection tubes, with use of the vacuum pump, until the follicle has completely collapsed.

The tube containing follicular fluid is then placed in a warming block in close proximity to the embryologist's workstation. At this point, good communication between the clinician, assisting nurse/healthcare assistant, and embryologist is essential (Figure 20.3). The embryologist must work carefully and efficiently to identify oocytes within

Figure 20.2 Ultrasound-guided transvaginal oocyte retrieval procedure Reproduced with permission of Mayo Foundation for Medical Education and Research. All rights reserved.

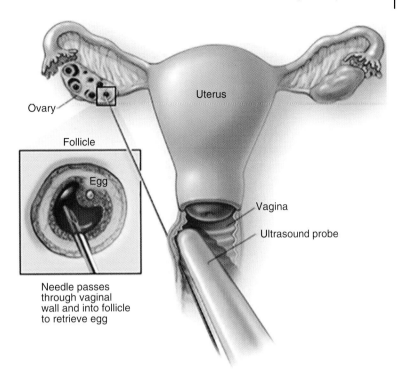

Figure 20.3 After each follicular aspiration, the theatre staff places the tube in a heated block. The embryologist collects the tube, recovers any oocytes present and places them in culture media. Reproduced with permission of the Association of Clinical Embryologists.

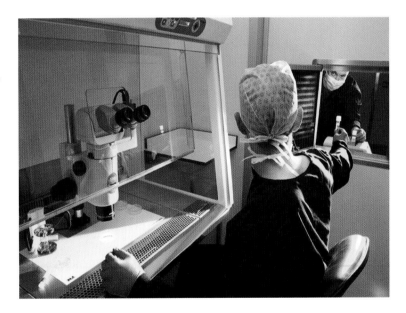

the follicular fluid and this should be the rate-determining step. If the clinician performs the TVOR too quickly, leading to several tubes of follicular fluid building up in the warming block, oocytes within the tubes will likely be subject to temperature fluctuations. Also, any blood within the tubes may begin to coagulate, making it very difficult to retrieve the oocytes. Care must be taken not to overfill the tubes so that the follicular fluid does not rest above the height of the warming block. If the female undergoing TVOR has very few follicles, the clinician may choose to wait after draining each follicle until the embryologist has confirmed the presence or absence of an oocyte. This will determine whether the clinician continues to flush a particular follicle or move on to the next.

Searching for Oocytes

To find oocytes within the follicular fluid, the embryologist first pours the fluid into Petri dishes that have been resting on the heated stage. Care is taken not to overfill the dishes as this can make it more difficult to visualize the oocytes (particularly in bloodier samples) and risks spillage. The oocyte–corona–cumulus complex (OCCC) can often be seen with the naked eye and the embryologist should first scan the dish to see if this is the case. Once observed, confirmation that there is an oocyte present is required with the use of a light microscope. If, at this point the oocyte is not obvious, spreading the OCCC is a good way to both verify the presence of an oocyte and assess its maturity (see Assessing Oocyte Maturity). This is done by picking up the OCCC using a glass pipette and then tipping the Petri dish slightly, creating an area at the top of the dish with a fine film of fluid (taking great care not to spill any follicular fluid). Placing the OCCC in this area whilst observing it via the light microscope, the embryologist should see the cumulus cells spread and an oocyte be revealed if present. Whilst handling oocytes, the embryologist should take care never to overstretch the OCCC as this could potentially lead to fracturing the zona surrounding the oocyte. If there are no OCCCs immediately visible to the naked eye, or those that were have been removed from the dish, the remaining fluid should be examined under the light microscope. The embryologist systematically observes the whole Petri dish, gently swirling or agitating the follicular fluid to reduce the chance of oocytes becoming lodged on the side of the Petri dish. Once fluid in a dish is deemed to be free of oocytes, it can be discarded in the appropriate clinical waste vessel.

Once identified, oocytes are usually washed through prewarmed handling media and placed in a holding dish, also containing handling media and overlaid with oil, which remains on the heated stage. If there is a particularly large number of oocytes being collected for a patient, the holding dish may become crowded and those oocytes collected first may have been on the heated stage for an extended period of time. In such cases, it is prudent to place these oocytes into the oocyte culture dish part way through the TVOR (e.g. when the clinician has completed collecting from one ovary and is moving to the next). Part of a laboratory's process validation for TVOR should include assessments of temperature stability in oocyte holding dishes over varying periods of time.

Follicular Fluid and Cysts

Follicular fluid can be identified by its straw-like colour. However, this is sometimes altered by the presence of blood during TVOR. One can also expect to observe sheets of granulosa and thecal cells along with the OCCC.

Certain types of ovarian cysts may be present at the time of oocyte collection, possibly as a direct result of ovarian stimulation, or as an underlying factor relating to subfertility. Simple follicular ovarian cysts are the most common, and are often associated with ovarian stimulation. They are harmless and contain clear, watery fluid, with few or no cells present.

Endometrioma are a type of cyst formed when endometrial tissue grows within the ovaries. They contain a thick, brown fluid, derived from old blood and hence are often referred to as chocolate cysts. Whilst oocytes do not form within endometrioma, this fluid should be examined as it may contain an oocyte from a previously drained follicle.

Preparing the Oocytes for Culture

Once the TVOR is complete and all the tubes containing follicular fluid have been checked, the oocytes collected must now be transferred to the oocyte culture dish. Each time oocytes are moved from one vessel to another, the embryologist must count the number present before and after the transfer, along with checking the patient details on both vessels match. At this point the oocytes are being transferred from Zwitterionic handling media to bicarbonate-buffered media. It is therefore important to wash the oocytes through pre-equilibrated bicarbonate-buffered media before placing them in their final culture drop/well.

Some clinics prefer to trim excess granulosa and cumulus cells from oocytes prior to placing them in culture. This is not necessary for oocytes that are intended for intracytoplasmic sperm injection (ICSI) as mechanical denudation of the oocytes will be performed before the injection procedure. This 'trimming' is done using sterile needles (usually of a fine gauge), attached to 1 mL or 2 mL syringes for stability, in a knife-and-fork-like fashion. Great care must be taken to stay away from the oocyte to avoid puncturing it or mechanical damage such as fracturing the zona. This method may also be applied during TVOR to dissect out oocytes that are found in tubes containing coagulated blood (see Problem Solving).

Assessing Oocyte Maturity

The developmental competence of an embryo depends on the nucleic and cytoplasmic maturity of the oocyte from which it is derived (Balaban et al. 2011). Retrieval of a mature cohort of preovulatory oocytes has been the aim of careful follicular monitoring throughout ovarian stimulation. Some IVF laboratories estimate the maturity of an oocyte based on the appearance of the OCCC at the time of retrieval. This is a subjective and often inaccurate method, and there is yet to be a worldwide consensus on the morphological grading of OCCCs and oocyte competence. In their 2003 study, Lin et al. use a grading system to estimate oocyte maturity based on the characteristics of the OCCC. This system broadly reflects those used in IVF laboratories around the world. Nucleic maturity of an oocyte can only be confirmed by the visualization of the first polar body. This is achieved by mechanical denudation of oocytes prior to ICSI on day 0 or at the fertilization check on day 1 post-IVF insemination.

The appearance of cumulus cells, level of elasticity between the cumulus cells, and relative expansion of the corona radiata cells can all be clues to the nucleic maturity of the oocyte. The greater the elasticity between the cumulus cells, the greater the spread that will be observed by the embryologist. This in turn leads to the oocyte being more easily observed using a light microscope. OCCCs with such behaviour are likely to contain an oocyte that is at the metaphase II stage in development and is considered mature. Mature oocytes are most commonly collected from follicles between 13 and 24 mm in size (Wittmaack et al. 1994). For immature oocytes (those at metaphase I or the germinal vesicle stages), the gaps between the cumulus cells are much tighter, as with those between the corona radiata and the oocyte. This leads to an overall much darker appearance to the OCCC and reduces the visibility of the oocyte with light microscopy. Immature oocytes are usually collected from the smaller follicles within the cohort (<13 mm). OCCCs can also be classed as postmature. In such complexes the cumulus cells can appear atretic with dark patches, giving a 'lace like' appearance. The oocyte within the complex is usually very easily observed. Such OCCCs most often come from larger follicles in cases of asynchronous follicular development. It may be the case that one or two follicles grow quickly, ahead of the main cohort, and are sacrificed in order to allow the larger group of follicles to reach the desired size, optimizing the number of mature oocytes collected. Postmature oocytes, whilst at the desired nucleic maturity (metaphase II), are aged and are likely to have poorer rates of normal fertilization and subsequent embryo development than their mature counterparts, collected at the appropriate developmental stage.

Whilst OCCC grading is an inaccurate method, it can be used as a useful tool for counselling those patients who are suspected of having a higher than normal rate of immature oocytes.

Problem Solving

Ovulation

As discussed earlier, the timing of TVOR is of the upmost importance in achieving collection of mature oocytes. If the TVOR is delayed for any reason, there is a risk oocytes may be lost via ovulation. With the use of transvaginal ultrasound, ovulation is indicated by the presence of several collapsed follicles and free fluid in the pouch of Douglas. At this point, it is possible for the clinician to collect fluid from the pouch of Douglas, which may contain the released oocytes. The embryologist should examine the fluid as described above.

When No Eggs Are Collected Unexpectedly

On rare occasions, it is possible that, despite apparently normal follicular development and having ruled out ovulation, no oocytes are collected. There is much debate in the literature surrounding empty follicle syndrome and whether cases observed are genuine (normal levels of oestradiol and appropriate serum levels of beta human chorionic gonadotropin (β-hCG) on the day of TVOR), or false (caused by human error, follicular dysfunction, low bioavailability of β-hCG, or pharmacological factors) (Deepika et al. 2015; Madani and Jahangiri 2015).

Prior to TVOR, the timing of the trigger injection should be confirmed as part of the admission process. Then, if a reasonable number of follicles have been drained from one ovary and no oocytes have been found, the embryologist must alert the clinician to this. Before moving on to the second ovary, the efficacy of the trigger should be investigated. If possible, the quickest way to do this, provided a β-hCG trigger was used, is a urinary pregnancy test. A positive result will be obtained if the trigger was administered correctly. Follow the directions of the pregnancy kit using the follicular fluid in place of urine. If β-hCG is not detected, it is possible to stop the TVOR and administer another trigger injection in an attempt to rescue any developing oocytes in the remaining follicles. A second TVOR should then be carried out approximately 36 h later (Ndukwe et al. 1997; Evbuomwan et al. 1999).

Oestradiol levels are positively correlated with follicular development and are often used to determine a female's risk of OHSS in the case of an elevated ovarian response. However, there are some instances in which, despite having many follicles, a patient has a lower than expected oestradiol level. Such patients often have fewer mature oocytes collected than predicted by folliculogram (Mittal et al. 2014). Hence, knowing a female's oestrogen level prior to TVOR can help manage patient expectations regarding the number of oocytes predicted for retrieval.

Blood Clots in Collection Tubes

As mentioned earlier, if the follicular fluid is contaminated with a large amount of blood, this blood can coagulate, forming a gelatinous mass within the collection tube. Normally, tubes containing follicular fluid are checked for the presence of oocytes in the order in which they were collected. If the embryologist notices that a tube is particularly bloody, this tube should be checked immediately, ahead of the others, to avoid coagulation. If coagulation occurs, the mass should be teased apart, very carefully, using fine gauge needles attached to 1 mL or 2 mL syringes, all the while looking down the microscope to ensure there is no damage to a OCCC that may be contained within.

Conclusion

This chapter has described the main areas relating to the safe collection and culture of oocytes, and some of the unforeseen issues that can occur during the process. Comprehensive monitoring during ovarian stimulation and strict adherence to timing of TVOR (after trigger injection administration) allows for the collection of as many mature oocytes as possible. Careful consideration must be given to the location and design of the area within which oocyte collection will take place. Extensive validation of the equipment and process should be carried out to ensure oocytes are collected and stored in an optimal environment. Fluctuations in temperature, pH and osmolality during the collection process can result in irreparable damage to oocytes. Care must also be taken during harvesting and handling to avoid any mechanical damage. Prior preparation and communication between the multidisciplinary team is key to an effective TVOR.

References

Balaban, B., Brison, D., Calderón, G. et al. (2011). The Istanbul consensus workshop on embryo assessment: proceedings of an expert meeting. Reprod BioMed Online 22: 632–646.

Deepika, K., Rathore, S., Garg, N. et al. (2015). Empty follicle syndrome: successful pregnancy following dual trigger. J Hum Reprod Sci 8: 170–174.

Dellenbach, P., Nissand, I, Moreau, L. et al. (1985). Transvaginal sonographically controlled follicle puncture for oocyte retrieval. Fertil Steril 44: 656–662.

Evbuomwan, I.O., Fenwick J.D., Shiels R. et al. (1999). Severe ovarian hyperstimulation syndrome following salvage of empty follicle syndrome: case report. Hum Reprod 14: 1707–1709.

Lin, Y.C., Chang, S.Y., Lan, K.C. et al. (2003). Human oocyte maturity in vivo determines the outcome of blastocyst development in vitro. J Assist Reprod Genet 20: 506–512.

Madani, T. and Jahangiri, N. (2015). Empty follicle syndrome: the possible cause of occurrence. Oman Med J 30: 417–420.

Mittal, S., Gupta, P., Malhotra N. et al. (2014). Serum estradiol as a predictor of success of in vitro fertilization. J Obstet Gynecol India 64: 124–129.

National Institute for Health and Care Excellence (2013). Fertility problems : assessment and treatment. Available from: https://www.nice.org.uk/guidance/cg156/chapter/recommendations (accessed 12 February 2018).

Ndukwe, G. Thornton, S. Fishel, S. et al. (1997). 'Curing' empty follicle syndrome. Hum Reprod 12: 21–23.

Pickering, S.J., Braude, P.R., Johnson, M.H. et al. (1990). Transient cooling to room temperature can cause irreversible disruption of the meiotic spindle in the human oocyte. Fertil Steril 54: 102–108.

Steptoe, P.C. and Edwards, R.G. (1970). Laparoscopic recovery of preovulatory human oocytes after priming of ovaries with gonadotrophins. Lancet 295(7649): 683–689.

Sun, X.-F., Wang, W.-H. and Keefe, D.L. (2004). Overheating is detrimental to meiotic spindles within in vitro matured human oocytes. Zygote 12: 65–70.

Swain, J.E. (2010). Optimizing the culture environment in the IVF laboratory: impact of pH and buffer capacity on gamete and embryo quality. Reprod BioMed Online 21: 6–16.

Swain, J.E., Cabrera, Zu, X. et al. (2012). Microdrop preparation factors influence culture-media osmolality, which can impair mouse embryo preimplantation development. Reprod BioMed Online 24: 142–147.

Wang, W.H., Meng, L., Hackett, R.J. et al. (2001). Limited recovery of meiotic spindles in living human oocytes after cooling-rewarming observed using polarized light microscopy. Hum Reprod 16: 2374–2378.

Will, M.A., Clark, N.A. and Swain, J.E. (2011). Biological pH buffers in IVF: help or hindrance to success. J Assist Reprod Genet 28: 711–724.

Wittmaack, F.M., Kreger, D.O., Blasco, L. et al. (1994). Effect of follicular size on oocyte retrieval, fertilization, cleavage, and embryo quality in in vitro fertilization cycles: a 6-year data collection. Fertil Steril 62: 1205–1210.

21

Sperm Preparation: Strategy and Methodology

Stephen Harbottle

Introduction

Since the pioneering work of Sir Robert Edwards, Patrick Steptoe, and Jean Purdy (Edwards et al.1969) in the latter half of the twentieth century, which culminated in the birth of the world's first test-tube baby, Louise Joy Brown on 25 July 1978, it has been clear that methodology must be developed and refined to prepare sperm for use in assisted reproduction technology (ART).

The need to separate spermatozoa from seminal plasma is fundamental to the *in vitro* fertilization (IVF), intracytoplasmic sperm injection (ICSI), or intrauterine insemination (IUI) processes as it allows sperm to capacitate and exhibit a hyperactivated pattern of activity which is an intrinsic expression of their fertilization ability (Mortimer 1991). Since a simple one stage 'washing' process was first described for human fertilization (Edwards et al. 1969), the process has been further refined through the additions of 'swim-up' (Lopata et al. 1978), two washes (Edwards et al. 1980), 'density gradient separation' (Pertoft et al. 1978), and a wash combined with a swim-up (Mahadevan and Baker 1984). What is both noticeable and interesting is that all of these techniques as described still make a valuable contribution to our laboratory processes today.

Despite the methodology adopted, the aim is consistent throughout our most modern laboratories; to remove the seminal plasma and other nonspematozoal seminal components and be left with a highly purified seminal fraction containing the highest possible population of highly motile and morphologically normal sperm for use in insemination or injection.

This chapter aims to provide an overview of the techniques currently available to clinical scientists in their tool kit of sperm preparation.

Sperm Separation Techniques: Why Do We Need Them?

Before we consider what we must do to prepare sperm we must consider why we must do it. Pivotal to this understanding is a realization that, under *in vivo* conditions, human semen would not find itself in the vicinity of an ovulated egg in the vestments of the Fallopian tubes. During its journey from the site of insemination (the vagina) through the challenging and hostile environment of the female reproductive tract, those sperm with the greatest fertilization potential are actively selected from those sperm with poor potential and the other nonsperm cellular and molecular components of the semen. Supported in their journey by cervical mucus, potentially fertile spermatozoa migrate to the site of conception and undergo the processes of capacitation, gaining a hyperactivated state of motility and the acrosome reaction, prior to finally making contact with the oocyte itself (Mortimer 1989).

The aim of any sperm preparation procedure is multifactorial:

- To extract a sperm population with improved sperm motility, sperm morphology, and DNA integrity.
- To remove seminal plasma, nonsperm cells, and other nonbeneficial seminal detritus.

Clinical Reproductive Science, First Edition. Edited by Michael Carroll.
© 2019 John Wiley & Sons Ltd. Published 2019 by John Wiley & Sons Ltd.
Companion website: www.wiley.com/go/carroll/clinicalreproductivescience

- To permit normal sperm function including capacitation without the induction of the acrosome reaction prematurely.
- To be time efficient and cost-effective.
- To resist the magnification of reactive oxygen species (ROS).
- To be nonreprotoxic and have no detrimental short- or long-lasting effects on the sperm harvested or on subsequent embryo or fetal development.

What Separation Techniques Are Available?

The widespread introduction of IVF procedures during the 1980s led to a rapid development of a range of deployable sperm preparation techniques as described previously. In general, the range of techniques available today can be summarized into four broad categories (for the purpose of this text, the author has given focus to those techniques most commonly practiced in ART laboratories today; it is accepted that other more 'niche' techniques may be encountered, particularly outside the UK by more adventurous readers):

1) Direct sperm washing
2) Sperm challenge separation (migration)
3) Density gradient centrifugation
4) Adaptive filtration.

These techniques are interchangeable to some extent and their main applications and benefits are briefly summarized in Table 21.1. The savvy clinical scientist will approach each sperm preparation without prejudice and will adapt their preparation strategy based on the quality of the sample observed to ensure that they take every step possible to maximize the quality of the resultant yield. A summary of the relative advantages and disadvantages of each technique is listed later in Table 21.3.

The Importance of Consideration of 'Reprotoxicity'

Sperm cells are highly sensitive to changes in temperature so great measures are taken to ensure that temperature control (and particularly prevention of temperature elevation) is maintained throughout the sperm preparation process. Historically, little attention has been afforded to the consumables and 'plastic ware' used during sperm preparation procedures and the direct effect this may have on the resultant sperm yield. 'Reprotoxicity', or the release of reprotoxic components or molecules into the IVF

Table 21.1 A summary of the four most commonly adopted sperm preparation techniques.

Sperm Preparation Method	Description and Principle	Outline of Procedure
Direct sperm washing	Simple means of removing seminal plasma without materially altering the characteristics of the sperm	Add of a volume of sperm wash culture media, centrifuge, remove supernatant and resuspend
Sperm challenge separation (swim-up)	Separates sperm based on motility with migration of highly motile sperm into a 'clean' and harvestable layer of culture media for insemination	Layer sperm wash media onto semen or sperm pellet. Incubate for 60 min. Harvest motile sperm from wash media layer
Density gradient centrifugation (DGC)	Selection by density using colloidal silica to trap low density cells whereas high density sperm with improved sperm function penetrate the column and form a pellet	Gradient media formed into two layers of different densities (high/low). Set up differential gradient column, usually either 90%/45% or 80%/40%. Centrifuge for 20 min at 300g followed by removal and washing of the pellet
Adaptive filtration	Pass prepared sperm exposed to a selection solution through an adaptive filter (e.g. magnetic) to further enhance yield quality	Using MACS as an example, coat with magnetic particles, pass through magnetic filtration field, harvest enhanced yield for treatment

culture system (Nijs et al. 2009) can result in a reduction in the efficacy of treatment or, in its most extreme case, a complete culture system failure. You may be further alarmed to discover that in an audit of IVF laboratory plastic ware of the 36 common types of laboratory consumable tested, 16 (36%) of them were reprotoxic to the IVF culture system (Nijs et al. 2009). It is for this reason that it is essential that our starting point for any ART procedure, including the preparation of sperm for treatment, is the production of the sample into a known nonreprotoxic container and its subsequent processing through a validated reprotoxin free chain of consumables to its final use in ART or cryopreservation.

Direct Sperm Washing

This process represents the most basic of sperm preparation techniques and has changed very little since it was first described by Edwards et al. for ART use in 1969 (Figure 21.1). Its usual application is when a sperm sample appears severely oligozoospermic or even cryptozoospermic. Working with consumables known to be nonreprotoxic, the strategy is to concentrate any spermatozoa present in the sample into a smaller and more workable volume, usually for ICSI treatment. The sample is pipetted into a nonreprotoxic conical tube and centrifuged at

$300\,g$ for $10-20\,\text{min}$. At the end of the centrifugation step the seminal supernatant is carefully removed and the pellet is resuspended in $2-3\,\text{mL}$ of a suitable culture media designed to sustain spermatozoal metabolism for an extended period of time (most if not all IVF culture media manufacturers produce such a medium which clinics choose based on personal preference). The tube is centrifuged for a further $10\,\text{min}$ at $300\,g$, the supernatant is again discarded and the small final volume of culture medium (usually $0.1-0.25\,\text{mL}$) is added prior to assessment for use in treatment.

The main disadvantage of this technique is, due to it being a 'concentrate everything you have' approach, the resultant sperm preparation is often hard to work with as all of the nonsperm cells and cellular debris are also collected. Allowing motile sperm time to swim out of the debris in an ICSI dish for $15-30\,\text{min}$ prior to an injection procedure is highly recommended.

Sperm Challenge Separation (The 'Swim-Up')

Separation by swim-up is in essence a sperm race, in that the principle is based entirely upon the selection of sperm based on their motility and nothing else. Progressive motility is clearly an essential trait a

Figure 21.1 Sperm washing. *Source:* Author's own design.

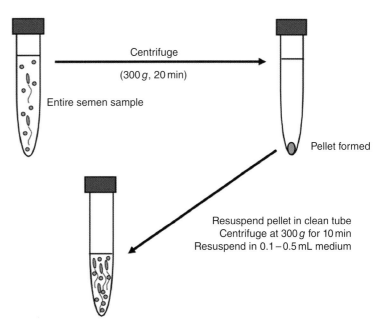

Entire semen sample

Centrifuge
$(300\,g, 20\,\text{min})$

Pellet formed

Resuspend pellet in clean tube
Centrifuge at $300\,g$ for $10\,\text{min}$
Resuspend in $0.1-0.5\,\text{mL}$ medium

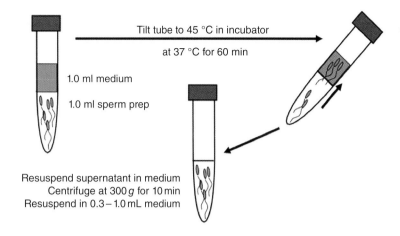

Tilt tube to 45 °C in incubator

at 37 °C for 60 min

1.0 ml medium

1.0 ml sperm prep

Resuspend supernatant in medium
Centrifuge at 300 *g* for 10 min
Resuspend in 0.3 – 1.0 mL medium

Figure 21.2 The swim-up procedure.
Source: Author's own design.

sperm capable of fertilizing an egg *in vivo* must possess, so this technique is firmly based on the functionality of reproduction and as such can be regarded as a more natural technique by comparison. That said, despite promising fertilization rates in early ART procedures in the tubal infertility population, case reports soon followed suggesting that more complex cases involving male factor, multifactorial, or idiopathic infertility could result in a failure of fertilization when using swim-up prepared sperm (Trounson et al. 1980; Yates et al. 1987). The technique is clearly of little value in cases of significant oligo- or asthenozoospermia as it will not serve to concentrate a final yield in the same way as the density gradient centrifugation or direct washing preparatory procedures, and therefore its role is somewhat niche in modern IVF practice with most clinics adopting the density gradient procedure as their front-line methodology. Swim-up may be deployed following density gradient as a further step to refine the final yield for use in IVF treatment. This is, however, time consuming and is not common practice, particularly in large and high-throughput ART service laboratories.

Working with neat semen rather than precentrifuged and pelleted semen is recommended to reduce the risk of process-induced ROS accumulation (Aitken and Clarkson 1988). Working with consumables and media known to be nonreprotoxic, the swim-up column can be prepared by either under-laying or over-laying 1.0 mL of semen against 1.0 mL of sperm culture medium, although most experienced operators would agree that the best differentiation is obtained by under-laying the semen once competence has been obtained. The preparation is then incubated at 35–37 °C for a period of 60 min before

the top (culture medium) fraction is harvested which, in theory, should contain the most motile fraction of the sample or at least a fraction with enhanced motility (Figure 21.2).

Care should be taken when harvesting the swim-up, particularly if the swim-up is performed with semen rather than prepared sperm post density gradient, as it is entirely possible to compromise the whole procedure with an accidental slip of the wrist by accidentally contaminating the yield fraction with seminal plasma and all the nonsperm cells and potential sources of ROS it contains. Harvesting should be performed with a clean pipette starting at the upper meniscus and aspirating gradually downwards until around 75% of the upper layer has been collected. This highly motile seminal fraction can then be resuspended in culture medium to adjust the concentration to the recommended range for IVF (5–20 million sperm per mL) or to a lower or higher concentration for ICSI or IUI.

Use of the Migration Sedimentation Chamber for Sperm Preparation

A more advanced sperm separation technique based on the principles of the swim-up is the migration sedimentation chamber (MSC, Research Instruments, UK). The MSC, as first described comprises of '…two built-in concentric tubes in which the progressive sperm 'jump over' the edge of the central tube. They then sediment at the bottom of the central conical tube where they can be collected by aspiration' (Tea et al. 1984).

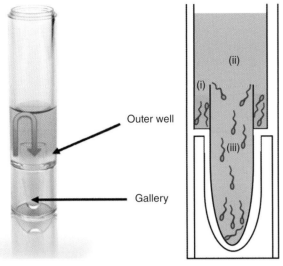

(i) Semen is placed in the wells

(ii) Culture media is added to the device gallery

(iii) Motile sperm migrate from the wells and sediment in the lower chamber.

Outer well

Gallery

Figure 21.3 The migration sedimentation chamber (MSC). Reproduced with permission of Research Instruments.

The MSC is, by comparison to other methodologies, noninvasive, particularly when compared with methodology dependent upon the use of centrifugation (Yener et al. 1990). Essentially the MSC method constitutes a swim-up technique combined with a sedimentation step. The external well of the MSC device is loaded with 400 μL of semen and 2 mL of culture medium is added to the device gallery. The device can then be incubated at 35–37 °C for 60 min before the motile fraction is carefully aspirated from the central gallery taking care not to disturb or accidentally harvest any of the semen from the outer well (Figure 21.3).

MSC sperm preparation, when compared to swim-up of neat or centrifuged and pelleted semen, demonstrated an improvement in the yield and the motility of the recovered sperm whilst the morphology remained unchanged (Ramos et al. 2015). Zavos et al. (2000) evaluated an alternate device, the Multi-ZSC (Biogen, Turkey) which deploys four tiered levels within a single MSC device for sperm preparation. Their study demonstrated that the device was effective in compartmentalizing sperm populations based on their motility and morphology and proposed that the device had a bright future by facilitating the selection of specific subpopulations of sperm for different clinical and research applications. A further study on the efficacy of the Multi-ZSC refuted some of these claims, showing that the yield was much reduced when compared to that published by

Zavos and that the morphometry of the sperm heads declined in the populations harvested from higher up the device (Lampiao and Plessis 2006). Limited further detail is available on the efficacy of MSC devices and they have not been integrated into routine clinical practice despite the early promise shown.

Density Gradient Separation

Density gradient separation of semen is the most commonly deployed method of sperm preparation used in the field of ART today (Figure 21.4). Two methods were developed, continuous and discontinuous density gradient centrifugation, both of which have been demonstrated to be effective in enhancing resultant motility and fertilization capacity as judged by the enhanced ability to penetrate zona-free hamster ova (Berger et al. 1985) as well as the morphology of the resultant sperm preparation (Pousette et al. 1986). To describe the difference between the two, continuous gradients represent a column constructed with a gradual and continuous increase in solution density from the top of the gradient to the bottom. By contrast, the discontinuous gradient is usually formed of two discreet and visible layers, normally one of 40–45% above and one of 80–90% of the density gradient solution. The requirement of continuous density gradient centrifugation for ultra-high centrifugation and the fact

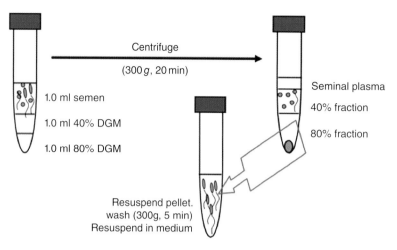

Figure 21.4 Density gradient centrifugation using density gradient medium (DGM).

that the two techniques produced comparable yields means that the discontinuous method is now predominantly used (Nieschlag and Behre 2001).

The process separates morphologically normal, motile sperm from the other cellular and noncellular components based on discrete differences in the density of individual cells using centrifugal force. It is well known and well recorded that the density of living spermatozoal cells differs from that of those that are dead or have degenerated (Nieschlag and Behre 2001).

'Percoll', a suspension of colloidal silica coated with polyvinylpyrrolidone (PVP) (Pertoft et al. 1978), was used in routine clinical practice internationally until late 1996 when its clinical use was suspended principally due to concerns over elevated endotoxin levels within the product which could result in significant inflammation in patients exposed to sperm prepared using the product.

In response to the removal of Percoll as the market leading sperm preparation product, other manufacturers brought to market products promising similar results based upon similar principles of density gradient separation. By basing the solutions (for example PureSperm, SpermGrad, Isolate, SilSelect) on low-toxicity, silane-coated silica particles adjusted for osmolarity with polysucrose (Henkel and Schill 2003), all of these products, unlike Percoll are approved for human use in ART.

A density gradient column is constructed in a non-reprotoxic conical centrifuge tube by preparing two solutions, a 40 or 45% and a 80 or 90% suspension of the density gradient solution, in an appropriate sperm culture medium. The two solutions are mixed thoroughly immediately prior to constructing the column to ensure homogeneity. One millilitre of the higher density layer is pipetted into the conical tube and overlaid with 1.0 mL of the lower density solution. If this is performed with care, the operator can visibly see the interface between the two solutions in the tube. If this interface is not visible, the column should be discarded and a second column constructed. One millilitre of liquefied semen is layered on the top of the density gradient column and the loaded column is centrifuged for 20 min at 300 g. During centrifugation, any cells contained within the semen will sediment at the very top of the density gradient column forming a visible raft as the top layer of the density gradient solution prevents penetration into the column of large nonsperm cells in the ejaculate.

Density gradients separate sperm based on an equilibrium whereby sperm density equals that of the gradient (Le Lannou and Blanchard 1988). Sperm are thus separated principally on the basis of differences in density (Bolton and Braude 1984). Spermatozoa with normal, ovoid heads present a dense and homogeneous nucleus when viewed in an electron microscope, whereas chromatin from atypical heads has a coarsely granular appearance with nuclear vacuoles of various sizes (Le Lannou and Blanchard 1988). Therefore, those sperm with well-packaged nuclear material have a higher density and are able to penetrate the higher density fraction of the column, collecting in a pellet in the very bottom of the conical tube.

Following centrifugation, the pellet can be harvested, washed and the highly motile fraction of sperm obtained used in ART. Great care must be taken when harvesting the pellet to prevent contamination with any of the cells trapped within the density gradient or the semen layer itself. To achieve best results, it is recommended to pipette away and discard the seminal layer, the top layer of the gradient, and the lower layer to well below the interface before harvesting the pellet with a clean pipette. The harvested pellet is resuspended in 3 mL of culture medium and recentrifuged at 300 g for a further 5 to 10 minutes in an attempt to wash away any remnants of the density gradient solution. The subsequent pellet is then re-suspended in a variable volume of culture medium to obtain a concentration of sperm appropriate for the intended ART (see Table 21.2) and is stored appropriately at room temperature prior to use.

The shrewd clinical scientist will be aware that the volume of density gradient solution used to construct the column can be varied to facilitate preparation of severely oligozoospermic samples. The 'mini-percoll' was proposed as an effective method to prepare oligozoospermic samples, resulting in a statistically significant improvement in the posttreatment seminal parameters of motility, progression, and proportion of normal forms as well as improved fertilization rates from IVF (Ord et al. 1990).

Which Technique is 'Better'?

In short, none. All have their advantages and disadvantages (Table 21.3) and all have their place in a well-constructed ART service. A meta-analysis of sperm preparation outcome data has demonstrated that no one technique can or should be recommended (Boomsma et al. 2007). Techniques can and should be combined to maximize quality or deployed individually where quantity is the limiting factor. For example, in patients with elevated ROS levels in the ejaculate or with proven or suspected genital tract inflammations, the conventional swim-up technique should certainly not be the method of choice, but rather more gentle methods like density gradient centrifugation or migration-sedimentation (Henkel and Schill 2003). Most laboratories will have a standard protocol for preparation of sperm, which may vary dependent upon the ART procedure being performed.

Storage of Sperm Preinsemination

Having taken great care to collect, process, and prepare a sperm preparation without causing it any harm, we must also take great care not to cause the sample any harm in the period of time between its preparation and its use in ART. One consideration we must make is whether to store the sample prior to use at 'room temperature' or at a known controlled temperature in a laboratory incubator. Progressive motility and morphology have been demonstrated to be significantly higher after incubation at room temperature compared with 35 °C in a laboratory incubator for 24 h. The proportions of acrosome-reacted, apoptotic, and dead spermatozoa were significantly lower in samples incubated for 24 h at room temperature compared with 35 °C in a laboratory incubator (Thijssen et al. 2014). In addition, it has been demonstrated that

Table 21.2 Recommended final sperm concentrations for different assisted reproductive treatment techniques.

ART Procedure	Recommended Sperm Concentration Range (M/mL)
IUI	>3
IVF	5–20
ICSI / IMSI	1–5[a]

[a] ICSI can be attempted with any concentration of sperm and in some cases the operator will be tasked with searching for individual sperm for extended periods of time to attempt to facilitate treatment. ICSI, intracytoplasmic sperm injection; IMSI, intracytoplasmic morphologically selected sperm injection; IUI, intrauterine insemination; IVF, *in vitro* fertilization.

Table 21.3 The advantages and disadvantages of the most common sperm preparation methods.

Procedure	Advantages	Disadvantages
Sperm washing	Inexpensive Quick Simple to perform	Concentrates cell debris Encourages ROS formation Resultant suspension often difficult to work with
Sperm challenge separation	Inexpensive Most 'natural' Simple to perform Delivers very pure suspension for treatment use Reduction in levels of ROS	Only suitable for highly motile, high concentration samples Lower yield than density gradient procedure Reduction in the proportion of normally chromatin condensed sperm
Density gradient separation	Effective even when sperm concentration is very low Yield is clean and highly motile Significant reduction in levels of ROS in yield	More expensive Greater skill required to construct effective column Increased risk of contamination if poorly conducted
Adaptive filtration	Effective reduction in sperm DNA damage incidence	Regarded as experimental Expensive Time consuming

ROS, reactive oxygen species.

incubation of sperm prior to treatment at 37 °C in a laboratory incubator causes a significant increase in the levels of DNA fragmentation within the prepared sperm over a 24 h period (Matsuura et al. 2010). It is therefore recommended to store sperm prior to insemination at room temperature.

Managing Sero-Discordancy During ART

Some people may request ART because of sero-discordancy within their relationship. The careful management of such cases is of critical importance to ensure that the risk of viral transmission to the partner and/or the resultant offspring is minimized (note the intentional use of the word 'minimized' as this technique offers no more than risk reduction). It is well reported that viruses can persist in cryostored material in a viable condition even after storage in liquid nitrogen (Tedder et al. 1995). A now universally accepted sperm washing procedure was published in 1992, which combines the density gradient and swim-up elements of sperm preparation into one comprehensive protocol.

Using this procedure, the authors reported a sero-conversion rate to partner or neonate of 0% and a pregnancy rate of 51.7% in 29 HIV-negative women inseminated with washed sperm from an HIV-positive partner (Semprini et al. 1992), and subsequently in the facilitation of ICSI treatment (Marina et al. 1998; Peeraer et al. 2004).

With developments in HIV virus research and improvements in highly active antiretroviral drug therapy (HAART), the management of sero-discordancy has shifted away from ART interventions where there is no identifiable fertility diagnosis, and the viral positive male partner is well controlled and HAART compliant. Furthermore, the National Institute for Health and Clinical Excellence (NICE) in their Fertility Guidance document, CG156, published in 2013, recommend that in cases where the HIV-positive man is well controlled, conception should be facilitated by natural intercourse limited to the time of ovulation, with the caveat that both partners are well counselled of the risks involved, no other infections are present, and the male partner has maintained an plasma HIV viral copy load of less than 50 copies/mL for the last 6 months (NICE 2013).

Offering ART to Men with Severe Asthenozoospermia or Necrozoospermia

It is uncommon but not unheard of for men to produce semen samples that contain no motile sperm (necrozoospermia). One example of a medical condition which causes necrozoospermia is Kartagener syndrome, an autosomal recessive genetic disease accounting for approximately 50% of cases of primary ciliary dyskinesia (Yan-Wei et al. 2014), in which most or all of the sperm will appear immotile. Other examples where motility may be significantly compromised are when using frozen/thawed samples or sperm which were retrieved surgically (or both!). Clearly, where motile sperm are not present, treatment which relies upon the ability of the sperm to migrate to the egg to effect fertilization, such as IVF or IUI, is not a viable option, and so ICSI treatment must be deployed. However, how can we determine if a sperm is dead or merely immotile and thus may yet possess fertilization potential?

There are two realistic alternatives to assist with this selection process. We must either reliably identify those sperm which are still viable (in such a way that it is reversible and does not render the sperm unusable) or we must stimulate the sperm in an attempt to rekindle some visible sign of motility. The hypo-osmotic swelling (HOS) test has become well established as an effective clinical tool since early reports of its use 20 years ago (Casper et al. 1996). The test relies on the ability of the tail of a viable sperm to visibly coil when exposed to a culture medium, which is hypo-osmotic, due to an influx of fluid into the tail, which causes the curvature. The effect is rapid, readily identifiable, indicative of vitality, and most importantly, reversible. The skilled operator need only harvest sperm which exhibit coiled tails (and, if numbers permit are also morphologically normal), return these sperm to isosmotic culture medium, and store them for subsequent ICSI treatment.

An alternative method adopts the use of stimulatory chemicals such as pentoxifylline, which serve to stimulate sperm motility without altering the sperm membrane structure (Henkel and Schill 2003). Exposure to pentoxifylline may, in some cases, result in sperm which otherwise appeared immotile regaining nonprogressive (and in some cases even progressive) motility. This methodology has been successfully deployed in ICSI treatment and live births following treatment have been reported (Terriou et al. 2000), although in the UK concerns remain over the use of pentoxifylline clinically as it is not licensed for IVF use.

Preparation of Surgically Retrieved Sperm

The different methodology for the harvesting and processing of sperm and testicular biopsies retrieved surgically from men with obstructive and nonobstructive azoospermia are described in Chapter 23.

It is important to prepare surgically retrieved sperm swiftly and appropriately to optimize yield for ART. Sperm collected surgically differ from those collected via ejaculation as the sperm themselves may lack motility at the time of aspiration and have not been exposed to the other components of semen including the contributions from the accessory glands in the male reproductive tract.

The overlying principle when preparing surgically recovered sperm is to maximize the motile sperm yield whilst reducing as much as practicable the numbers of nonsperm cells. It is highly likely that during the process, any sperm aspirated surgically (or obtained following the processing of testicular tissue), will be harvested along with a significant population of red blood cells. The presence of red blood cells not only represents a challenge from the point of view of debris but also increases the chance and frequency of sperm-to-sperm adherence post-preparation and of the formation of aggregation and 'rafting' in the resultant sperm preparation. Depending on the volume and concentration of sperm harvested and the amount of nonsperm contamination in the aspirates, swim-up, density gradient separation, and basic sperm washing all have a place when preparing the sample for ART use; it is the role of the experienced clinical scientist to best deploy the techniques to obtain the best results.

In circumstances where there is a high level of debris in the final sample it is recommended to pipette the sperm into an ICSI injection dish 15–30 min prior to injection to allow migration of the most motile (and thus desirable) sperm from any debris towards the outer meniscus of the sperm catching drop which is usually formed of polyvinylpyrrolidone (PVP).

Future Methodologies for Sperm Preparation and Selection

Little has functionally changed in the science of sperm selection since the processes of sperm preparation by swim-up and density gradient were first reported in the mid to late twentieth century. Recent technological advances have, however, resulted in the emergence of novel methodologies for selection of sperm which may, for the first time in over 50 years, represent a significant step forwards in practice when coupled with modern ART options.

Magnetic Activated Cell Sorting

Magnetic activated cell sorting (MACS) technology (Figure 21.5) can be used to actively select against sperm demonstrating signs of or a predisposition towards apoptosis. The macromolecule Annexin V is known to bind to receptors on the heads of apoptotic or periapoptotic sperm and, by exposing a suspension of sperm to magnetic particles coated in Annexin V then passing the sperm through a column containing a ferromagnetic matrix, in the presence of a powerful magnetic field, the apoptotic sperm can be removed from the sample (de Vantéry Arrighi et al. 2009).

The resultant sperm preparation can then be adjusted to the required concentration for the relevant ART procedure and used for insemination purposes. It has been proposed that MACS technology confers an improvement in clinical pregnancy rate (Gil et al. 2013) when compared with preparation of sperm by density gradient separation alone and that the levels of DNA fragmented sperm present in the final sperm preparation are reduced (Polak de Fried and Denaday 2010).

Hyaluronan Binding Assay

There is evidence in the literature to suggest that sperm with the greatest capacity to fertilize the egg

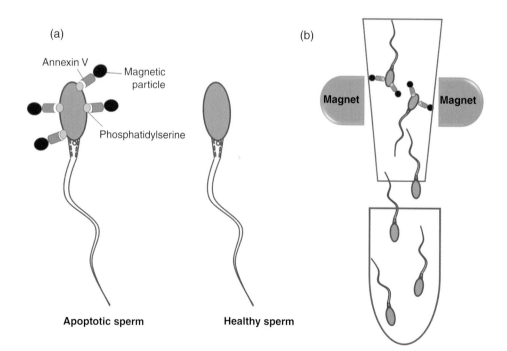

Figure 21.5 Magnetic activated cell sorting. (a) Apoptotic or periapoptotic sperm bind to the Annexin V-coated magnetic beads. No binding occurs in healthy sperm. (b) Separation of sperm is achieved by passing the sperm mix through a magnetic column. Apoptotic sperm are retained while healthy sperm pass though *Source:* Image courtesy of Ana-Maria Tomova.

and form a healthy pregnancy will adhere to hyaluronan *in vitro*. By exposing sperm to a dish coated in hyaluronan during an ICSI procedure, sperm which bind to hyaluronan can be preferentially selected for injection. It is hypothesized that that selection of sperm for injection using HA binding prior to ICSI has beneficial effects on clinical outcomes compared with standard ICSI (Witt et al. 2016).

Intracytoplasmic Morphologically Selected Sperm Injection

First described by in 2002 by Bartoov et al., intracytoplasmic morphologically selected sperm injection (IMSI) uses the motile sperm organelle morphological examination (MSOME) technique to assess individual sperm according to their ultramorphology at a magnification of up to 7000 times (Figure 21.6). At such magnification, vacuolation of the nuclear envelope of the sperm is readily observable and sperm can be categorized into four categories (I, II, III and IV) as described by Vanderzwalmen et al. (2008).

Early published evidence and meta-analyses suggested significant improvements in blastocyst development, pregnancy, and implantation rates when IMSI was performed using sperm types I and II (Bartoov et al. 2003; Souza Setti et al. 2010), although a later meta-analysis demonstrated no effect on live birth and miscarriage rates (Teixeira et al. 2013), recommending that further well-constructed prospective randomized controlled trials are required to draw any robust conclusions. There is also limited evidence to suggest that vacuolation of the nuclear area of the sperm head is linked to sperm DNA fragmentation (Wilding et al. 2011) and studies are ongoing to determine if such a link can be validated as this would represent a significant breakthrough in sperm selection for ART.

Conclusion

There are a multitude of alternate strategies the clinical scientist can deploy to prepare sperm for ART and the techniques can be combined to further enhance results. The clinical scientist will ensure they are skilled in a number of different techniques and will realize that a dynamic and somewhat pragmatic approach should be adopted to each individual sperm preparation procedure. The ultimate aim of sperm preparation is to take a semen sample, do it no harm during collection and processing, and produce a sperm preparation which is of as high a quality as is possible from the raw material provided. As any adept clinical scientist will tell you, this will on occasion involve thinking on your feet and being creative. Should you double up and perform two density gradient columns to increase the yield where concentration is low but volume is high? Should you use swim-up following density gradient separation where yield is high but motility could still be improved? Should you spin the entire sample down and resuspend in culture medium when only one

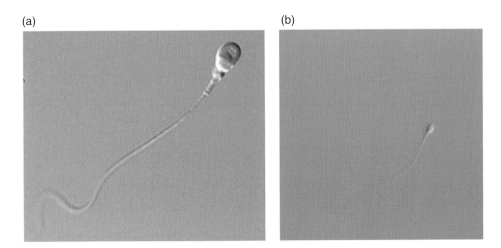

(a) (b)

Figure 21.6 (a) IMSI vs (b) ICSI assessment of sperm. *Source:* Author's own photographs.

single twitching sperm was seen on an entire glass slide? What is certain is without skill and familiarity in the techniques described in this chapter you will not be best equipped to ensure that your patients receive the best possible chances of a successful outcome to their ART treatment under your care.

References

Aitken, R. and Clarkson, J. (1988). Significance of reactive oxygen species and antioxidants in defining the efficacy of sperm preparation techniques. J Androl 9: 376–376.

Bartoov, B., Berkovitz, B., Eltes, F. et al. (2002). Real-time fine morphology of motile human sperm cells is associated with IVF-ICSI outcome. J Androl 23: 1–8.

Bartoov, B., Berkovitz, A., Eltes, F. et al. (2003). Pregnancy rates are higher with intracytoplasmic morphologically selected sperm injection than with conventional intracytoplasmic injection. Fertil Steril 80: 1413–1419.

Berger, P. Marrs, R. and Moyer, D. (1985). Comparison of techniques for selection of motile spermatozoa. Fertil Steril 43: 268–273.

Bolton, V. and Braude, P. (1984). Preparation of human spermatozoa for in vitro fertilization by isopycnic centrifugation on self generating density gradient. Arch Androl 13: 167–176.

Boomsma, C.M., Heineman, M.J., Cohlen, B.J. et al. (2007). Semen preparation techniques for intrauterine insemination. Cochrane Database Syst Rev CD004507.

Casper, R.F., Meriano, J.S., Jarvi, K.A, et al. (1996). The hypo-osmotic swelling test for selection of viable sperm for intracytoplasmic sperm injection in men with complete asthenozoospermia. Fertil Steril 65: 972–976.

de Vantéry Arrighi, C., Lucas, H., Chardonnens, D. et al. (2009). Removal of spermatozoa with externalized phosphatidylserine from sperm preparation in human assisted medical procreation: effects on viability, motility and mitochondrial membrane potential. Reprod Biol Endocrinol 7: 1.

Edwards, R.G., Bavister, B.D. and Steptoe, P.C. (1969). Early stages of fertilization in vitro of human oocytes matured in vitro. Nature 221: 632–635.

Edwards, R.G., Steptoe, P.C. and Purdy, J.M. (1980). Establishing full term human pregnancies using cleaving embryos grown in vitro. Br J Obstet Gynaecol 87: 737–756.

Gil, J., Sar-Shalom, V., Melendez Sivira, Y. et al. (2013). Sperm selection using magnetic activated cell sorting (MACS) in assisted reproduction: a systematic review and meta-analysis. Assist Reprod Genet 30: 479–485.

Henkel, R.A. and Schill, W.B. (2003). Sperm preparation for ART. Reprod Biol Endocrinol 1: 108–129.

Lampiao, F. and Du Plessis, S. (2006). Comparing the Multi-ZSC one-step standardized swim-up method to the double-wash swim-up method with regard to the effects of sperm separation on morphology, head morphometry, and acrosome reaction inducibility. Fertil Steril 86: 739–741.

Le Lannou, D. and Blanchard Y. (1988). Nuclear maturity and morphology of human spermatozoa selected by Percoll density gradient centrifugation or swim-up procedure. J Reprod Fertil 84: 551–556.

Lopata, A., Brown, J.B., Leeton, J.F. et al. (1978). In vitro fertili- zation of preovulatory oocytes and embryo transfer in infer- tile patients treated with clomiphene and human chorionic gonadotropin. Fertil Steril 30: 27–35.

Mahadevan, M. and Baker, G. (1984). Assessment and preparation of semen for in vitro fertilization. In: *Clinical In Vitro Fertilization* (ed. C. Wood and A. Trounson), 83–97. Berlin: Springer-Verlag.

Marina, S., Marina, F., Alcolea, R. et al. (1998). Pregnancy following intracytoplasmic sperm injection from an HIV-1-seropositive man. Hum Reprod 13: 3247–3239.

Matsuura, R., Takeuchi, T. and Yoshida, A. (2010). Preparation andincubation conditions affect the DNA integrity of ejaculated human spermatozoa. Asian J Androl 12: 753–759.

Mortimer, D. (1989). Sperm transport in the human female reproductive tract. In: *Oxford Reviews of Reproductive Biology*, Volume 5 (ed. C.A. Finn), 30. Oxford: Oxford University Press.

Mortimer, D. (1991). Sperm preparation techniques and iatrogenic failures of in-vitro fertilisation. Hum Reprod 6: 173–176.

National Institute for Health and Care Excellence (NICE) (2013). Fertility problems: assessment and treatment, 1.3.10. https://www.nice.org.uk/guidance/cg156/ (accessed 12 February 2018).

Nijs, M., Franssen, K., Cox, A. et al. (2009). Reprotoxicity of intrauterine insemination and in vitro fertilization-embryo transfer disposables and products: a 4-year survey. Fertil Steril 92: 527–535.

Nieschlag, E. and Behre, H. (2001). *Andrology: Male Reproductive Health and Dysfunction*, 2nd edn, 350–351. Berlin: Springer.

Ord, T., Patrizio, P., Marello, E. et al. (1990). Mini-Percoll: a new method of semen preparation for IVF in severe male factor infertility. Hum Reprod 5: 987–989.

Peeraer, K., Nijs, M., Raick, D. et al. (2004). Pregnancy after ICSI with ejaculated immotile spermatozoa from a patient with immotile cilia syndrome: a case report and review of the literature. Reprod Biomed Online 9: 659–663.

Pertoft, H., Laurent, T., Låås, T. et al. (1978). Density gradients prepared from colloidal silica particles coated by polyvinylpyrrolidone (Percoll). Analyt Biochem 88: 271–282.

Polak de Fried, E. and Denaday. F. (2010). Single and twin ongoing pregnancies in two cases of previous ART failure after ICSI performed with sperm sorted using annexin V microbeads. Fertil Steril 94:15–18.

Pousette, A., Akerlöf, E., Rosenborg, L. et al. (1986). Increase in progressive motility and improved morphology of human spermatozoa following their migration through Percoll gradients. Int J Androl 9: 1–13.

Ramos, V.B., Cipriani Dda, C., Araújo, E.S. et al. (2015). Sperm selection using three semen processing techniques. JBRA Assist Reprod 19: 223–226.

Semprini, A.E., Levi-Setti, P., Bozzo, M. et al. (1992). Insemination of HIV-negative women with processed semen of HIV-positive partners. Lancet 340(8831):1317–1319.

Souza Setti, A., Ferreira, R.C., Paes de Almeida Ferreira Braga, D. et al. (2010). Intracytoplasmic sperm injection outcome versus intracytoplasmic morphologically selected sperm injection outcome: a meta-analysis. RBM Online 21: 450–455.

Tea, N.T., Jondet, M. and Scholler, R. (1984). A 'migration-gravity sedimentation' method for collecting motile spermatozoa from human semen. In: In *Vitro Fertilization, Embryo Transfer and Early Pregnancy. Studies in Fertility, Vol. 1* (ed. R.F. Harrison, J. Bonnar and W. Thompson), 117–120. Dordrecht: Springer.

Tedder, R.S., Zuckerman, M.A., Brink, N.S. et al. (1995). Hepatitis B transmission from contaminated cryopreservation tank. Lancet 346(8968): 137–140.

Teixeira, D.M., Barbosa, M.A.P., Ferriani, R.A. et al. (2013). Regular (ICSI) versus ultra-high magnification (IMSI) sperm selection for assisted reproduction. Cochrane Database of Systematic Reviews 7: CD010167.

Terriou, P., Hans, E., Giorgetti, C. et al. (2000). Pentoxifylline initiates motility in spontaneously immotile epididymal and testicular spermatozoa and allows normal fertilization, pregnancy, and birth after intra-cytoplasmic sperm injection. J Assist Reprod Genet 17: 194–199.

Thijssen, A., Klerkx, E., Huyser, C. et al. (2014). Influence of temperature and sperm preparation on the quality of spermatozoa. RBM Online 28: 436–442.

Trounson, A.O., Leeton, J.F, Wood, C. et al. (1980). The investigation of idiopathic infertility by in vitro fertilization. Fertil Steril 34: 431–438.

Vanderzwalmen, P., Hiemer, A., Rubner, P. et al. (2008). Blastocyst development after sperm selection at high magnification is associated with size and number of nuclear vacuoles. RBM Online 17: 617–627.

Wilding, M., Coppola, G., di Matteo, L. et al. (2011). Intracytoplasmic injection of morphologically selected spermatozoa (IMSI) improves outcome after assisted reproduction by deselecting physiologically poor quality spermatozoa. J Assist Reprod Genet 28: 253–262.

Witt, K.D., Beresford, L., Bhattacharya, S., et al. (2016). Hyaluronic Acid Binding Sperm Selection for assisted reproduction treatment (HABSelect): study protocol for a multicentre randomised controlled trial. BMJ Open 6:.e012609.

Yan-Wei, S., Lu, D. and Ping, L. (2014). Management of primary ciliary dyskinesia/Kartagener's syndrome in infertile male patients and current progress in defining the underlying genetic mechanism. Asian J Androl 16: 101–106.

Yates, C.A. and De-Kretser, D.M. (1987). Male-factor infertility and in vitro fertilization. J In Vitro Fert Embryo Transf 4: 141–147.

Yener, C., Mathur, S. and Parent B. (1990). Comparison of two sperm preparation techniques using automated sperm motion analysis: migration sedimentation versus swim-up. Arch Androl 25: 17–20.

Zavos, P.M., Abou-Abdallah, M., Aslanis, P. et al. (2000). Use of the Multi-ZSC one-step standardized swim-up method: recovery of high-quality spermatozoa for intrauterine insemination or other forms of assisted reproductive technologies. Fertil Steril 74: 834 –835.

22

Diagnostic Semen Analysis: Uncertainty, Clinical Value, and Recent Advances

Mathew Tomlinson

What is Semen Analysis?

A diagnostic semen analysis is a systematic microscopic examination of a number of semen parameters, which if performed correctly should have a degree of clinical value. Clinical value in this sense means that testing provides a general indication of a man's reproductive health as well as his approximate chance of fatherhood. It is, however, not an exact science and semen parameters can only be considered as broad prognostic indicators as indicated by Table 22.1. Furthermore, as successful natural and assisted conception are both multifactorial, what the semen analysis is not capable of is accurate prediction of the chance of pregnancy. Information gained from the average testing procedure should, however, help the medical and scientific team to establish: (i) why the patient and his partner have not conceived and (ii) identify the most appropriate treatment (Table 22.1).

Standardization, Limitations, and Uncertainty in Routine Semen Analysis

The relationships between measures of semen quality and the chance of conception has been a controversial subject for decades. Although it is clear that there exist strong associations between natural or assisted conception and the number and motility of sperm, and there exist certain morphological defects, which lead to infertility, significant uncertainty is associated with the measurement of semen parameters. There are a number of clear factors which seem to either suggest or contribute to this uncertainty:

- The numerous confounding factors which contribute to success/failure of conception, even more so where assisted conception is concerned.
- Semen analysis in many centres lacks quality and standardization despite the best efforts of bodies such as the World Health Organization (WHO 1992, 1999, 2010).
- Methods, the application of these methods, and indeed the level of training varies significantly between centres.
- Procedural factors (external influences) are not always controlled for in order to make sense of any result.

Uncertainty in relation to laboratory testing simply means the existence of doubt or level of error associated with a particular measurement or result. An essential component of the laboratory accreditation process (ISO15189, International Standard Organization 2012) is to ensure that methods are 'fit for purpose' and involves assessment and reporting on the level of uncertainty associated with the outcome of any test. Unfortunately, the entire process of diagnostic semen analysis, from specimen collection and transport, to testing, and finally to issuing a report, is prone to error and therefore has associated levels of uncertainty (discussed at length in Tomlinson 2016). This must, where possible, be controlled for in order to gain sensible information for the testing process.

Clinical Reproductive Science, First Edition. Edited by Michael Carroll.
© 2019 John Wiley & Sons Ltd. Published 2019 by John Wiley & Sons Ltd.
Companion website: www.wiley.com/go/carroll/clinicalreproductivescience

Table 22.1 Information provided by the semen analysis.

Aspect of Semen Analysis	Likelihood
Man has sperm or no sperm (sterility v. fertility)	*****
Man has ejaculatory functional defect	****
Sperm have motility	*****
Degree of motility (swimming speed)	**
Sperm parameters within the reference range	***
Sperm meet predefined criteria for correct shape/size	***
Sperm are capable of fertilization/pregnancy	**

Table 22.2 Sperm concentration in consecutive samples in 625 men.[a]

	First Sample	Second Sample	Consistency (%)
Azoospermia	20	19	95
Oligozoospermia	220	194	88
Normozoospermia	386	411	94

[a] M.J. Tomlinson, unpublished data.

Sources of Uncertainty – Biological Variability?

It has long been assumed that an individual's semen quality often varies from sample to sample and in extreme cases, from normal to having parameters in the pathological range. If this was the case it would significantly reduce the clinical value of any single test. Intersample variation is subject to differences in the degree of sexual abstinence, specimen collection methods, or indeed quality assurance in relation to sperm concentration assessment (Francavilla et al. 2007). This was confirmed by data from our own laboratories where two samples were routinely collected from each patient, 10 weeks apart, with all men adhering to the same specimen acceptance criteria. Between sample sperm concentration was relatively stable with regard to overall diagnosis. Table 22.2 shows that of the 625 men producing a 'normal' sperm count (at the time $>20 \times 10^6$/mL), 386 (62%) in their first sample, 411 also produced a normal sperm count on their second visit (93% agreement). Of the 220 men who were oligozoospermic in their first sample, 194 would receive the same diagnosis the second time around (88% agreement), and of the 20 men who were azoospermic, 19 also had no sperm in the second sample (95% agreement) (Table 22.2).

This demonstrates that the overall 'diagnostic uncertainty' or error due to biological variation is perhaps less than has been described previously and can be reduced by implementing recommended laboratory methods and proper training of staff. Perhaps with tighter control and examination of 'total sperm output' as opposed to concentration, even more consistency between samples may be achievable. Despite this data, repeating semen analysis would remain a sensible course of action where abnormalities are detected.

Sources of Uncertainty – Pre-Examination

Information has to be sufficiently instructive to ensure that the patient collects the specimen using an appropriate method (masturbation or, in exceptional cases, intercourse using a silastic sheath), after the appropriate period of sexual abstinence, using the correct container. The specimen must be delivered to the laboratory in a suitable condition for testing, i.e. external influences on sperm quality have been minimized (WHO 2010; Mortimer et al. 2013). The next key stage is specimen reception, which acts as a gateway to the laboratory and ensures that its 'specimen acceptance' criteria are complied with, i.e. that the patient has followed the instructions provided and has collected a complete sample. Moreover, the specimen reception is often the first (and only) point of contact with the laboratory and often the only opportunity for the patient's identity to be confirmed 'beyond reasonable doubt'. It is worth bearing in mind at this stage that a laboratory can have the most rigorous testing and quality assurance procedures in place, but if the patient is misidentified, the test becomes not only wasteful but potential misleading or even harmful.

Essentially there are four phases of the pre-examination process, which require laboratory control: (i) specimen request; (ii) information/instruction to the patient; (iii) sample collection; (iv) delivery and specimen reception. The key areas of provision of instruction for semen analysis clearly differ from other areas of laboratory medicine in that sample quality is highly dependent on both the duration of sexual abstinence, duration and quality of sexual stimulation at collection, and the delay between collection and analysis (Björndahl et al. 2010). The first and last of these three aspects therefore require careful control but are highly dependent on patient compliance with the instructions provided. A further consideration is the need to minimize the risk of exposure to either extremes of temperature or sperm toxicants. Control is achieved in part by giving specific instruction, but also important is the use of specimen containers as well as other laboratory plastics (pipettes, tips, tubes) which have batch traceability and have been toxicity tested on sperm. Unnecessary delays in testing are likely to have an effect on 'time-dependent' semen parameters such as motility and agglutination. As motility could become significantly reduced and agglutination could increase, laboratories should comment on results obtained from samples that do not conform to the requirements for collection and handling, and clearly declare how the lack of compliance influences the interpretation of results.

Sources of Uncertainty – Examination Process

As the vast majority of semen samples contain an extremely heterogeneous cohort of sperm in terms of their function and morphology, the key to any sperm quality test is firstly to obtain a well-mixed sample. If homogenization is hampered by high viscosity or heavy agglutination/aggregation then a reliable result is less likely. Performing multiple measures (multiple sampling) and taking a mean measurement, or indeed using an enzyme digester such as chymotrypsin to treat samples prior to measuring sperm concentration, can help reduce error. Secondly, regardless of the parameter under examination, the uncertainty due to sampling error should be minimized by assessing larger numbers of sperm. Four hundred sperm per testing procedure should be viewed as the acceptable

minimum, reducing sampling error to below 5% (WHO 2010). Lastly, the testing methods themselves must satisfy some very basic criteria in order to be of clinical value and have little associated uncertainty including:

- Validity: evidence that its use relates to a clinical picture.
- Reliability: technique achieves the right answer.
- Repeatability: repeat testing achieves the same answer.
- Reproducibility: different individuals achieve the same answer.

Sperm Concentration

Several publications have shown that sperm concentration measurements are highly dependent on the method used (Ginsburg and Armant 1990; Mahmoud et al. 1997; Bailey et al. 2007; Kirkman-Brown and Björndahl 2009). However, demonstration of method reliability currently requires a demonstration of parity with the haemocytometer as the current gold standard until such time as a new standard is shown to be more reliable and reproducible. Although aimed at improving standardization further, the highly prescriptive approach to haemocytometer use described in the latest WHO (2010) manual is an acknowledgement that the method can also be prone to error. The WHO protocol has been refined over the years to improve consistency further by suggesting that: pipette tips are wiped prior to dispensing semen; the chamber is loaded quickly before sperm have time to settle out of suspension; the number of sperm counted is increased and repeated if two sides of the chamber do not agree. All are all sensible control measures but are by no means a foolproof guarantee that an error cannot be made. In fact, the estimation of any sperm parameter is susceptible to the errors associated with a lack of homogeneity. Thorough sample mixing and homogenization is therefore critical for accuracy and precision but it is not necessarily always possible. The haemocytometer is particularly susceptible if the sample is viscous and/or agglutinated and cannot be accurately diluted or homogenized. A sensible measure in cases where homogenization is deemed unlikely is to inform the requesting clinician and offer a repeat test.

Alternatives to the haemocytometer have been available for many years, especially several that profess to allow enumeration of sperm whilst still motile. These are marketed as either a specialist reusable sperm counting chamber, e.g. Horwell® (Horwell Ltd, London, UK) or Makler® (Sefi Medical Instruments, Haifa, Israel), or a disposable slide with a fixed coverslip which has a known chamber depth of 20 μm, e.g. Leja® (Gynotec Malden, Nieuw-Vennep, the Netherlands), CellVision® (CellVision, Heerhugowaard, the Netherlands), or Microcell® (Conception Technologies, San Diego, CA, USA). Results with the Horwell® and Makler® chambers are reported as being inconsistent and unreliable (relative to the haemocytometer), with the former giving significant overestimations and the latter giving both over- and underestimations (Shiran et al. 1995; Mahmoud et al. 1997; Bailey et al. 2007). Although popular in an *in vitro* fertilization (IVF) setting because of their convenience, one-step methods such as these introduce errors associated with estimating numbers of 'moving sperm' and have therefore found parity with the haemocytometer difficult to achieve. Figure 22.1 summarizes the most commonly used methods for the assessment of sperm concentration, highlighting how they are generally used and general advantages and disadvantages of each.

Chamber/method	Diluted/undiluted	Advantages	Disadvantages
1. Haemocytometer 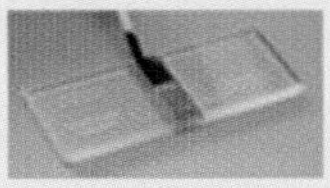	Fixed/diluted	Evidence base/validation Reliable Sperm immobilized	Inaccurate for viscous samples Dilution and mathematics prone to error Time consuming EQA results show wide variability
2. Horwell® 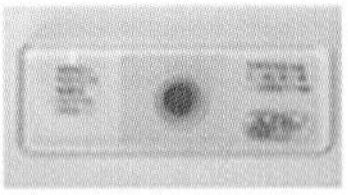	Undiluted	Simple, rapid	Relies on enumeration of motile sperm Little or no validation Overestimates relative to 1
3. Makler® 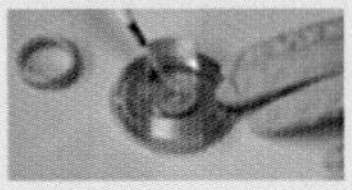	Undiluted	Simple, rapid	Enumeration of motile sperm Results variable and ureliable with both under- and overestimation published Relatively poor validation
4. Microcell®/Leja® 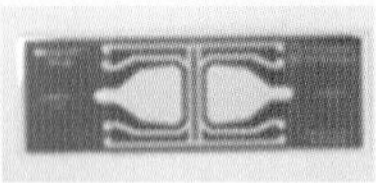	Undiluted or fixed/diluted	Simple, rapid	Enumeration of motile sperm Underestimates relative to 1 Reliable if sample fixed/diluted (Bailey et al. 2007) Cumbersome calculations
5. CASA 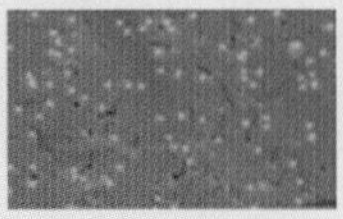	Undiluted or diluted	Rapid Simultaneous assessment of count/motility/velocity Relatively good validation Reproducibility and removal of human error	Tends to underestimate (relative to 1.) Some (older) systems unable to remove debris or nonsperm cells Relies on slide 4

Figure 22.1 Alternative methods used for assessing sperm concentration.

Sperm Motility

The difficulty in providing reliable manual estimates of sperm motility has been acknowledged for many years. Apart from the consensus view of the WHO, the industry lacks a 'gold standard' methodology, which would form the basis of any validation exercise, or calibration material that could be used to train scientific staff. The grading of sperm swimming speed 'by eye' is highly subjective. Even the experienced operator cannot avoid focusing on a moving object or studying the field for several minutes during which time many sperm will have entered the field and left. This leaves only the immotile fraction enumerated with any accuracy and an overcounting of motile sperm, which is compounded in samples with higher density and high velocity sperm (Tomlinson et al. 2010). This can easily be demonstrated by comparing motility scored directly from the microscope with that obtained from a time-limited video loop where the percentage progression is usually significantly lower. Indeed, if the author was to make any recommendation for improving the reliability of manual assessments it would be to create video clips of between one and two seconds and estimate the motility from these instead of the microscope. The advantage of automated systems is that they estimate motility usually for 0.5 to one second; any longer and too many sperm will have left or entered the field, distorting the proportion of immotile to motile sperm. It is interesting that the WHO (2010) has now abandoned the grading of sperm into four categories (a, b, c, d) in favour of the simpler alternative which considers both progressive grades (a and b) together, apparently for no other reason than its relative technical simplicity. However, many believe that although this move reduces uncertainty in the mind of the operator it will reduce clinical relevance of manual sperm motility assessment, since sperm velocity has been repeatedly demonstrated to be of more significance than simple progression (Barratt et al. 1992; Larsen et al. 2000; Garrett et al. 2003; Björndahl, 2010; Barratt et al. 2011).

Another fundamental issue associated with motility measurement is the failure of many laboratories to use any sort of temperature control. Sperm velocity and therefore the degree of progression is highly temperature dependent and will fluctuate greatly from room temperature to measurement at $37\,^{\circ}$C. Table 22.3 shows the shift, not in progression, but from percent grade b to percent grade a in response to increasing temperature, which not only illustrates how sensitive sperm are to temperature but also how this effect would be missed if only progression was measured.

Sperm Morphology

Sperm morphology analysis has been surrounded by controversy for many years and possibly more than any other semen parameter. Like motility it is subject to human perception and interpretation but unlike motility, which has an obvious function, there exists little evidence to demonstrate conclusively exactly which sperm shapes or sizes are compatible with fertility. Published data on the definition of

Table 22.3 Mean sperm count and motility parameters for 25 samples analysed first at room temperature (19–23 °C) and using a heated microscope stage (36–37 °C). Parameters were compared by Student's *t*-test after log transformation.

	Cold (19–23 °C)					Warm (36–37 °C)				
	Count (millions)	Grade a (%)	Grade b (%)	pm	Velocity	Count (millions)	Grade a (%)	Grade b (%)	pm	Velocity
Mean	44.38	20.5[a]	22.0[a]	46.1	20.3[a]	45.1	28.9	14.1	46.6	28.3
Min	13	5	9	18	15.2	13	7	5	12	21.5
Max	95	58	30	77	29	89	64	24	84	40.7

[a] P < 0.001 Warm versus cold. pm, progressive motility.

'normal' or 'ideal' are derived from associations between populations of sperm found in the female reproductive tract and either natural or assisted conception (Mortimer and Menkveld 2001). Sperm found in cervical mucus or close to the site of fertilization are significantly more homogeneous than those in semen, yet fundamentally there is no certainty that only 'normal' sperm can fertilize. Conversely, we cannot be sure that sperm with defects (either subtle or less subtle) are incapable of achieving fertilization unless the defect is clearly likely to have an effect on sperm function, e.g. absence of acrosome or tail. Fundamentally, this is because the assays used to measure sperm morphology are performed on sperm whose functional capacity remains largely unknown. This leads to a number of unanswerable questions, which exacerbate any associated uncertainty, i.e. the sperm may be labelled morphologically 'normal', but how do we know that the sperm was also motile or otherwise functionally competent. Conversely, a morphologically borderline sperm form or one considered to have a less than 'ideal' shape may well be very capable of swimming the length of the female reproductive tract and possessing the necessary characteristics to complete fertilization. Morphology assessment is recommended using fixed sperm, usually stained with the Papanicoloau (Pap) or Diff Quik stains (Figure 22.2). The trend is currently to report the percentage of normal forms only and score those sperm according to 'strict criteria' based on the original data by Kruger et al. (1986) and discussed at

length in Mortimer and Menkveld (2001). The fundamental difference from the previous system requires the technician to categorize any sperm that does not meet these criteria (including borderline sperm) as 'abnormal'.

This in itself creates uncertainty since the 'borderline' form could easily be incorrectly classified due to: individuals having slight differences in interpretation; creation of artefacts by fixation and processing; or an inability to see sperm adequately it they adhere to artefacts such as debris or nonsperm cells (Boersma et al. 2001; Rothman et al. 2013). As a consequence of strict scoring and the adaptation of laboratories to current methods, the average number of 'normal' sperm per sample has become significantly reduced and has lowered the recognized reference range for the 'fertile' population. The WHO (2010) have adopted the 'strict morphology' assessment, suggesting a reference limit of 4%, derived from the fifth centile of a population of fertile couples conceiving within 12 months. However, modern laboratories should be aware that the clinical studies which were used to underpin the 'strict philosophy' were based on remarkably low numbers of patients and did not use the most robust or highly successful IVF system. Moreover, they have never been adequately reproduced and indeed more recent and more powerful data suggests that the reporting of the percentage of normal forms according to strict criteria is of little or no clinical value (Hotaling et al. 2011; Van der Hoven et al. 2015).

With this in mind, it is difficult to offer the andrology laboratory an alternative other than to suggest that morphological criteria associated with more certainty should be the focus. A limited number of morphological defects are most definitely associated with aberrant sperm function and laboratories will not be forgiven for failure to recognize them. These include: globozoospermia (absence of acrosome); absence of a normal tail ('stump tail'); multiple tails (both affecting motility); multiple heads; amorphous (which may affect motility and DNA structure) (Figure 22.3). Examination and recording of defects which are the result of 'strict' scoring, such as subtle changes in size, shape, or a blemish (some of which could be artefacts), will remain controversial and associated with uncertainty until such a time that morphology can be more definitively related to function.

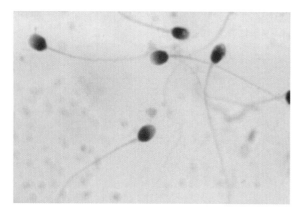

Figure 22.2 Sperm morphology fixed and stained using Papanicoloau.

Figure 22.3 Sperm defects which could be classified as 'high risk': (a) Globozoospermia. (b) 'Stump' tails. (c) Multiple tails. (d) Multiple head and tails (conjoined).

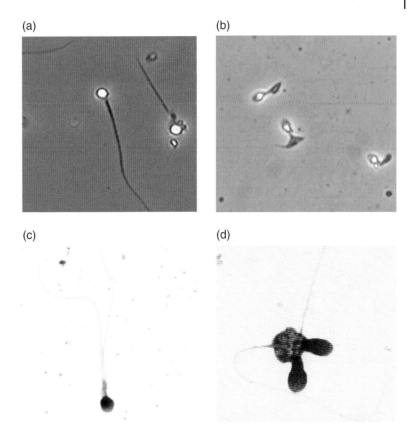

Computer-Assisted Semen Analysis (CASA)

The idea of a computer-assisted system that provides basis semen analysis data more quickly, more reliably, and more reproducibly than can be achieved manually is clearly an attractive one. If it is validated against a reliable standard then the advantages in terms of consistency are clear. Computer algorithms are more likely to give comparable data between technicians or between laboratories. Unfortunately, adoption of such systems has not been straightforward, with early systems proving to be quite 'clunky', inaccurate, and provided sperm kinetic parameters that had little clinical value, which failed to gain the confidence of the market.

More recently, systems have been developed which are more user-friendly and have slowly gained acceptance. However, the majority of laboratories continue to resist change and find it difficult to relinquish their well-established manual methods even if they are prone to error and associated with

uncertainty. This is perhaps understandable when early CASA systems failed to show anywhere near parity with the haemocytometer for concentration and were prone to missing sperm, detecting debris and nonsperm cells. Despite providing intricate motility parameters, if sperm detection itself was a fundamental problem, then confidence in the measurements would be low. Sperm detection with CASA is something of a compromise and depends on how the computer algorithms deal with different-sized objects. If any objects are allowed to be detected, then all sperm may be recognized but so too will nonsperm cells and debris. Restricting detection to objects of sperm size does not account for variation of head size and changing image quality due to the optical properties of seminal fluid from different patients. To overcome the problem of distinguishing sperm from nonsperm cells, more recent systems such as the SCA® (sperm class analyzer) from Microptic (Barcelona, Spain) and the SAMi CASA system (Staffordshire, UK) provide an intuitive solution, allowing editing of the captured sperm screen (Figure 22.4) to ensure that (i) only sperm are detected and (ii) missed sperm can be replaced which gives a more reliable sperm concentration and one which is in line with the haemocytometer (Tomlinson et al. 2010). Moreover, if object identification can be considered more accurate then it stands to reason that the ratio of motile to immotile objects will also be classified with more reliability.

Semen parameters based on sperm kinetics were developed partly in response to the interest in CASA in the early 1990s and used as either an adjunct to semen analysis or to study sperm hyperactivation. A number of sperm motion parameters which cannot be measured manually were permitted by video frame analysis, such as lateral head displacement (ALH) and beat cross frequency (BCF), and three different measures of sperm velocity: path velocity (VAP), curvilinear velocity (VCL), and straight-line velocity (VSL) velocity (Figure 22.5). Sperm hyperactivation, which it is postulated occurs as part of the capacitation process, has been defined using thresholds for these parameters but to date its

clinical relevance remains uncertain, especially in the human (Zhu et al. 1994; Mortimer 1997). Since the measurement of sperm kinetics is a product of the use of CASA systems, and ultimately the

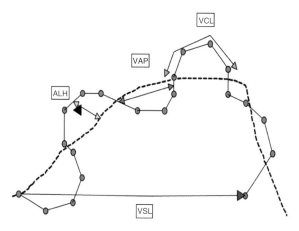

Figure 22.5 Schematic of sperm kinetic parameters permitted by CASA analysis. ALH, lateral head displacement; VAP, path velocity; VCL, curvilinear velocity; VSL, straight-line velocity.

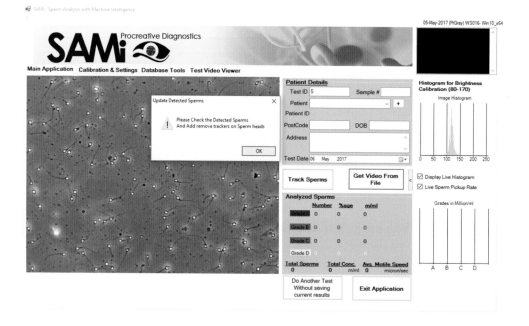

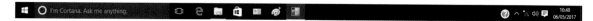

Figure 22.4 Editing using the SAMi system – nonsperm objects are normally excluded based on size. Objects detected in error and can be deleted at this stage (insert).

values obtained from each machine will differ depending on the video frame rate employed or duration of tracking, justification for the routine measurement of for example ALH or BCF is difficult. However, sperm velocity is a different matter and in general appears to be correlated with an improved chance of conception, either naturally (Barratt et al. 1992) or through assisted reproductive techniques (Marshburn et al. 1992; Larsen et al. 2000; Garrett et al. 2003). Deciding which particular estimate of velocity is the most biologically relevant is difficult, bearing in mind that the variations in what should be a simple distance/time calculation are only permitted because of the intricacies of the algorithms used in the various CASA devices. The distance travelled for VSL is the end-point minus the start point so can only truly represent distance/time if the sperm are travelling in straight lines, since a sperm following a curved trajectory could be misrepresented (Figure 22.5).

VAP is a smoothed average path velocity and VCL is probably the best reflection of distance travelled over time since it takes into account each video data point. Both represent sperm swimming speed adequately and moreover give a more objective value than is possible by any manual motility analysis. However, in general, longer sperm tracking and higher frame rates are preferable, but this is always a compromise since tracking sperm for much longer than one second reduces the number of sperm which

may be analysed in a single field of view. Systems which track for less than one second and at a frame rate of 25–30 Hz will capture a large number of sperm in a given field, but the sperm track will be short and have a 'smoothed' appearance. Others which track for longer and at a higher frame rate will capture fewer sperm per analysis but their trajectories may more accurately reflect a true pattern of motion (Figure 22.6). Importantly, from a clinical laboratory perspective, objective assessment of sperm velocity and motility in a large population of sperm can only be permitted using a CASA instrument and takes on even more significance when the current guidance for manual assessment is considered.

CASA and Sperm Morphology

Sperm morphology modules have been offered by CASA manufacturers for more than 20 years but laboratories remain sceptical regarding its role in routine semen analysis, possibly even more so than with sperm concentration and motility. Users are perhaps right to remain cautious especially since (as discussed earlier) the definitions employed for normal and abnormal sperm are associated with such a high level of uncertainty that by automating the process, the end result might well be a more consistent outcome but one which could be consistently incorrect. There are no data which supports

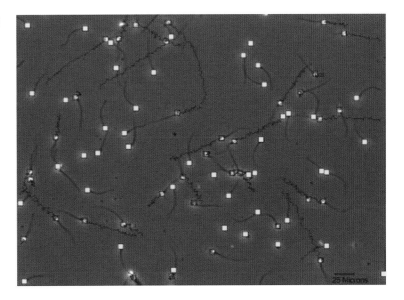

Figure 22.6 Tracked sample showing sperm swimming at speeds of up to 75–80 μm per second.

automated sperm morphology analysis in favour of manual analysis and in many cases automation of analysis at high power (x 1000) can take longer than a manual test. Until the definition of what is considered 'normal' and how 'borderline' forms should be managed is fully understood by the andrology industry then there is little or no advantage to automating the process.

Optional Tests (Antisperm Antibodies and DNA Fragmentation)

The use of the term 'optional' is not necessarily to belittle the importance of these perhaps more difficult to measure sperm characteristics, but simply to demonstrate that many bodies including the WHO, ASRM (American Society for Reproductive Medicine), and ESHRE (European Society for Human Reproduction and Embryology) consider them to be more peripheral or nonroutine. Both are associated with a lack of consensus regarding the most appropriate testing regime and their exact relationship with the success or failure of either natural or assisted conception (Barratt et al. 2010; Zini et al. 2011; Tomlinson et al. 2013).

Rumke and Hellinga (1959) first described the existence of antibodies to sperm in the 1950s and despite a flurry of research activity in the 1980s and 1990s, for many laboratories, antisperm antibody (ASA) measurement is becoming almost redundant. There remains little evidence for a direct association between fertilization failure at IVF, or pregnancy failure due to ASA, independent of other sperm factors such as motility and/or agglutination. One of the few meta-analyses performed on the subject by Zini et al. (2011) considered 10 IVF and six intracytoplasmic sperm injection (ICSI) studies which met their inclusion criteria and failed to find any significant link between the presence or level of ASAs and pregnancy. However, they did concede that the most commonly used laboratory methods (immunobead test or SpermMar test (Fertipro, Beernem, Belgium)) were crude at best and were unable to determine the exact function of the immunoglobulin being detected. This should serve as a key message and is applicable to all testing procedures that if the test itself is 'surrounded by uncertainty' then so will the clinical answers provided by that test. There is no standardized 'gold standard' ASA method and inconsistency in interpretation of the various tests based on an indirect test prompted the UKNEQAS scheme to abandon its EQA (external quality assessment) antibody scheme some years ago. Until such time that a properly validated, reliable, and reproducible test can be produced, routine ASA testing is unlikely to be recommended.

DNA fragmentation testing by one of a number of semi-established methods is routinely offered in many laboratories and at least some of these appear to offer information relating to events upstream of fertilization, which may add to the value of the more conventional parameters. However, the arguments in favour of routine DNA damage testing either over traditional semen parameters or as an additional independent parameter remain difficult to interpret. In one of the few meta-analyses available, Zini et al. (2008) examined a total of 808 IVF and 741 ICSI cycles from 11 studies and showed a consensus association between DNA damage and pregnancy loss but not fertilization or pregnancy. Another analysis by Simon et al. (2014) is slightly more positive showing that sperm DNA damage measured by COMET and TUNEL assays were associated with fertilization rate, embryo quality, and implantation rate and may therefore add significant information to the semen analysis. What is clear from the available evidence is that amongst the available tests (COMET; Sperm Chromatin Structure Assay (SCSA®); Terminal deoxynucleotidyl transferase-mediated fluorescein-dUTP Nick End Labelling (TUNEL); Sperm Chromatin Dispersion (SCD) or HALO test) none can be considered a 'gold standard'. Moreover, only two of these assays (HALO and TUNEL) are suitable for routine testing in the average andrology laboratory as they are available in kit form and do not require specialist equipment. The position of the ESHRE (European Society for Human Reproduction and Embryology) SIGA (specialist interest group in andrology) supports the idea that a more robust test is required before it can be used routinely (Barratt et al. 2010; Tomlinson et al. 2013). Until such time that data generated in one centre are adequately reproduced in another using the same method and there is consensus on how patients with an adverse result should be managed, DNA fragmentation assays will continue to be viewed with a healthy level of scepticism.

Conclusion: Clinical Value of Semen Analysis

Bearing in mind the previous discussion on uncertainty, it is perhaps not surprising that the clinical value of semen analysis is a controversial subject area and that many studies do not agree with each other. Tomlinson et al. (2013) provide a basic overview of the potential 'confounding factors' in a single IVF sample, which also contribute to outcome. Although not an exhaustive list, semen variables (concentration, motility, morphology, and volume) represented only 13% (4 of 30) amongst a list of both clinical and embryological parameters deemed to contribute to a positive outcome, so it is perhaps no wonder that it is difficult to know answers to questions such as: what is the minimum or optimum number of morphologically normal or progressively motile sperm required to result in pregnancy? The answer will never be very precise until such time that semen analysis is able to combine analysis of these primary parameters with more detailed tests of sperm function and integrity. The answer may be slightly more straightforward when discussing either artificial insemination or natural conception since without the intervention of the embryology lab, the level of 'confounding variables' is a magnitude lower. Therefore, in their recent review Tomlinson et al. (2013) concluded that the average semen analysis was simply not sufficiently sensitive for a suitable threshold or 'cut off' for suitability for IVF to be decided, and the simple answer was that for IVF, semen quality was below that required for IUI (intrauterine insemination) or natural conception. Furthermore, and for the same reasons, ICSI was required when it was considered high risk to contemplate IVF with any given sample.

Because of the level of laboratory uncertainty and the lack of suitable trials, only very large studies or a 'body of evidence' based on similar studies would seem to carry sufficient weight for the laboratory community to take notice. Despite the average ejaculate containing in excess of 60 million sperm and some many more, a number of notable studies have demonstrated that as few as 5 million motile sperm are required for a reasonable chance of success through IUI (Wainer et al. 2004; Van Weert et al. 2004; Badawy et al. 2009; Merviel et al. 2010; Tomlinson et al. 2013). Moreover, the extensive studies commissioned by the WHO prior to the latest edition of the semen analysis manual (WHO 2010) in many ways parallel this number, having provided the latest reference range from the fifth centile of: sperm concentration 15×10^6/mL; progression 32%; and normal forms 4% (Cooper et al. 2009). Taking the WHOs own data, most couples with $>5 \times 10^6$ motile sperm would seem to belong to the 'fertile' as opposed to the 'subfertile' category. The question remains, however: does the evidence point towards a 5 million motile sperm threshold because it represents a real biological optimum or is it simply because below this level, semen analysis is simply too insensitive to detect a lower threshold. Until laboratory semen analysis becomes more reliable and is associated with a lower degree of uncertainty, we will not know.

Conflict of Interest Declaration

The author of this article is a part-time co-director of Procreative Diagnostics, a company involved in the research, development, and commercialization of a novel CASA system.

References

Badawy, A., Elnashar, A. and Eltotongy, M. (2009). Effect of sperm morphology and number on success of intrauterine insemination. Fertil Steril 91: 777–781.

Bailey, E., Fenning, N.R., Chamberlain, S. et al. (2007). Validation of sperm counting methods using Limits of Agreement. J Androl 28: 364–373.

Barratt, C.L., Björndahl, L., Menkveld, R. et al. (2011). ESHRE special interest group for andrology basic semen analysis course: a continued focus on accuracy, quality, efficiency and clinical relevance. Hum Reprod 26: 3207–3212.

Barratt, C.L.R., Tomlinson, M.J. and Cooke, I.D. (1992). Prognostic significance of computerized motility analysis for in vivo fertility. Fertil Steril 60: 520–525.

Barratt, C.L., Aitken, R.J., Bjorndahl, L. et al. (2010). Sperm DNA: organization, protection and vulnerability: from basic science to clinical applications–a position report. Hum Reprod 25: 824–838.

Barratt, C.L.R., Tomlinson, M.J. and Cooke, I.D. (1992). Prognostic significance of computerized motility analysis for in vivo fertility. Fertil Steril 60: 520–525.

Björndahl, L. (2010). The usefulness and significance of assessing rapidly progressive spermatozoa. Asian J Androl 12: 33–35.

Björndahl, L., Mortimer, D., Barratt, C.L. et al. (2010). *A Practical Guide to Basic Laboratory Andrology*, 1st edn. Cambridge: Cambridge University Press.

Boersma, A., Rasshofer, R. and Stolla, R. (2001). Influence of sample preparation, staining procedure and analysis conditions on bull sperm head morphometry using the morphology analyser integrated visual optical system Reprod Domest Anim 236: 222–229.

Cooper, T.G., Noonan, E., von Eckardstein, S. et al. (2009). World Health Organization reference values for human semen characteristics. Hum Reprod Update 16: 231–245.

Francavilla, F., Barbonetti, A., Necozione, S. et al. (2007). Within-subject variation of seminal parameters in men with infertile marriages. Int J Androl 30: 174–181.

Garrett, C., Liu, D.Y., Clarke, G.N. et al. (2003). Automated semen analysis: 'zona pellucida preferred' sperm morphometry and straight-line velocity are related to pregnancy rate in subfertile couples. Hum Reprod 18: 1643–1649.

Ginsburg, K.A. and Armant, D.R. (1990). The influence of chamber characteristics on the reliability of sperm concentration and movement measurements obtained by manual and videomicrographic analysis Fertil Steril 5: 882–887.

Hotaling, J.M., Smith, J.F., Rosen, M. et al. (2011). The relationship between isolated teratozoospermia and clinical pregnancy after in vitro fertilization with or without intracytoplasmic sperm injection: a systematic review and meta-analysis. Fertil Steril 95: 1141–1145.

ISO15189, International Standard Organization 2012 (https://www.ukas.com/services/accreditation-services/medical-laboratory-accreditation-iso-15189/)

Kirkman-Brown, J. and Björndahl, L. (2009). Evaluation of a disposable plastic Neubauer counting chamber for semen analysis. Fertil Steril 91: 627–631.

Kruger, T.F., Menkveld, R., Stander, F.S. et al. (1986). Sperm morphologic features as a prognostic factor in in vitro fertilization. Fertil Steril 46: 1118–1123.

Larsen, L., Scheike, T., Jensen, T.K. et al. (2000). A computer–assisted semen analysis parameters as predictors for fertility of men from the general population. The Danish First Pregnancy Planner Study Team. Hum Reprod 15: 1562–1567.

Mahmoud, A.M., Depoorter, B., Piens, N. et al. (1997). The performance of 10 different methods for the estimation of sperm concentration Fertil Steril 68: 340–345

Marshburn, P.B., McIntire, D., Carr, B.R. et al. (1992). Spermatozoal characteristics from fresh and frozen donor semen and their correlation with fertility outcome after intrauterine insemination. Fertil Steril 58: 179–186.

Merviel, P., Heraud, M.H., Grenier, N. et al. (2010). Predictive factors for pregnancy after intrauterine insemination (IUI): an analysis of 1038 cycles and a review of the literature. Fertil Steril 93: 79–88.

Mortimer, S.T. (1997). A critical review of the physiological importance and analysis of sperm movement in mammals. Hum Reprod 3: 403–439.

Mortimer, D. and Menkveld, R. (2001). Sperm morphology assessment–historical perspectives and current opinions. J Androl 22: 192–205.

Mortimer, D., Barratt, C. L., Björndahl, L. et al. (2013) What should it take to describe a substance or product as 'sperm-safe'. Hum Reprod Update 19(Suppl 1): i1–45; 306–311.

Rothmann, S.A., Bort, A.M., Quigley, J. et al. (2013). Sperm morphology classification: a rational method for schemes adopted by the world health organization. Methods Mol Biol 927: 27–37.

Rumke, P. and Hellinga, G. (1959). Autoantibodies against spermatozoa in sterile men. Am J Clin Pathol 32: 357–363.

Shiran, E., Stoller, J., Blumenfeld, Z. et al. (1995). Evaluating the accuracy of different sperm counting chambers by performing strict counts of photographed beads. J Assist Reprod Genet 12: 434–442.

Simon, L., Liu, L., Murphy, K. et al. (2014). Comparative analysis of three sperm DNA damage assays and sperm nuclear protein content in couples undergoing assisted reproduction treatment. Hum Reprod 29: 904–917.

Tomlinson, M.J. (2016). Uncertainty of measurement and clinical value of semen analysis: has standardisation through professional guidelines helped or hindered progress? Andrology 4: 763–770.

Tomlinson, M.J., Lewis, S. and Morroll, D. (2013). Sperm quality and its relationship to natural and assisted conception: British Fertility Society Guidelines for Practice. Hum Fertil 16: 175–193.

Tomlinson, M.J., Naeem, A., Jayaprakasan, K. et al. (2010). Validation of a novel computer assisted sperm analysis (CASA) system employing multi-target tracking algorithms. Fertil Steril 93: 1911–1920.

van den Hoven, L., Hendriks, J.C, Verbeet, J.G. et al. (2015). Status of sperm morphology assessment: an evaluation of methodology and clinical value. Fertil Steril 103: 53–58.

Van Weert, J.M., Repping, S., Van Voorhis, B.J. et al. (2004). Performance of the postwash total motile sperm count as a predictor of pregnancy at the time of intrauterine insemination: a meta-analysis. Fertil Steril 82: 612–620.

Wainer, R., Albert, M., Dorion, A. et al. (2004). Influence of the number of motile spermatozoa inseminated and of their morphology on the success of intrauterine insemination. Hum Reprod 19: 2060–2065.

World Health Organization (1987, 1992, 1999). *WHO Laboratory Manual for the Examination of Human Semen and Semen-Cervical Mucus Interaction*, 2nd, 3rd and 4th edn. Press syndicate of the University of Cambridge.

World Health Organization (2010). *WHO Laboratory Manual for the Examination and Processing of Human Semen*, 5th edn. Geneva: World Health Organization Press.

Zhu, J.J. Pacey, A.A., Barratt, C.L. et al. (1994). Computer-assisted measurement of hyperactivation in human spermatozoa: differences between European and American versions of the Hamilton-Thorn motility analyser. Hum Reprod 9: 456–462.

Zini, A., Boman, J.M., Belzile, E. et al. (2008) Sperm DNA damage is associated with an increased risk of pregnancy loss after IVF and ICSI: systematic review and meta-analysis. Hum Reprod 23: 2663–2668.

Zini, A., Lefebvre, J., Kornitzer, G. et al. (2011). Anti-sperm antibody levels are not related to fertilization or pregnancy rates after IVF or IVF/ICSI. J Reprod Imm 88: 80–84.

23

Surgical Sperm Retrieval

Muhammad A. Akhtar, Elizabeth Hester, Solmaz Gul Sajjad, and Yasmin Sajjad

Introduction

Surgical management of male infertility, including surgical sperm retrieval (SSR), has greatly improved treatment outcomes for those affected. Around 5% of men suffer with infertility, presenting as either azoospermia, in which no sperm is found in the semen, or oligozoospermia, which is a decreased sperm count with other semen parameters (shape, motility) also frequently altered (Rittenberg and El‐Toukhy 2010). The former, more severe finding may have an obstructive or nonobstructive aetiology (Raheem and Ralph 2011).

Obtaining sperm through methods of SSR and using it to attempt conception through intracytoplasmic sperm injection (ICSI) has widened the scope for the success of assisted reproduction (Silber et al. 1994; Devroey et al. 1995). SSR includes either obtaining sperm from epididymis in men with obstructive azoospermia, or obtaining testicular biopsies in men with both obstructive and nonobstructive azoospermia. Laboratories analyse the tissue for the presence of viable sperm and then use cryopreservation if feasible, for use in assisted reproductive treatment.

As with all scientific advances, the benefits of treating previously incurable infertility through assisted conception must be weighed up against the drawbacks, not least the risk of hereditary conditions being passed down unimpeded to the next generation (Hansen et al. 2002; Schieve et al. 2002)

Whilst other surgical treatment for male infertility exists, this chapter will focus on SSR as a management method for azoospermic patients, and will discuss the different methods of SSR and any pre‐ or postoperative considerations.

Azoospermia

Azoospermia affects 15% of the infertile male population. It is defined as the presence of no sperm in the semen (Jarow et al. 1989). Two semen analyses should be performed to confirm this according to NICE fertility guidelines (NICE 2013).

Obstructive Azoospermia

Obstructive azoospermia (OA) is usually due to mechanical obstruction, mostly in the reproductive ductal system, rather than defective sperm production. Therefore, sperm can be effectively retrieved from the epididymi (Goldstein and Tanrikut 2006). OA may result from epididymal, vasal, or ejaculatory duct pathology. OA may be acquired or congenital, i.e. present from birth. Cystic fibrosis is a common cause of OA due to congenital bilateral absence of vasa deferentia (Anguiano et al. 1992; Chillon et al. 1995). Cystic fibrosis carrier status in either partner may produce consequences for the next generation; therefore, genetic counselling is offered (Sharlip et al. 2002). Acquired causes could be due to infections, iatrogenic injury, or injuries such as testicular torsion which can cause tubular blockage in the testes. Acquired obstructive conditions are often due to bacterial infections such as sexually transmitted or urinary tract infections, which cause scarring and blockage of the epididymis. Vasectomy and other surgical procedures in the inguinal region, such as hernia repair and orchidopexy, can also damage the vas deferens (Baker and Sabanegh 2013).

Investigative findings in cases of OA can depend on the underlying pathology; for example, absent

Clinical Reproductive Science, First Edition. Edited by Michael Carroll.
© 2019 John Wiley & Sons Ltd. Published 2019 by John Wiley & Sons Ltd.
Companion website: www.wiley.com/go/carroll/clinicalreproductivescience

vasa deferentia indicate a diagnosis of congenital bilateral absence of vasa deferentia (Schlegel 2004). Characteristic semen parameters with elements of epididymal sclerosis may be seen. However, scrotal ultrasound scans, hormone profiles (follicle stimulating hormone (FSH), luteinizing hormone (LH), testosterone, and inhibin), and testicular volume will be universally normal (Esteves et al. 2011b).

Nonobstructive Azoospermia

Nonobstructive azoospermia (NOA) is generally considered a nonmedically manageable cause of male infertility. These patients, who constitute up to 10% of all infertile men, have abnormal spermatogenesis as the cause of their azoospermia. The establishment of *in vitro* fertilization using ICSI as a standard treatment modality has resulted in a number of these men successfully fathering a child through surgically retrieved sperm from the testis. NOA is caused by faulty sperm production; therefore, more complex retrieval techniques have to be employed, compared with epididymal retrieval for OA (Lopushnyan and Walsh 2012). Coexisting chromosomal (e.g. Klinefelter syndrome) or systemic disorders may become apparent during investigations for male infertility (Kamischke et al. 2003; Weber 2006).

Diagnostic criteria for NOA may include reduced testicular volume ($<10\,cm^3$), loss of testicular resilience on palpation, and flat epididymis. Some men may have a history of cryptorchidism. In contrast to the normal investigation results in OA, patients with NOA have increased FSH levels, although testosterone and oestradiol levels may remain within a normal range. Palpation may reveal epididymal flattening and reduced testicular volume. Table 23.1 compares the characteristics of OA and NOA.

Use of SSR to Treat Azoospermia

It is thought that more than half of the infertile male population with azoospermia could be treated surgically (Esteves et al. 2011a) in order to increase the chance of achieving fatherhood. SSR, in combination with ICSI, using sperm obtained from testicular tissue together with an oocyte (Palermo et al. 1992; Silber et al. 1995), allows couples affected by azoospermia to conceive using autologous gametes, rather than be limited to the options of sperm donation or adoption as was previously the case (Lopushnyan and Walsh 2012).

Preparation for SSR

Hormone Profile

After the initial history and examination have been completed, certain investigations are necessary prior to surgery. In order to determine an obstructive or nonobstructive cause for azoospermia and thereby select the appropriate surgical technique, semen analysis and blood tests for a hormone profile must be carried out. The hormone levels of interest are:

- FSH
- LH
- Testosterone and sex hormone binding globulin (SHBG)
- Prolactin
- Inhibin (Schlegel 2004).

Table 23.1 Comparison of characteristics of obstructive vs nonobstructive azoospermia.

	Obstructive azoospermia	Non-obstructive azoospermia
Cause	Mechanical obstruction in ductal system	Faulty sperm production in testes
Hormone profile	Normal FSH, LH, testosterone and inhibin	Raised FSH Normal testosterone and oestradiol
Testicular palpation	Absent vasa deferentia Epididymal thickening	Epididymal flattening Reduced testicular tone
Testicular volume	Normal	Reduced

FSH, follicle-stimulating hormone; LH, luteinizing hormone.

Karyotyping

Karyotype analysis is important in infertile males, especially those with NOA or an especially low sperm count. Y chromosome abnormalities, namely deletions of sperm production genes (in the AZF region on Y chromosome) are more common in azoospermic men. (De Braekeleer and Dao 1991; Samli et al. 2006). Klinefelter syndrome, inversions, and translocations also show increased prevalence in the infertile population (Practice Committee ASRM 2008a). Determining the type of abnormality found during karyotype analysis can help predict the likelihood of viable sperm being found in the testes on retrieval (Brandell et al. 1998; Krausz et al. 2000; Hopps et al. 2003).

As previously mentioned, use of assisted reproductive technology such as ICSI may lead to undesirable genetic material being passed through to future generations (Kent-First et al. 1996). Therefore, karyotype testing and genetic counselling are advised prior to offering any assisted conception treatment.

Scrotal Ultrasound Scanning

It is important to assess the scrotum and its contents in azoospermic men using scrotal ultrasound scanning (USS), not only to assess testicular volume (Ammar et al. 2012) but also to screen for the presence of testicular tumours, which infertile men are at greater risk of developing (Walsh et al. 2009).

Further efforts should be made to offer scrotal USS to the following groups of men:

- Patients who have undergone previous open testicular SSR and are planning a subsequent attempt,
- Patients with an abnormal testicular examination.
- Patients for whom a testicular examination was not possible. e.g. due to high body mass index.
- Patients with a history of and/or treatment for undescended testes.
- Patients who have undergone testicular surgery,

Anaesthetic Considerations

Due to the sensitive nature of SSR and the accompanying patient unease, most operations are carried out using general or regional anaesthetic, especially for open approaches (men with NOA). Alternative strategies to this include inducing anaesthesia using spinal or epidural methods, which may be employed if a patient cannot tolerate general anaesthetic, or spermatic cord block combined with anaesthesia to the surrounding cutaneous regions. Pain can be controlled by local nerve block.

Methods of SSR

Using surgical retrieval, sperm from testicular tissue can be used either fresh or cryopreserved for ICSI treatment. Future repeat attempts may be carried out if care and attention is taken to preserve the integrity of the testes (Esteves et al. 2013).

SSR techniques vary depending on whether the cause of azoospermia is obstructive or nonobstructive, as the type of azoospermia determines the site used. In cases of OA, epididymal retrieval, known as percutaneous epididymal sperm aspiration (PESA), is attempted first, unless epididymal pathology inhibits this. Failure of epididymal retrieval warrants progress to testicular retrieval. Testicular sperm retrieval is always used in cases of NOA. Testicular volume and FSH levels can be used to predict presence of viable sperm in the retrieved testicular tissue (Bromage et al. 2007).

The surgical approach, as well as the site of retrieval, varies with different techniques. Sperm can be retrieved percutaneously or by using an open approach, with the possibility of enhancing either method further using microscopic surgery (Silber et al. 1994; Craft et al. 1995; Okada et al. 2002). Table 23.2 summarizes the different techniques for OA and NOA and the different possible approaches.

Methods for Obstructive Azoospermia

Epididymal retrieval techniques will usually be attempted first in cases of OA. Testicular extraction is performed if the former method fails to yield any viable sperm (Esteves et al. 2011b).

Table 23.2 Types of azoospermia and appropriate sperm retrieval methods.

Obstructive azoospermia	Epididymal retrieval	Percutaneous epididymal sperm aspiration (PESA)
		Microsurgical epididymal sperm aspiration (MESA)
	Testicular retrieval (after failed epididymal retrieval)	Testicular sperm aspiration (TESA)
		Testicular fine needle aspiration (TEFNA)
		Testicular sperm extraction Single or multiple biopsies (TESE)
Nonobstructive azoospermia	Epididymal retrieval	N/A
	Testicular retrieval	Testicular sperm aspiration (TESA)
		Testicular fine needle aspiration (TEFNA)
		Testicular sperm extraction Single or multiple biopsies (TESE)
		Micro-surgical testicular sperm extraction (micro-TESE)

Epididymal Retrieval Methods
PESA
Method: The surgeon inserts a 26 gauge needle through the scrotum into the epididymis, located by testicular palpation: 0.1 mL of clear fluid is aspirated by creating a vacuum inside a 1 mL tuberculin syringe (first by drawing back the plunger, then alternately advancing and withdrawing the needle inside the epididymis) (Figure 23.1). Alternate PESA sites within the epididymis may be used for repeat attempts should the primary aspirate yield no viable sperm, determined by microscopic examination of the harvested fluid in culture medium.

Advantages:

- First-line treatment for OA that is incurable through reconstruction.
- Fast operation and can be performed multiple times at multiple sites.
- Comparatively noninvasive.

Disadvantages:

- Local complications at aspiration site, e.g. haematoma.

- Primary attempt may not produce acceptable sperm yield, leading to repeat PESA or other retrieval technique, e.g. testicular methods (Lopushnyan and Walsh 2012).
- Quality of sperm retrieved is not as good as microsurgical epididymal sperm aspiration.

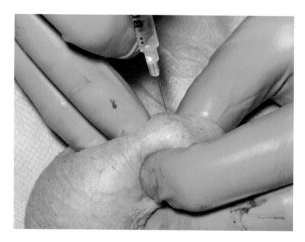

Figure 23.1 PESA with a needle into the epididymis.

Microsurgical Epididymal Sperm Aspiration

Method: The second of the epididymal retrieval methods, in comparison to PESA, microsurgical epididymal sperm aspiration (MESA) is an open procedure as opposed to a percutaneous technique. Using microsurgical instruments, sperm are extracted from tubules through epididymal aspiration. The surgeon accesses the tubules by inserting a microscope through a small horizontal incision in the scrotal and epididymal tissue (Esteves et al. 2013). Much like with PESA, sperm-containing fluid is aspirated through a needle into culture medium, which is then analysed in a laboratory to determine viable sperm content and multiple epididymal sites can be used if the primary yield is unacceptable (Esteves et al. 2011b).

Advantages:

- Yields are adequate sperm for frozen storage.
- Greater sperm yield than PESA (Lopushnyan and Walsh 2012).
- Quality of sperm retrieved is superior compared to PESA, as selection of better quality sperm by visualization is possible.

Disadvantages:

- Complex microsurgical skills needed in comparison to PESA.
- Expensive in comparison to PESA.

Testicular Retrieval Methods

Testicular Sperm Aspiration – Including Testicular Fine Needle Aspiration

Method: Testicular sperm aspiration (TESA) is a percutaneous procedure much like PESA. However, the needle is passed through the scrotum into the upper testis (to avoid the testicular artery), rather than into the epididymis. Again, as in PESA, sperm-containing tissue is extracted into a syringe, which is then analysed for viable sperm. A variety of needles can be used: wide bore needles, fine needles for testicular fine needle aspiration (TEFNA) originally used to investigate azoospermia (Turek et al. 1997), or biopsy needles which produce a core of tissue sample (Morey et al. 1993). TESA is indicated in OA should attempts to retrieve sperm through epididymal methods either not have been possible, or have yielded no sperm.

Advantages:

- Percutaneous procedure, therefore does not carry the risk of open procedures.
- Complications linked to general naesthesia are eliminated, as TESA can be carried out under local anaesthetic.

Disadvantages:

- Chance of complications such as haematoma and testicular atrophy.

Testicular Sperm Extraction – Uni- And Multifocal

Method: Compared with TESA, testicular sperm extraction (TESE) is an open procedure rather than a percutaneous technique. Inside both testes, sperm are retrieved by creating either single or multiple incisions in the tunica albuginea, (Figures 23.2 and 23.3). Sperm-containing testicular tissue is extracted using scissors and can then be used for azoospermia investigations as well as for assisted reproduction treatment use. Failure of PESA or TESA is an indication for TESE amongst obstructive azoospermic males.

Advantages:

- Greater sperm yield than TESA.
- Multifocal TESE increases yield further as more of the testicle is taken as a sample (Lopushnyan and Walsh 2012).

Disadvantages:

- Open procedures are higher risk than percutaneous procedures.
- Chance of vasculature damage during operation.
- Multifocal TESE excises more tissue therefore negatively affects sperm production.

Methods for NOA

Epididymal retrieval methods are not attempted for males with NOA; only testicular techniques are used.

Testicular Retrieval Methods

The following methods are used for first-line treatment in nonazoospermic men and are described in detail in the previous section:

- Testicular Sperm Aspiration (TESA).
- Testicular Sperm Extraction (TESE).

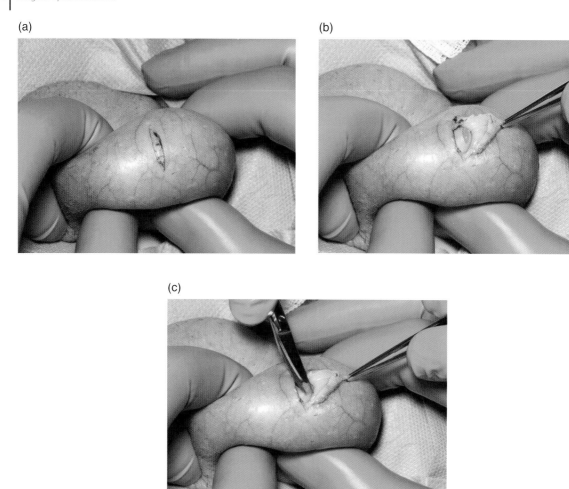

Figure 23.2 Unifocal open TESE. (a) Single incision on each testicle exposing tunica vaginalis. (b) Single incision on each testicle, exposing the spermatic tubule for biopsy. (c) Extraction of testicular tissue using surgical scissors.

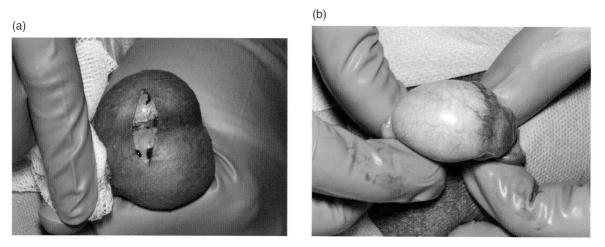

Figure 23.3 Multifocal open TESE. (a) Midline scrotal incision for scrotal exploration. (b) Testicle after scrotal exploration.

(c)

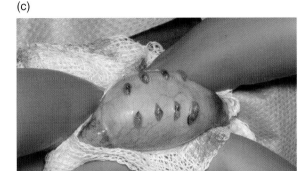

(d)

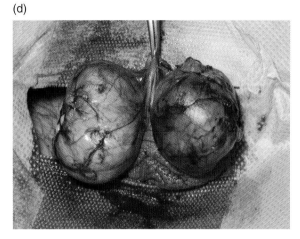

Figure 23.3 (Continued) (c) Multiple incisions on tunica albuginea on the testicle showing spermatic tubules. (d) Scrotal septum held showing both testicles after TESE.

Microsurgical Testicular Sperm Extraction

Method: Like MESA, microsurgical testicular sperm extraction (micro-TESE) is an open procedure performed through a scrotal incision using a microscope to aid operating and visualize a high level of detail (Esteves et al. 2013). The procedure involves a 3–4 cm incision in the midline of the scrotum, whilst the patient is under general anesthetic. The incision is used to open the testes for observation under a high-powered microscope with a magnification of x 30–40. The surgeon uses the microsurgical tools to select subjectively the most sizeable or swollen seminiferous tubules for extraction, which are then analysed in the laboratory for viable sperm yield (Esteves et al. 2011b). Once the sample has been retrieved, a fine suture is used to close the testes under the operating microscope. This procedure is then repeated on the other side. Micro-TESE leaves the patient with a small suture resulting in little or no scarring, and minimal amounts of pain. The multilayered closing technique is used to ensure that the patient has a reduced risk of infection or bleeding postsurgery.

Micro-TESE was developed as a means of minimizing testicular trauma by combining a less invasive approach with an open excisional biopsy, using optical magnification to pinpoint zones of active spermatogenesis. Micro-TESE is thought to have a high sperm retrieval rate and a lower risk of postoperative complications. The advantage of using micro-TESE is that it allows identification of the larger, opaque tubules that are presumed to contain more germ cells with active spermatogenesis. From a study performed by Ghalyanini et al. showing the comparison between conventional TESE and micro-TESE, it was seen that micro-TESE managed to avoid haematoma, fibrosis, and androgen decline (Ghalayini et al. 2011).

Advantages:

- High magnification visualization allows for selection of tubules estimated to yield the greatest number of sperm – desirable characteristics include increased size and pale colour.
- Micro-TESE allows for a high yield of sperm from small extraction samples due to tubule selection; therefore, there is a lower chance of negatively affecting sperm production in the already small testes of NOA men.

Disadvantages:

- Complex microsurgical skills needed in comparison to TESE.
- Expensive in comparison to TESE.

SSR Aftercare

Postoperative Considerations

Immediate Postoperative Period

- A genital branch of genitofemoral nerve block is recommended for postoperative pain relief.
- A scrotal support dressing is applied to reduce the risk of haematoma and bruising.

Up to 24 Hours Postprocedure

- Patients should be informed of risk of bruising, discomfort, or swelling (Esteves et al. 2011b) and advised to keep scrotal support in place for 24h minimum (Figure 23.4).
- Patients are counselled to restrain from ejaculation and strenuous physical activity for approximately 7–10 days
- As SSR is performed as day case surgery, patients may return home 4–5h postoperation. However, patients may not leave unaccompanied.

Up to One Week Postprocedure

- Depending on the retrieval method used, patients should rest after surgery:
  - 48h is suggested for open retrievals.
  - At least 24h for percutaneous retrievals.
- Keep wound site clean and dry.
- Oral pain relief can be taken up to 5 days postoperation. Pain should improve within a week (Esteves et al. 2011b).
- However, use of scrotal supports during this time decreases risk of long-term pain.
- Resume normal daily life, but avoid sexual intercourse, sports, and intense physical activity for 10 days (Esteves et al. 2013).

Complications

Following sperm retrieval, the risk of complications differs according to the surgical approach used. SSR is generally thought to be low risk. However, possible postoperative complications include infection, haematoma, hydrocele, and pain (Schiff et al. 2005; Silber 2000):

- Complications are less common using the micro-TESE method compared with TESE (Schlegel 1999; Donoso et al. 2007; Turunc et al. 2010), due to microscopic visualization and therefore avoidance of testicular vasculature (Esteves et al. 2013).
- Risks of haematoma and reduced testicular testosterone production accompany TESE procedures, especially when greater quantities of tissue are excised (Ramasamy et al. 2005; Carpi et al. 2009).
- Open retrieval methods generate decreased haematoma risk, compared with percutaneous methods (Rosenlund et al. 1998; Practice Committee ASRM 2008b)
- Complications due to general anaesthetic should also be considered.

Complications can be followed up with scrotal ultrasound scans in the postoperative period to ensure resolution.

Follow-Up

Recovery, discussions surrounding assisted reproduction treatment following successful sperm retrieval, or counselling concerning the next steps should the operation have yielded no sperm will all take place at the 2-week follow-up appointment. It is recommended that repeat procedures be avoided by appropriate surgical technique selection in the first instance. However, if a secondary retrieval is necessary, hormone profile investigations should be repeated and a scrotal ultrasound scan requested.

Conclusion

The field of male infertility is changing and evolving as we become more aware of its importance in reproductive medicine and surgery. SSR can benefit men with both OA and NOA as many retrieval techniques now exist, varying in site and surgical approach used. Thus, patients can be considered on

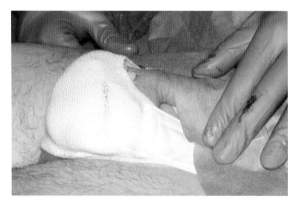

Figure 23.4 Scrotal support after TESE surgery.

a case-by-case basis, with the most appropriate retrieval method selected to bring about the greatest potential for sperm yield. Following successful retrieval, assisted reproduction treatments such as ICSI can be used to achieve a clinical pregnancy.

Microscopic methods of sperm retrieval are promising techniques as they reduce complications such as testicular atrophy and bleeding, and produce higher quality sperm yield due to the ability to visualize and excise specific lucrative testicular tissue. However, although these techniques will be used more frequently in the future, there are disadvantages to overcome such as cost and the need to train operators to a high standard.

Acknowledgements

Dr P.N. Schlegel, Cornell Medical Centre, USA.

References

Ammar, T., Sidhu, P.S. and Wilkins, C.J. (2012). Male infertility: the role of imaging in diagnosis and management. Br J Radiol 85: S59–68.

Anguiano, A., Oates, R.D., Amos, J.A. et al. (1992). Congenital bilateral absence of the vas deferens. A primarily genital form of cystic fibrosis. JAMA 267: 1794–1797.

Baker, K. and Sabanegh, E. Jr. (2013). Obstructive azoospermia: reconstructive techniques and results. Clinics (Sao Paulo) 68(Suppl 1): 61–73.

Brandell, R.A., Mielnik, A., Liotta, D. et al. (1998). AZFb deletions predict the absence of spermatozoa with testicular sperm extraction: preliminary report of a prognostic genetic test. Hum Reprod 13: 2812–2815.

Bromage, S.J., Falconer, D.A., Liebermann, B.A. et al. (2007). Sperm retrieval rates in subgroups of primary azoospermic males. Eur Urol 51: 534–540.

Carpi, A., Sabanegh, E. and Mechanick, J. (2009). Controversies in the management of nonobstructive azoospermia. Fertil Steril 91: 963–970.

Chillon, M., Casals, T., Mercier, B. et al. (1995). Mutations in the cystic fibrosis gene in patients with congenital absence of the vas deferens. N Engl J Med 332: 1475–1480.

Craft, I., Tsirigotis, M., Bennett, V. et al. (1995). Percutaneous epididymal sperm aspiration and intracytoplasmic sperm injection in the management of infertility due to obstructive azoospermia. Fertil Steril 63: 1038–1042.

De Braekeleer, M. and Dao, T.N. (1991). Cytogenetic studies in male infertility: a review. Hum Reprod 6: 245–250.

Devroey, P., Liu, J., Nagy, Z. et al. (1995). Pregnancies after testicular extraction (TESE) and intracytoplasmic sperm injection (ICSI) in non-obstructive azoospermia. Hum Reprod 10: 1457–1460.

Donoso, P., Tournaye, H. and Devroey, P. (2007). Which is the best sperm retrieval technique for non-obstructive azoospermia? A systematic review. Hum Reprod Update 13: 539–549.

Esteves, S.C., Miyaoka, R. and Agarwal, A. (2011a). Surgical treatment of male infertility in the era of intracytoplasmic sperm injection – new insights. Clinics (Sao Paulo) 66: 1463–1478.

Esteves, S.C., Miyaoka, R. and Agarwal, A. (2011b). Sperm retrieval techniques for assisted reproduction. Int Braz J Urol 37: 570–583.

Esteves, S.C., Miyaoka, R., Orosz, J.E. et al. (2013). An update on sperm retrieval techniques for azoospermic males. Clinics (Sao Paulo) 68(Suppl 1): 99–110.

Ghalayini, I.F., A-Ghazo, M.A, Hani, O.B. et al. (2011). Clinical comparison of conventional testicular sperm extraction and microdissection techniques for non-obstructive azoopsermia. J Clin Med Res 3: 24–131.

Goldstein, M. and Tanrikut, C. (2006). Microsurgical management of male infertility. Nat Clin Pract Urol 3: 381–391.

Hansen, M., Kurinczuk, J.J., Bower, C. et al. (2002). The risk of major birth defects after intracytoplasmic sperm injection and in vitro fertilization. N Engl J Med 346: 725–730.

Hopps, C.V., Mielnik, A., Goldstein, M. et al. (2003). Detection of sperm in men with Y chromosome microde- letions of the AZFa, AZFb, and AZFc regions. Hum Reprod 18: 1660–1665.

Jarow, J.P., Espeland, M.A. and Lipshultz, L.I. (1989). Evaluation of the azoospermic patient. J Urol 142: 62–65.

Kamischke, A., Baumgardt, A., Horst, J. et al. (2003). Clinical and diagnostic features of patients with suspected Klinefelter syndrome. J Androl 24: 41–48.

Kent-First, M.G., Kol, S., Muallem, A. et al. (1996). The incidence and possible relevance of Y-linked microdeletions in babies born after intracytoplasmic sperm injection and their infertile fathers. Mol Hum Reprod 2: 943–950.

Krausz, C., Quintana-Murci, L. and McElreavey, K. (2000). Prognostic value of Y deletion analysis. What is the clinical prognostic value of Y chromosome microdeletion analysis? Hum Reprod 15: 1431–1434.

Lopushnyan, N.A. and Walsh, T.J. (2012). Surgical techniques for the management of male infertility. Asian J Androl 14: 94–102.

Morey, A.F., Deshon, G.E., Jr., Rozanski, T.A. et al. (1993). Technique of biopty gun testis needle biopsy. Urology 42: 325–326.

NICE (2013). Fertility: assessment and treatment of people with fertility problems. Clinical Guideline 156. http://guidance.nice.org.uk/CG156.

Okada, H., Dobashi, M., Yamazaki, T. et al. (2002). Kamidono S. Conventional versus microdissection testicular sperm extraction for nonobstructive azoospermia. J Urol 168: 1063–1067.

Palermo, G., Joris, H. and Devroey, P. et al. (1992). Pregnancies after intracytoplasmic injection of single spermatozoon into an oocyte. Lancet 340(8810): 17–8

Practice Committee of American Society for Reproductive Medicine in collaboration with Society for Male Reproduction and Urology (2008a). Evaluation of the azoospermic male. Fertil Steril 90(5 Suppl): S74–77.

Practice Committee of American Society for Reproductive Medicine in collaboration with Society for Male Reproduction and Urology (2008b). The management of infertility due to obstructive azoospermia. Fertil Steril 90(5 Suppl): S121–124.

Raheem, A. and Ralph D. (2011). Male infertility: causes and investigations. Trends Urol Men's Health 2: 8–11.

Ramasamy, R., Yagan, N. and Schlegel, P.N. (2005). Structural and functional changes to the testis after conventional versus microdissection testicular sperm extraction. Urology 65: 1190–1194.

Rittenberg, V. and El-Toukhy, T. (2010). Medical treatment of male infertility. Hum Fertil (Camb)13: 208–216.

Rosenlund, B., Westlander, G., Wood, M. et al. (1998). Sperm retrieval and fertilization in repeated percutaneous epididymal sperm aspiration. Hum Reprod 13: 2805–2807.

Samli, H., Samli, M.M., Solak, M. et al. (2006). Genetic anomalies detected in patients with non-obstructive azoospermia and oligozoospermia. Arch Androl 52: 263–267.

Schieve, L.A., Meikle, S.F., Ferre, C. et al. (2002). Low and very low birth weight in infants conceived with use of assisted reproductive technology. N Engl J Med 346: 731–737.

Schiff, J.D., Palermo, G.D., Veeck, L.L. et al. (2005). Success of testicular sperm injection and intracytoplasmic sperm injection in men with Klinefelter syndrome. J Clin Endocr Metab 90: 6263–6267.

Schlegel, P.N. (1999). Testicular sperm extraction. microdissection improves sperm yield with minimal tissue excision. Hum Reprod 14: 131–135.

Schlegel, P.N. (2004). Causes of azoospermia and their management. Reprod Fertil Dev 16: 561–572.

Sharlip, I.D., Jarow, J.P., Belker, A.M. et al. (2002). Best practice policies for male infertility. Fertil Steril 77: 873–882.

Silber, S.J. (2000). Microsurgical TESE and the distribution of spermatogenesis in non-obstructive azoospermia. Hum Reprod 15: 2278–2284.

Silber, S.J., Devroey, P., Tournaye, H. et al. (1995). Fertilizing capacity of epididymal and testicular sperm using intracytoplasmic sperm injection (ICSI). Reprod Fertil Dev 7: 281–292, discussion 292–293.

Silber, S.J., Nagy, Z.P., Liu, J. et al. (1994). Conventional in-vitro fertilization versus intracytoplasmic sperm injection for patients requiring microsurgical sperm aspiration. Hum Reprod 9: 1705–1709.

Turek, P.J., Cha, I. and Ljung, B.M. (1997). Systematic fine-needle aspiration of the testis. correlation to biopsy and results of organ "mapping" for mature sperm in azoospermic men. Urology 49: 743–748.

Turunc, T., Gul, U., Haydardedeoglu, B. et al. (2010). Conventional testicular sperm extraction combined with the microdissection technique in nonobstructive azoospermic patients: a prospective comparative study. Fertil Steril 94: 2157–2160.

Walsh, T.J., Croughan, M.S., Schembri, M. et al. (2009). Increased risk of testicular germ cell cancer among infertile men. Arch Intern Med 169: 351–356.

Weber, R. (2006). Endocrine factors. In: *Andrology for the Clinician*. (ed. W.-B. Schill, F.H. Comhaire, and T. Hargreave T.). Berlin: Springer.

24

In Vitro Fertilization and Intracytoplasmic Sperm Injection

Bryan Woodward

Introduction

Historically, many methods have been employed to achieve fertilization *in vitro* (see Table 24.1). Nowadays, two insemination methods are in common use in *in vitro* fertilization (IVF) laboratories: conventional IVF insemination and intracytoplasmic sperm injection (ICSI) (Figure 24.1)

Conventional IVF insemination relies on free-swimming progressively motile sperm being able to penetrate the cumulus cells that surround the oocyte and bind to the zona pellucida (ZP) before entering the oocyte cytoplasm. Prepared sperm are added to the media containing the cumulus-oocytes-complexes (COCs) using a micropipette and sterile tip (Figure 24.2). This method enables a calculated concentration of progressively motile sperm/mL to be added to each COC (Box 24.1).

By contrast, ICSI involves the injection of a single sperm directly into the cytoplasm of the oocyte. ICSI bypasses the problems of sperm having to independently pass through the cumulus cell, bind to the ZP, and penetrate the oolemma. Performance of ICSI requires a high level of micromanipulation skills to ensure that the sensitive oocyte is not damaged by the procedure, since injection involves piercing the membrane of the oocyte and aspiration of the cytoplasm into the injection pipette.

IVF or ICSI: The Dilemma

If there is a sufficient number of highly progressive motile sperm of good morphology in the pre- and post-preparation, then the chances of fertilization following conventional IVF insemination should theoretically be high. However, it should be noted that low fertilization, and even complete failure of fertilization, may result even when the sperm quality is good. Frapsauce et al. (2009) estimated that despite normal sperm parameters, 5% of IVF attempts result in an unpredicted failure of fertilization, with 56% of cases having no obvious oocyte anomaly other than a complete lack of ZP–sperm binding. In such instances, the cause of failed fertilization cannot be ascertained without cytogenetic analysis of the unfertilized oocyte (see Table 24.2).

In Europe, there is a marked variation in the relative proportions of IVF and ICSI procedures. According to a report in 2013 from the European IVF-Monitoring (EIM) Consortium for the European Society of Human Reproduction and Embryology (ESHRE), the difference seems to be related to geographic distribution. IVF remains the dominant technology in several countries from northern and eastern Europe (Denmark, Finland, Iceland, Ireland, Kazakhstan, Lithuania, Romania, Russia, Sweden, and the Netherlands). Whilst, in contrast, most countries from western and central Europe (Germany, Italy, Spain, Austria, and Switzerland) use ICSI for over 75% of cases (Ferraretti et al. 2013).

A review by Palermo et al. (2015) showed that ICSI does not yield higher pregnancy rates than IVF but acts as a normalizer of fertilization, mollifying absent or low fertilization. These conclusions are supported by another study which showed that when compared with conventional IVF insemination, ICSI was not associated with improved post-fertilization reproductive outcomes, irrespective of male factor infertility diagnosis (Boulet et al. 2015).

Clinical Reproductive Science, First Edition. Edited by Michael Carroll.
© 2019 John Wiley & Sons Ltd. Published 2019 by John Wiley & Sons Ltd.
Companion website: www.wiley.com/go/carroll/clinicalreproductivescience

Table 24.1 Insemination techniques used to cause fertilization *in vitro*.

Technique	Abbreviation	Description of Technique
Conventional *in vitro* fertilization insemination	Conventional IVF insemination	Motile sperm are added to media containing oocytes
Subzonal insemination	SUZI	Several motile sperm are injected into the perivitelline space
High insemination concentration	HIC	A higher than conventional concentration of motile sperm are added to media containing oocytes
Laser assisted IVF	LA-IVF	A laser is used to cause several ablations completely through the zona pellucida (ZP). Conventional IVF then takes place
Intracytoplasmic sperm injection	ICSI	A single sperm is microinjected directly into the cytoplasm of the oocyte

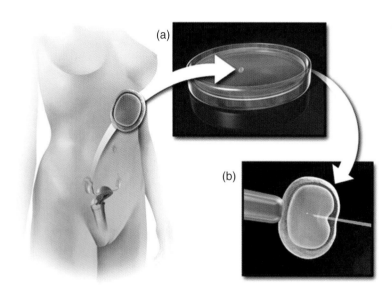

Figure 24.1 Assisted reproductive fertilization *in vitro* techniques. After oocyte retrieval, fertilization is accomplished by (a) insemination or (b) intracytoplasmic sperm injection. *Source*: Blausen Medical – Wikimedia

However, some clinics prefer to reduce the risk of a failed fertilization and therefore promote frequent use of ICSI rather than IVF. This is despite the additional risks associated with the ICSI procedure.

Timing of Insemination

The timing of fertilization is based on the time when the oocytes are considered to be at their most competent level in terms of meiotic and cytoplasmic maturity. At this stage, the oocytes should be most receptive to sperm penetration and the fertilization process. Prior to collection, the oocytes mature *in vivo* during ovarian stimulation. When the follicles reach the desired size, an injection of human chorionic gonadotrophin (hCG) or GnRH agonist is administered to provide the final maturation 'trigger'. The hCG injection is intended to mimic the surge of luteinizing hormone that takes place in the natural menstrual cycle. The oocyte collection takes place around 36 h after the hCG trigger. The oocytes are thought to be most competent around 4 h later.

Traditionally, the insemination time is usually based on the number of hours elapsed from the time of administration of the hCG trigger injection (hours post-hCG), rather than the time from oocyte retrieval. If oocyte collection takes place at around 36 hours post-hCG, then the insemination takes place at around 40 h post-hCG.

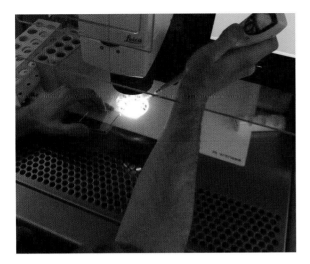

Figure 24.2 Insemination technique. Prepared sperm are added to the wells or droplets using a micropipette. Image courtesy of Assisted Conception Suite, Glasgow Royal Infirmary, Glasgow, UK

Individual clinics may set their own variation in the standard timings, which may also need to take into account the workload of the theatre and lab (i.e. the number of cases to be dealt with, and the number of staff available to perform them). The embryology team may also need to adjust the timing of insemination due to anticipated difficulty with ICSI cases. For example, to perform ICSI on a difficult case (e.g. twenty metaphase II oocytes with very poor quality sperm derived from testicular surgery) will take longer than a simpler case (e.g. three metaphase II oocytes with good quality sperm). The start time for the former insemination may be brought forward as a result. The embryologist should keep a record of the time of insemination in the embryology notes. For ICSI, this should include the start and end time of the injection procedure.

Box 24.1   Calculating the number of sperm for conventional IVF insemination.

Method 1

For a post-preparation sample, with a concentration of C (million/mL) and a motility of M (% progressively motile), the insemination volume can be calculated using the equation below. This will give an insemination concentration of 100 000 progressively motile sperm in a volume of 0.5 mL media. It should be noted that the insemination will be approximate, since the media volume will have changed with the addition of the cumulus-oocyte-complexes

$$\text{Volume to inseminate}\,(\mu L) = 100/C \times M$$

Method 2

For a post-preparation sample, with a concentration of C (million/mL), a motility of M (% progressively motile) and morphology of I (% ideal forms), the insemination volume can be calculated using the equation below. This will give an insemination concentration of 100 000 progressively motile sperm in a volume of 0.65 mL media.

$$\text{Volume to inseminate}\,(\mu L) = 65/Y$$

Where $Y = C \times M \times I$

Table 24.2 Reasons for failed fertilization after conventional IVF insemination where good sperm quality was observed pre- and post-preparation.

Observation	Possible Reason	Possible Gamete at Fault	
		Sperm	Oocyte
No sperm attached to ZP, no PN, 1 PB	Failure of sperm to penetrate cumulus	Y	N
	Failure of sperm to bind to ZP	Y	Y
Sperm attached to ZP, no PN, 1 PB	Failure of sperm to penetrate ooplasm	Y	Y
Sperm attached to ZP, no PN, 2 PB	Failure of sperm chromatin to decondense in ooplasm	Y	N

PB, polar body; PN, pronuclei; ZP, zona pellucida.

Table 24.3 Equipment needed for conventional *in vitro* fertilization (IVF) insemination and intracytoplasmic sperm injection (ICSI).

	IVF	ICSI
Equipment	Hotblock (to keep sperm warm)	Inverted microscope with Hoffman modulation contrast and heated stage (on which to perform ICSI)
	Micropipette (to add sperm)	Micromanipulation equipment (syringes, tubing, pipette holders, X-Y-Z controllers)
	Stereomicroscope and heated stage (on which to perform insemination)	Micropipette (to add sperm)
	Inverted microscope with Hoffman modulation contrast and heated stage (to observe sperm movement in the dish immediately postinsemination)	Hotblock (to keep sperm warm)
Consumables	Pipette tips (to add sperm)	Denudation pipettes (to transfer oocytes)
	Dishes (for incubation of cumulus-oocyte-complexes and sperm)	Pipette tips (to add sperm)
		Dishes (low lipped) (for ICSI)
		Holding pipette
		Injection pipette
		Dishes (for washing oocytes post-ICSI)

Note all manipulations should take place on a heated stage to maintain the gametes at 37 °C. Dish type has not been specified, as it is the choice of the individual laboratory.

The equipment required for conventional IVF insemination and ICSI is listed in Table 24.3.

Conventional IVF Insemination

Prior to conventional IVF insemination, the COCs should be transferred to the dishes in which the insemination will take place. The prepared sperm sample should be incubated and equilibrated to the same temperature (37 °C) and gas/pH levels of the media containing the COCs. Many laboratories use the same media for the prepared sperm sample and the COC culture to ensure there are no differences in media constituents, pH, and osmolality.

The number of sperm to be inseminated should already have been calculated, along with the required volume of the post-preparation (see Box 24.1). These figures should be sufficient to maximize the chance of fertilization. A too high concentration risks an increased chance of polyspermy and also compromised embryo development due to the high levels of free radicals introduced with high sperm numbers. Typically, a sperm concentration of 100×10^6/mL is

recommended, although this can be as low as 20×10^6/mL or as high as 300×10^6/mL.

For the actual insemination process, a sterile tip should be fitted to a micropipette, set to the required insemination volume. The sperm sample should be removed from the incubator, and placed in a hotblock. The COC dish should be removed from the incubator and placed on a heated stage in a laminar flow hood.

In many countries, it is mandatory to perform a double identity check at the time of the insemination procedure. This involves both the embryologist and a witness checking that the oocytes and sperm belong to the same patients beyond a shadow of a doubt. The development of fail-safe mechanisms to prevent assisted reproductive technology (ART) mix-ups is critical (de los Santos and Ruiz 2013).

The required volume of sperm should then be taken up into the pipette tip and gently dispensed into the media containing the COCs. The insemination should be directed away from the COCs, to allow the dispensed sperm to then swim towards the oocytes. In theory, this allows the better swimming sperm to reach the oocyte first.

Once all COCs in a dish have been inseminated, it is recommended that the media is observed under a higher magnification, such as x400 on an inverted microscope, to check that the sperm are swimming optimally and starting to penetrate the cumulus cells. The dish is then be returned to the incubator where it should remain until the time of the fertilization check, 16–18 h later. The insemination time, the concentration of progressively motile sperm inseminated, and the names of the embryologist and witness should be recorded in the embryology notes.

Different laboratories have variations on the conventional IVF insemination technique. These may include: adding the sperm to a separate insemination dish and then adding the COCs; inseminating in large volumes or droplets; and adjusting the time of coincubation of gametes, such that the COCs are removed to a fresh dish a short time after insemination (Guo et al. 2012). The short insemination time remains controversial as one study highlighted that a 1-h gamete exposure decreased the fertilization rate and did not improve embryo quality compared with a standard 18-h insemination procedure (Barraud-Lange et al. 2008).

ICSI Procedure

The success of the clinical ICSI technique was first reported in 1992 by a group from Brussels (Palermo et al. 1992) and the process has since been described in detail in the published literature (e.g. Ebner et al. 2001). Anecdotally, some believe that ICSI may have taken place by accident during a subzonal insemination (SUZI) procedure, with a needle 'slip' such that the oocyte was penetrated and the sperm injected. However, such a tale is unlikely, since the ICSI process had been occurring in animals for many years before 1992. The first live offspring conceived by ICSI were reported for the frog, when four normal frogs resulted from 562 oocytes injected with sperm (Brun 1974).

However, it is fortuitous that ICSI is such a success in human oocytes, since the majority of animal species experience low success rates. Membrane damage and lysis during injection has been reported for rodents, e.g. the mouse (Hu et al. 2012). Furthermore, in many other species the sperm cannot fully decondense after injection, e.g. the cow (Arias et al. 2014).

Preparation of Oocytes for ICSI

Removal of Cumulus-Corona Cells

Denudation refers to the process by which the cumulus and corona cells that surround the oocyte are removed. This enables embryologists to visualize the oocyte and oolemma in detail during the ICSI procedure. Ebner et al. (2006) suggested that incomplete denudation of oocytes prior to ICSI may enhance embryo quality and blastocyst development. This team therefore recommended that some cumulus cells should be left on the ZP to protect the oocyte at the time of ICSI, rather than perform a complete denudation. However, it is necessary that a sufficient amount of cytoplasm is clearly visible to allow for accurate assessment of pronuclei (PN) number when it comes to checking fertilization status post-ICSI.

Denudation usually involves a combination of chemical (using hyaluronidase) and mechanical (using pipettes) processing. The duration of exposure to hyaluronidase (30 s) and concentration (40–80 IU) should be kept to a minimum, as excessive exposure to the acid may damage oocyte ultrastructure (De Vos et al. 2008). Hyaluronidase concentration in ready-to-use media for cumulus cell removal is generally 80 IU/mL, but a diluted concentration of 30–40 IU/mL may be preferred.

The hyaluronidase should be warmed to 37 °C (no gas is needed) prior to use. Droplets of hyaluronidase can be prepared under oil, with wash droplets of buffered media (e.g. HEPES or MOPS) included in the same dish (see Figure 24.3). COCs should be transferred to the hyaluronidase using a sterile Pasteur pipette. They should be gently mixed with the hyaluronidase by flushing up and down the pipette. This process should loosen and removed the majority of cumulus cells, such that the oocytes usually remain with a few layers of more tightly-bound cumulus cells attached. The oocytes should then be transferred to wash droplets for further denudation.

Once in the wash droplets, denudation pipettes of decreasing lumen diameter (290 μm, 190 μm, 155 μm, and 135 μμm) should be used to remove further cumulus. Dedicated pipettes and pipette holders specifically designed for oocyte/embryo handling should be used. Care should be taken to avoid oocyte damage by too vigorous pipetting or from a pipette diameter which is too small.

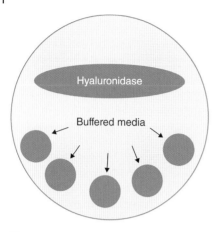

Figure 24.3 Setting up a dish for oocyte denudation. The denudation dish consists of one large droplet of hyaluronidase and several smaller droplets of buffered medium. The cumulus-oocyte-complexes are initially transferred to the hyaluronidase droplets using a sterile Pasteur pipette. Once the majority of the cumulus has been removed, each oocyte with its remaining layers of cumulus cells is transferred to a wash droplet.

The denuded oocytes should then be washed in pre-equilibrated culture media and incubated prior to ICSI. The maturation status of oocytes can be assessed at this time.

Injection Procedure

ICSI practitioners must be fully familiar with the micromanipulation equipment to be used (Figure 24.4). Different types of micromanipulators are available for IVF clinics, including electronic and hydraulic joysticks, and air or oil-accentuated syringes (see 'Troubleshooting ICSI Procedures' in Elder et al. 2015).

Rather than providing a detailed description of the ICSI procedure, a few important points will now be discussed. For example, it is essential that each oocyte should be firmly secured using a holding pipette, such that its position is safely fixed throughout the injection process. If the oocyte is not securely fixed, the oocyte can move as a result of the injection process, which increases the risk of oocyte damage. Traditionally the polar body (PB) was recommended to be positioned at 6 or 12 o'clock (Van Steirteghem et al. 1993), since this aimed to direct the path of the injection pipette at the furthest distance from the presumed position of the metaphase II spindle (Nagy et al. 1995). However, the precise position of the PB has since been shown to be less relevant (Woodward et al. 2008), provided it is positioned away from the direct pathway of the injection pipette. Sperm can be injected either head-first or tale-first, although the former may allow for better visualization (Woodward et al. 2005). Finally, it is essential that a breach of the oolemma is observed before proceeding with the sperm injection (see Figure 24.5).

Other parameters to consider include:

1) The equipment: all ICSI practitioners should be fully familiar with the working of the ICSI

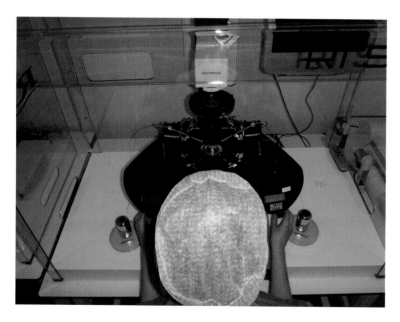

Figure 24.4 The intracytoplasmic sperm injection (ICSI) station or rig. The ICSI rig is a microscope with micromanipulation station containing a holding micropipette and an injection micropipette. Image courtesy of Assisted Conception Suite, Glasgow Royal Infirmary, Glasgow, UK.

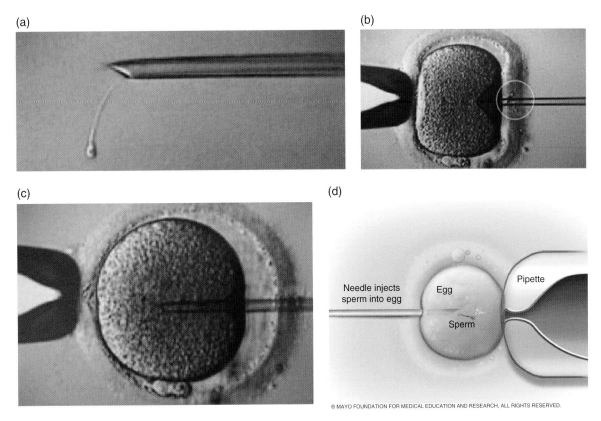

(a)

(b)

(c)

(d)

Needle injects
sperm into egg

Egg

Pipette

Sperm

Figure 24.5 The intracytoplasmic sperm injection (ICSI) procedure. Sperm are firstly captured, immobilized, and aspirated slowly into the injection pipette (a). The micropipette containing the sperm is then moved towards the oocyte, which is secured by the holding pipette. The injection micropipette is inserted through the zona pellucida, where the sperm is positioned near the tip of the micropipette (b, circle). The injection pipette pierces the oolemma, and the sperm is injected in to the centre of the oocyte (c). The injection pipette is then gently withdrawn and the oocyte released. Schematic depiction of ICSI (d). *Source:* (a), (b) and (c) https://commons.wikimedia.org; (d) reproduced with permission of Mayo Foundation for Medical Education and Research. All rights reserved.

equipment being used. If a laboratory has more than one rig, a record of which station was used should be made, as they may vary in performance even if the equipment is the same make/model.

2) The operator: not all ICSI practitioner perform ICSI at the same speed. According to the ESHRE Guidelines for Best Practice in IVF Laboratories (2015), the duration of sperm localization, immobilization, and injection should be minimal.

3) The conditions: all oocytes should be maintained at 37 °C and the correct pH/osmolality in the droplets throughout the time of the ICSI procedure. It may be necessary to adjust the number of oocytes placed in each ICSI dish according to the skill level of the embryologist (see point 1) and the difficulty of the case, to ensure *in vitro* conditions are not compromised.

4) The sperm quality: if the sperm is not easy to locate then this will add time to the capture problems. Records should be kept if there are problems with sperm immobilization or morphology (sometimes sperm are not easily immobilized, or only grossly abnormal-shaped sperm are available).

5) The oocyte quality: oocyte dysmorphisms may exist, e.g. variation in ZP thickness/regularity, perivitelline space (PVS) size, oolemma flexibility, cytoplasmic granularity, presence of smooth endoplasmic reticulum aggregates, etc. The timing of the ICSI procedure may be reduced by assessing and segregating the metaphase II oocytes prior to transfer to the ICSI dish, rather than transferring all oocytes and assessing at the time of ICSI. Any immature oocytes can be reassessed once the ICSI of all metaphase II oocytes

has been completed. However, it should be noted that such oocytes may not necessarily be at metaphase II if they have only recently extruded a PB.

6) Failed injection: if the sperm is observed to not enter the ooplasm, and thus ends up in the PVS, this oocyte should be reinjected only once all other oocytes have been through the ICSI procedure, and preferably at a different position. This allows the oolemma time to recover prior to another physical breach.

After ICSI, all injected oocytes should be washed in pre-equilibrated media, prior to transfer to the culture dish. The dish should then be returned to the incubator until the time of the fertilization check. The insemination time should be recorded, including the start and end of the procedure. The timing is important, as an unnecessary delay may negatively affect the chances of fertilization. The name of the practitioner and the witness, and micromanipulation station (if more than one) should also be recorded in the embryology notes. At the end of the procedure, both the holding and injection pipettes should be discarded into clinical waste dedicated to sharps disposal, prior to setting up fresh sterile pipettes for the next ICSI procedure.

PVP or not PVP? That is the question

Viscous substances such as polyvinylpyrrolidone (PVP) can be used to facilitate the handling and immobilization of sperm for ICSI. However, a Japanese group has expressed concern that PVP is harmful and should not be used (Kato and Nagao, 2012). They have demonstrated that PVP causes significant damage to sperm membranes (as detected by transmission electron microscopy) and also that PVP remains locally within ICSI-derived embryos during the early developmental period. Both factors could detrimentally affect the viability of embryos derived from ICSI using PVP. They suggest that, with experience, it is possible to immobilize sperm using a lower concentration of PVP solution or even use PVP-free media, which would negate any concerns.

Selecting Oocytes for ICSI

A range of oocytes can be collected from patients following ovarian stimulation. Even fertile female donors can produce oocytes with a variety of

dysmorphism, as evidenced by the wide range of chromosome abnormalities in the embryos derived from young oocyte donors (Munné et al. 2006).

An Alpha-ESHRE Consensus was published in 2011, which proposed oocytes with two distinct dysmorphisms should not be inseminated: giant oocytes and oocytes with the presence of smooth endoplasmic reticulum aggregates (SERa) in the cytoplasm (Alpha and ESHRE 2011). If giant oocytes are collected, they should not be selected for ICSI, as there is a very high risk that they will be aneuploid, even if only one PB is observed. Similarly, SERa has been reported to be associated with adverse outcomes, although healthy babies have been born from oocytes presenting the SERa dysmorphism (Van Beirs et al. 2015). If such dysmorphisms exist, patients should be correctly informed that there is a decreased chance of pregnancy.

The appearance of all oocyte dysmorphisms should be recorded on the embryology notes, so that the fertilization status, embryo development, and fate can be traced for each oocyte. Oocyte quality can be additionally assessed prior to ICSI by using computerized polarization microscopy, which allows digital imaging of birefringent structures such as the ZP and meiotic spindle (Dib et al. 2013). The level of birefringence may then be used to help grade oocyte quality and help predict the developmental potential of an embryo that subsequently develops. However, others have questioned the usefulness of this technology (Swiatecka et al. 2014).

Immature oocytes should not be injected. Oocytes at the germinal vesicle stage, when matured *in vitro*, have a high aneuploidy rate and low developmental potential. Oocytes at the metaphase I stage may be cultured for a few hours to achieve maturation (first PB extrusion) *in vitro*. In such a case, ICSI should be performed at least 2 h after PB extrusion (Balakier 2004; Montag et al. 2006).

Selecting Sperm For ICSI

Sperm morphology is accepted as the best predictor of fertilization potential, and hence ICSI practitioners aim to select live sperm based on appearance where possible (Li et al. 2014). Enhanced sperm observation with higher-resolution microscopy, such as the intracytoplasmic morphologically selected sperm injection (IMSI) technique, is used by some laboratories, although the benefit of IMSI as a routine treatment is questionable (Ebner et al. 2014).

Globozoospermia is a rare and poorly understood condition, whereby sperm are round-headed and lack an acrosome. Globospermic samples are generally considered unable to fertilize using ICSI, unless the oocyte is artificially activated postinjection. Case reports are now emerging which describe ICSI for globozoospermia combined with oocyte activation by calcium ionophore, resulting in the birth of healthy babies (e.g. Karaca et al. 2015).

Other methods to help select the best sperm for ICSI include use of polarization microscopy to measure partial head birefringence (Vermey et al. 2015) and hyaluronic acid binding methods (e.g. using commercial media such as SpermSlow® and specially treated dishes such as PICSI®). However, there is still insufficient evidence to conclude if any of these advanced sperm selection techniques should be recommended for use in routine clinical practice (McDowell et al. 2014).

If sperm are not motile, as seen in semen samples from men suffering from immotile cilia syndrome, a vitality test can be used to select viable sperm at the time of injection. An example is the hypo-osmotic swelling test (HOS) which can be used to identify viable sperm from a pool of immotile sperm. Healthy live births have been reported following HOS combined with ICSI (e.g. Peeraer et al. 2004).

Fertilization Assessment

The Optimal Time to Perform Fertilization Assessment

Following conventional IVF insemination, the gametes are normally coincubated for 16–18 h before the oocytes are assessed to see if fertilization has taken place. The oocytes need to be denuded from the remaining cumulus cells, which should have been loosened by the sperm. The denuded oocytes should be washed in fresh pre-equilibrated medium prior to evaluation.

Following ICSI, if time-lapse imaging has been used, then the exact time of any PN formation can be observed from the stored images. If not, then the oocytes need to be assessed at 16–18 h after ICSI.

Oocytes need to be examined in detail for the presence and number of PN and polar bodies. Fertilization assessment should be performed under high magnification (at least x 200), using an inverted microscope equipped with Hoffman optics or equivalent. Again, if oocytes have been incubated in a time-lapse incubator, then the assessment of the images may be performed without the need to remove the dish.

As well as assessing PN number and position (abuttal), the morphological status of each oocyte should be recorded. Normally fertilized (2PN) oocytes should be transferred into new dishes with pre-equilibrated fresh culture medium. 2PN oocytes resulting from ICSI can remain in culture in the same dish or be moved to new dishes according to laboratory policy.

Normal Fertilization

According to the Alpha-ESHRE Consensus (2011), a good quality, normally fertilized oocyte has 2PN juxtaposed and centrally positioned, and 2PBs (Alpha and ESHRE 2011). PN should ideally be comparable in size, with any clear size differences recorded, as any asymmetry may influence selection. The PN position within the cytoplasm (central/peripheral) and degree of abuttal should also be noted.

Some laboratories also look at the distribution, position, and number of nuclear precursor bodies within the PN. Braga et al. (2013) have shown that different PN features may influence further embryo development, especially the quality of the blastocyst. This group has demonstrated an association between PN and blastocyst morphology which may be used as a prognostic tool for implantation. However, others consider nucleoli scoring to be less predictive of embryo viability, when compared with embryo morphokinetics (Aguilar et al. 2014)

The presence of a halo (movement of organelles away from the oolemma) and the PB number should also be noted, alongside any unusual features (e.g. abnormal oocyte shape, ZP thickness/evenness, clusters of cytoplasmic granularity, a large PVS size, etc.).

Failed fertilization

If no PN are observed, this usually indicates failed fertilization. This can be confirmed if only one PB is present. If failed fertilization occurs, the ZP should be observed to see if there is any sperm–ZP binding. If this is absent, then failed fertilization is most likely. Such oocytes can be observed for a further 24 h to see if fertilization takes place later. If an embryo forms, then a transfer can be considered, as pregnancies have arisen from such events (Feenan and Herbert 2006). It is recommended that such embryos are cultured for 5 days to the blastocyst stage *in vitro* to provide assurance of developmental competence.

If oocytes do fail to fertilize after conventional IVF insemination, some countries allow 'rescue ICSI', whereby the oocytes are subjected to ICSI despite having already been coincubated with motile sperm. Rescue ICSI can result in the delivery of healthy newborns, although the pregnancy rates are low (Beck-Fruchter et al. 2014). Other researchers have analysed the clinical and economic worth of rescue ICSI and have found the cost-effectiveness of the procedure in terms of total fertilization failure to be worthwhile (Shalom-paz et al. 2011).

Following a failed fertilization cycle, the options for a future treatment cycle include: increasing the insemination number for IVF insemination, ICSI, or use of donor gametes. ICSI is often the more popular option, as it maintains the genetic make-up of the couple.

Abnormal Fertilization

Oocytes with >2PN should be immediately discarded and not used for treatment under any circumstance since an additional set of chromosomes exists within the zygote. Diandric triploidy results from two haploid sperm or a single diploid sperm fertilizing the oocyte, resulting in 3PN and 2PN respectively. In the latter case, the male PN will be larger than the female PN as it is diploid. This scenario emphasizes the need to assess PN size and symmetry, to assist in identifying possible abnormalities. Digynic triploidy may occur after ICSI due to nonextrusion of the second PB, such that 3PN form (Rosenbusch 2008).

Oocytes displaying 1PN may have undergone activation rather than fertilization. Pregnancies have been reported from the transfer of embryos derived from 1PN oocytes (Feenan and Herbert, 2006). However, other laboratories prefer not to take any risk, and allow all embryos derived from 1PN oocytes to perish.

Conclusion

This chapter has outlined how oocytes are fertilized *in vitro* via conventional IVF and ICSI, and how fertilization assessments are subsequently carried out in the IVF laboratory. For further information, atlases on embryology such as the *Atlas of Oocytes, Zygotes and Embryos in Reproductive Medicine* (Elder et al. 2012) are recommended. Such an atlas provided numerous images of oocytes and zygotes, demonstrating the variation of dysmorphisms and types of fertilization that result in the human.

References

Alpha Scientists in Reproductive Medicine and ESHRE Special Interest Group of Embryology (2011). The Istanbul consensus workshop on embryo assessment: proceedings of an expert meeting. Hum Reprod 26: 1270–1283.

Aguilar, J., Motato, Y., Escribá, M.-J. et al. (2014). The human first cell cycle: impact on implantation. Reprod Biomed Online 28: 475–484.

Arias, M.E., Sánchez, R., Risopatrón, J. et al. (2014). Effect of sperm pretreatment with sodium hydroxide and dithiothreitol on the efficiency of bovine intracytoplasmic sperm injection. Reprod Fertil Dev 26: 847–854.

Balakier, H. (2004). Time-dependent capability of human oocytes for activation and pronuclear formation during metaphase II arrest. Hum Reprod 19: 982–987.

Barraud-Lange, V., Sifer, C., Pocaté, K. et al. (2008). Short gamete co-incubation during in vitro fertilisation decreases the fertilisation rate and does not improve embryo quality: a prospective auto controlled study. J Assist Reprod Genet 25: 305–310.

Beck-Fruchter, R., Lavee, M., Weiss, A. et al. (2014). Rescue intracytoplasmic sperm injection: a systematic review. Fertil Steril 101: 690–698.

Boulet, S.L, Mehta, A., Kissin, D.M. et al. (2015). Trends in use of and reproductive outcomes associated with intracytoplasmic sperm injection. JAMA 313: 255–263.

Braga, D.P., Setti, A.S., Figueira, R. de C. et al. (2013). The combination of pronuclear and blastocyst morphology: a strong prognostic tool for implantation potential. J Assist Reprod Genet 30: 1327–1332.

Brun, R.B. (1974). Studies on fertilisation in Xenopus laevis. Biol Reprod 11: 513–551.

de los Santos, M.J. and Ruiz, A. (2013). Protocols for tracking and witnessing samples and patients in assisted reproductive technology. Fertil Steril 100: 1499–1502.

De Vos, A., Van Landuyt, L., Van Ranst, H. et al. (2008). Randomized sibling-oocyte study using recombinant human hyaluronidase versus bovine-derived Sigma hyaluronidase in ICSI patients. Hum Reprod 23: 1815–1819.

Dib, L.A., Araújo, M.C., Giorgenon, R.C. et al. (2013). Noninvasive imaging of the meiotic spindle of in vivo matured oocytes from infertile women with endometriosis. Reprod Sci 20: 456–462.

Ebner, T., Moser, M., Sommergruber, M. et al. (2006). Incomplete denudation of oocytes prior to ICSI enhances embryo quality and blastocyst development. Hum Reprod 21: 2972–2977.

Ebner, T., Shebl, O., Oppelt, P. and Mayer, R.B. (2014). Some reflections on intracytoplasmic morphologically selected sperm injection. Int J Fertil Steril 8: 105–112.

Ebner, T., Yaman, C., Moser, M. et al. (2001). A prospective study on oocyte survival rate after ICSI: influence of injection technique and morphological features. J Assist Reprod Genet 18: 623–628.

Elder K, Van den Bergh M and Woodward BJ (2015). *Troubleshooting and Problem Solving in The IVF Laboratory*. Cambridge: Cambridge University Press.

ESHRE Guideline Group on Good Practice in IVF Labs, De los Santos MJ, Apter S, Coticchio G et al. (2015). Revised guidelines for good practice in IVF laboratories (2015). Hum Reprod 31: 685–686.

Feenan, K. and Herbert, M. (2006). Can 'abnormally' fertilized zygotes give rise to viable embryos? Hum Fertil 9: 157–169.

Ferraretti, A.P., Goossens, V., Kupka, M. et al. (2013). Assisted reproductive technology in Europe, 2009: results generated from European registers by ESHRE. Hum Reprod 28: 2318–2331.

Frapsauce, C., Pionneau, C., Bouley, J. et al. (2009). Unexpected in vitro fertilisation failure in patients with normal sperm: a proteomic analysis. Gynecol Obstet Fertil 37: 796–802.

Guo, H., Yang, J., Zhang, C. et al. (2012). Analysis of clinical data of patients with different outcomes after short-time insemination. Andrologia 44(Suppl 1): 667–671.

Hu, L.L., Shen, X.H., Zheng, Z. et al. (2012). Cytochalasin B treatment of mouse oocytes during intracytoplasmic sperm injection (ICSI) increases embryo survival without impairment of development. Zygote 20: 361–369.

Karaca, N., Akpak, Y.K., Oral, S. et al. (2015). A successful healthy childbirth in a case of total globozoospermia with oocyte activation by calcium ionophore. J Reprod Fertil 16: 116–120.

Kato, Y. and Nagao, Y. (2012). Effect of polyvinylpyrrolidone on sperm function and early embryonic development following intracytoplasmic sperm injection in human assisted reproduction. Reprod Med Biol 11: 165–176.

Li, B., Ma, Y., Huang, J. et al. (2014). Probing the effect of human normal sperm morphology rate on cycle outcomes and assisted reproductive methods selection. PLoS One 9: e113392.

McDowell, S., Kroon, B., Ford, E. et al. (2014). Advanced sperm selection techniques for assisted reproduction. Cochrane Database Syst Rev 10: CD010461.

Montag, M., Schimming, T., van der Ven, H. (2006). Spindle imaging in human oocytes: the impact of the meiotic cell cycle. Reprod Biomed Online 12: 442–446.

Munné, S., Ary, J., Zouves, C. et al. (2006). Wide range of chromosome abnormalities in the embryos of young egg donors. Reprod Med Online 12: 340–346.

Nagy, Z.P., Liu, J., Joris, H. et al. (1995). The influence of the site of sperm deposition and mode of oolemma breakage at intracytoplasmic sperm injection on fertilisation and embryo development rates. Hum Reprod 10: 3171–3177.

Palermo, G., Joris, H., Devroey, P. et al. (1992). Pregnancies after intracytoplasmic injection of single spermatozoon into an oocyte Lancet 340(8810): 17–18.

Palermo, G.D., Neri, Q.V. and Rosenwaks, Z. (2015). To ICSI or not to ICSI. Semin Reprod Med 33: 92–102.

Peeraer, K., Nijs, M., Raick, D. et al. (2004). Pregnancy after ICSI with ejaculated immotile spermatozoa from a patient with immotile cilia syndrome: a case report and review of the literature. Reprod Biomed Online 9: 659–663.

Rosenbusch, B.E. (2008). Mechanisms giving rise to triploid zygotes during assisted reproduction. Fertil Steril 90: 49–55.

Shalom-paz, E., Alshalati, J., Shehata, F. et al. (2011). Clinical and economic analysis of rescue intracytoplasmic sperm injection cycles. Gynecol Endocrinol 27: 993–996.

Swiatecka, J., Bielawski, T., Anchim, T. et al. (2014). Oocyte zona pellucida and meiotic spindle birefringence as a biomarker of pregnancy rate outcome in IVF-ICSI treatment. Ginek Pol 85: 264–271.

Van den Bergh, M., Elder, K. and Ebner, T. (2012). *Atlas of Oocytes, Zygotes and Embryos in Reproductive Medicine*. Cambridge: Cambridge University Press.

Van Beirs, N., Shaw-Jackson, C., Rozenberg, S. et al. (2015). Policy of IVF centres towards oocytes affected by Smooth Endoplasmic Reticulum aggregates: a multicentre survey study. J Assist Reprod Genet 32: 945–950.

Van Steirteghem, A.C., Nagy, Z., Joris, H. et al. (1993). High fertilisation and implantation rates after intracytoplasmic sperm injection. Hum Reprod 8: 1061–1066.

Vermey, B.G., Chapman, M.G., Cooke, S. et al. (2015). The relationship between sperm head retardance using polarized light microscopy and clinical outcomes. Reprod Biomed Online 30: 67–73.

Woodward B.J., Montgomery, S.J., Hartshorne, G.M. et al. (2008). Spindle position assessment prior to ICSI does not benefit fertilisation or early embryonic potential. Reprod Biomed Online 16: 232–238.

Woodward, B.J., Campbell, K.H.S. and Ramsewak, S.S. (2005). A comparison of headfirst and tailfirst microinjection of sperm at intracytoplasmic sperm injection. Ferti Steril 89: 711–714.

25

Morphological Assessment of Embryos in Culture

J. Diane Critchlow

Why Do We Select Embryos?

The purpose of embryo selection is to improve live birth rates per egg collection by maximizing use of all embryos with implantation potential, but to achieve low multiple pregnancy rates by reducing the number of fresh embryos transferred (Pandian et al. 2013). Selection of spare embryos for cryostorage and use in future cycles increases cumulative live birth rates (Glujovsky 2012).

Routine or 'conventional' embryo assessment is currently focused mainly on morphological criteria and cleavage rate during development. This is performed noninvasively at several predetermined microscopic evaluations during removal of the embryos from the incubator and continues to be the most widespread system in use (Gianaroli et al. 2000; Magli et al. 2012). However, this process may result in detrimental environmental stress and provides only a brief snapshot of embryo development. It must also be remembered that despite the best efforts of embryologists to select an embryo for transfer with the most potential, the process of implantation includes several factors that may not be directly related to the embryo, including receptivity of the endometrium (Evans et al. 2014). The ability of alternative screening technologies (preimplantation genetic screening (PGS), metabolomics, proteomics) has been evaluated in recent years, but has not yet superseded routine morphology assessment (Gleicher et al. 2014; Vergouw et al. 2014). Most recently, use of time-lapse imaging (TLI) with formulation of morphokinetic algorithms to assess embryos has produced higher implantation rates

(Meseguer et al. 2011; Basile et al. 2015), but improvements may be the result of undisturbed culture reducing embryo stress.

In the UK, it is policy for all clinics to reduce multiple birth rates to below 10% (HFEA) and the NICE Fertility Guidelines (2013) recommend elective single embryo transfer (eSET) in women who have at least one 'top quality' embryo. However, the lack of standardized embryo morphology grading systems in assisted reproductive technology clinics worldwide has made the definition of embryo 'quality' and comparison of studies very difficult. Recently, there has been a move towards standardization of grading schemes internationally (Cutting et al. 2008; Vernon et al. 2009; Racowsky et al. 2010; Alpha/ESHRE Istanbul Consensus 2011; Pons et al. 2014) and the development of external quality assessment (EQA) schemes (UK NEQAS) to assess interlaboratory performance and reduce operator subjectivity. However, while there is a certain amount of agreement on what constitutes a 'top quality' or a 'poor' embryo, it is more difficult to find a consensus between laboratories when attempting to evaluate intermediate quality embryos. The latter may be deselected from clinical use and yet may have implantation potential (Kirkegaard et al. 2014).

A Cochrane data review (Pandian et al. 2013) revealed that there is no evidence of a significant difference in the cumulative live birth rate when a single cycle of double embryo transfer is compared with repeated eSETs (fresh and frozen cycles), particularly in younger women. Improvement in cryostorage techniques and frozen embryo success rates seems to be leading to a change in thinking and

Clinical Reproductive Science, First Edition. Edited by Michael Carroll.
© 2019 John Wiley & Sons Ltd. Published 2019 by John Wiley & Sons Ltd.
Companion website: www.wiley.com/go/carroll/clinicalreproductivescience

questioning of embryo selection methods in fresh cycles (Gleicher et al. 2015). Extended culture to the blastocyst stage, rather than earlier cleavage stage transfer, has become increasingly integrated into routine clinical practice by many assisted reproductive technology centres worldwide. The 'deselection' of embryos by extended culture or by grading as 'unsuitable' for cryostorage may lead to loss of embryos which may have implantation potential. Indeed, an earlier Cochrane review showed that cumulative pregnancy rates from embryos transferred on Day 3 significantly outperformed transfers at blastocyst stage (Glujovsky et al. 2012). In the light of current information regarding possible compromised endometrial quality in stimulated cycles (Shapiro et al. 2011), there is strong evidence to suggest that IVF outcomes can be improved with the adoption of 'freeze-all' or elective frozen embryo transfer (eFET) strategies (Evans et al. 2014; Roque et al. 2015). There is also evidence for improved neonatal outcomes in frozen cycles (Imudia et al. 2014). This may lead to a different emphasis being placed on embryo assessment and selection, particularly in fresh cycles.

This chapter will review the most widely used embryo assessment methods using morphological parameters at defined stages of culture postinsemination. Photomicrographic illustrations have not been included, but can be found in a recent extensive review (Magli et al. 2012).

Conventional Morphology Assessment

Assessment of Zygotes and Cleavage Stage Embryos

The most widely used morphological parameters have been cell number/rate of embryo development, cell size/cleavage evenness, and cell fragmentation. However, it will become clear in the sections below that assessment of each of these parameters can be subjective and interrelated. For example, large anuclear fragments may be mistaken for cells, which will in turn affect the accuracy of cell count, degree of fragmentation, and assessment of cell size/ cleavage evenness. Nevertheless, early embryo selection based on morphology assessment improves

implantation and pregnancy rates (De Placido et al. 2002; Vernon et al. 2009; Machtinger and Rackovsky 2013). Analysis of pronuclear (PN) morphology after fertilization and multinucleation (MN) scoring at the 2–4-cell stage has also been widely used.

Pronuclear/Zygote Grading

The process of fertilization involves an ordered series of morphological changes that affect the appearance of the one cell zygote (Edwards and Beard 1999). Assessment at the zygote stage is also useful in countries where legislation requires that only a limited number of embryos may continue in culture prior to embryo transfer (Zollner et al. 2002; Senn et al. 2006); embryos considered to have the best implantation potential after PN grading are cultured for transfer and sibling zygotes are cryostored.

PN scoring involves assessment of the alignment of the PN and the number and relative position of the nucleolar precursor bodies (NPBs) in the PN. The most established methods of PN analysis have been described as Patterns 0–5 (Tesarik et al. 2000) and by Z scores 1–4 (Scott 2003), but with much variation between clinics. According to the Alpha/ESHRE Istanbul Consensus (2011), three grades for PN scoring are based on the morphology of NPBs and PNs: (1) symmetrical; (2) non-symmetrical and; (3) abnormal (Table 25.1). As the processes associated with fertilization by IVF insemination lag behind fertilization using ICSI (Nagy et al. 2003), PN

Table 25.1 Grading scheme for pronuclear stage embryo assessment (Alpha/ESHRE Istanbul Consensus 2011).

Grade	Rating	Description
1	Symmetrical	Zygotes presenting with equal numbers and size of NPBs, either aligned at the junction between PNs or scattered in both PNs.
2	Nonsymmetrical	Comprises all other patterns including peripherally localized PNs.
3	Abnormal	Single NPB or total absence of NPBs.

NPB, nucleolar precursor bodies; PN, pronuclei.

grading must be performed at a standardized time relative to insemination time, i.e. 17 + 1 h postinsemination (Alpha/ESHRE Istanbul Consensus 2011).

The value of PN scoring has been debated, with some studies showing a prognostic effect (Tesarik et al. 2000; Balaban et al. 2004; Zamora et al. 2011) and a correlation with aneuploidy (Gianaroli et al. 2003; Edirisinghe et al. 2005), or no prognostic value (James et al. 2006; Nicoli et al. 2010; Weitzman et al. 2010; Berger et al. 2014).

One of the main limitations of assessing the highly dynamic PN formation is having to use single and static observations. TLI systems may now be used to help define the timing for zygote assessment and the dynamic changes that occur, although the concept is not new (Payne et al. 1997). This may provide more information to solve discrepancies in the literature (Nicoli et al. 2013).

Early Cleavage Check

Checking embryos again on Day 1 (Table 25.2) for the time of syngamy (disappearance of PN) and first cleavage has been used by some laboratories as an additional tool in selecting embryos with high implantation potential and decreased chromosomal anomalies (Lawler et al. 2007; Hammoud et al. 2008).

Early cleaving embryos have been reported to divide more evenly, which has been correlated with a lower incidence of chromosomal errors (Hardarson et al. 2001), and in eSETs with higher clinical pregnancy rates (Salumets et al. 2003), although precocious embryo development (cleavage earlier than 20 h postinsemination) gave a poorer prognosis. Although a recent review found no value in an early cleaving check (de los Santos et al. 2014), the use of TLI may prove a particularly powerful tool to assess early cleavage and subtle morphological changes without removal from the incubator (Lemmen et al. 2008). The visualization of anomalous events with TLI such as direct cleavage and reverse cleavage previously not possible with conventional static microscopy may be useful as deselection criteria. Direct cleavage has been shown to be associated with very low implantation rates (1.2%) in embryos dividing from one to three cells in less than 5 h (Rubio et al. 2012a).

Day 2 and Day 3 Stage Embryos

Morphological evaluation at cleavage stages has traditionally formed the basis for determining embryo quality, with the first live birth reported following transfer at this stage (Steptoe and Edwards 1978). Recommended timings for assessment are shown in Table 25.3. Blastocyst stage transfer after extended culture to Day 5/6 was less common until culture media systems were improved. Routine use of PGS for IVF/ICSI cycles to deselect aneuploid cleavage stage embryos has been shown to be unreliable and even reduce pregnancy rates (Gleicher and Barad 2012) due to mosaicism of embryos at this stage. The following parameters are currently most widely used in Day 2 and Day 3 grading schemes.

Cell Number/Cleavage Rate

The single most important indicator of embryo viability is the occurrence of cellular division. The ideal cleavage was found to be four cells on Day 2 and eight cells on Day 3, with a markedly lower implantation potential for embryos below that and, to a lesser degree above that (Holte et al. 2007) and is in general agreement with previous observations (Van Royen et al. 1999; Magli et al. 2001). A correlation

Table 25.2 Recommended timings for early cleavage stage (Day 1) embryo assessment (Alpha/ESHRE Istanbul Consensus 2011).

Observation	Timing (Hours Postinsemination)	Expected Stage of Development
Syngamy check	23 ± 1 h	Up to 50% in syngamy (up to 20% at the two-cell stage)
Early cleavage check	26 ± 1 h post-ICSI 28 ± 1 h post-IVF	Two-cell stage

ICSI, intracytoplasmic sperm injection; IVF, *in vitro* fertilization.

Table 25.3 Recommended timings for cleavage stage Day 2 and Day 3 embryo assessment (Alpha/ESHRE Istanbul Consensus 2011).

Observation	Timing (Hours Postinsemination)	Expected Stage Of Development
Day 2 assessment	44 ± 1 h	Four-cell stage
Day 3 assessment	68 ± 1 h	Eight-cell stage

between 'normal cell number' and chromosomal constitution has also been reported (Almeida and Bolton 1996; Magli et al. 2007).

Fragmentation

Mitotic division of embryos can lead to externalization of parts of the cell cytoplasm, resulting in the presence of anuclear fragments surrounded by a plasma membrane (Antczak and van Blerkom 1999). Presence of fragmentation is common in human embryos and assessment has been used in almost all embryo scoring systems. Severe fragmentation of the embryo is associated with poor prognosis (Ziebe et al. 1997; Van Royen et al. 1999, 2001).

As well as the percentage of fragmentation in the embryo, fragment size and distribution has been shown to correlate with the probability of implantation (Alikani et al. 2000; Ebner et al. 2001; Van Blerkom et al. 2001). However, it is often unclear how to differentiate fragments from cells and then estimate the relative proportion of the embryo that is fragmented. Large fragments, sometimes resembling whole cells, often distributed randomly, are associated with uneven cells and produced a low implantation rate in some studies (Alikani and Cohen 1995). The loss of important cytoplasmic content, such as cell organelles, proteins, or mRNA may leave cells in largely fragmented embryos too small to be biologically competent (Johansson et al. 2003; Hnida et al. 2004).

The size of fragmented cells has been defined as <45 mm in diameter for Day 2 embryos, and <40 mm in diameter for Day 3 embryos (Johansson et al. 2003; Alpha/ESHRE Istanbul Consensus 2011). As mentioned earlier, these findings may influence scoring criteria; embryos previously scored with uneven-sized cells might now be scored as partially fragmented embryos. However, it is not easy to measure the size of fragments routinely, and use of TLI may reduce subjectivity.

The presence of small, scattered fragments (10–20%) does not appear to impair further development (Van Royen et al. 1999; Hardarson et al. 2001; Racowsky et al. 2003) and these may disappear through lysis or resorption during culture (Hardarson et al. 2001). Thus, a low degree of fragmentation may be normal and may suggest apoptotic elimination of selected cells in an effort to restore or maintain viability when anomalies are present (Ziebe 1997; Alikani et al. 2000).

It is also possible that these fragments are generated during successive divisions and are simply a product of imperfect cytokinesis rather than a specific anomaly.

Cell Size/Cleavage Evenness

When undergoing the first mitotic cell divisions, a zygote cleaving synchronously and symmetrically will present two, four, or eight cells of a similar size. Cells of equal size appear to be another indicator of implantation potential (Steer et al. 1992; Hardarson et al. 2001; Hnida et al. 2004; Paternot et al 2013). For all other early cleavage stages of three, five, six, seven, and nine cells, a size difference in the cells would be expected as the cleavage phase has not been completed (Scott 2001; Magli et al. 2012).

Several studies have identified the phenomenon of uneven cleavage leading to unequal cell size, and this is commonly found in IVF embryos. Unevenly sized cells have also been shown to have an increased prevalence of chromosomal abnormalities (Hardarson et al. 2001; Magli et al. 2001: Ziebe et al. 2003), including multinucleation (Hardarson et al. 2001). The latter study suggested that early cleavage may be hindered by the presence of aneuploidy delaying the cell cycle. This impairment may also be due to uneven distribution of proteins, mRNA, mitochondria, and furthermore may possibly disturb the polarized allocation of certain proteins and genes in both oocytes and embryos (Antczak and Van Blerkom 1999).

However, there are difficulties with routine microscopic assessment as cells scored as unevenly cleaved may actually be large anucleate fragments. As mentioned above in the section on fragmentation, embryos with uneven-sized cells might be scored as partially fragmented embryos and vice-versa. This will in turn also affect the reliability of the cell count assessment, e.g. an embryo scored as an uneven eight-cell may actually be a fragmented six-cell embryo. TLI may be used as a tool to improve reliability of assessment allowing quantitative measurement.

Multinucleation

A cell containing more than a single interphase nucleus, is defined as being multinucleated (MN) and considered abnormal. A negative impact on the implantation potential of MN embryos has been observed (Van Royen et al. 2003; Saldeen and

Sundstrom, 2005) and has been correlated with a high degree of chromosomal aberration (Kligman et al. 1996; Hardarson et al. 2001) with MN cells being significantly larger than nonnucleated cells (Hnida et al. 2004).

However, it was shown that among embryos in which both cells were bi- or multinuclear at the two-cell stage, 30% had only mononuclear cells following cleavage (Staessen and Van Steirteghem 1998). Thus, some MN cells still seem to be able to cleave normally (Meriano et al. 2004).

Factors that have been suggested to affect the rate of MN include culture media (Winston et al. 1991), and poor temperature control especially in relation to oocyte retrieval (Pickering et al. 1990). Different mechanisms leading to MN cells have been suggested including the dissociation of karyokinesis from cytokinesis, partial fragmentation of the nucleus, or defective migration of chromosomes at mitotic anaphase (Munne and Cohen 1993; Staessen and Van Steirteghem 1998). Fluorescence *in situ* hybridization (FISH) demonstrated that all these mechanisms may be involved.

Grading Schemes for Selection of Cleavage Stage Embryos

In the UK, a standardized grading scheme (Cutting et al. 2008; Table 25.4) is used by the External Quality Assessment Scheme (UK NEQAS) for Embryology, launched in 2009. This grading scheme was presented

Table 25.4 UK National Grading Scheme for Day 2 and Day 3 cleavage stage embryo assessment.

	Blastomere Number
Blastomere size	4 = regular, even division 3 = <20% difference (blastomere diameter) 2 = 20–50% difference 1 = >50% difference (after Hardarson et al. 2001)
Fragmentation	4 = <10% fragmentation by volume 3 = 10–20% 2 = 20–40% 1 = >50% (after van Royen et al. 2003)

Example: The grade is recorded as [cell number] c (size/fragmentation); therefore, a four-cell embryo with slightly uneven cell division (~10% difference in cell size) and around 30% fragmentation by volume will be scored 4c(3/2).
Source: Cutting et al. (2008).

Table 25.5 Amended UK National Grading Scheme for Day 2 and Day 3 cleavage stage embryo assessment (ACE 2017).

Grades	Blastomere Size	Fragmentation
4	Same as ideal stage specific embryo[a]	<10%
3	Stage specific size for majority of blasts (i.e. slightly uneven sizes)	10–20%
2	Majority of blasts different sizes	20–50%
1	Not stage specific	>50%

[a] See Figure 25.1.

in 2011 at the Istanbul Consensus meeting by Daniel Brison and endorsed the NICE Fertility Guidelines (2013). The grading scheme has recently been reviewed by an ACE working party in consultation with the ACE membership and UK NEQAS Reproductive Science (Critchlow et al. 2016). The amended grading scheme was released by ACE in January 2017 and adopted by the UK NEQAS Scheme for Embryology in April 2017. ACE and NEQAS have agreed that all embryos should be graded in a stage-specific way (Table 25.5). This is particularly relevant for those embryos that are naturally asynchronous, such as those with three, five and seven blastomeres.

An explanation of stage-specific grading for cleavage stage embryos is:

An optimal Day 2 embryo (Grade 1: 44 + 1 h postinsemination) would have four equally sized mononucleated cells in a three-dimensional tetrahedral arrangement, with <10% fragmentation. An optimal Day 3 embryo (68 + 1 h postinsemination) would have eight equally sized mononucleated cells, with <10% fragmentation (Alpha/ESHRE Istanbul Consensus 2011; Table 25.6).

Assessment of Day 4, 5 and 6 Stage Embryos

Day 4 Embryo Assessment

Assessment on Day 4 has not been commonly used for embryo selection, although grading systems have been described (Tao et al. 2002; Feil et al. 2008; Alpha/ESHRE Istanbul Consensus 2011). Early compaction appears to be a good prognosticator for

Table 25.6 Grading scheme for Day 2 and Day 3 cleavage stage embryo assessment (Alpha/ESHRE Istanbul Consensus 2011).

Grade	Rating	Description
1	Good	<10% fragmentation, stage specific cell size, no multinucleation
2	Fair	Up to 25% fragmentation, stage specific cell size for the majority of cells, no multinucleation
3	Poor	Severe fragmentation (>25%), cell size not stage specific, evidence of multinucleation

implantation (Tao et al. 2002; Skiadas et al 2006; Le Cruguel 2013) and use of TLI may prove useful. An optimal embryo at this stage (92 ± 2 h postinsemination) would be compacted or compacting, and have entered into a fourth round of cleavage. Compaction should include virtually all the embryo volume (Alpha/ESHRE Istanbul Consensus 2011).

Day 5 and 6 Blastocyst Assessment
The following morphology parameters have been included in most grading schemes:

- Expansion of the blastocoel cavity
- Inner cell mass (ICM)
- Trophectoderm (TE).

Transferring embryos at the blastocyst stage is the most biologically correct stage for embryos to be in the uterus, as earlier stages are naturally in the Fallopian tube. Embryonic genome activation has occurred and two different cell types can be examined providing additional information for the embryologist, particularly when selecting for eSET (Gardner and Balaban 2006) The extent to which the trophectoderm develops will reflect the embryo's ability to attach and implant in the endometrium, while development of the inner cell mass is crucial for the development of the fetus itself (Kovacic et al. 2004).

With improvement in culture media systems, the utilization of blastocyst stage embryo transfer has become much more widespread (Gleicher et al. 2015). Early studies reported that fewer chromosomally abnormal embryos reached blastocyst stage (Magli et al. 2001), but later little correlation between blastocyst morphology and chromosomal abnormalities was found (Fragouli et al. 2012; Schoolcraft et al. 2010). While higher rates of chromosome abnormalities have been found in blastocysts developing from embryos that had poor Day 3 morphology (Bielanska et al. 2002; Hardarson et al. 2003), another study found that 65% of mosaic blastocysts had good morphology (Bielanska et al. 2005). Thus, extended culture does not appear to be an appropriate tool to screen against chromosomal abnormalities (Gleicher et al. 2015).

An improved method of PGS using TE biopsy was proposed as part of routine IVF (Fragouli and Wells 2012; Rubio et al. 2012b), and produced further support for blastocyst culture. However, currently available data do not demonstrate outcome improvements for routine cycles (Gleicher and Barad 2012; Gleicher et al 2014). It is also important that the endometrium is receptive at the time of embryo transfer since a recent study found 30% of euploid blastocysts failed to implant highlighting that factors other than those relating to the embryo need to be considered to ensure success.

The disadvantages of extended culture to blastocyst couples, particularly for couples who have a high number of good quality embryos, include a lower rate of spare embryos available for cryostorage. For patients with low numbers of embryos, there may be poor survival to blastocyst stage. Furthermore, there is no evidence that an embryo that does not develop *in vitro* between Day 3 and Day 5 would not have done so *in vivo* after replacement at the cleavage stage (Vajta et al. 2010). Epigenetic risks have also been associated with prolonged maintenance of embryos *in vitro* (Chason et al. 2011).

A Cochrane data review (Glujovsky et al. 2012) provided evidence that there was a small significant difference in live birth rates in favour of blastocyst transfer compared with cleavage stage transfer. However, cumulative clinical pregnancy rates from cleavage stage (derived from fresh and thaw cycles) resulted in higher clinical pregnancy rates than from blastocyst cycles. As slower growing or poorer morphology blastocysts are usually deselected and discarded they result in fewer cryostored embryos after extended culture. Nevertheless, slow blastocysts vitrified on Day 6 appear to give good results in frozen embryo replacement cycles when transferred on Day 5 (Sunkara et al. 2010).

Grading Schemes for Selection of Blastocyst Stage Embryos

The UK standardized grading scheme (Cutting et al. 2008; Table 25.7) is used by the UK NEQAS Scheme for Embryology and endorsed by the NICE Fertility Guidelines (2013) and has recently been reviewed by an ACE working party in consultation with the ACE membership and UK NEQAS Reproductive Science (Critchlow et al. 2016; Table 25.8). The amended grading scheme was released by ACE in January 2017 and adopted by the UK NEQAS Scheme for Embryology in April 2017 (Figure 25.1). With the amended grading scheme there is a reduction in ICM grading from five grades to four (A–D or 4–1)

Table 25.7 UK National Grading Scheme for Day 5 blastocyst stage embryo assessment based on that originally developed by Gardner and Schoolcraft (1999) and developed further by Stephenson et al. (2007).

Stage of Development	Grade	Description
Expansion status	6	Hatched
	5	Hatching
	4	Expanded (blastocoel volume larger than early embryo)
	3	Full blastocyst (blastocoel fills embryo)
	2	Blastocyst (blastocoel >50% volume of embryo)
	1	Early blastocyst (blastocoel <50% volume of embryo
Inner cell mass (ICM)	5	ICM prominent (easily discernible, tightly adhered, compacted cells)
	4	ICM cells less prominent (cells less compacted and larger in size, loosely adhered)
	3	Very few cells visible (cells similar to TE cells)
	2	ICM cells degenerate/necrotic
	1	No ICM cells
Trophectoderm	3	Continuous layer small identical cells
	2	Fewer, larger cells, not continuous
	1	Sparse cells, large/flat/degenerate

TE, trophectoderm.

Table 25.8 Amended UK National Grading Scheme for blastocyst stage embryo assessment (ACE 2017).

Expansion Score	Expansion Status	ICM/TE score*	Inner Cell Mass (ICM)	Trophectoderm (TE)
6	Hatched blastocyst (the blastocyst has evacuated the ZP)			
5	Hatching blastocyst (trophectoderm has started to herniate through ZP)			
4	Expanded (blastocoel volume larger than the embryo, with thinning of ZP)	A	ICM prominent, easily seen, tightly adhered compacted cells	Continuous layer of small identical cells
3	Full blastocyst (blastocoel completely fills embryo)	B	ICM less prominent (cells appear compacted and larger in size, loosely adhered)	Fewer cells with gaps, not continuous
2	Blastocyst (blastocoel >50% volume of embryo)	C	Very few cells visible (cells similar to TE)	Fewer small cells with large cells, not continuous
1	Early blastocyst (blastocoel <50% volume of embryo)	D	No visible cells or visible cells are degenerate or necrotic	Sparse cells, large/flat/degenerate

ZP, zona pellucida.

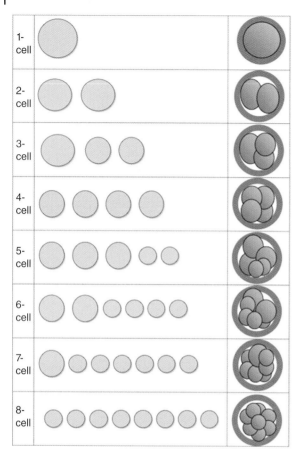

Figure 25.1 Cell sizes in idealized embryos.

energy utilization through the sodium/potassium ATPases on the basolateral membrane of the TE and formation of effective tight junctions between TE cells to form a barrier (Watson et al. 2004).

Time Lapse Imaging (TLI)

Morphokinetic and Morphometric Embryo Assessment

A review of the parameters assessed with TLI and the formulation of morphokinetic algorithms to assess embryo quality is outside the realm of this chapter and the full benefit of the technology and its place among other embryo screening tools remains to be determined (Kovacs 2014).

The main advantage of TLI is continuous, noninvasive embryo observation without the need to remove the embryo from optimal culturing conditions. The extra information provided on the cleavage pattern, morphological changes, and embryo development dynamics not available with routine morphology grading, may improve selection of embryos and the concept is not new (Payne et al. 1997). In addition, quantitative morphometric assessment, e.g. measurement of cell size, is possible (Paternot et al. 2013)

Recent use of this technology has shown improved implantation rates (Rubio et al. 2014; Basile et al 2015), but whether morphokinetic algorithms could ever replace human decision making when selecting embryos for transfer or cryostorage is questionable (Kaser and Racowsky 2014). Kirkehaard et al. (2014) did not find any significant differences in the morphokinetics of embryos that implanted and those that failed to implant in their study population, highlighting the danger that embryos with potential but with a poor algorithm score may be discarded.

At present, morphokinetic data is used mainly in combination with and to support the conventional morphological parameters described previously (Kovacs 2014). Perhaps the use of TLI with algorithms may make deselection more reliable, so fewer embryos with implantation potential are discarded and more embryos are selected for cryostorage and future use.

and an increase in TE grading from three to four (A–D or 4–1) (Figure 25.2). The grading scheme for blastocysts proposed at the Istanbul Consensus in 2011 is shown in Table 25.9.

An optimal embryo at this developmental stage (116 + 2 h) will be a fully expanded through to hatched blastocyst with an ICM that is prominent, easily discernible and consisting of many cells, with the cells compacted and tightly adhered together, and a TE that comprises many cells forming a cohesive epithelium. While the ICM has a high prognostic value for implantation and fetal development, a functional TE is also essential. Grading expansion is important as a reflection of embryo competence as production of the cavity requires both extensive

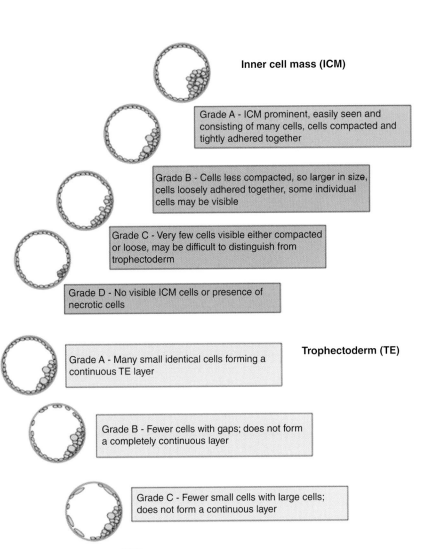

Inner cell mass (ICM)

Grade A - ICM prominent, easily seen and consisting of many cells, cells compacted and tightly adhered together

Grade B - Cells less compacted, so larger in size, cells loosely adhered together, some individual cells may be visible

Grade C - Very few cells visible either compacted or loose, may be difficult to distinguish from trophectoderm

Grade D - No visible ICM cells or presence of necrotic cells

Trophectoderm (TE)

Grade A - Many small identical cells forming a continuous TE layer

Grade B - Fewer cells with gaps; does not form a completely continuous layer

Grade C - Fewer small cells with large cells; does not form a continuous layer

Grade D - Very few cells or degenerate cells

Figure 25.2 Amended UK National Grading Scheme for blastocyst stage embryo assessment (ACE 2017).

Table 25.9 Grading scheme for Day 5 blastocyst stage embryo assessment (Alpha/ESHRE Istanbul Consensus 2011).

	Grade	Rating	Description
Stage of development	1		Early
	2		Blastocyst
	3		Expanded
	4		Hatched/Hatching
Inner cell mass	1	Good	Prominent, easily discernible, with many cells that are compacted and tightly adhered
	2	Fair	Easily discernible with many cells loosely group together
	3	Poor	Difficult to discern with few cells
Trophectoderm	1	Good	Many cells forming a cohesive epithelium
	2	Fair	Few cells forming a loose epithelium
	3	Poor	Very few cells

Conclusion

The most widely used morphological parameters to select embryos for transfer are: (i) cell number/rate of embryo development, cell size/cleavage evenness, cell fragmentation and multinucleation for cleavage for Day 2 to Day 3 stage embryos; (ii) blastocyst expansion, ICM and TE assessment for Day 5 stage embryos; and (iii) PN grading at fertilization check, particularly if embryos are selected for further culture or cryostorage on Day 1. At present, it is useful to adopt a published consensus grading system with defined parameters and standardized times postinsemination for assessment wherever possible, which will allow more meaningful comparison of studies. Participation in interlaboratory EQA schemes and within-laboratory quality control is also recommended.

The use of TLI technology enables semiquantitative evaluation of embryo morphology and developmental kinetics, to support decisions made with conventional morphology assessment (Kovacs 2014). It may also reduce some of the subjectivity and interoperator variability associated with conventional assessment and should be beneficial in terms of undisturbed culture conditions.

Finally, the main aim of embryo selection is to improve live birth rates per egg collection, by maximizing use of all embryos with implantation potential, but with correspondingly low multiple pregnancy rates. This may ultimately involve using bespoke culture and embryo selection strategies for individual patients, giving the best cumulative pregnancy rates by including frozen embryo replacement cycles where possible. Embryo selection using current methods, particularly extended culture and alternative methods (including -omics and even routine PGS at cleavage stage), has led to the possible deselection embryos considered to be 'intermediate' or 'poor' quality, but which still may have implantation potential (Gleicher et al. 2015). It is also important to ensure that embryo transfer is performed when the endometrium is optimal for implantation (Evans et al. 2014). Use of individualized strategies, taking into account patient fertility history and possible tests for endometrial receptivity, may range from 'freeze all' cycles at PN stage with subsequent frozen embryo replacements, to eSET after fresh blastocyst transfer.

References

ACE (2017). UK NEQAS Scheme for Embryology. http://www.cmft.nhs.uk/ukneqasrepsci.aspx)

Alpha Scientists in Reproductive Medicine and ESHRE Special Interest Group of Embryology (2011). The Istanbul consensus workshop on embryo assessment: proceedings of an expert meeting Hum Reprod 26: 1270–1283.

Alikani, M. and Cohen, J. (1995). Patterns of cell fragmentation in the human embryo. J Assist Reprod Genet 12: 28S.

Alikani, M., Calderon, G., Tomkin, G. et al. (2000). Cleavage anomalies in early human embryos and survival after prolonged culture in-vitro. Hum Reprod 15:2634–2643.

Almeida, P.A. and Bolton, V.N. (1996). The relationship between chromosomal abnormality in the human preimplantation embryo and development in vitro. Reprod Fertil Dev 8: 235–241.

Antczak M, Van Blerkom J. (1999). Temporal and spatial aspects of fragmentation in early human embryos: possible effects on developmental competence and association with the differential elimination of regulatory proteins from polarized domains. Hum Reprod 14: 429–447.

Balaban, B., Yakin, K., Urman, B. et al. (2004). Pronuclear morphology predicts embryo development and chromosome constitution. Reprod Biomed Online 8: 695–700.

Basile, N., Vime, P., Florensa, M. et al. (2015). The use of morphokinetics as a predictor of implantation: a multicentric study to define and validate an algorithm for embryo selection. Hum Reprod 30: 276–283.

Berger, D., Zapantis Merhi, Z., Younger, J. et al. (2014). Embryo quality but not pronuclear score is associated with clinical pregnancy following IVF. Assist Reprod Genet 31: 279–283.

Bielanska, M., Tan, S.L. and Ao, A. (2002). Chromosomal mosaicism throughout human preimplantation embryo development in vitro:

incidence, type and relevance to embryo outcome. Hum Reprod 17: 413–419.

Bielanska, M., Jin, S., Bernier, M. et al. (2005). Diploid-aneuploid mosaicism in human embryos cultured to the blastocyst stage. Fertil Steril 84: 336–342.

Chason, R.J., Csokmay, J., Segars, J.H. et al. (2011). Environmental and epigenetic effects upon preimplantation embryo metabolism and development. Trends Endocrinol Metab 22: 412–420.

Critchlow, J.D, Horne, G., Goddard, P. et al. (2016). Development of an external quality assessment (EQA) scheme for embryo morphology using the UK standard embryo grading scheme. 32nd Annual Meeting of ESHRE, Helsinki, Finland.

Cutting, R., Morroll, D., Roberts, S.A. et al., BFS and ACE (2008). Elective single embryo transfer: guidelines for practice British Fertility Society and Association of Clinical Embryologists. Hum Fertil 11: 131–146.

de los Santos, M.J., Arroyo, G., Busquet, A. et al., ASEBIR Interest Group in Embryology. (2014). A multicenter prospective study to assess the effect of early cleavage on embryo quality, implantation, and live-birth rate. Fertil Steril 101: 981–987.

De Placido, G., Wilding, M., Strina, I. et al. (2002). High outcome predictability after IVF using a combined score for zygote and embryo morphology and growth rate. Hum Reprod 17: 2402–2409.

Ebner, T., Yaman, C, Moser M et al. (2001). Embryo fragmentation in vitro and its impact on treatment and pregnancy outcome. Fertil Steril 76: 281–285.

Edwards, R.G. and Beard, H.K. (1999). Hypothesis: sex determination and germline formation are committed at the pronuclear stage in mammalian embryos. Mol Hum Reprod 5: 595–606.

Edirisinghe, W.R., Jemmott, R., Smith, C. et al. (2005). Association of pronuclear Z score with rates of aneuploidy in in-vitro fertilised embryos. Reprod Fertil Dev 17: 529–534.

Evans, J., Hannan, N.J., Edgell, T.A. et al. (2014). Fresh versus frozen embryo transfer: backing clinical decisions with scientific and clinical evidence. Hum Reprod Update 20: 808–821.

Feil, D., Henshaw, R.C. and Lane, M. (2008). Day 4 embryo selection is equal to Day 5 using a new embryo scoring system validated in single embryo transfers. Hum Reprod 7: 1505–1510.

Fragouli, E. and Wells, D. (2012). Aneuploidy screening for embryo selection. Semin Reprod Med 30: 289–301.

Gardner, D.K. and Schoolcraft, W.B. (1999). Culture and transfer of human blastocysts. Curr Opin Obstet Gynecol 11: 307–311.

Gardner, D.K. and Balaban, B. (2006). Choosing between day 3 and day 5 embryo transfers. Clin Obstet Gyn 49: 85–92.

Gianaroli, L., Plachot, M. and Magli, M.C. (2000). Atlas of embryology. Hum Reprod 15: 79.

Gianaroli, L., Magli, M.C., Ferraretti, A.P. et al. (2003). Pronuclear morphology and chromosomal abnormalities as scoring criteria for embryo selection. Fertil Steril 80: 341–349.

Gleicher, N. and Barad, D.H. (2012). A review of, and commentary on, the ongoing second clinical introduction of preimplantation genetic screening (PGS) to routine IVF practice. J Assist Reprod Genet 29: 1159–1166.

Gleicher, N., Kushnir, V.A. and Barad, D.H. (2014). Preimplantation genetic screening (PGS) still in search of a clinical applications: a systematic review. Reprod Biol Endocrinol 12: 22.

Gleicher, N., Kushnir, V.A. and Barad, D.H. (2015). Is it time for a paradigm shift in understanding embryo selection? Reprod Biol Endocrinol 13: 3.

Glujovsky, D., Blake, D., Farquhar, C. et al. (2012). Cleavage stage versus blastocyst stage embryo transfer in assisted reproductive technology. Cochrane Database Syst Rev 11: 7.

Hammoud, I., Vialard, F., Casasnovas, P. et al. (2008). How viable are zygotes in which the PN are still intact at 25 h? Impact on the choice of embryo for transfer. Fertil Steril 90: 551–556.

Hardarson, T., Hanson, C., Sjögren A et al. (2001). Human embryos with unevenly sized blastomeres have lower pregnancy and implantation rates: indications for aneuploidy and multinucleation. Hum Reprod 16: 313–318.

Hardarson T, Caisander C, Sjögren A et al. (2003). A morphological and chromosomal study of blastocysts developing from morphologically suboptimal human preembryos compared to control blastocysts. Hum Reprod 18: 399–407.

HFEA http://hfeaarchive.uksouth.cloudapp.azure.com/www.hfea.gov.uk/Multiple-births-after-IVF.html

Hnida, C., Engenheiro, E. and Ziebe, S. (2004). Computer-controlled, multilevel, morphometric analysis of blastomere size as biomarker of fragmentation and multinuclearity in human embryos. Hum Reprod 19: 288–293.

Holte, J., Berglund, L., Milton, K. et al. (2007). Construction of an evidence-based integrated morphology cleavage embryo score for implantation potential of embryos scored and transferred on day 2 after oocyte retrieval. Hum Reprod 22: 548–557.

Imudia A., Goldman, R.H., Awonugaet, A.O. et al. (2014). The impact of supraphysiologic serum estradiol levels on peri-implantation embryo development and early pregnancy outcome following in vitro fertilization cycles. J Assist Reprod Genet 31: 65–71.

James, A.N., Hennessy, S., Reggio, B. et al. (2006). The limited importance of pronuclear scoring of human zygotes. Hum Reprod 21: 1599–1604.

Johansson, M., Hardarson, T. and Lundin, K. (2003). There is a cut off limit in diameter between a blastomere and a small anucleate fragment. J Assist Reprod Genet 20: 309–313.

Kaser, D.J. and Racowsky, C. (2014). Clinical outcomes following selection of human preimplantation embryos with time-lapse monitoring: a systematic review. Hum Reprod 20: 617–631.

Kirkegaard, K., Campbell, A., Agerholm, I. et al. (2014). Limitations of a time-lapse blastocyst prediction model: a large multicentre outcome analysis. Reprod Biomed Online 29: 156–158.

Kligman, I., Benadiva, C., Alikani, M. et al. (1996). The presence of multinucleated blastomeres in human embryos is correlated with chromosomal abnormalities. Hum Reprod 11: 1492–1498.

Kovacic, B., Vlaisavljevic, V., Reljic, M. et al. (2004). Developmental capacity of different morphological types of day 5 human morulae and blastocysts. Reprod Biomed Online 8: 687–694.

Kovacs, P. (2014). Embryo selection: the role of time-lapse monitoring Reprod Biol Endocrinol 12: 124.

Le Cruguel, S., Ferré-L'Hôtellier, V., Morinière, C. et al. (2013). Early compaction at day 3 may be a useful additional criterion for embryo transfer. J Assist Reprod Genet 30: 683–690.

Lawler, C., Baker, H.W.G. and Edgar, D.H. (2007). Relationships between timing of syngamy, female age and implantation potential in human in vitro-fertilised oocytes. Reprod Fertil Dev 19: 482–487.

Lemmen, J.G., Agerholm, I. and Ziebe, S. (2008). Kinetic markers of human embryo quality using time-lapse recordings of IVF/ICSI-fertilized oocytes. Reprod Biomed Online 17: 385–391.

Machtinger, R. and Racowsky, C. (2013). Morphological systems of human embryo assessment and clinical evidence. Reprod Biomed Online 26: 210–221

Magli, M.C., Gianaroli, L., Ferraretti, A.P. (2001). Chromosomal abnormalities in embryos. Mol Cell Endocrinol 183: 29–34.

Magli, M.C., Gianaroli, L., Ferraretti, A.P. et al. (2007). Embryo morphology and development are dependent on the chromosomal complement. Fertil Steril 87: 534–540.

Magli, C., Jones, G. M., Lundin, K. et al. and The Special Interest Group on Embryology (2012). Atlas of Human Embryology: from Oocytes to Preimplantation Embryos. Hum Reprod 27(Suppl 1).

Meriano, J., Clark, C., Cadesky, K.et al. (2004). Binucleated and micronucleated blastomeres in embryos derived from human assisted reproduction cycles. Reprod Biomed Online 9: 511–520.

Meseguer, M., Herrero, J., Tejera, A. et al. (2011). The use of morphokinetics as a predictor of embryo implantation. Hum Reprod 26: 2658–2671.

Munne, S. and Cohen, J. (1993). Unsuitability of multinucleated human blastomeres for preimplantation genetic diagnosis. Hum Reprod 8: 1120–1125.

Nagy, Z.P., Dozortsev, D., Diamond, M. et al. (2003). Pronuclear morphology evaluation with subsequent evaluation of embryo morphology significantly increases implantation rates. Fertil Steril 80: 67–74.

National Institute for Health and Care Excellence (2013). https://www.nice.org.uk/guidance/cg156

Nicoli, A., Capodanno, F., Moscato, L. et al. (2010). Analysis of pronuclear zygote configurations in 459 clinical pregnancies obtained with assisted reproductive technique procedures. Reprod Biol Endocrinol 8: 77.

Nicoli, A., Palomba, S., Capodanno, F. et al. (2013). Pronuclear morphology evaluation for fresh in vitro fertilization (IVF) and intracytoplasmic sperm injection (ICSI) cycles: a systematic review. J Ovar Res 6: 64.

Pandian, Z., Marjoribanks, J., Ozturk, O. et al. (2013). Number of embryos for transfer following in vitro fertilisation or intra-cytoplasmic sperm injection. Cochrane Satabase Syst Rev 29: 7.

Paternot, G., Debrock, S., De Neubourg, D. et al. (2013). Semi-automated morphometric analysis of human embryos can reveal correlations between total embryo volume and clinical pregnancy. Hum Reprod 28: 627–633.

Payne, D., Flaherty, S.P., Barry, M.F. et al. (1997).Preliminary observations on polar body extrusion and pronuclear formation in human oocytes using time-lapse video cinematography. Hum Reprod 12: 532–541.

Pickering, S.J., Braude, P.R, Johnson, M.H. et al. (1990). Transient cooling to room temperature can cause irreversible disruption of the meiotic spindle in the human oocyte. Fertil Steril 54: 102–108.

Pons, M.C., de los Santos, M.J., Múgica, A. et al. ASEBIR Embryology Interest Group: (2014). Multicenter study to validate the ASEBIR criteria for the early assessment of day + 3 embryo morphology and its relationship with the live birth rate. Med Reprod Embriol Clin 1: 50–55.

Racowsky, C., Combelles, C.M., Nureddin, A. et al. (2003). Day 3 and day 5 morphological predictors of embryo viability. Reprod Biomed Online 6: 323–331.

Racowsky, C., Vernon, M., Mayer, J. et al. (2010). Standardization of grading embryo morphology J Assist Reprod Genet 27: 437–439.

Roque, M., Valle, M., Guimarães, F., et al. (2015). Freeze-all policy: fresh vs. frozen-thawed embryo transfer. Fertil Steril 103:1190–1193.

Rubio, I., Kuhlmann, R., Agerholm, I., Kirk, J. et al. (2012a). Limited implantation success of direct-cleaved human zygotes: a time-lapse study. Fertil Steril 98: 1458–1463.

Rubio, C., Rodrigo, L., Mir, P. et al. (2012b). Use of array comparative genomic hybridization (array-CGH) for embryo assessment: clinical results. Fertil Steril 99: 1044–1048.

Rubio, I., Galán, A., Larreategui, Z. et al. (2014). Clinical validation of embryo culture and selection by morphokinetic analysis: a randomized, controlled trial of the EmbryoScope. Fertil Steril 102: 1287–1294.

Saldeen, P. and Sundström, P. (2005). Nuclear status of four-cell preembryos predicts implantation potential in in vitro fertilization treatment cycles. Fertil Steril Sep 84: 584–589.

Salumets, A., Hydén-Granskog, C, Mäkinen S et al. (2003). Early cleavage predicts the viability of human embryos in elective single embryo transfer procedures. Hum Reprod 18: 821–825.

Schoolcraft, W.B., Fragouli, E., Stevens, J. et al. (2010). Clinical application of comprehensive chromosomal screening at the blastocyst stage. Fertil Steril 94: 1700–1706.

Scott, L. (2001). Oocyte and embryo polarity. Semin Reprod Med 18: 171–183.

Scott, L. (2003). Pronuclear scoring as a predictor of embryo development. Reprod Biomed Online 6: 201–14.

Senn, A., Urner, F., Chanson, A. et al. (2006). Morphological scoring of human pronuclear zygotes for prediction of pregnancy outcome. Hum Reprod 21: 234–239.

Shapiro, B.S., Daneshmand, S.T., Garner, F.C. et al. (2011). Evidence of impaired endometrial receptivity after ovarian stimulation for in vitro fertilization: a prospective randomized trial comparing fresh and frozen-thawed embryo transfer in normal responders. Fertil Steril 96: 344–348.

Skiadas, C.C., Jackson, K.V. and Racowsky, C. (2006). Early compaction on day 3 may be associated with increased implantation potential. Fertil Steril 86: 1386–1391

Staessen, C. and Van Steirteghem, A.(1998). The genetic constitution of multinuclear blastomeres and their derivative daughter blastomeres. Hum Reprod 13: 1625–1631.

Steer, C.V., Mills, C.L., Tan, S.L. et al. (1992). The cumulative embryo score: a predictive embryo scoring technique to select the optimal number of embryos to transfer in an in-vitro fertilization and embryo transfer programme. Hum Reprod 7: 117–119.

Stephenson, E.L., Braude, P.R. and Mason, C. (2007). International community consensus standard for reporting derivation of human embryonic stem cell lines. Regen Med 2: 349–362.

Steptoe, P.C. and Edwards, R.G. (1978). Birth after the reimplantation of a human embryo. Lancet 2: 366.

Sunkara, S.K., Siozos, A., Bolton, V.N. et al. (2010). The influence of delayed blastocyst formation on the outcome of frozen-thawed blastocyst transfer: a systemic review and metanalysis. Hum Reprod 25: 1906–1915.

Tao, J., Tamis R., Fink, K. et al. 2002). The neglected morula/compact stage embryo transfer. Hum Reprod 17: 1513–1518.

Tesarik, J., Junca, A.M., Hazout, A. et al. (2000). Embryos with high implantation potential after intracytoplasmic sperm injection can be recognized by a simple, non-invasive examination of pronuclear morphology. Hum Reprod 15: 1396–1399.

UK NEQAS http://www.cmft.nhs.uk/saint-marys/our-services/ukneqasrepsci.aspx

Vajta, G., Rienzi, L., Cobo, A, et al. (2010). Embryo culture: can we perform better than nature? Reprod Biomed Online 20: 453–469.

Van Blerkom, J., Davis, P. and Alexander, S. (2001). A microscopic and biochemical study of fragmentation phenotypes in stage-appropriate human embryos. Hum Reprod 16: 719–729.

Van Royen, E., Mangelschots, K., De Neubourg, D. et al. (1999). Characterization of a top quality embryo, a step towards single-embryo transfer. Hum Reprod 14: 2345–2349.

Van Royen, E., Mangelschots, K., De Neubourg, D. et al. (2001). Calculating the implantation potential of day 3 embryos in women younger than 38 years of age: a new model. Hum Reprod 16: 326–332.

Van Royen, E., Mangelschots, K., Vercruyssen, M. et al. (2003). Multinucleation in cleavage stage embryos. Hum Reprod 18: 1062–1069.

Vergouw, C.G., Heymans, M.W., Hardarson, T. et al. (2014). No evidence that embryo selection by near-infrared spectroscopy in addition to morphology is able to improve live birth rates: results from an individual patient data meta-analysis. Hum Reprod 29: 455–461.

Vernon, M.W., Stern, J.E., Ball, G.D. et al. (2009). Utility of the national embryo morphology data collected by SART: correlation between morphologic grade and live birth rate. Fertil Steril 92(Suppl.): S164.

Watson, A.J., Natale, D.R. and Barcroft, L.C. (2004). Molecular regulation of blastocyst formation. Anim Reprod Sci 82–83: 583–592.

Weitzman, V.N., Schnee-Riesz, J., Benadiva, C et al. (2010). Predictive value of embryo grading for embryos with known outcomes. Fertil Steril 93: 658–662.

Winston, N.J., Braude, P.R., Pickering, S.J. et al. (1991). The incidence of abnormal morphology and nucleocytoplasmic ratios in 2-, 3- and 5-day human pre-embryos. Hum Reprod 6: 17–24.

Zamora, R.B., Sánchez RV, Pérez JG et al. (2011). Human zygote morphological indicators of high rate of arrest at the first cleavage stage. Zygote 19: 339–344.

Ziebe, S., Petersen, K., Lindenberg, S. et al. (1997). Embryo morphology or cleavage stage: how to select the best embryos for transfer after in-vitro fertilization. Hum Reprod 12: 1545–1549.

Ziebe, S., Lundin, K., Loft, A. et al. for the CEMAS II and III Study Group. (2003). FISH analysis for chromosomes 13, 16, 18, 21, 22, X and Y in all blastomeres of IVF pre-embryos from 144 randomly selected donated human oocytes and impact on pre-embryo morphology. Hum Reprod 18: 2575–2581.

Zollner, U., Zollner, K.P., Hartl, G. et al. (2002). The use of a detailed zygote score after IVF/ICSI to obtain good quality blastocysts: the German experience. Hum Reprod 17: 1327–33.

26

In Vitro Culture of Gametes and Embryos – The Culture Medium

Robbie Kerr

Introduction

Historical Development of Embryo Culture Media

Following the pioneering work of Ludwig and Ringer almost 150 years ago, the first tissue culture media were developed from simple salts solutions based on the chemical properties of blood serum and were able to support the beating frog heart *in vitro* (Ringer 1882; Ringer 1883). This simple medium was composed of sodium chloride (NaCl), potassium chloride (KCl), calcium chloride (CaCl$_2$), and sodium bicarbonate (NaHCO$_3$). Known as Krebs–Ringer bicarbonate (KRB), it was discovered by the accidental addition of tap water to culture medium being developed for another study by Ringer's assistant Carl Ludwig. They discovered that the key component in tap water which was critical to maintaining a regular heartbeat *in vitro* was CaCl$_2$. In 1907, Locke and Rosenheim made further modifications to Ringer's saline by the addition of 11.1 mM glucose to study the perfused rabbit heart (Locke and Rosenheim 1907). Further modifications were made by the addition of sodium dihydrogen phosphate (NaH$_2$PO$_4$), magnesium chloride (MgCl$_2$), increasing the concentration of NaHCO$_3$ to provide extra buffering capacity (Tyrode 1910), and increasing the concentration of NsHCO$_3$, coupled with the removal of glucose from the formulation (Krebs and Henseleit 1932), to form the basis of Krebs–Ringer bicarbonate solution which, when gassed with 5% CO$_2$ in air or nitrogen is still used to regulate pH in many culture media.

The first recorded culture of mammalian embryos was by Brachet in 1912 in the rabbit, followed by studies on the culture of rabbit embryos using a variety of poorly defined culture media, such as coagulated blood plasma (Lewis and Gregory 1929). In 1941, the first successful culture of mouse embryos on a blood clot was reported (Khul 1941). However, In 1949 John Hammond, considered the father of embryo culture, made a significant breakthrough when he reported the culture of mouse embryos from the four-cell stage through to the blastocyst stage in a medium based on Krebs–Ringer solution but supplemented with glucose and 5% egg white (Hammond 1949). In this seminal work Hammond demonstrated that glucose was essential for compaction and development to the blastocyst stage, a discovery that sparked significant research to model mammalian preimplantation development *in vitro*.

In 1956, an elegant study by Wesley Whitten showed that 90% of eight-cell mouse embryos could develop to the blastocyst stage in media based on Krebs–Ringer solution supplemented with 5.55 mM glucose, penicillin, and streptomycin and replacing egg white as a protein source with bovine serum albumin (BSA) (Whitten 1956). The development of Whitten's media was followed by a major breakthrough in 1958 when McLaren and Biggers reported the first successful live births following the transfer of mouse blastocysts derived by culture from the eight-cell stage in Whitten's medium (McLaren and Biggers 1958). At the time this development opened 'Pandora's box' in terms of primary scientific research and clinical medicine and was one the key events which lead to human *in vitro* fertilization (IVF) becoming a reality with the birth of Louise Brown in 1978 (Steptoe and Edwards 1978).

Significant developments in embryo culture took place at this time including the addition of lactate to facilitate culture of mouse embryos from the two-cell stage to the blastocyst stage (Whitten 1957). However, this feat could not be reproduced with pronuclear stage embryos, which led to the identification of the 'two-cell block' in preimplantation mouse embryos. With the exception of some inbred and F1 strains (Brinster 1963; Brinster 1968; Whittingham, 1971), one-cell mouse embryos exhibit a 'two-cell block' to development *in vitro*, whereby they undergo a single cleavage division and arrest at the two-cell stage. Further refinements to Whitten's media were used to improve the effectiveness of culture from the two- and eight-cell stages to the blastocyst stage which included the addition of phosphenolpyruvate, pyruvate, lactate, and oxaloacetate (Brinster 1963; Brinster 1968; Whittingham 1971). The development of both Brinster's medium and Whitten's M16 medium were significant developments but neither could overcome the two-cell block in the mouse, a phenomenon replicated in other mammalian species at differing cell stages, and which is known to coincide with the activation of the embryonic genome in each species studied (Rieger et al. 1992). The first reported evidence of the two-cell block being successfully overcome in outbred strains was reported in 1989 when Chatot et al. showed that a high lactate to pyruvate ratio with the addition of 0.1 mM ethylenediaminetetraacetic acid (EDTA) to Brinster's medium, alongside the removal of glucose, could support development from zygote to morula stage. However, culture to the blastocyst stage could only be achieved through the addition of glucose at the three- to four-cell stage (Chatot et al. 1989) (see Table 26.1 for a summary).

Back to Nature: The Refinement of Embryo Culture Medium

Throughout the 1970s and 1980s a major focus of research on the culture of mammalian embryos was centred on refining the composition of media to mimic more closely the environment found in the female reproductive tract. This so called 'back to nature' concept is based on the principle that the differences in the composition of the oviductal and uterine fluids that exist throughout the reproductive cycle may reflect the varying metabolic needs of the embryo during early development (Leese 1998). David Gardner developed sequential media for human embryos using the principles, in part, of the *back to nature* concept, specifically for pyruvate lactate and glucose in the human oviduct and uterus (Gardner et al. 1996; Gardner and Leese 1990). The remaining part of the concept relied on mouse experiments, which may not be directly comparable to the environment in which the human embryo exists *in vivo*. Controversially, it was suggested that to truly optimize embryo culture, sequential media were required which would meet the changing environments and requirements of the early embryo (Gardner and Leese 1990). The hypothesis was that five distinct media would be required for true sequential culture (Leese, 1995; Biggers and Summers 2008):

1) Oocyte aspiration media to mimic human follicular fluid.
2) Oocyte incubation and maturation media based on the composition of the fluid from the ampulla of the Fallopian tube postovulation.
3) Fertilization media which corresponds to the fluid from the ampullary–isthmic junction postcoitus.
4) Preimplantation culture media based on oviductal fluid composition postfertilization.
5) Embryo transfer media similar to that observed in the uterine lumen on Day 5 postinsemination.

One of the fundamental issues with this approach to culture media was that the composition of the oviduct and uterine fluids is highly variable and prone to sampling errors in both human and mouse studies (Summers and Biggers 2003). Furthermore, measurement of the composition of fluids from the female reproductive tract are not a true reflection of the microenvironments to which the embryo is exposed and represent only the overall composition. It is also of note that the environment to which embryos are exposed *in vitro* differs from that *in vivo*. Embryos cultured *in vitro* are exposed to a relatively large volume of media in which nutrients are depleted over time and lactate and ammonia concentrations increase. However, *in vivo* embryos exist in a dynamic environment where contact with

Table 26.1 Back to nature: the refinement of embryo culture medium.

Year	Discovery	Author
1561	First correct anatomical description of the Fallopian tube	G. Fallopius
1677	Discovery of mammalian spermatozoa	A. Van Leeuwenhoek
1797	Recovery of embryos from rabbit Fallopian tube	W.C. Cruikshank
1827	Identification of an egg in a mammalian ovarian follicle	K.E. Von Baer
1890	Understanding that fertilization requires the fusion of one sperm with one egg in sea urchin, rabbits and starfish	O. Hertwik (sea urchin) E. Van Beneden (rabbit) H. ol (starfish)
1890	First documented embryo transfer in rabbits	W. Heape
1912	First documented culture of mammalian embryos (rabbits)	A. Brachet
1930	First published experiments on IVF carried out in rabbits	G. Pincus
1932	'Brave New World' was published by Aldous Huxley. Realistically describing the technique of IVF as we know it	A. Huxley
1944	First attempted at IVF using human oocytes	J. Rock and M. Menkin
1949	Retrieval and successful culture of mouse oocytes	J. Hammond Jr
1949	Successful development of culture medium to support development of mouse embryos from eight-cell to blastocyst stage	J. Hammond Jr
1951	Capacitation in spermatozoa	M.C. Chang; C.R. Austin
1958	Successful embryo transfer of mouse blastocysts to a recipient female followed by birth of live young	A. McLaren and J.D. Biggers
1959	Unequivocal demonstration of IVF in the rabbit	M.C. Chang
1963	Development of culture media to support culture of mouse embryos from two-cell to blastocyst stage	R.L. Brinster
1969	Successful fertilization of the human oocyte *in vitro*	R.G. Edwards, B.D. Bavister and P.C. Steptoe
1972	Successful cryopreservation of mouse embryos	I. Wilmut, D.G. Whittingham
1976	Development of the first specific culture medium to reflect the follicular, tubal, and uterine environments of the sheep, rabbits, and humans	Y. Menezo
1976	First human IVF pregnancy (ectopic)	P.C. Steptoe and R.G. Edwards
1978	Birth of the world's first child from IVF (Louise Brown)	P.C. Steptoe and R.G. Edwards

IVF, *in vitro* fertilization.

maternal tissue and reduced levels of fluid lead to a rapid exchange of nutrients, gases, and waste products. These differences will undoubtedly give rise to different stresses on the developing embryo in the laboratory than those found *in vivo*.

A major advance in the design of embryo culture media was the use of an industrial modelling system known as simplex optimization to determine the optimal concentration of each individual component of the culture media (Lawitts and Biggers 1991a,b).

In a series of complex and lengthy experiments they generated a base culture medium based on M16 and CZB medium containing defined concentrations of NaCl, KCl, KH_2PO_4, $MgSO_4$, lactate, pyruvate, and glucose using BSA as a protein source. Using this base medium a series of media were developed, each with an elevated concentration of a single component. These media were tested for their ability to sustain the development of mouse embryos from the zygote to the blastocyst stage and a computer model was used to optimize each component. This approach required several thousand mouse embryos per optimization, making it impossible as a means for optimizing a medium for human IVF. Nevertheless, through this work the authors discovered that high levels of NaCl, pyruvate, KH_2PO_4, and glucose were detrimental to mouse embryo development while low levels of NaCl and corresponding low osmolarity were able to overcome the two-cell block in the mouse. Building on these findings, it was subsequently shown that by increasing the concentration of KCl to 2.5 mM improved blastocyst formation rates (Erbach et al. 1994), which reflected the K^+ content of the oviductal fluid. This media, known as KSOM, became the cornerstone of many developments and modifications in culture media over the coming years and through various modifications was shown to support cattle, rabbit, rhesus monkey, porcine, rat, and critically, human embryos (Biggers 1998). However, it should be appreciated that the original optimization was performed in mouse embryos.

On reviewing the historical development of embryo culture media it becomes apparent that the human embryo has a capacity to adapt to a variety of culture environments due to a high degree of 'plasticity' in the early embryo, as first suggested by Anne McLaren in 1972. However, adaptation by an embryo to suboptimal conditions is not without cost in terms of reduced viability. The more an embryo has to adapt to its environment the more its viability is compromised. Strict control of the components that make up all embryo culture media is therefore imperative. A discussion of these components follows, although it is important to note that this is not exhaustive as IVF culture media contain a huge variety of components, not all of which are fully declared in the published formulations.

Salts and Osmolality

All commercially available embryo culture media share the same inorganic ions (Na^+, K^+, Cl^-, Ca^{2+}, Mg^{2+}, SO_4^{2-}, and in some cases PO_4^{2-}) (Biggers 1998). The use of these salts in media formulation can be traced back to the original KRB. Patrick Quinn devised the first commercial medium specifically for human embryo culture, known as 'human

tubal fluid' (HTF) in 1985. The name, however, was a misnomer, since the concentrations of salts used were not taken from fluid collected from human Fallopian tubes, but were based on those for mouse embryo culture such as M16 and Whitten's media, with the exception of Mg^{2+} and PO_4^{2-} which were at much lower concentrations in Quinn's HTF (Quinn et al. 1985a,b). These days a wide array of both single-step and sequential culture media are available. However, historically a direct comparison was difficult as most commercial media are proprietary formulations. Recently, through the use of high purity liquid chromatography and mass spectrometry, two studies have analysed the formulations of several commercially available sequential and single-step culture systems (Morbeck et al. 2014; Morbeck et al. 2017). These studies confirm that several media do contain salt concentrations similar to those observed in the original SOM and KSOM formulations (Lawitts and Biggers 1991a). Inorganic ions serve a variety of roles in cell function. One such function is in maintaining an intracellular environment in which K^+ concentrations are high and Na^+ concentrations are low (Kaplan 2002). This distribution is largely mediated by the Na^+,K^+-ATPase (sodium pump) enzyme and is crucial to maintain the cell membrane potential, which indirectly provides an energy source for numerous 'electrogenic' transporters critical for the transport of metabolites and amino acids as well as the regulation of intracellular pH (Baltz and Zhou 2012). The concentration of inorganic ions is fundamental to the regulation of the external and internal osmolality of the early embryo. Osmolality is a measure of the total osmotic pressure in a solution (osmol/kg).

Osmolarity is closely connected with the regulation of cell volume as mammalian cells control cellular volume by adjusting intracellular concentrations of osmotically active solutes to regulate osmotic pressure (Hallows and Knauf 1994; Hallows et al. 1994). The influx of osmolytes raises intracellular pressure, which in turn causes an increase in cell volume, whereas an efflux of osmolytes leads to a reduction in cell volume. The early embryo is extremely sensitive to increases in external osmolarity as evidenced during the development of KSOM media that had a significantly lower osmolarity (250 mOsM) than that of M16 and CZB media (290 mOsM and 275 mOsM respectively). The addition of NaCl to

KSOM to raise the osmolarity to levels similar to that seen in M16 and CZB was sufficient to initiate the two-cell block in mouse embryo development (Hadi et al. 2005; Wang et al. 2005).

Why do preimplantation embryos show improved development in low osmolarity? One possibility is that such conditions mimic the low osmolarity present in the female tract. However, this is unlikely as analysis of mouse, rat, and porcine oviductal fluid showed a range of osmolarities from 290 to 310 mOsM (Waring, 1976; Collins and Baltz 1999; Li et al. 2007). It was also shown in a series of experiments at higher osmolarity, blocks to embryo development could be avoided through the addition of any of the following organic osmolytes: amino acids or amino acid derivatives such as glutamine, glycine, proline, betanine, and β-alanine (Van Winkle et al., 1990; Lawitts and Biggers 1991b; Hammer and Baltz 2003). Indeed, glycine has been shown to be the principle organic osmolyte used by the preimplantation embryo as the high affinity glycine transporter GLYT1 is expressed and active in mouse embryos until the four-cell stage and regulates the accumulation of glycine in the early embryo (Steeves et al. 2003). Furthermore, GLYT1 is also expressed in human embryos indicating a similar role (Hammer et al., 2000). GLYT1, however, cannot regulate the uptake of betaine and proline which are regulated by SIT1 which is also active in the early embryo and appears to work in tandem with GLYT1 as betaine is accumulated at lower levels than glycine in the early embryo (Anas et al. 2008). These findings were consistent with the hypothesis that the preimplantation embryo maintains cellular volume via mechanisms similar to those observed in somatic cells. However, unlike somatic cells the levels of inorganic ions required to maintain normal cell volume can exert a negative effect on development such that the early embryo can replace a portion of these with organic osmolytes (Van Winkle et al. 1990).

Energy Sources and Metabolites

During the first 6 days of development *in vivo,* the human preimplantation embryo most likely exists in a constantly changing microenvironment, containing a variety of nutrients as it grows from fertilization through to the blastocyst stage. However, this cannot be confirmed since the microenvironment cannot be sampled and, thinking logically, the environment in the oviduct should, one imagines, be focused in maintaining homeostasis and minimizing variation. The key stages in the early development of the embryo include rapid early mitotic cleavage divisions to the eight-cell stage in the absence of cellular growth as a consequence of a reduction in cellular biomass through reducing blastomere size with each division. This is followed by compaction of the early embryo and the formation of gap and tight junctions between the cells of the early embryo to facilitate cell to cell communication and nutrient exchange during the process of blastocyst formation during which the first major event of cellular differentiation occurs giving rise to two distinct cell populations; the trophectoderm and the inner cell mass. During this stage, major increases in protein synthesis and increased metabolic activity are evident. With regard to energy sources and metabolites, we can ask: (i) how does the preimplantation embryo regulate these processes?; (ii) what are the metabolic requirements of the embryo during this time?; (iii) what nutrients are required in a culture medium?

In the early cleavage stages of development, genetic control of the embryo relies mainly on maternal mRNA stores prior to activation of the embryonic genome between the four- and eight-cell stage in the human embryo. During early cleavage, metabolic activity is low compared with that required for blastocyst formation activation when metabolic activity increases significantly (Leese 1991; Leese 1995).

The major nutrients available to the early embryo *in vivo* are: (i) pyruvate; (ii) lactate; (iii) glucose; (iv) amino acids; and (v) endogenous triglyceride. The role of amino acids as nutrients in embryo culture media are mainly discussed later. In the female reproductive tract, namely the oviduct and uterus, the embryo is exposed to differing concentrations of pyruvate, lactate, and glucose (Table 26.2). Pyruvate and lactate concentrations are relatively high in the early cleavage stages of development in the human oviduct before falling significantly during compaction and blastocyst formation in the uterus (Gardner et al. 1996). The importance of pyruvate as an energy source for the cleavage stage embryos was first established in the 1960s and 1970s (Biggers and Stern 1973). The early embryo generates adenosine

Table 26.2 The differing metabolic requirements of the embryo as it develops in the female tract based on the analysis of the oviductal and uterine fluids. As the embryo develops low glucose combined with high pyruvate and lactate is required during the cleavage stages in the oviduct, switching to high glucose and low pyruvate and lactate as the embryo undergoes compaction and blastulation prior to implantation in the uterus.

Site	Pyruvate (mM)	Lactate (mM)	Glucose (mM)
Oviduct	0.32	10.5	0.50
Uterus	0.10	5.87	3.15

triphosphate (ATP) through oxidative phosphorylation of pyruvate and lactate and amino acids such as aspartate and glutamine (Leese and Barton 1985; Gardner et al. 1996; Lane and Gardner 2005). However, excess concentrations of lactate can alter the rate of pyruvate oxidation in the cell, which in turn affects the availability of NAD^+ and NADH, and of ATP production. For this reason, both pyruvate and lactate are key components of all commercial culture media with the balance of these nutrients being critical due to their ability to sustain the metabolism and viability of the developing embryo.

In common with the situation observed *in vivo* some commercial sequential IVF media such as the G series™ (Vitrolife, Göteborg, Sweden) have pyruvate and lactate concentrations which are higher in the cleavage stage medium compared with levels in the blastocyst stage medium, with the ratio of pyruvate to lactate being optimized to avoid negative effects from the impact of lactate on the regulation of redox potential. This is not always the case, as in other systems such SAGE Quinn's Advantage™ (Origio, Målov, Denmark) and Sydney IVF™ (Cook Medical, Bloomington, IN, USA) the difference in lactate between the stage one and stage 2 media is less pronounced (Morbeck et al. 2014). To date several studies have assessed the uptake of pyruvate in relation to pregnancy and blastocyst formation rates. Embryos that develop to the blastocyst stage show increased pyruvate uptake between Days 2.5 and 4.5, whereas those arrested at cleavage stages had significantly lower pyruvate uptake. Interestingly, polyspermic and parthenogenetic embryos also had lower pyruvate uptakes at later stages indicating the impaired developmental

potential of these embryos (Hardy et al. 1989b). These findings were further supported in a study where the levels of pyruvate and glucose uptake, and lactate production in embryos which arrested were below those which developed normally (Gott et al. 1990). Furthermore, culture of embryos in pyruvate-free medium resulted in developmental arrest in the majority of cleavage-stage embryos and those that did reach the blastocyst stage showed significantly reduced metabolic activity during the morula to blastocyst stage transition (Conaghan et al. 1993a). These studies were limited to the assessment of the levels of uptake of pyruvate with a view to its potential as a biomarker of developmental potential. It is important to consider the metabolic fate of pyruvate, as high uptake may indicate inappropriate or inefficient use of an energy substrate in the developing embryo (Zander-Fox and Lane 2012). A recent retrospective study has proposed that there may actually be a threshold at which overconsumption of pyruvate exerts a negative effect. In this study, the authors proposed the existence of a "Goldilocks zone", or as it is known in Sweden, of lagom meaning 'just the right amount' within which embryos with maximum developmental potential can be classified (Leese et al. 2016).

Another energy substrate common to all commercial culture media is glucose. As with pyruvate and lactate the embryo's demand for this key substrate appears to change throughout development (Table 26.2). Glucose is present in the female reproductive tract secretions at levels between 0.5 mM and 3.15 mM dependent on location, and the species and glucose transporters are present in both human and mouse embryos. Glucose is the primary energy source for the generation of ATP in almost all mammalian somatic cells via glycolysis, which converts glucose to pyruvate, generating two ATP molecules. Pyruvate is then converted to acetyl-CoA which via the tricarboxylic acid cycle is oxidized to produce CO_2 and H_2O in the mitochondria and an additional 32 molecules of ATP.

Historically, it was suggested in some studies that glucose is toxic during *in vitro* culture prior to activation of the embryonic genome, and glucose and phosphate together may inhibit development of the early embryo (Chatot et al. 1989). Moreover, the same authors showed that complete removal of glucose from the culture media is not beneficial for embryo development either. High glucose levels may exert a negative effect on development of the early embryo through increased free radical formation and impairment of mitochondrial function (Pampfer 2000), indicating that high external concentrations of glucose in simple culture media are toxic rather than glucose itself. The key question was one of toxicity versus consumption. Some of the initial animal studies have shown that the two-cell mouse embryo cannot use glucose as an energy substrate and is dependent upon pyruvate and lactate at this stage (Biggers and Stern 1973). However, in contrast to this, the eight-cell mouse embryos can develop to the blastocyst stage in media supplemented with glucose alone (Leese and Barton 1985; Gardner et al. 1996; Lane and Gardner 2005). Other studies have suggested that glucose is essential for blastocyst development in the mouse (Martin and Leese 1995). In the human embryo, the situation is similar to that observed in the mouse, with uptake of glucose being low during the early cleavage stages but increasing significantly postembryonic genome activation, and reaching maximal levels during blastocyst development (Hardy et al. 1989b; Gott et al. 1990). Furthermore, arrested human embryos are unable to switch from a pyruvate/lactate-based metabolism to glucose on Day 4 when compared with those which reach the blastocyst stage (Gott et al., 1990; Gardner et al. 2001). Moreover, elevated levels of glucose uptake in human embryos correlates with improved blastocyst quality on Days 5 and 6 (Gardner et al. 2001). Critically, glucose uptake has been correlated with increased pregnancy rates in both human and mouse embryos with those blastocysts that had elevated glucose uptake (Gardner et al. 1996). Once again it may be that the 'Goldilocks principle' also applies here and that there is a threshold at which glucose consumption is optimal for embryo development (Leese et al. 2016).

Amino Acids

Although there is no increase in protein content during the transition from the zygote to the early blastocyst, there is a continual turnover of amino acids in early development (Sellens et al. 1981). Amino acids also function as energy substrates and have a number of specialized roles. For example,

they function as osmolytes (Dumoulin et al. 1997; Dawson et al. 1998), antioxidants (Nasr-Esfahani et al. 1992), and regulators of pH (Edwards et al. 1998; Lane and Gardner 2005). Amino acids can be classified as either essential or nonessential: essential amino acids are those obtained from the diet which cannot be synthesized *de novo*, whereas nonessential amino acids are those are those synthesized by the cells themselves (Table 26.3). It is of note that under certain circumstances or disease states a subgroup of nonessential amino acids exist, classified as conditionally essential amino acids (Reeds 2000). In the case of the early embryo these distinctions are largely irrelevant as *in vivo* the embryo would be exposed to a full complement of amino acids derived from the secretions of the female reproductive tract.

Amino acids have been shown to be essential for blastocyst development in both rabbit (Daniel and Krishnan 1967) and mouse (Gardner and Lane 1993; Lane and Gardner 1994). Early studies in the mouse showed that blastocyst formation rates were significantly improved in the mouse when embryos were cultured only in the presence of nonessential amino acids. Furthermore, embryos cultured in these conditions also showed higher implantation rates if transferred at the cleavage stage, whereas embryos cultured to the blastocyst stage showed higher implantation rates when all 20 amino acids were used.

These studies demonstrate that the early embryo has differing requirements for amino acids dependent upon its stage of development, similar to its requirements for glucose. In human embryos, it was shown that the addition of either glutamine or taurine could increase blastocyst formation rates (Gardner and Lane 1993: Lane and Gardner 1994). These experiments were carried out in the absence of glucose so one possible explanation for this is that glutamine, in conjunction with pyruvate, was being used as the primary energy source in these studies. Further studies showed that medium supplemented with nonessential amino acids up to Day 3 followed by blastocyst culture in medium containing all 20 amino acids significantly increased blastocyst formation rates (Devreker et al. 2001).

Further studies in human embryos have shown that amino acid utilization is indicative of embryo viability. The amino acid turnover of individual donated human embryos, carried out by high

Table 26.3 Classification of essential nonessential and conditionally essential amino acids.

Essential	Nonessential	Conditionally Essential
Histidine	Alanine	Arginine
Isoleucine	Arginine	Cysteine
Leucine	Asparagine	Glutamine
Lysine	Aspartic acid	Glycine
Methionine	Cysteine	Proline
Phenylalanine	Glutamic acid	Serine
Threonine	Glutamine	Tyrosine
Tryptophan	Glycine	
Valine	Proline	
	Serine	
	Tyrosine	

performance liquid chromatography (HPLC), demonstrated that those embryos which go onto form a blastocyst showed different patterns of amino acid utilization compared with those that arrested (Houghton et al. 2002). It was determined that those embryos reaching the blastocyst stage consumed more leucine, and fluctuations in the levels of alanine, arginine, glutamine, methionine, and aspargine were related to blastocyst formation. Subsequently, a follow-up study on the spent culture media of embryos cultured to the two-cell stage in an IVF programme showed that asparagine, glycine, and leucine were all significantly associated with clinical pregnancy and live birth rates (Brison et al. 2004). Other studies have also shown amino acid turnover differs in male and female bovine embryos (Sturmey et al. 2010), with aneuploidy (Picton et al. 2010), and DNA damage (Sturmey et al. 2009). Furthermore, the uptake of amino acids by blastocysts that result in a pregnancy has been shown to correlate with increased levels glucose uptake in the same embryos (Gardner and Wale, 2013). Despite substantial evidence that the addition of amino acids to embryo culture media can exert a positive effect on embryo development, concerns do exist in relation to the accumulation of toxic ammonium, a product of spontaneous breakdown of amino acids in the culture medium (Gardner and Lane 1993). This breakdown is more pronounced at the temperatures commonly used for embryo incubation, so thought should be given to the storage, handling, and incubation times of media containing amino acids. This is of particular relevance with the move to back to single-step culture (discussed later in the chapter).

Macromolecules and Growth Factors

The majority of commercial culture media used in IVF are supplemented with a source of protein and in some cases nonprotein macromolecules or recombinant products. The most common supplement used is human serum albumin (HSA). Historically, serum was required to aid proliferation and cell attachment. However, due to significant batch-to-batch variation and potential adverse effects on development, it was discontinued. During the 1980s, the use of BSA, human fetal cord serum, or maternal serum was widespread. However, once again significant batch-to-batch variation was an issue (Pool 2004). In the quest for more stable culture conditions, the use of HSA has become virtually universal in IVF, although the use of recombinant HSA to reduce batch-to-batch issues has never been implemented fully in the clinical setting. The use of HSA and other supplements are not without issues. Almost all commonly used supplements carry a risk of potential disease transmission due to their origin (i.e. human blood), such as prion or viral contamination, although this is minimized through heat treatment. The role of protein supplementation varies throughout development from simple lubrication of sperm movement in insemination media (Lane et al. 2001) to replacing the protective effects of the cumulus cells in oocytes stripped for intracytoplasmic sperm injection in handling media (Alvarez and Storey 1995). Albumin has multiple physiological functions in cleavage and blastocyst stage embryo culture, such as: a chelator of heavy metals; a free radical scavenger; a pH and osmotic regulator; for stabilization of the cell membranes; for inhibition of lipid peroxidation; as a growth factor carrier; as a surfactant; and as a nutrient (Otsuki et al. 2013). Its role as a growth factor carrier is of particular interest as *in vivo* human embryos are exposed to numerous growth factors ranging from those produced by the embryo itself to those produced in the oviduct and the endometrium. These growth factors will act on receptors expressed by the embryo to exert antiapoptotic effects and increase developmental rates (Hardy et al. 1989a; Hardy and Spanos 2002). For this reason, *in vitro* protein supplementation of culture media is critical since it will facilitate the binding of such growth factors and their release during the culture period. There is a significant body of evidence on the effects of addition or removal of growth factors from the culture environment and the effects on embryo development. To date, many different growth factors have been evaluated which includes epidermal growth factor (EGF) (Khamsi et al. 1996), leukaemia inhibitory factor (LIF) (Dunglison et al. 1996), Insulin-like growth factor I (IGF-I) (Lighten et al. 1998), platelet-derived growth factor (PDGF) (Lopata and Oliva 1993), heparin-binding epidermal growth factor (HB-EGF) (Martin et al. 1998), and granulocyte-macrophage colony stimulating factor (GM-CSF) (Ziebe et al. 2013). These growth factors, singly, or in some cases, in combination (Ziebe et al. 2013) have been shown to improve developmental rates in cell numbers, blastocyst formation, and implantation rates to varying degrees. However, it is important to note that growth factors can also exert a negative effect on embryo development and that in many studies the concentrations used have been far removed from the physiological concentrations the developing embryo would be exposed to *in vivo*. For example, the culture of human embryos in media supplemented with IGF-I, LIF, or HBEGF, are known to stimulate the development found that different gene expression profiles were evident in each group (Yu et al. 2012). Moreover, the addition of growth factors to culture media may increase developmental rates which may not necessarily be advantageous since there is evidence that IVF culture may cause imprinting errors in the early embryo (Kimber et al. 2008). Furthermore, the addition of growth factors may alter the apoptosis pathway, which is vital in ensuring the early embryo can cope with abnormal cell development (Bolton et al. 2016). To date, the most promising data on growth factor supplementation has come from GM-CSF supplementation. GM-CSF is expressed in the female reproductive tract (Dudley et al. 1990; Zhao and Chegini 1994; Zhao et al. 1995). Preimplantation human embryos express GM-CSF receptors (Sjoblom et al. 2002) and expression of GM-CSF is reduced in those patients who exhibit recurrent miscarriage (Perricone et al. 2003).

A multicentre double-blind randomized controlled trial (RCT) reported no increase in aneuploidy or mosaicism in human embryos cultured with or without GM-CSF (Agerholm et al. 2010). The use of GM-CSF has also shown to increase pregnancy rates in several human studies. However, in a multicentre double-blind RCT this was found to be limited to a subgroup of patients with at least one previous miscarriage (Ziebe et al. 2013). Thus, although such studies are promising, further research is needed to evaluate the benefits of growth factor supplementation of IVF culture media.

A further well characterized macromolecule commonly used as a supplement in IVF culture media is hyaluronan, a major glycosaminoglycan present in the follicular, oviductal, and uterine fluids (Dyrlund et al. 2015). Receptors for hyaluronan are expressed by both the preimplantation embryo from the oocyte through to the blastocyst stage and the endometrium (Behzad et al. 1994; Campbell et al. 1995). The synthesis of hyaluronan increases dramatically on the day of implantation and decreases to basal levels by the following day, strongly suggesting a crucial role in the implantation process (Carson et al. 1987; Zorn et al. 1995). A Cochrane review of the evidence to support the addition of hyaluronan to IVF culture media confirmed improved pregnancy rates and live birth rates although only six of the 16 RCTs in the review reported on live birth (Bontekoe et al. 2010; Bontekoe et al. 2014). In 2014 a follow-up Cochrane report compiled data from 17 publications (>3800 transfers), 16 of which studied hyaluronan. It was found that there was a positive treatment effect for all 16 studies investigating the effect of hyaluronan on live birth rates (Bontekoe et al. 2014). With regard to the mode of action, the potential beneficial effect of hyaluronan may be mediated by several mechanisms, ranging from improved cell–cell adhesion and cell–matrix adhesion during implantation (Turley and Moore, 1984) to receptor-mediated biological function by the hyaluronan receptors expressed by the blastocyst stage embryo (Campbell et al. 1995). Furthermore, in the endometrium its expression is limited to the late secretory phase during which implantation takes place (Yaegashi et al. 1995). Furthermore, the bovine preimplantation embryo also expresses RHAMM/IHABP, another type of hyaluronan receptor on the embryo surface at the time of implantation (Stojkovic et al. 2003). It should be noted that very little mechanistic data exists in the case of the human embryo, therefore data on the benefits of its use should be interpreted with a note of caution.

In conclusion, when deciding on embryo culture media it is essential that laboratories consider the individual components of the media and their interactions. However, this is a challenge due to the lack of studies on the human embryo and the overreliance on animal models. In general terms, a simple well-defined presupplemented medium with the required quality control would be preferred over complex media with aftermarket supplementation.

Single-step and Sequential Culture Systems

There are two major schools of thought on the most effective way to culture human zygotes to the blastocyst stage: single-step versus sequential medium. In the case of single-step medium, the embryos are cultured from the day of fertilization in the same culture medium with or without a medium change on Day 3. In sequential systems one medium is used from the zygote to cleavage stage, after which the embryos are transferred to a second medium claimed to meet the embryo's developmental requirements up to the blastocyst stage.

These two systems are based around two differing hypotheses: in the case of the single-step system the hypothesis is 'let the embryo choose', whereas with the sequential system the 'back to nature' hypothesis is key. Both systems will be discussed in detail in the following sections. However, it should be noted at the outset that both of these concepts may be flawed, as some would argue that the embryo 'will always choose' in the case of single step, and as discussed earlier the 'back to nature concept' is only based on the concentrations of glucose, lactate and pyruvate rather than the actual composition of human oviductal fluid.

Single-Step Culture Systems

In the previous sections of this chapter we have outlined the history of modern culture media development and defined some of the key components the culture media including glucose, amino acids,

salts, protein sources, and macromolecules. To date, however, a major limitation in the development of culture media is the ability to perform large empirical studies on the human embryo to optimize culture conditions. For this reason, the majority of commercial media have been derived from mouse models and the process of simplex optimization; interestingly, the basic principles of low sodium and low osmolarity from the mouse model are not consistent in all commercial media (Morbeck et al. 2014; Morbeck et al. 2017). In the case of the sequential culture system, the primary data used in its development was derived from sampling of both the Fallopian and uterine fluids throughout the menstrual cycle (Gardner and Lane 1996). However, as discussed previously the composition of these fluids may not actually accurately represent the microenvironment which surrounds the embryo *in vivo* as they do not reflect the potential interactions between the embryo and the maternal tissue. Furthermore, such studies can be impacted by sampling errors as noted previously (Summers and Biggers 2003). Interestingly, several studies in the mouse model have shown that varying glucose levels exert no effect on development (Summers et al. 1995). Further studies in the mouse have shown that no significant differences in either blastocyst formation, hatching, or cell numbers were evident comparing single-step with sequential culture (Biggers et al. 2005). More recent studies on human embryos now support increased rates of blastocyst formation. However, no significant differences in pregnancy rates were evident suggesting that the use of single-step culture is as effective as sequential culture (Reed et al. 2009; Sepulveda et al. 2009; Summers et al. 2013; Costa-Borges et al. 2016).

The use of single-step culture media also provides several practical advantages for the embryos and the embryologist, notably a reduction in stress on the embryo associated with changing medium on Day 3 and removal of the risk for potential osmotic shock by moving the embryo from solution to another. By contrast, sequential media do not mimic the situation *in vivo* where the embryo exists in a dynamic environment, where changes will be gradual; instead, the embryo experiences a swift change from one media to another *in vitro*. In practical terms, the use of single-step media reduces the number of media required, thus simplifying inventory control and traceability. Furthermore, the use of a single-step system is less labour intensive for the embryologist and can provide significant cost savings.

Sequential Culture Systems

Sequential culture systems are founded on the basis of the 'back to nature' hypothesis in that they provide a culture environment which is believed to be closer to that in which the embryo exists *in vivo* by providing a culture environment which meets the specific need of the embryo at each developmental stage. Sequential media were first used in the early days of IVF in the form of Earl's or KRB, supplemented with 8% serum or albumin to facilitate fertilization, followed by more complex media such as Hams F10 supplemented with higher levels of albumin or serum and glutamine for culture to the cleavage stages. Many of the commercially available sequential media systems used in clinics today such as the G-Series™ (Vitrolife), SAGE Quinn's Advantage™ (Origio) and Sydney IVF™ (Cook Medical) were based on three distinct media. Firstly, to facilitate fertilization a media with little glucose was used, followed by a second media for culture to Day 3 which contained lactate, nonessential amino acids, and pyruvate (as opposed to glucose as this was considered to be toxic during the early cleavage stages). The final media was to facilitate blastocyst growth and expansion that contained glucose, essential and nonessential amino acids, and vitamins amongst other components (Barnes et al. 1995; Gardner and Lane 1997; Devreker et al. 2001).The current crop of single-step media still use a specific media for fertilization due to differing requirements of the zygote and the early embryo, but use a single media until Days 5 and 6 with or without the need to refresh the media on Day 3 in contrast to the sequential system.

The components of these media have been discussed in detail previously in this chapter so the key question for the IVF laboratory is which is better? This is not a straightforward question to answer, as there is limited hard evidence to suggest that one system is superior to another. Those who are advocates of the 'back to nature approach' would argue that a single-step media may have harmful effects on the embryo due to the build-up of ammonia and exposure of the embryo to nonphysiological levels of glucose. Furthermore, the sequential system alleviates these issues through changing the media and better reflects the *in vivo* environment by mirroring the cyclical changes in concentrations of glucose, lactate, and the metabolic needs for higher glucose and pyruvate levels at the blastocyst stage (Conaghan et al. 1993b; Gardner and Lane 1997). However, there is no solid evidence for their use over single-step systems (Basile et al. 2013; Summers et al. 2013; Hardarson et al. 2015). Those who advocate the 'let the embryo choose' approach argue that changing the culture media introduces an unnecessary stress on the embryo and that sequential media may not accurately reflect the ever changing *in vivo* environment as evidence from the mouse would suggest (Summers et al. 1995). In fact, the choice for many laboratories will be based on their own experience and the practicalities of which system works best for them. Indeed, with the increasing use of time lapse and the morphometrics of embryo development to aid embryo selection, the use of single-step culture increasingly makes sense for the IVF laboratory and has shown to produce comparable results to sequential media in multiple laboratories.

Conclusion

In summary, IVF culture media have improved significantly since the early days of Brinster's and Whitten's media. However, it is clear that all aspects of the currently available IVF culture media could be further refined. Recent improvements have in part been facilitated through better quality control of the manufacturing process and the components used rather than as a result of a better understanding of the needs of embryos. One issue is the inability to study embryo-derived proteins accurately due to background noise from the vast numbers of nondeclared proteins in the current crop of single-step or sequential media (Mantikou et al. 2013). There is general agreement across the sector that the IVF laboratory must have better control of the composition of culture media to reduce culture-induced stress on the embryo. Such goals can only be achieved via a coordinated strategy of primary research in both animal and clinical models involving both academic and commercial partners.

References

Agerholm, I., Loft, A., Hald, F. et al. (2010). Culture of human oocytes with granulocyte-macrophage colony-stimulating factor has no effect on embryonic chromosomal constitution. Reprod Biomed Online 20: 477–484.

Alvarez, J.G. and Storey, B.T. (1995). Differential incorporation of fatty acids into and peroxidative loss of fatty acids from phospholipids of human spermatozoa. Mol Reprod Dev 42: 334–346.

Anas, M.K., Lee, M.B., Zhou, C. et al. (2008). SIT1 is a betaine/proline transporter that is activated in mouse eggs after fertilization and functions until the 2-cell stage. Development 135: 4123–4130.

Baltz, J.M. and Zhou, C. (2012). Cell volume regulation in mammalian oocytes and preimplantation embryos. Mol Reprod Dev 79: 821–831.

Barnes, F.L., Crombie, A., Gardner, D.K. et al. (1995). Blastocyst development and birth after in-vitro maturation of human primary oocytes, intracytoplasmic sperm injection and assisted hatching. Hum Reprod 10: 3243–3247.

Basile, N., Morbeck, D., Garcia-Velasco, J. et al. (2013). Type of culture media does not affect embryo kinetics: a time-lapse analysis of sibling oocytes. Hum Reprod 28: 634–641.

Behzad, F., Seif, M.W., Campbell, S. and Aplin, J.D. (1994). Expression of two isoforms of CD44 in human endometrium. Biol Reprod 51: 739–747.

Biggers, J.D. (1998). Reflections on the culture of the preimplantation embryo. Int J Dev Biol 42: 879–884.

Biggers, J.D., Mcginnis, L.K. and Lawitts, J.A. (2005). One-step versus two-step culture of mouse preimplantation embryos: is there a difference? Hum Reprod 20: 3376–3384.

Biggers, J.D. and Stern, S. (1973). Metabolism of the preimplantation mammalian embryo. Adv Reprod Physiol 6: 1–59.

Biggers, J.D. and Summers, M.C. (2008). Choosing a culture medium: making informed choices. Fertil Steril 90: 473–483.

Bolton, H., Graham, S.J., Van Der Aa, et al. (2016). Mouse model of chromosome mosaicism reveals lineage-specific depletion of aneuploid cells and normal developmental potential. Nat Commun 7: 11165.

Bontekoe, S., Blake, D., Heineman, M.J. et al. (2010). Adherence compounds in embryo transfer media

for assisted reproductive technologies. Cochrane Database Syst Rev CD007421.

Bontekoe, S., Heineman, M.J., Johnson, N. et al. (2014). Adherence compounds in embryo transfer media for assisted reproductive technologies. Cochrane Database Syst Rev CD007421.

Brinster, R.L. (1963). A method for in vitro cultivation of mouse ova from two-cell to blastocyst. Exp Cell Res 32: 205–208.

Brinster, R.L. (1968). In vitro culture of mammalian embryos. J Anim Sci 27(Suppl 1): 1–14.

Brison, D.R., Houghton, F.D., Falconer, D. et al. (2004). Identification of viable embryos in IVF by non-invasive measurement of amino acid turnover. Hum Reprod 19: 2319–2324.

Campbell, S., Swann, H.R., Aplin, J.D. et al. (1995). CD44 is expressed throughout pre-implantation human embryo development. Hum Reprod 10: 425–430.

Carson, D.D., Dutt, A. and Tang, J.P. (1987). Glycoconjugate synthesis during early pregnancy: hyaluronate synthesis and function. Dev Biol 120: 228–235.

Chatot, C.L., Ziomek, C.A., Bavister, B.D. et al. (1989). An improved culture medium supports development of random-bred 1-cell mouse embryos in vitro. J Reprod Fertil 86: 679–688.

Collins, J.L. and Baltz, J.M. (1999). Estimates of mouse oviductal fluid tonicity based on osmotic responses of embryos. Biol Reprod 60: 1188–1193.

Conaghan, J., Handyside, A.H., Winston, R.M. et al. (1993a). Effects of pyruvate and glucose on the development of human preimplantation embryos in vitro. J Reprod Fertil 99: 87–95.

Conaghan, J., Hardy, K., Handyside, A.H. et al. (1993b). Selection criteria for human embryo transfer: a comparison of pyruvate uptake and morphology. J Assist Reprod Genet 10: 21–30.

Costa-Borges, N., Belles, M., Meseguer, M. et al. (2016). Blastocyst development in single medium with or without renewal on day 3: a prospective cohort study on sibling donor oocytes in a time-lapse incubator. Fertil Steril 105: 707–713.

Daniel, J.C., Jr. and Krishnan, R.S. (1967). Amino acid requirements for growth of the rabbit blastocyst in vitro. J Cell Physiol 70: 155–160.

Dawson, K.M., Collins, J.L. and Baltz, J.M. (1998). Osmolarity-dependent glycine accumulation indicates a role for glycine as an organic osmolyte in early preimplantation mouse embryos. Biol Reprod 59: 225–232.

Devreker, F., Hardy, K., Van Den Bergh, M. et al. (2001). Amino acids promote human blastocyst development in vitro. Hum Reprod 16: 749–756.

Dudley, D.J., Mitchell, M.D., Creighton, K. et al. (1990). Lymphokine production during term human pregnancy: differences between peripheral leukocytes and decidual cells. Am J Obstet Gynecol 163: 1890–1893.

Dumoulin, J.C., Van Wissen, L.C., Menheere, P.P. et al. (1997). Taurine acts as an osmolyte in human and mouse oocytes and embryos. Biol Reprod 56: 739–744.

Dunglison, G.F., Barlow, D.H. and Sargent, I.L. (1996). Leukaemia inhibitory factor significantly enhances the blastocyst formation rates of human embryos cultured in serum-free medium. Hum Reprod 11: 191–196.

Dyrlund, T.F., Kirkegaard, K., Poulsen, E.T. et al. (2015). Unconditioned commercial embryo culture media contain a large variety of non-declared proteins: a comprehensive proteomics analysis. Hum Reprod 29: 2421–2430.

Edwards, L.J., Williams, D.A. and Gardner, D.K. (1998). Intracellular pH of the mouse preimplantation embryo: amino acids act as buffers of intracellular pH. Hum Reprod 13: 3441–3448.

Erbach, G.T., Lawitts, J.A., Papaioannou, V.E. et al. (1994). Differential growth of the mouse preimplantation embryo in chemically defined media. Biol Reprod 50: 1027–1033.

Gardner, D.K. and Lane, M. (1993). Amino acids and ammonium regulate mouse embryo development in culture. Biol Reprod 48: 377–385.

Gardner, D.K. and Lane, M. (1996). Alleviation of the '2-cell block' and development to the blastocyst of CF1 mouse embryos: role of amino acids, EDTA and physical parameters. Hum Reprod 11: 2703–2712.

Gardner D.K. and Lane, M. (1997). Culture and selection of viable blastocysts: a feasible proposition for human IVF? Hum Reprod Update 3: 367–382.

Gardner, D.K., Lane, M., Calderon, I. et al. (1996). Environment of the preimplantation human embryo in vivo: metabolite analysis of oviduct and uterine fluids and metabolism of cumulus cells. Fertil Steril 65: 349–353.

Gardner, D.K., Lane, M., Stevens, J. et al. (2001). Noninvasive assessment of human embryo nutrient consumption as a measure of developmental potential. Fertil Steril 76: 1175–1180.

Gardner, D.K. and Leese, H.J. (1990). Concentrations of nutrients in mouse oviduct fluid and their effects on embryo development and metabolism in vitro. J Reprod Fertil 88: 361–368.

Gardner, D.K. and Wale, P.L. (2013). Analysis of metabolism to select viable human embryos for transfer. Fertil Steril 99: 1062–1072.

Gott, A.L., Hardy, K., Winston, R M. et al. (1990). Non-invasive measurement of pyruvate and glucose uptake and lactate production by single human preimplantation embryos. Hum Reprod 5: 104–108.

Hadi, T., Hammer, M.A., Algire, C. et al. (2005). Similar effects of osmolarity, glucose, and phosphate on cleavage past the 2-cell stage in mouse embryos from outbred and F1 hybrid females. Biol Reprod 72: 179–187.

Hallows, K.R. and Knauf, P.A. (1994). Regulatory volume decrease in HL-60 cells: importance of rapid changes in permeability of Cl- and organic solutes. Am J Physiol 267: C1045–C1056.

Hallows, K.R., Restrepo, D. and Knauf, P.A. (1994). Control of intracellular pH during regulatory volume decrease in HL-60 cells. Am J Physiol 267: C1057–1066.

Hammer, M.A. and Baltz, J.M. (2003). Beta-alanine but not taurine can function as an organic osmolyte in preimplantation mouse embryos cultured from fertilized eggs. Mol Reprod Dev 66: 153–161.

Hammer, M.A., Kolajova, M., Leveille, M. et al. (2000). Glycine transport by single human and mouse embryos. Hum Reprod 15: 419–426.

Hammond, J., Jr. (1949). Recovery and culture of tubal mouse ova. Nature 163: 28.

Hardarson, T., Bungum, M., Conaghan, J. et al. (2015). Noninferiority, randomized, controlled trial comparing embryo development using media developed for sequential or undisturbed culture in a time-lapse setup. Fertil Steril 104: 1452–9, e1–4.

Hardy, K., Handyside, A.H. and Winston, R.M. (1989a). The human blastocyst: cell number, death and allocation during late preimplantation development in vitro. Development 107: 597–604.

Hardy, K., Hooper, M.A., Handyside, A.H. et al. (1989b). Non-invasive measurement of glucose and pyruvate uptake by individual human oocytes and preimplantation embryos. Hum Reprod 4: 188–191.

Hardy, K. and Spanos, S. (2002). Growth factor expression and function in the human and mouse preimplantation embryo. J Endocrinol 172: 221–236.

Houghton, F.D., Hawkhead, J.A., Humpherson, P.G. et al. (2002). Non-invasive amino acid turnover predicts human embryo developmental capacity. Hum Reprod 17: 999–1005.

Kaplan, J. H. (2002). Biochemistry of Na,K-ATPase. Annu Rev Biochem 71: 511–535.

Khamsi, F., Armstrong, D. T. and Zhang, X. (1996). Expression of urokinase-type plasminogen activator in human preimplantation embryos. Mol Hum Reprod 2: 273–276.

Khul, W. (1941). Untersuchungen uber die cytodynamik der furchung und fruhentwicklung des eis der weissen maus. Abb Senchenb Naturforsch Ges 456: 1–17.

Kimber, S.J., Sneddon, S.F., Bloor, D.J. et al. (2008). Expression of genes involved in early cell fate decisions in human embryos and their regulation by growth factors. Reproduction 135: 635–647.

Krebs, A. and Henseleit, K. (1932). Untersuchungen uber die Harnstoffbildung im teirkoper. Z Phys Chem 210: 33–66.

Lane, M. and Gardner, D. K. (1994). Increase in postimplantation development of cultured mouse embryos by amino acids and induction of fetal retardation and exencephaly by ammonium ions. J Reprod Fertil 102: 305–312.

Lane, M. and Gardner, D. K. (2005). Mitochondrial malate-aspartate shuttle regulates mouse embryo nutrient consumption. J Biol Chem 280: 18361–18367.

Lane, M., Hooper, K. and Gardner, D. K. (2001). Effect of essential amino acids on mouse embryo viability and ammonium production. J Assist Reprod Genet 18: 519–525.

Lawitts, J.A. and Biggers, J.D. (1991a). Optimization of mouse embryo culture media using simplex methods. J Reprod Fertil 91: 543–556.

Lawitts, J.A. and Biggers, J.D. (1991b). Overcoming the 2-cell block by modifying standard components in a mouse embryo culture medium. Biol Reprod 45: 245–251.

Leese, H.J. (1991). Metabolism of the preimplantation mammalian embryo. Oxf Rev Reprod Biol 13: 35–72.

Leese, H. J. (1995). Metabolic control during preimplantation mammalian development. Hum Reprod Update 1: 63–72.

Leese, H.J. (1998). Human embryo culture: back to nature. J Assist Reprod Genet 15: 466–8.

Leese, H.J. and Barton, A.M. (1985). Production of pyruvate by isolated mouse cumulus cells. J Exp Zool 234: 231–236.

Leese, H.J., Guerif, F., Allgar, V. et al. (2016). Biological optimization, the Goldilocks principle, and how much is lagom in the preimplantation embryo. Mol Reprod Dev 83: 748–754.

Lewis, W.H. and Gregory, P.W. (1929). Cinematographs of living developing rabbit-eggs. Science 69: 226–229.

Li, R., Whitworth, K., Lai, L. et al. (2007). Concentration and composition of free amino acids and osmolalities of porcine oviductal and uterine fluid and their effects on development of porcine IVF embryos. Mol Reprod Dev 74: 1228–1235.

Lighten, A.D., Moore, G.E., Winston, R.M. et al. (1998). Routine addition of human insulin-like growth factor-I ligand could benefit clinical in-vitro fertilization culture. Hum Reprod 13: 3144–3150.

Locke, F.S. and Rosenheim, O. (1907). Contributions to the physiology of the isolated heart: The consumption of dextrose by mammalian cardiac muscle. J Physiol 36: 205–220.

Lopata, A. and Oliva, K. (1993). Chorionic gonadotrophin secretion by human blastocysts. Hum Reprod 8: 932–938.

Mantikou, E., Youssef, M.A., Van Wely, M. et al. (2013). Embryo culture media and IVF/ICSI success rates: a systematic review. Hum Reprod Update 19: 210–220.

Martin, K.L., Barlow, D.H. and Sargent, I.L. (1998). Heparin-binding epidermal growth factor significantly improves human blastocyst development and hatching in serum-free medium. Hum Reprod 13: 1645–1652.

Martin, K.L. and Leese, H.J. (1995). Role of glucose in mouse preimplantation embryo development. Mol Reprod Dev 40: 436–443.

Mclaren. A. and Biggers, J. D. (1958). Successful development and birth of mice cultivated in vitro as early as early embryos. Nature 182: 877–878.

Morbeck, D. E., Baumann, N. A. and Oglesbee, D. (2017). Composition of single-step media used for human embryo culture. Fertil Steril 107: 1055–1060.

Morbeck, D.E., Krisher, R.L., Herrick, J.R. et al. (2014). Composition of commercial media used for human embryo culture. Fertil Steril 102: 759–766. e9.

Nasr-Esfahani, M.H., Winston, N.J. and Johnson, M.H. (1992). Effects of glucose, glutamine, ethylenediaminetetraacetic acid and oxygen tension on the concentration of reactive oxygen species and on development of the mouse preimplantation embryo in vitro. J Reprod Fertil 96: 219–231.

Otsuki, J., Nagai, Y., Matsuyama, Y. et al. (2013). The redox state of recombinant human serum albumin and its optimal concentration for mouse embryo culture. Syst Biol Reprod Med 59: 48–52.

Pampfer, S. (2000). Peri-implantation embryopathy induced by maternal diabetes. J Reprod Fertil (Suppl) 55: 129–139.

Perricone, R., De Carolis, C., Giacomelli, R. et al. (2003). GM-CSF and pregnancy: evidence of significantly reduced blood concentrations in unexplained recurrent abortion efficiently reverted by intravenous immunoglobulin treatment. Am J Reprod Immunol 50: 232–237.

Picton, H.M., Elder, K., Houghton, F.D. et al. (2010). Association between amino acid turnover and chromosome aneuploidy during human preimplantation embryo development in vitro. Mol Hum Reprod 16: 557–569.

Pool, T.B. (2004). Development of culture media for human assisted reproductive technology. Fertil Steril 81: 287–289.

Quinn, P., Kerin, J.F. and Warnes, G.M. (1985a). Improved pregnancy rate in human in vitro fertilization with the use of a medium based on the composition of human tubal fluid. Fertil Steril 44: 493–498.

Quinn, P., Warnes, G.M., Kerin, J.F. et al. (1985b). Culture factors affecting the success rate of in vitro fertilization and embryo transfer. Ann NY Acad Sci 442: 195–204.

Reed, M.L., Hamic, A., Thompson, D.J. et al. (2009). Continuous uninterrupted single medium culture without medium renewal versus sequential media culture: a sibling embryo study. Fertil Steril 92: 1783–1786.

Reeds, P. J. (2000). Dispensable and indispensable amino acids for humans. J Nutr 130: 1835S–1840S.

Rieger, D., Loskutoff, N.M. and Betteridge, K.J. (1992). Developmentally related changes in the metabolism of glucose and glutamine by cattle embryos produced and co-cultured in vitro. J Reprod Fertil 95: 585–595.

Ringer, S. (1882). Concerning the Influence exerted by each of the constituents of the blood on the contraction of the ventricle. J Physiol 3: 380–393.

Ringer, S. (1883). A further contribution regarding the influence of the different constituents of the blood on the contraction of the heart. J Physiol 4: 29–42.

Sellens, M.H., Stein, S. and Sherman, M.I. (1981). Protein and free amino acid content in preimplantation mouse embryos and in blastocysts under various culture conditions. J Reprod Fertil 61: 307–315.

Sepulveda, S., Garcia, J., Arriaga, E. et al. (2009). In vitro development and pregnancy outcomes for human embryos cultured in either a single medium or in a sequential media system. Fertil Steril 91: 1765–1770.

Sjoblom, C., Wikland, M. and Robertson, S.A. (2002). Granulocyte-macrophage colony-stimulating factor (GM-CSF) acts independently of the beta common subunit of the GM-CSF receptor to prevent inner cell mass apoptosis in human embryos. Biol Reprod 67: 1817–1823.

Steeves, C.L., Hammer, M.A., Walker, G.B. et al. (2003). The glycine neurotransmitter transporter GLYT1 is an organic osmolyte transporter regulating cell volume in cleavage-stage embryos. Proc Natl Acad Sci USA 100: 13982–13987.

Steptoe, P.C. and Edwards, R.G. (1978). Birth after the reimplantation of a human embryo. Lancet 2, 366.

Stojkovic, M., Krebs, O., Kolle, S. et al. (2003). Developmental regulation of hyaluronan-binding protein (RHAMM/IHABP) expression in early bovine embryos. Biol Reprod 68: 60–66.

Sturmey, R.G., Bermejo-Alvarez, P., Gutierrez-Adan, A. et al. (2010). Amino acid metabolism of bovine blastocysts: a biomarker of sex and viability. Mol Reprod Dev 77: 285–296.

Sturmey, R.G., Hawkhead, J.A., Barker, E.A. et al. (2009). DNA damage and metabolic activity in the preimplantation embryo. Hum Reprod 24: 81–91.

Summers, M.C., Bhatnagar, P.R., Lawitts, J.A. et al. (1995). Fertilization in vitro of mouse ova from inbred and outbred strains: complete preimplantation embryo development in glucose-supplemented KSOM. Biol Reprod 53: 431–437.

Summers, M.C. and Biggers, J.D. (2003). Chemically defined media and the culture of mammalian preimplantation embryos: historical perspective and current issues. Hum Reprod Update 9: 557–582.

Summers, M.C., Bird, S., Mirzai, F.M. et al. (2013). Human preimplantation embryo development in vitro: a morphological assessment of sibling zygotes cultured in a single medium or in sequential media. Hum Fertil 16: 278 285.

Turley, E. and Moore, D. (1984). Hyaluronate binding proteins also bind to fibronectin, laminin and collagen. Biochem Biophys Res Commun 121: 808–814.

Tyrode, M. (1910). The mode of action of some purgative salts. Arch Int Pharmacodyn Ther 20: 205–223.

Van Winkle, L.J., Haghighat, N. and Campion E. (1990). Glycine protects preimplantation mouse conceptuses from a detrimental effect on development of the inorganic ions in oviductal fluid. J Exp Zool 253: 215–219.

Wang, F., Kooistra, M., Lee, M. et al. (2005). Mouse embryos stressed by physiological levels of osmolarity become arrested in the late 2-cell stage before entry into M phase. Biol Reprod 85: 702–713.

Waring, D.W. (1976). Rate of formation and osmolality of oviductal fluid in the cycling rat. Biol Reprod 15: 297–302.

Whitten, W.K. (1956). Culture of tubal mouse ova. Nature 177: 96.

Whitten, W. K. (1957). Culture of tubal ova. Nature 179: 1081–1082.

Whittingham, D.G. (1971). Culture of mouse ova. J Reprod Fertil Suppl 14: 7–21.

Yaegashi, N., Fujita, N., Yajima, A. et al. (1995). Menstrual cycle dependent expression of CD44 in normal human endometrium. Hum Pathol 26: 862–865.

Yu, Y., Yan, J., Li, M. et al. (2012). Effects of combined epidermal growth factor, brain-derived neurotrophic factor and insulin-like growth factor 1 on human oocyte maturation and early fertilized and cloned embryo development. Hum Reprod 27: 2146–2159.

Zander-Fox, D. and Lane, M. (2012). Media composition: energy sources and metabolism. Methods Mol Biol 912: 81–96.

Zhao, Y. and Chegini, N. (1994). Human fallopian tube expresses granulocyte-macrophage colony stimulating factor (GM-CSF) and GM-CSF alpha and beta receptors and contain immunoreactive GM-CSF protein. J Clin Endocrinol Metab 79: 662–665.

Zhao, Y., Rong, H. and Chegini, N. (1995). Expression and selective cellular localization of granulocyte-macrophage colony-stimulating factor (GM-CSF) and GM-CSF alpha and beta receptor messenger ribonucleic acid and protein in human ovarian tissue. Biol Reprod 53: 923–930.

Ziebe, S., Loft, A., Povlsen, B.B. et al. (2013). A randomized clinical trial to evaluate the effect of granulocyte-macrophage colony-stimulating factor (GM-CSF) in embryo culture medium for in vitro fertilization. Fertil Steril 99: 1600–1609.

Zorn, T.M., Pinhal, M.A., Nader, H.B. et al. (1995). Biosynthesis of glycosaminoglycans in the endometrium during the initial stages of pregnancy of the mouse. Cell Mol Biol 41: 97–106.

27

Incubators in the Assisted Reproductive Technology Laboratory

Louise Hyslop

Introduction

Incubators have a critical role in providing a stable environment for optimal embryo development within the *in vitro* fertilization (IVF) laboratory. To this end, incubators regulate the temperature, gas concentration, and humidity. Initially, IVF laboratories only had the option of large single chamber incubators designed for larger scale tissue culture. Nowadays there is an increasing range of benchtop and time-lapse incubators designed specifically for gamete and embryo culture. Closed systems for gamete and embryo culture which also facilitate manipulation have been developed as an alternative to stand-alone incubators and IVF workstations. This chapter will outline the main features to consider when selecting between the varieties of incubators available on the market.

Incubator Types

Single Chamber Incubators

Single chamber incubators were designed for large scale tissue culture with flasks rather than the small dishes used in IVF laboratories for gamete and embryo culture. Nevertheless, this style of incubator is currently the most widely used in UK IVF laboratories (Bolton et al. 2014). These incubators are available in a wide range of chamber volumes from approximately 20 to 200 litres (Figure 27.1).

The large capacity for multiple patients also makes them a popular choice as a back-up incubator and/or a separate location for equilibration of culture dishes. It is not within the scope of this chapter to compare manufacturers and incubator models. The main incubator features which regulate the gas concentration, temperature, and humidity will be discussed with the advantages and disadvantages of each.

Benchtop Incubators

Benchtop incubators have been designed specifically for the culture of gametes and embryos in IVF laboratories. An increasing number of IVF laboratories have introduced them for embryo culture but usually in combination with another incubator type (Bolton et al. 2014). These incubators usually have more than one chamber with a volume of less than 1 litre (Figure 27.2).

The small chamber size restricts the maximum number of patient dishes but the smaller incubator footprint allows laboratories to have more than one benchtop incubator in the same space required for a single large chamber incubator.

Time-lapse Incubators

Standard morphology assessment provides only snapshots at specific time points during the dynamic embryo development process. Time-lapse systems take digital images of embryos at set intervals and can provide information that can be missed with

(a) (b)

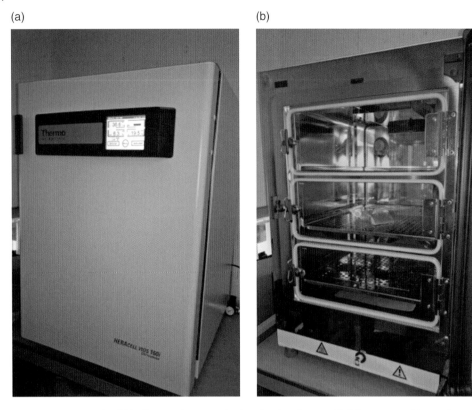

Figure 27.1 Example of (a) a large volume single chamber incubator with (b) segmented inner door to reduce gas loss in a single chamber incubator.

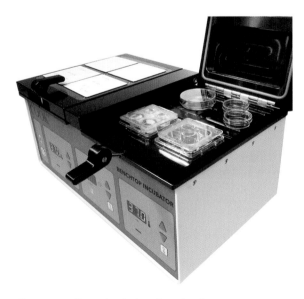

Figure 27.2 Example of a benchtop incubator.
Reproduced with permission of Cook Medical, Bloomington, Indiana, USA.

standard morphological assessment, such as the presence of multinucleation. Additional features provided by time-lapse imaging include timing of cell divisions, cell division patterns, and intervals between cleavage cycles (Figure 27.3).

Two different types of time-lapse system have been developed:

- Time-lapse camera that can be placed into most existing incubators, for example Primo Vision™ (Vitrolife, Göteborg, Sweden) and EEVA™ (Auxogyn, Menlo Park, CA, USA) systems.
- Combined time-lapse camera and incubator such as the Embryoscope™ (Vitrolife), Miri TL® (Esco, Egaa, Denmark) and Geri (Genea Biomedx, Sydney, Australia) systems.

Currently, there are five time-lapse systems available (Table 27.1).

Noninvasive time-lapse monitoring in combination with the use of single-step medium reduces the

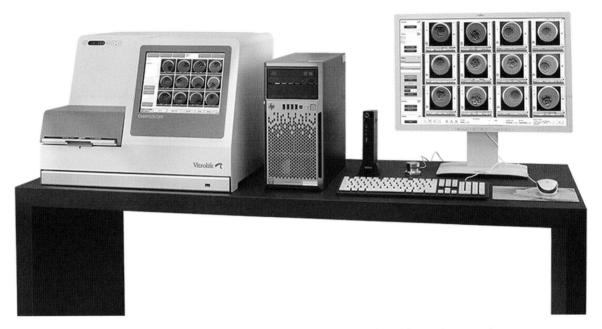

Figure 27.3 Embryoscope™ time-lapse system. Reproduced with permission of Vitrolife, Göteburg, Sweden.

Table 27.1 Comparison of commercially available time-lapse systems.

	Primo Vision™	EEVA™	Embryoscope™	Miri TL®	Geri
Type of system	Standalone camera that can be placed in standard incubator	Standalone camera that can be placed in standard incubator	Combined camera/incubator	Combined camera/incubator	Combined camera/incubator
Incubator design	User defined	User defined	Single chamber incubator for up to six Embryoslides®	Benchtop incubator with six separate chambers	Benchtop incubator with six separate chambers
Illumination	Bright field, green LED (550 nm)	Dark field, red LED (625 nm)	Bright field, red LED (635 nm)	Bright field, red LED (635 nm)	Bright field, orange LED (591 nm)
Maximum number of focal planes	11	1	17 but reduced depending upon frequency of image capture	7	11
Frequency of image capture	From 5 minutes	5 minutes	From 10 minutes	5 minutes	5 minutes
Maximum number of embryos per dish	16 – Primo Vision embryo culture dish	12 – EEVA dish	12 - Embryoslide®	14 – CultureCoin culture dish	16 – Geri dish
Embryo culture	Group	Group	Single	Single	Single
Total number of embryos monitored	96	48	72	84	96

need to expose the embryos to atmospheric conditions and the associated fluctuations in temperature and pH. Single-step culture media that does not require a medium change on Day 3 is commercially available, therefore the embryos can remain undisturbed for up to 5 days in an environmentally controlled environment. Numerous studies have been published with time-lapse monitoring safety data because a primary concern was the frequent exposure to light. Randomized controlled trials (RCTs) have shown no benefit to embryo quality of undisturbed culture in a time-lapse incubator with frequent image capture versus a conventional incubator. The first Cochrane systematic review of time-lapse systems for embryo incubation and assessment concluded that no clear evidence existed of a difference in clinical outcome between time-lapse systems and conventional incubation (Armstrong et al. 2015).

Further prospective RCTs are required to demonstrate if undisturbed culture in addition to the morphology and developmental kinetic data from time-lapse monitoring can identify the embryos with the highest implantation potential. The time-lapse images are assessed either by an embryologist or some systems have cell tracking software algorithms to evaluate morphokinetic parameters.

Closed Systems for Micromanipulation and Culture

Closed systems provide a stable environmentally controlled environment for culture and all manipulations from egg collection to embryo transfer. Integration of the incubators into the enclosed workstations ensures the embryos are not exposed to atmospheric conditions and the environment is stable because the incubators do not need to recover following door opening. The enclosed workstations have CO_2 and temperature controls to allow manipulations in bicarbonate-buffered media without the drop in temperature and gradual increase in pH which occur whilst manipulating in conventional open-fronted cabinets (Hyslop et al. 2012).

There are currently two closed systems commercially available: VitroSafe (Vitro Safe Systems, Glossop, UK) and Ac-tive® IVF (Ruskinn, Bridgend,

UK). The use of these truly closed systems from egg collection to embryo transfer has been associated with an increase in blastocyst development and implantation rate (Hyslop et al. 2012). Prospective randomized controlled trials are required to compare these closed systems to the standard open workstations in combination with either standalone incubators or time-lapse monitoring.

An additional benefit of the closed system is during the training of inexperienced operators, where manipulation times will be longer during the initial training period but the environmental control protects the embryos.

Main Incubator Features to Consider When Selecting an Incubator

CO_2 Regulation

Precise and reliable regulation of CO_2 is a critical function of incubators. This is determined by the type of gas sensor used to monitor CO_2: thermal conductivity (TC) or infrared (IR). CO_2 readings by TC sensors are influenced by the relative humidity. After door opening, the relative humidity needs to stabilize before the CO_2 concentration can be accurately determined and adjusted back to the desired set point. IR sensors function independently of the relative humidity, and therefore the CO_2 recovery time is faster compared with TC sensor incubators. Whilst IR sensors are more costly and have shorter lifespans, they are often the preferred option in IVF laboratories because of quicker CO_2 recovery. Incubator companies are continually trying to design incubators with faster gas recovery and to this end a new TC sensor has been designed with humidity compensation. The CO_2 measurement is unaffected by changes in humidity so the incubator is able to recover faster following a door opening. The recovery time is still slightly slower than IR sensor incubators, but the new TC sensor is more economical, has a long service life, and can remain *in situ* during heat sterilization of the incubator.

It is important to note that the set point for CO_2 should be determined by the target pH of the medium used for embryo culture, particularly since the altitude of the clinic influences the required CO_2 level in the incubator. As the altitude increases the atmospheric pressure decreases and therefore a higher CO_2 concentration is required to obtain sufficient pressure to equilibrate the embryo culture medium.

O_2 Regulation

Production of reactive oxygen species (ROS) has been demonstrated to impact embryo development negatively (Guérin et al. 2001). One mechanism to reduce the formation of ROS is by culture in an environment of low oxygen, which more closely resembles the O_2 concentration *in vivo* (Yedwab et al. 1976; Byatt-Smith et al. 1991). Numerous studies have investigated whether embryo culture in reduced oxygen can improve clinical outcome but initially the data appeared to be conflicting. Meta-analysis and further subgroup analysis have shown that clinical outcome is improved with embryo culture in reduced oxygen in combination with blastocyst stage transfer (Meintjes, 2009; Waldenstrom et al. 2009; Kovacic et al. 2010) but not cleavage stage transfer (Meintjes 2009; Kovacic et al. 2010).

The two most common O_2 sensors in IVF incubators to achieve 5% O_2 are zirconium and galvanic/fuel-cell sensors. The galvanic cell is a diffusion-limited metal/air battery which has a finite lifespan and needs replacing more frequently than zirconia cells. Whilst zirconia cells are more expensive, the speed of response is quicker in comparison and so they have become the preferred option.

Incubator Gas Recovery

The recovery timing is determined not only by the gas sensors but the incubator volume. Larger volume incubators usually have the option of segmented inner doors to reduce gas loss (Figure 27.1). At the other extreme of volume are the increasing number of benchtop incubators with multiple separate chambers designed specifically for IVF laboratories. The small chamber volume of less than a litre allows

for fast gas recovery. Alternatively, cylinders of premixed gas can be used to provide accurate gas concentrations and speed up recovery time following door opening.

Temperature Control

Maintaining the optimal temperature for embryo culture is crucial for meiotic spindle integrity and reducing environmental stress (Wang et al. 2001; Sun et al. 2004). Careful consideration is therefore required when choosing between incubators with different heating mechanisms. There are three main types of heating mechanism employed:

1) Water-jacketed.
2) Direct-heated.
3) Direct heat transfer by contact of the incubator surface with the culture dish.

Historically, water-jacketed incubators are renowned for temperature stability. They are able to retain heat longer during door openings and power failure, although the speed of recovery is slowest out of the three incubator types. These incubators are heavier due to the water jacket and more complex to maintain to ensure that no contamination originates from the jacket water. To reduce cross-contamination, direct-heated incubators are available without air circulating fans and are still able to warm up quickly. The fastest recovery is achieved by direct heat transfer in benchtop incubators designed specifically for IVF laboratories. However, these benchtop incubators lose heat immediately if there is power loss and therefore it is essential to have at least a battery backup or alternatively an uninterruptible power supply.

When purchasing a new incubator, it is important to consider not only the speed of temperature recovery but also temperature uniformity, to provide consistent results irrespective of location within the chamber. Regardless of the heating mechanism and presence of a fan there can be temperature gradients across surfaces and between shelves. Laboratories should evaluate temperature variations and optimize incubator management to deal with any hot or cold spots.

Humidity

Humidity is required to minimize evaporation of media, although it may not be an essential requirement in some IVF laboratories that use an oil overlay. There are three main types of humidification systems employed:

1) Passive humidification: evaporation of a water reservoir usually located in the base of the incubator. This water reservoir must be replaced regularly otherwise it could become a potential source of contamination.
2) Semiactive humidification: inlet gases are prehumidified by being bubbled through an external water reservoir.
3) Active humidification: water vapour is injected into the chamber under the control of a continuously monitoring humidity sensor.

A side-effect of high humidity is condensation, which can be a breeding ground for microbial contamination. To minimize condensation on the inner segmented doors, some incubators have a heated outer door.

Other Considerations When Selecting an Incubator

Independent Monitoring

The capacity to perform independent 24-h monitoring of incubator conditions is an important feature. To achieve this there are numerous alarm systems which can monitor the temperature and gas concentrations and alert on-call staff if any parameters fall outside specified limits. The minimal chamber volume of benchtop incubators is beneficial to reduce the recovery timing following door opening, but in some incubators is too small to allow the use of accurate independent CO_2 sensors. Irrespective of this design deficit, these benchtop incubators are becoming widely used with additional measures to reduce the risk of lack of 24-h gas monitoring. Unfortunately, additional measures cannot identify out-of-hours issues and a major incident was reported to the Human Fertilisation and Embryology Authority in 2014 (www.hfea.gov.uk).

Quality Control

Quality control checks are more difficult to perform in benchtop incubators because of the small chamber size. Some manufacturers have incorporated measuring and sampling ports into the design to assist with temperature and gas concentration measurements. For pH measurement there are various options, including semimicro/micro pH electrodes. A blood gas analyser is an option but it is expensive.

Cost

The cost of purchase, usage, and maintenance should be considered because it varies with incubator design and sensors selected for gas regulation.

Future Developments

Permeable medical devices have been developed for *in vivo* culture of embryos. The device, loaded with inseminated eggs or embryos, is inserted into the uterus. The porous device allows fertilization and embryo development to occur in a dynamic microenvironment with cross-talk between the developing embryos and endometrium. Whilst *in vivo* culture reduces the exposure of the embryos to synthetic *in vitro* culture conditions it should be noted that fertilization and early cleavage stage embryo development in the uterus is not physiological. After removal of the device the embryos are retrieved and cultured *in vitro* until selection for transfer. A pilot study demonstrated that it is feasible to culture embryos *in vivo* (Blockeel et al. 2009). A prospective RCT is required to compare the impact on sibling embryo development of conventional *in vitro* culture versus *in vivo* culture and quality as only a limited number of patients were included in this study.

Conclusion

Optimal embryo development is dependent upon providing a stable culture environment and so incubator selection is a critical decision for the

IVF laboratory. There is no consensus on which is the best incubator design for optimal embryo culture. Therefore, the main incubator features covered in this chapter should to be considered during the decision process. Other considerations include incubator capacity and available laboratory space.

References

Armstrong, S., Arroll, N., Cree, LM. et al. (2015). Time-lapse systems for embryo incubation and assessment in assisted reproduction. Cochrane Database Syst Rev 2: CD011320.

Blockeel, C., Mock, P., Verheyen, G. et al. (2009). An in vivo culture system for human embryos using an encapsulation technology: a pilot study. Hum Reprod 24: 790–796.

Bolton, V., Cutting, R., Clarke, H. et al. (2014). ACE consensus meeting report: Culture systems. Hum Fertil 17: 239–251.

Byatt-Smith, J.G., Leese, H.J. and Gosden, R.G. (1991). An investigation by mathematical modelling of whether mouse and human preimplantation embryos in static culture can satisfy their demands for oxygen by diffusion. Hum Reprod 6: 52–57.

Guérin, P., El Mouatassim, S. and Ménézo, Y. (2001). Oxidative stress and protection against reactive oxygen species in the pre-implantation embryo and its surroundings. Hum Reprod Update 7: 175–189.

Human Fertilization and Embryology Authority (2014). Incidents case study: a cautionary tale on the use of benchtop incubators.

Hyslop, L., Prathalingam, N., Nowak, L. et al. (2012). A novel isolator-based system promotes viability of human embryos during laboratory processing. PLoS One 7: e31010.

Kovacic, B., Sajko, M.C. and Vlaisavljević, V. (2010). A prospective, randomized trial on the effect of atmospheric versus reduced oxygen concentration on the outcome of intracytoplasmic sperm injection cycles. Fertil Steril 94: 511–519.

Meintjes, M., Chantilis, S.J., Douglas, J.D. et al. (2009). A controlled randomized trial evaluating the effect of lowered incubator oxygen tension on live births in a predominantly blastocyst transfer program. Hum Reprod 24: 300–307.

Sun, X.F., Wang, W.H. and Keefe, D.L. (2004). Overheating is detrimental to meiotic spindles within in vitro matured human oocytes. Zygote 12: 65–70.

Waldenström, U., Engström, A.B., Hellberg, D. et al. (2009). Low-oxygen compared with high-oxygen atmosphere in blastocyst culture, a prospective randomized study. Fertil Steril 91: 2461–2465.

Wang, W.H., Meng, L., Hackett, R.J., et al. (2001). Limited recovery of meiotic spindles in living human oocytes after cooling-rewarming observed using polarized light microscopy. Hum Reprod 16: 2374–2378.

Yedwab, G.A., Paz, G., Homonnai, T.Z. et al. (1976). The temperature, pH, and partial pressure of oxygen in the cervix and uterus of women and uterus of rats during the cycle. Fertil Steril 27: 304–309.

28

Embryo Transfer Techniques and Improving Embryo Implantation Rates

Rachel Cutting

Introduction

Since the advent of *in vitro* fertilization (IVF) there have been many advances in ovarian stimulation regimens and laboratory conditions which have led to the complex process of IVF employed worldwide today. Although technological advances in the laboratory have improved embryo viability and increased knowledge of endometrial receptivity has been gained, embryo transfer is still a critical limiting technique in an IVF cycle. Meldrum et al. as early as 1987, highlighted that a meticulous embryo transfer technique is essential for a successful programme. However, despite its clear importance, the technique itself remains relatively unchanged and although millions of babies have been born worldwide, across Europe pregnancy rates per embryo transfer still remain around 32% (Ferraretti et al. 2013), with lack of implantation attributed to poor uterine receptivity, poor quality embryos, or the embryo transfer technique (Brown et al. 2010). In recent years, in an attempt to improve implantation rates, focus has been on adjuncts to treatment around the time of embryo transfer, either through patient medication or modifications to procedures in the laboratory. This chapter aims to review the technique of embryo transfer and discuss the additional factors which can influence implantation rates.

Embryo Transfer Technique

The paucity of published material on embryo transfer techniques should not detract from the importance of the procedure and it is clear that to maximize implantation rates, embryos should be transferred back to the uterus in a gentle and atraumatic manner (Schoolcraft et al. 2001), minimizing the chance of inducing uterine contractions (Frydman, 2004). Reviewing the literature, it is reported that technically challenging embryo transfers reduce the chance of pregnancy (Englert et al. 1986; Tomas et al. 1998) with use of a tenaculum, touching the fundus, and blood on the catheter being ranked highly as factors affecting successful outcomes (Kovacs 1999). Other factors, such as the presence of mucus on the catheter, are thought to reduce implantation rates by either plugging the end of the catheter or introducing contamination into the endometrial cavity. Therefore, removal of cervical mucus prior to the catheter being inserted is recommended (Schoolcraft et al. 2001). Two meta-analyses/systematic reviews show that higher pregnancy rates are achieved using soft catheters compared with hard catheters (Abou-Setta et al. 2005; Buckett 2006). Figures 28.1 and 28.2 show a two-part catheter, with an inner and outer part. The outer introducer can be placed in position before the embryos are loaded into the inner catheter.

Christianson et al. (2014) conducted a worldwide survey focused on how the embryo catheter was loaded and different embryo transfer techniques, which included responses from 265 centres in 71 countries. Common practices amongst clinics included prewashing the embryo transfer catheter (82%), preference for the use of a catheter marked for ultrasound view (42%), and use of a different embryo transfer media (42%). A wide variation of transfer medium was used. The most commonly reported method for loading the catheter was medium–air–embryo–air–medium (42%) with the

Clinical Reproductive Science, First Edition. Edited by Michael Carroll.
© 2019 John Wiley & Sons Ltd. Published 2019 by John Wiley & Sons Ltd.
Companion website: www.wiley.com/go/carroll/clinicalreproductivescience

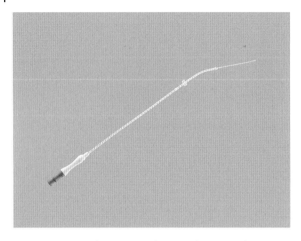

Figure 28.1 Guardia access catheter with inner and outer catheter. Reproduced with permission of Cook Medical, Bloomington, Indiana, USA.

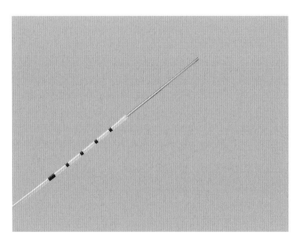

Figure 28.2 The two-part catheter. Reproduced with permission of Cook Medical, Bloomington, Indiana, USA.

final volume of the catheter up to 0.3 mL in 68% of centres (Figure 28.3). The use of air bubbles aids visualization under ultrasound guidance and may protect the embryos from trauma (Christianson et al. 2014). However, some reports are contradictory and postulate that air bubbles can be detrimental. Ebner et al. (2001) reported that low transfer volume (<10 μL) and air bubbles have a negative effect on outcome. Embryos were retained in the catheter for longer than 60 seconds in only 9% of centres and 100% of centres checked the catheter for retained embryos after the procedure.

Where embryos are deposited in the uterus can affect outcome (Figure 28.4). Touching the fundus reduces pregnancy rates (Schoolcraft et al. 2001) and

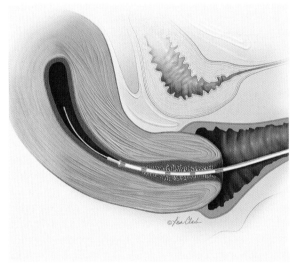

Figure 28.4 Uterine embryo transfer. *Source:* © 2013 Lisa Clarke courtesy of Cook Medical, Bloomington, Indiana, USA.

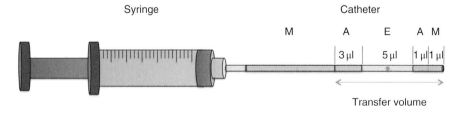

M: Medium
A: Air
E: Embryo (s)

Figure 28.3 Embryo transfer loading.

if embryos are deposited less than 5 mm from the fundus, this can increase the risk of ectopic pregnancy (Nazari et al. 1993). The use of ultrasound to visualize the embryo transfer catheter as it traverses the cervical canal, internal os, and enters the uterine cavity allows the embryos to be deposited accurately at a defined distance from the fundus allowing for variations in cervical length, uterine size, and position to be taken into account. Many IVF centres routinely perform ultrasound-guided embryo transfers, as evidence suggests improvement in clinical pregnancy rates using ultrasound rather than just 'clinical touch' (Abou-Setta 2012). The update of the 2007 Cochrane review in 2010 included 17 randomized trials and demonstrated significantly higher pregnancy rates with ultrasound guidance, but no difference in live birth rates (Brown et al. 2010). However, the authors did note that this finding should be interpreted with caution due to heterogeneity of the trials. Visualization of the catheter tip rather than introducing the catheter blindly into the uterine cavity has several benefits. Not only does it allow the catheter tip to be accurately positioned, it also minimizes endometrial trauma by preventing the catheter either indenting or embedding in the endometrium (Woolcott and Stanger 1997). Avoiding trauma to the endometrium is thought to decrease myometrial contractions, which are associated with reduced implantation rates (Fanchin et al. 1998). Several catheters are now echogenic, which enhances ultrasound visualization (Figure 28.5).

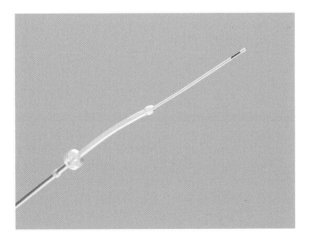

Figure 28.5 Catheter with echogenic tip. Reproduced with permission of Cook Medical, Bloomington, Indiana, USA.

Endometrial Thickness and Pattern

Measurement of the thickness of endometrium in the midsagittal plane via transvaginal ultrasound is a standard method used as an indicator for endometrial receptivity (Wu et al. 2014). A 2014 systematic review and meta-analysis showed that although endometrial thickness cannot be used to predict IVF outcome in terms of occurrence (pregnant versus not pregnant), it could be used to indicate the probability of implantation occurring (Kasius et al. 2014). The analysis found that the probability of pregnancy was significantly lower in the group with thin endometrium ($\leq$7 mm), although it is difficult to explain the reason for this finding due to limited research. It has, however, been suggested that in thin endometrium, oxygen concentrations are increased in basal layer endometrium, which negatively impacts on implantation (Casper 2011). Further research, however, is required using molecular tools to provide more information on the link between thin endometrium and endometrial receptivity. Endometrial pattern is also currently used as a measure of endometrial receptivity and although this could not be included in the meta-analysis due to a lack of consistency in the classification systems for endometrial patterns, several studies have found a relationship between pattern and outcome (Dechaud et al. 2008; Chen 2010; Kuc et al. 2011). Although some studies contradict this (Detti et al. 2011), a study including 1933 women undergoing IVF treatment found a significantly reduced implantation and pregnancy rate in cycles where a triple-line endometrial pattern (Figure 28.6) was not observed on the day of human chorionic gonadotropin (hCG) administration (Zhao 2012). The group concluded that combined endometrial thickness and pattern could not predict the outcome of IVF-embryo transfer when endometrial thickness was <7 mm or >14 mm, while a triple-line pattern with a moderate endometrial thickness appeared to be associated with higher pregnancy rates.

Endometrium Receptivity

The findings that lower pregnancy rates are achieved in stimulated IVF cycles compared with natural cycles in ovum donation cycles have led to further

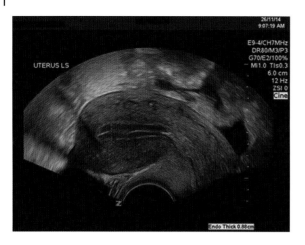

Figure 28.6 A triple line endometrium.

studies looking at the effect of controlled ovarian stimulation on endometrial receptivity. Investigations using microarray technology have compared endometrial gene expression profiles during the implantation window in a woman's stimulated and preceding natural cycle. The study found more than 200 genes showed a differential expression of more than threefold when the stimulated and natural cycles were compared (Horcajasdas et al. 2005). Haouzi et al. (2012) also described how different gene and protein-expression profiles may play a critical role in endometrial receptivity in natural and stimulated cycles.

Recently, there has been much interest in the effect of elevated progesterone on cycle outcome. Studies have shown that elevated progesterone levels on the day of hCG administration negatively affect pregnancy rates (Bosch et al. 2010; Xu et al. 2012). A systematic review and meta-analysis of more than 60 000 cycles concluded that elevated levels of progesterone on the day of hCG administration was associated with reduced pregnancy rates in fresh cycles (Venetis et al. 2013). However, the effect seems to be linked with endometrial receptivity rather than an effect on embryo quality, as live birth rates from frozen embryo cycles with elevated progesterone in the associated stimulation cycle (in which the embryos are created) are not affected (Lahoud et al. 2012). Further studies have shown that in patients with elevated progesterone levels (>1.5 ng/mL) on the day of hCG administration there is a shift in endometrial gene expression from the prereceptive to the receptive stage, which suggests accelerated endometrium maturation (Haouzi 2014). However, it is unclear whether this advancement in maturation reduces endometrial receptivity, as study of receptivity biomarkers did not show a change. Further research is therefore required to determine if it is the receptivity which is affected, or a desynchronized cross-talk between the embryo and endometrium due to the acceleration of endometrial maturation (Haouzi et al. 2014).

Embryo Transfer Media

Advances in embryo culture medium has seen the development of specific embryo transfer medium containing adherence compounds. One of these components is hyaluronic acid, a natural macromolecule which is present abundantly in the human endometrium and has been seen to increase around the time of implantation in mice studies (Carson et al. 1987). Although the exact mechanisms are unknown, it is proposed that hyaluronic acid may have direct and indirect effects on the embryo and implantation potential (Urman et al. 2008). These effects include an increase in cell–cell adhesions and cell–matrix adhesions to facilitate the apposition and attachment of the blastocyst (Gardener et al. 1999). Hyaluronic acid may also be receptor-mediated as the primary receptor for hyaluronic acid is CD44, which is expressed on the preimplantation embryo (Campbell et al. 1995) and endometrial stroma (Behzad et al. 1994). The viscous property of the transfer medium might enhance the embryo transfer process (Simon et al. 2003). Two randomized controlled trials in 2006 and 2008 showed hyaluronic acid-enriched transfer media have a positive effect (Valajerdi et al. 2006; Urman et al. 2008). This was followed by a Cochrane review in 2010 which concluded that there was an overall increase of 8% in clinical pregnancy rates when adherence compounds were added to the embryo transfer medium. However, there was no evidence of an increase in the number of live births (Bontekoe et al. 2010). The update in 2014 still found that the use of functional concentrations of hyaluronic acid in transfer media improved clinical pregnancy and live birth rates but suggested that the evidence was only of moderate quality

(Bontekoe et al. 2014). More recently, further randomized controlled studies have contradicted previous positive findings and have suggested that for cleavage stage embryos, hyaluronic acid-enriched transfer media have no advantage (Safari et al. 2014) and clinical pregnancy rates, implantation, and delivery rates do not differ significantly when cycles with advanced maternal age, previous IVF failures, low oocyte number, or poor embryo quality were compared (Fancsovits et al. 2015).

Blastocyst Transfer

There have been many factors which have led to the increased use of blastocyst transfer in IVF programmes, including improvements in culture systems and the requirement to reduce multiple birth rates. The potential advantages of extending culture include the improved selection of viable embryos to increase implantation rates. The benefits of blastocyst transfer have been well documented and the most recent systematic review provides evidence that there is a small significant improvement in live birth rates in favour of blastocyst transfer (Day 5 to 6) compared with cleavage stage transfer (Day 2 to 3) (Glujovsky et al. 2012). However, cumulative clinical pregnancy rates from cleavage stage embryos (derived from fresh and thaw cycles) resulted in higher clinical pregnancy rates than from blastocyst cycles (Glujovsky et al. 2012). The increased implantation rates from blastocyst transfer are not only thought to be due to improved embryo selection but also due to better synchronization of embryo development with the female tract as, *in vivo*, the preimplantation embryo resides in the Fallopian tube until Day 4 (Croxatto et al. 1978).

Endometrial Injury

Complex interaction between the embryo and endometrium is required for implantation to occur and despite the advances in assisted reproductive technology little is known of the exact mechanisms involved. However, recently it has been postulated that inducing injury to the endometrium (either by scratching the lining of the endometrium using a biopsy tube or by telescopic investigation of the uterus using a camera, known as hysteroscopy) in the month preceding a treatment cycle can improve success rates (Shohayeb and El-Khayat 2012). The local injury induces secretions of cytokines and growth factors (Basak et al. 2002), and upregulates the gene expression profile related to increased endometrial receptivity (Kalma et al. 2009). The main focus of this research has been with patients with recurrent implantation failure. A recent meta-analysis and systematic review suggested that inducing injury in the cycle preceding treatment improved pregnancy outcomes (Potdar et al. 2012). However, although a further meta-analysis showed that clinical pregnancy was significantly higher after endometrial injury in both the randomized and nonrandomized studies, the improvement did not reach statistical significance in the randomized study which reported live birth rates (El-Toukhy et al. 2012). More recently, the effect of endometrial injury has been reported in unselected IVF patients (Yeung et al. 2014). In this study, endometrial injury did not improve ongoing clinical pregnancy rates and subgroup analysis actually found that women who had at least one previous failed transfer had a decreased pregnancy rate. This highlights that further robust randomized studies are required to not only reach a consensus on when the optimum time to induce injury is but also to determine which groups of patients, if any, should have this procedure.

Luteal Support

For many years it has been acknowledged that the luteal phase in a stimulated IVF cycle is disrupted, which necessitates the need for a strategy to overcome this defect to allow for implantation to occur successfully. It is proposed that the reason for the defect is due to the supraphysiological oestrogen levels from multifollicular development which causes negative feedback on the hypothalamic–pituitary axis to inhibit luteinizing hormone (LH) secretion (Humaidan et al. 2012). The rise in LH commences the process of ovulation and the transformation from the follicular to luteal phase in which the follicle becomes a corpus luteum (Leth-Moller et al. 2014). LH then acts on the granulosa cells to produce progesterone which induces the secretory transformation of the endometrium (van der Linden et al. 2011). The lack of LH therefore shortens the luteal phase and reduces the chance of implantation (van der Linden et al. 2011). Once implantation occurs, secretion of hCG by the embryo acts on the corpus luteum to produce progesterone until the placenta takes over production of the steroid hormones (Leth-Moller et al. 2014). Whilst there is therefore a consensus that luteal support is required in an IVF cycle, there is debate over the most effective luteal support regimen to use (Gizzo et al. 2014).

Current options for luteal support include progesterone, administered either intramuscularly, orally, vaginally (Leth-Moller et al. 2014), or subcutaneously (Baker et al. 2014). hCG can also be used due to its similarity to LH (Leth-Moller et al. 2014). However, a recent worldwide internet-based survey, which included responses from 408 centres in 82 countries, showed a more consistent approach with 80% of cycles commencing luteal support on the day of egg collection, 77% of cycles using a vaginal progesterone as a single agent, and in 72% of cycles luteal support was administered until 8–10 weeks of gestation (Vaisbuch et al. 2014). Although there is little evidence to suggest extension of luteal support beyond biochemical pregnancy, many centres continue until the twelfth week of gestation and beyond (Russel et al. 2014).

Recently there has been a shift to use an agonist instead of hCG to trigger patients prior to egg collection as this regimen can lead to a significant reduction in the incidence of ovarian hyperstimulation syndrome (OHSS) (Leth-Moller et al. 2014). However, to achieve acceptable implantation rates a modified luteal support regime is required. This modified regime includes the use of either recombinant LH or progesterone/oestradiol (Leth-Moller et al. 2014), or supplementing the luteal phase with a single dose of 1500 IU hCG at egg collection (Humaidin et al. 2012). Alternatively, all embryo(s) may be frozen and replaced in a subsequent cycle.

A recent systematic review suggested a significant effect in favour of synthetic progesterone over micronized progesterone (Leth-Moller et al. 2014) with the recommendation to avoid the use of hCG to minimize OHSS and the finding that the addition of oestrogen to a luteal support regime has no added benefit. Further research to optimize luteal support is still required. Furthermore, in some cases luteal support does not correct the luteal defect and a freeze-all (where all the embryos are cryopreserved), and transfer in a natural or modified natural cycle may improve the chance of implantation (Check 2012).

Postembryo Transfer Interventions

It has been observed that embryos, after being deposited in the uterus, can move or be expelled due to several factors including peristalsis and contractions, low site of deposition, and negative pressure generated when removing the embryo transfer catheter (Abou-Setta et al. 2014). One posttreatment intervention which is advised in some centres is bed rest immediately following embryo transfer. However, a 2014 systematic review found that there is insufficient evidence to support any specific length of time for women to remain recumbent, if at all, following embryo transfer. Other postembryo transfer interventions which were reviewed included the use of fibrin sealants added to the embryo transfer fluid and the use of mechanical pressure to close the cervical canal following embryo transfer, neither of which showed any positive benefit (Abou-Setta et al. 2014).

Conclusion

Despite advances in IVF treatment, success rates remain relatively low and whilst the majority of cycles result in embryo transfer only a small proportion result in a live birth. Acknowledging that embryo transfer is a vital step is key for a successful IVF programme. Whilst there are many variables influencing whether implantation occurs, such as patient age, embryo quality, and uterine factors, the aim should be to optimize and standardize the embryo transfer procedure to minimize the chance of this being a limiting factor in the process. Effective training and ongoing competency assessment should be in place for both embryologists and the operator (clinicians and nurses) and an annual review to assess clinical pregnancy rates and ectopic pregnancy rates per operator should be conducted. Recently, strategies such as adopting a freeze-all policy to optimize the chance of implantation occurring have been suggested and further research should be conducted to ensure evidence-based guidelines can be produced.

References

Abou-Setta, A.M., Peters, L.R., D'Angelo, A. et al. (2014). Post-embryo transfer interventions for assisted reproduction technology cycles. Cochrane Database Syst Rev 8: CD006567.

Abou-Setta, A. (2012). Ultrasound guided embryo transfer (abdominal/vaginal): an evidence-based evaluation. In: *Practical Manual of In Vitro Fertilisation*, 571–574. Berlin: Springer.

Abou-Setta, A.M., Al-Inany, H.G., Mansour, R.T. et al. (2005). Soft versus firm embryo transfer catheters for assisted reproduction: a systematic review and meta-analysis. Hum Reprod 20: 114–121.

Baker, V.L., Jones, C.A., Doody, K. et al. (2014). A randomized, controlled trial comparing the efficacy and safety of aqueous subcutaneous progesterone with vaginal progesterone for luteal phase support of in vitro fertilization. Hum Reprod 29: 2212–2220.

Basak, S., Dubanchet, S., Zourbas, S. et al. (2002). Expression of pro-inflammatory cytokines in mouse blastocysts during implantation: modulation by steroid hormones. Am J Reprod Immunol 47: 2–11.

Behzad, F., Seif, M.W., Campbell, S. et al. (1994). Expression of two isoforms of CD44 in human endometrium. Biol Reprod 51: 739–747.

Bontekoe, S., Blake, D., Heineman, M.J. et al. (2010). Adherence compounds in embryo transfer media for assisted reproductive technologies. Cochrane Database Syst Rev 7: CD007421.

Bontekoe, S., Heineman, M.J., Johnson, N. et al. (2014). Adherence compounds in embryo transfer media for assisted reproductive technologies. Cochrane Database Syst Rev 2: CD007421.

Bosch, E., Labarta, E., Crespo, J. et al. (2010). Circulating progesterone levels and ongoing pregnancy rates in controlled ovarian stimulation cycles for in vitro fertilization: analysis of over 4000 cycles. Hum Reprod 25: 2092–2100.

Brown, J. Buckingham, K., Abou-Setta, A. et al. (2010). Ultrasound versus clinical touch for catheter guidance during embryo transfer in women. Cochrane Database Syst Rev: CD006107.

Buckett, W. (2006). A review and meta-analysis of prospective trials comparing different catheters used for embryo transfer. Fertil Steril 85: 728–734.

Campbell, S., Swann, H., Aplin, J.D. et al. (1995). CD44 is expressed throughout pre-implantation human embryo development. Hum Reprod 10: 425–430.

Carson, D.D., Dutt, A, Tang, J. (1987). Glycoconjugate synthesis during early pregnancy: hyaluronate synthesis and function. Dev Biol 120: 228–325.

Casper, R.F. (2011). It's time to pay attention to the endometrium. Fertil Steril 3: 519–521.

Check, J.H. (2012). Luteal phase support for in vitro fertilisation-embryo transfer – present and future methods to improve successful implantation. Clin Exp Obstet Gynecol 39: 422–428.

Chen, S.L., Wu, F.R., Luo, C. et al. (2010). Combined analysis of endometrial thickness and pattern in predicting outcome of in vitro fertilisation and embryo transfer: a retrospective cohort study. Reprod Biol Endocrinol 8: 30.

Christianson, M., Zhao, Y., Shoham, G. et al. (2014). Embryo catheter loading and embryo culture techniques: results of a worldwide web-based survey. J Assist Reprod Genet 31: 1029–1036.

Croxatto, H.B., Ortiz, M.E., Díaz, S. et al. (1978). Studies on the duration of egg transport by the human oviduct. II. Ovum location at various intervals following luteinizing hormone peak. Am J Obstet Gynecol 132: 629–634.

Dechaud, H., Bessuelle, E., Bousquet, P.J. et al. (2008). Optimal timing of ultrasonographic and doplar evaluation of uterine receptivity to implantation. Reprod Biomed Online 16: 3368–3375.

Detti, L., Saed, G.M., Fletcher, N.M. et al. (2011). Endometrial morphology and modulation of hormone receptors during ovarian stimulation for assisted reproductive technology cycles. Fertil Steril 95: 1073–1081.

Ebner, T., Yaman, C., Moser, M. et al. (2001) The ineffective loading process of the embryo transfer catheter alters implantation and pregnancy rates. Fertil Steril 76: 630–632.

El-Toukhy, T., Sunkara, S., and Khalaf, Y. (2012). Local endometrial injury and IVF outcome: a systematic review and meta-analysis. Reprod Biomed Online 25: 345–354.

Englert, Y., Puissant, F., Camus, M. et al. (1986). Clinical study on embryo transfer after human in vitro fertilisation. J In Vitro Fertil Embryo Transfer 3: 243–246.

Fanchin, R., Righini, C., Olivenness, F. et al. (1998). Uterine contractions at the time of embryo transfer alter pregnancy rates after in vitro fertilisation. Hum Reprod 13: 1968–1974.

Fancsovits, P., Lehner, A., Murber, A. et al. (2015). Effect of hyaluronan-enriched embryo transfer medium on IVF outcome: a prospective randomized clinical trial. Arch Gynecol Obstet 291: 1173–1179.

Farraretti, A., Goossens, V, Kupka, M. et al. (2013). European IVF-Monitoring (EIM) Consortium for European Society of Human Reproduction and Embryology (ESHRE). Assisted reproductive technology in Europe 2009: results generated from European registers by ESHRE. Hum Reprod 28: 2318–2311.

Frydman, R. (2004). Impact of embryo transfer techniques on implantation rates. J Gynecol Obstet Biol Reprod 33: S36–39.

Gardener, D.K., Rodriegez-Martinez, H. and Lane, M. (1999). Fetal development after transfer is increased by replacing protein with the glycosaminoglycan hyaluronan for mouse embryo culture and transfer. Hum Reprod 14: 2575–2580.

Gizzo, S., Andrisani, A., Esposito, F. et al. (2014). Which luteal phase support is better for each IVF stimulation protocol to achieve the highest pregnancy rate? A superiority randomized clinical trial. Gynecol Endocrinol 30: 1–7.

Glujovsky, D., Blake, D., Farquhar, C. et al. (2012). Cleavage stage versus blastocyst stage embryo transfer in assisted reproductive technology. Cochrane Database Syst Rev 7: CD002118.

Haouzi, D., Bissonnette, L., Gala, A. et al. (2014). Endometrial receptivity profile in patients with premature progesterone elevation on the day of HCG administration. Biomed Res Int 951937.

Haouzi, D., Dechaud, H., Assou, S et al. (2012). Insights into human endometrial receptivity from transcriptomic and proteomic data. Reprod Biomed Online 1: 23–34.

Horcajadas, J.A., Riesewijk, A., Polman, J. et al. (2005). Effect of controlled ovarian hyperstimulation in IVF on endometrial gene expression profiles. Mol Hum Reprod 11: 195–205.

Humaidan, P., Papanikolaou, E.G., Kyrou, D. et al. (2012). The luteal phase after GnRH-agonist triggering of ovulation: present and future perspectives. Reprod Biomed Online 24: 134–141.

Kalma, Y., Granot, I., Gnainsky, Y. et al. (2009). Endometrial biopsy-induced gene modulation: first evidence for the expression of bladder-transmembranal uroplakin 1b in human endometrium. Fertil Steril 91: 1042–1049.

Kasius, A., Smit, J.G., Torrence, H.L. et al. (2014). Endometrial thickness and pregnancy rates after IVF: a systematic review and meta-analysis. Hum Reprod Update 20: 530–541.

Kovacs, G.T. (1999). What factors are important for successful embryo transfer after in vitro fertilisation? Hum Reprod 14: 590–592.

Kuc, P., Kuzcynska, A., Topczewska, M. et al. (2011). The dynamics of endometrial growth and the triple layer appearance in three different controlled ovarian hyperstimulation protocols and their influence on IVF outcomes. Gynecol Endocrinol 11: 867–873.

Lahoud, R., Kwik, M., Ryan, J. et al. (2012). Elevated progesterone in GnRH agonist down regulated in vitro fertilisation (IVFICSI) cycles reduces live birth rates but not embryo quality. Arch Gynecol Obstet 285: 535–540.

Leth-Moller, K., Hammer Jagd, S. and Humaidan, P. (2014). The luteal phase after GnRHa trigger-understanding an enigma. Int J Fertil Steril 8: 227–234.

Meldrum, D.R., Chectkowski, R., Steingold, K.A. et al. (1987). Evolution of a highly successful in vitro fertilisation embryo transfer program. Fert Steril 48: 86–93.

Nazari, A., Askari, H.A., Check, J.H. et al. (1993). Embryo transfer technique as a cause of ectopic pregnancy in in vitro fertilisation. Fertil Steril 60: 919–921.

Potdar, N., Gelbaya, T. and Nardo, L.G. (2012). Endometrial injury to overcome recurrent embryo implantation failure: a systematic review and meta-analysis. Reprod Biomed Online 25: 561–571.

Russell, R., Kingsland, C., Alfirevic, Z. et al. (2014). Duration of luteal support after IVF is important, so why is there no consistency in practice? The results of a dynamic survey of practice in the United Kingdom. Hum Fertil (Camb) 13: 1–5.

Safari, S., Razi, M.H., Safari, S. et al. (2014). Routine use of EmbryoGlue® as embryo transfer medium does not improve the ART outcomes. Arch Gynecol Obstet 291: 433–437.

Schoolcraft, W., Surrey, E. and Gardener, D. (2001). Embryo transfer: techniques and variables affecting success. Fertil Steril 76: 863–870.

Shohayeb, A. and El-Khayat, W.D (2012). Does a single endometrial biopsy regimen (S-EBR) improve ICSI outcome in patients with repeated implantation failure? A randomised controlled trial. Eur J Obstet Gynecol Reprod Biol 164: 176–179.

Simon, A., Safran, A., Revel, A. et al. (2003). Hyaluronic acid can successfully replace albumin as the sole macromolecule in a human embryo transfer medium. Fertil Steril 79: 1434–1438.

Tomas, C., Tapanainen, J. and Martikainen, H. (1998). The difficulty of embryo transfer is an independent variable for predicting pregnancy in in vitro fertilisation treatments [Abstract. Fertil Steril 70(Suppl 1): S433.

Urman, B., Yakin, K., Ata, B. et al. (2008). Effect of hyaluronan-enriched transfer medium on implantation and pregnancy rates after day 3 and day 5 embryo transfers: a prospective randomized study. Fertil Steril 90: 604–612.

Valojerdi, M.R., Karimian, L., Yazdi, P.E. et al. (2006). Efficacy of a human embryo transfer medium: a prospective, randomized clinical trial study. J Assist Reprod Genet 23: 207–212.

van der Linden, M., Buckingham, K., Farquhar, C. et al. (2011). Luteal phase support for assisted reproduction cycles. Cochrane Database Syst Rev 10: CD009154.

Vaisbuch, E., de Ziegler, D., Leong, M. et al. (2014). Luteal-phase support in assisted reproduction treatment: real-life practices reported worldwide by an updated website-based survey. Reprod Biomed Online 28: 330–335.

Venetis, C.A., Kolibianakis, E.M., Bosdou, J.K. et al. (2013). Progesterone elevation and probability of pregnancy after IVF: a systematic review and meta-analysis of over 60 000 cycles. Hum Reprod Update 19: 433–457.

Woolcott, R. and Stanger, J. (1997). Potentially important variables identified by transvaginal ultrasound-guided embryo transfer. Hum Reprod 12: 963–966.

Wu, Y., Gao, X., Lu, X et al. (2014). Endometrial thickness affects the outcome of in vitro fertilisation and embryo transfer in normal responders after GnRH antagonist administration. Reprod Biol Endocrinol 12: 96–100.

Xu, B., Li, Z., Zhang, H. et al. (2012).Serum progesterone level effects on the outcome of in vitro fertilization in patients with different ovarian response: an analysis of more than 10,000 cycles. Fertil Steril 97: 1321–1327.e1–4.

Yeung, T.W., Chai, J., Li, R.H. et al. (2014) The effect of endometrial injury on ongoing pregnancy rate in unselected subfertile women undergoing in vitro fertilization: a randomized controlled trial. Hum Reprod 29: 2474–2481

Zhao, J., Zhang, Q. and Li, Y. (2012). The effect of endometrial thickness and pattern measured by ultrasonography on pregnancy outcomes during IVF-ET cycles. Reprod Biol Endocrinol 28: 100.

29

Cryopreservation of Gametes and Embryos

Tope Adeniyi

Introduction: A Brief History of Gamete Cryopreservation

Cryopreservation can be defined as the process by which living cells, tissues, and organs are preserved in a stable or viable state with the use of appropriate cryoprotecting agents (CPA) at extremely low temperatures. The application of cryopreservation procedures was first reported as early as the sixteenth century (Sherman 1954; Sherman 1963) and by Spallanzani, a renowned Italian physiologist, who attempted to cryopreserve semen using snow in 1776. In 1949, Polge et al. reported an accidental, albeit, significant breakthrough in the process of cryopreservation when they discovered the potent cryoprotective potential of glycerol at extremely low temperatures in an attempt to successfully cryopreserve mammalian sperm (Polge et al. 1949). A growing interest in the field of cryobiology led several subsequent researchers to confirm that sperm cells can be frozen and thawed successfully; these findings were consistent and reproducible (Lovelock 1953; Bunge et al. 1954; Lovelock and Polge 1954; Sherman 1954; Mackenzie and Luyet 1967). Nevertheless, cryopreservation of both male and female gametes in assisted reproductive treatment (ART) remains an area of ongoing research to further improve current outcomes and to also ensure that the procedure is safer for patients and the children born through ART.

Principles of Cryopreservation

The process of gamete cryopreservation has evolved progressively over the last two centuries and its application has been embraced within animal breeding, conservation programmes, and human medicine, including ART. The cryopreservation procedures of ART involve exposure to CPA, cooling of gametes and embryos, storage at extremely low temperatures (-196 °C), and thawing or warming.

Water is the universal solvent and a major component of all living cells. Water also presents the potential for formation of dangerous ice crystals as the surrounding environment is super-cooled, at temperatures below freezing point. Earlier investigations by Mazur described the association between the formation of ice crystals at low temperatures in a super-cooled solution and its effects on biological cells (Mazur 1963). Following these investigations, the initial stages of freezing essentially involve the gradual removal of water molecules from within the intracellular environment to avoid cryoinjury or damage due to the formation of ice crystals inside the cell. The formation of ice crystals inside a cell can be avoided with the use of appropriate CPA, which safely dehydrates the cell as a result of the osmotic gradient created between the internal cellular environment and the external environment (freezing solution). This facilitates the movement of water molecules from inside the cell by osmosis

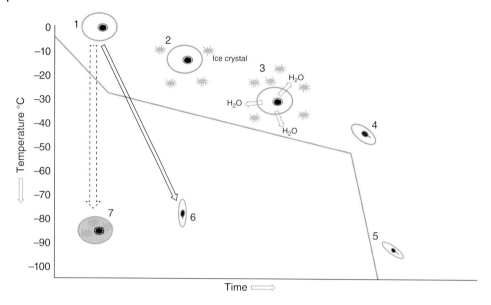

Figure 29.1 Cryopreservation. (1) Cells prepared for cryopreservation are placed in a cryomedium containing cryoprotectant. (2) As the temperature decreases, ice crystals form in the extracellular media, (3) which subsequently increase solute concentration causing osmotic dehydration. (4) Cells continue to shrink while losing intracellular water. (5) Successful cryopreservation is achieved with little or no ice crystal formation. (6) Vitrification of cells is carried out in medium with very high concentrations of cryoprotectant, thus minimizing any cryodamage. (7) In the absence of any cryoprotectant, the formation of intracellular ice crystals will damage cellular structures, ultimately killing the cells.

outward across the cell membrane into the external cellular environment until equilibrium is reached. Subsequently, as the temperature of the surrounding environment continues to decrease, formation of ice begins to spread in the external environment. This concentrates the solute and the freezing solution becomes viscous, inevitably initiating the migration or removal of possible residual water molecules from inside the cell into the external environment and inducing changes in cell volume as the cell begins to shrink during the process of cryopreservation (Figure 29.1). However, it is important to note that the complete or partial removal of excessive water molecules beyond what cells can tolerate for viability and membrane integrity can also be detrimental to cell survival.

Leibo et al. demonstrated that the rate of ice crystal formation during freezing is dictated by the cooling rate and the permeability of the given cell membrane to water molecules (Leibo et al. 1978; Leibo 1984). These findings have been shown to be very critical to the survival of any biological cell. Therefore, it is essential for the optimum cooling rate to be adequate and slow enough to allow the progressive withdrawal of water molecules from inside the cell so that excessive residual water molecules, which can form harmful intracellular ice crystals as the temperature decreases, are not trapped inside the cell. Similarly, if the cooling rate is too fast this may not allow appropriate migration of water molecules from inside the cell into the external environment, resulting in the formation of ice crystals within the intracellular environment causing cryodamage to cellular organelles. However, the avoidance of harmful ice crystals at this initial stage does not completely circumvent this problem, as recrystallization of ice has been shown to occur during thawing (Mazur 1990; Mazur and Kleinhans 2008; Mazur 2010). Therefore, the use of an appropriate combination of either permeating or nonpermeating cryoprotectants at a safe concentration is critical to avoiding rapid rehydration of the cell, which eventually causes the cell membrane to rupture. Despite these challenges, human gametes and embryos have been safely and successfully cryopreserved for more than 35 years with arguably optimized procedures (Bagchi et al. 2008; Aflatoonian et al. 2010; Argyle et al. 2016). However, for effective cryopreservation it is important to avoid or mini-mize deleterious conditions associated with cryo-preservation, which can be achieved through the following approaches: (i) use CPA to maintain cel-lular membrane fluidity and stability during osmo-sis; (ii) eliminate or reduce the formation of harmful intracellular and extracellular ice crystals; (iii) sub-stitute intracellular water molecules with CPA and; (iv) reduce cellular toxicity of CPA at high or low temperatures. Adhering to these practices can significantly reduce the impact of osmotic shock and cryoinjury and increased freeze–thaw survival rates for gametes and embryos in ART (Edgar et al. 2009; Wennerholm et al. 2009; Edgar and Gook 2012; Kopeika et al. 2015).

Permeating and Nonpermeating Cryoprotectants in ART

Routinely, cryopreservation media used in ART involves the use of cryoprotectants and can be classified into two different groups based on the mechanism of action during cryopreservation: (i) permeating and (ii) nonpermeating cryoprotectants.

The effectiveness of permeating cryoprotectants such as glycerol, dimethyl sulfoxide (DMSO), 1,2-propandiol (PROH), and ethylene glycol in prevent-ing or minimizing cryoinjury can be attributed to the high membrane permeability of these cryopro-tectants and their ability to displace water mole-cules from the intracellular environment, in addition to stabilizing the concentration of harmful electrolytes within intracellular spaces. On the con-trary, nonpermeating cryoprotectants such as sucrose, trehalose, polyvinylpyrrolidone (PVP), and lactose are unable to permeate cell membranes due their large molecular weight and size. Hence, they facilitate significantly the withdrawal of water mol-ecules from the intracellular environment via an osmotic gradient, in addition to reducing the risks of formation of harmful intracellular ice crystals. However, both groups of cryoprotectants may indi-rectly inflict cryoinjuries or osmotic shock on human reproductive gametes and embryos (Szurek and Eroglu 2011; Vanderzwalmen et al. 2013). Identification of the appropriate concentration, the type of cryoprotectants, and the cooling/warming

rates have been identified as some of the initial challenges of cryopreservation especially vitrifica-tion procedures (Lovelock 1953; Edgar et al. 2009; Edgar and Gook 2012).

Freezing Media and Cryopreservation in ART

The pioneering works of Polge et al. (1949) con-firmed the ability of specific compounds to protect sperm cells from osmotic shock or cryoinjury at extremely low temperatures. Moreover, the discov-ery of the cryoprotective properties of glycerol and the use of similar CPA has now become routine practice in cryobiology. The unique properties of CPA to facilitate a chain of both physical and chemi-cal events that allow for successful cryopreservation and storage of reproductive cells at extremely low temperatures and viability upon thawing include the following: high solubility in water, membrane per-meability, and low toxicity at low temperatures (Lovelock 1953; Lovelock and Polge 1954; Kopeika et al. 2015). In an attempt to minimize the potential damage associated with cryopreservation, freezing media used in ART for cryopreservation of gametes routinely contains permeating and nonpermeating CPA, physiological buffer, human serum albumin and inhibitors of apoptosis such as vitamin E, mela-tonin, and ascorbic acid.

The primary objective of cryopreservation media used in ART is to reduce the risks of cellular damage whilst ensuring cell survival and viability postcryo-preservation. Therefore, the composition of cryo-preservation media is arguably critical to gamete survival as cryopreservation procedures are associ-ated with nonphysiological chemical and physical changes which may compromise cell survival and normal cellular and gamete development after thaw-ing or warming (Aye et al. 2010; de Menorval et al. 2012). Unfortunately, detailed compositions of most commercially available human embryo cryopreser-vation media have not been properly documented by some manufacturers (Harper et al. 2012; Sunde and Balaban 2013). This lack of proper documenta-tion and transparency has raised significant con-cerns among leading researchers in ART and some professional bodies such as the European Society of

Human Reproduction and Embryology (ESHRE) and Alpha Scientists in Reproductive Medicine (Magli et al. 2008; Balaban et al. 2012). Nonetheless, available knowledge on the basic principles of cryobiology and the role/function of each essential component suggests the following as the basic composition of cryopreservation media.

Cryoprotecting Agents

Cryoprotecting agents (permeating and nonpermeating) primarily protect gametes from cryopreservation-related osmotic shock, which may result in cellular damage or injuries. Briefly, permeating cryoprotectant such as ethylene glycol penetrates the cell and displaces water molecules, and also forms a stable hydrogen bond with intracellular residual water molecules. This event significantly lowers the freezing point of water molecules and reduces the formation of deleterious ice crystals. Similarly, nonpermeating CPA such as sucrose and trehalose withdraw water molecules from the intracellular environment via an osmotic gradient. This prevents the risks of formation of harmful ice crystals during cryopreservation. Gametes cryopreservation media used in ART routinely contain a combination of appropriate concentrations of permeating and nonpermeating cryoprotectants. This combination reduces the risks of cytotoxicity of cryoprotectants and ice crystal formation, or recrystallization within the intracellular environment of the gametes during freezing, thawing, and warming (Vanderzwalmen et al. 2013; Kopeika et al. 2015).

Inhibitor of Apoptosis

Cryopreservation procedures are often associated with oxidation stress arising from Reactive Oxygen Species (ROS). These are free radicals with a potentially harmful impact that may compromise sperm function, survival, and viability as a result of impaired structural and DNA damage following cryopreservation (Said et al. 2010). Impaired membrane integrity or mechanical damages as result of ROS, osmotic shock, or cryoprotectant toxicities have been linked with reduced sperm motility, and poor oocyte and embryo survival and development (Martinez-Burgos et al. 2011). Hence supplementation of cryopreservation media with the appropriate

concentration of antioxidants has been shown to facilitate successful freezing and thawing of human reproductive gametes and embryos (Lane et al. 2002; Taylor et al. 2009). Antioxidants (enzymes and non-enzymes) are essential inhibitors of apoptosis and potential DNA damage. In fact, the addition of anti-oxidants such as vitamin E (α-tocopherol), ascorbic acid, selenium, and ubiquinones to cryopreservation and culture media used in ART have been advocated in order to reduce the impact of the *in vitro* culture environment and micromanipulation-related damage (Taylor et al. 2009; Agarwal et al. 2014; Amidi et al. 2016). According to Agarwal et al. (2014) evidence suggesting the efficacies of antioxidants in oocyte and embryo cryopreservation procedures may be apparent. However, the establishment of this evidence following a large and properly designed randomized controlled clinical trial remains essential in ART.

Salts

The appropriate concentration of a suitable salt remains an essential component of cryopreservation media and various micromanipulation media used in ART. However, sodium (Na^+) is thought to cause significant damage to the cell membrane and its integrity, as the removal of the high cellular concentration of sodium salts is energy dependent via the sodium pump. This critical energy dependent procedure may be significantly disrupted during cryopreservation, which may compromise cell survival. An experimental study by Toner et al. showed that mouse oocytes failed to survive the thawing procedure in a hypertonic sodium chloride (NaCl) solution supplemented with phosphate buffered saline solution without a cryoprotecting agent (Toner et al. 1993). Although, this observation may be different in the presence of a cryoprotecting agent (Arcarons et al. 2016), nonetheless this experimental study by Toner et al. suggested that an isotonic solutions of NaCl may not be adequate in preventing cell lysis. Unpublished data involving the use of choline chloride as a substitute for sodium chloride showed a contrary observation as the majority of oocytes remained intact at room temperature following thawing in the absence of a cryoprotectant (Stachecki et al. 1998; Gardner et al. 2007; Lin et al. 2009). A related case report (Quintans et al. 2002) involving the successful live birth of two babies, used a media in which NaCl was substituted by choline chloride (ChCl). This clinical evidence suggested that cryopreservation media with low Na^+ concentration might be a more beneficial component in the media. Unlike Na^+, choline salts are nonmembrane penetrating cations which efficiently remain in the external environment preventing the influx of cations into the intracellular environment during freezing and thawing (Stachecki et al. 1998).

Buffers

pH buffers such as 3-(N-morpholino) propanesulfonic acid (MOPS) and 4-(2-hydroxyethyl)-1-piperazine-ethane sulfonic acid (HEPES) are very critical chemical substances with unique abilities to stabilize changes in pH which may be associated with *in vitro* culture or gamete handling outside the incubator environment such as the cryopreservation procedures of ART. Alteration in pH levels arising from changes in temperature and osmolarity in the immediate environment of the gamete is often associated with cryopreservation. Biological pH buffers are essential in providing a relatively stable physiological pH environment (pH 6–8) for most gamete micromanipulation procedures (Will et al. 2011). Furthermore, this role is critical as nonphysiological pH may compromise gamete membrane integrity, normal embryo development, and post-thaw sperm motility.

Macromolecules

The inclusion of protein molecules in the form of Human Serum Albumin (HSA) enhances the viscosity of the cryopreservation media. Important macromolecules such as antifreeze proteins provide an additional source of cryoprotection by reducing the growth and formation of ice crystals during the cooling stages of cryopreservation procedures. Also, they assist in limiting the impact of osmotic shock experienced by cells and gametes during cryopreservation (Elliott et al. 2017). Furthermore, macromolecules such as glycoproteins are effective in protecting cell surfaces during cryopreservation in addition to facilitating appropriate gamete and embryo handling which prevents gametes and embryos from sticking to plastic wares and carrier devices during macromanipulation.

Cryopreservation Media and Related Challenges

Human sperm freezing media used in ART are essentially formulated for the maintenance and preservation of sperm function and viability, and DNA integrity for continuity of progeny. These are critical objectives which facilitate optimum sperm survival after cryopreservation with significant impact on sperm functional viability, motility, and treatment outcomes (Amidi et al. 2016). In severe conditions, these cryopreservation related changes may culminate in cell death by apoptosis or total loss of sperm motility (Said et al. 2010). Also, potential deviations from sperm cryopreservation procedures may compromise the ability of the human sperm to successfully activate the metaphase II (MII) oocyte for normal fertilization to occur (Ducibella et al. 2002; Ozil et al. 2005; Gardner et al. 2007).

A similar observation has been reported in several experimental studies involving cryopreservation (vitrification) of mouse and human MII oocytes, and subsequent normal embryo development (Ducibella et al. 2002; Gardner et al. 2007; Larman et al. 2007a). These studies highlight the importance of oocyte activation and fertilization processes as a prerequisite to normal gametes and embryo development and how susceptible these critical processes may become to the elements of cryopreservation. Nonetheless, current cryopreservation media used in ART remain efficient, yielding acceptable survival and clinical pregnancy rates with successful live births (Boldt 2011; Cobo et al. 2014; Nagy et al. 2016). The presence of Ca^{2+} in cryopreservation media has been implicated in premature cortical granule exocytosis leading to hardening of the zona pellucida (ZP) (Larman et al. 2006). However, this challenge may be circumvented by the intracytoplasmic sperm injection (ICSI) procedure. Nonetheless, the use of Ca^{2+}-free cryopreservation media in ART has been advocated due to concern over premature ZP hardening and potential parthenogenetic activation of the oocyte (Larman et al. 2004; Ozil et al. 2005). Several studies have also reported cryopreservation-related changes to the oocyte's spindle structure and integrity, thickening of the ZP, repositioning of the polar body, and chromosome misalignment (Larman et al. 2007b; Cobo et al. 2008c; Bromfield et al. 2009). Some of these changes are often irreversible and may be partly responsible for suboptimal fertilization outcomes or complete fertilization failure occasionally observed with frozen–thawed oocytes (Larman et al. 2007a). Regardless of these observations it remains plausible if these observations are the result of the physical and chemical changes associated with cryopreservation procedures or a product of a specific component of the cryopreservation media (Katz-Jaffe et al. 2008; Larman et al. 2011). However, available clinical data obtained from ART cryopreservation procedures remains reassuring despite the association of these potentially detrimental impacts with the cryopreservation procedure (Cobo and Diaz 2011; Garcia-Velasco et al. 2013; Wennerholm et al. 2013).

Gamete and Embryo Cryopreservation

Oocyte Cryopreservation

In 1986 Chen reported the first successful cryopreservation of the human MII oocyte using the traditional/slow method of cryopreservation (Chen 1986). This report led to a successful clinical pregnancy and a twin live birth. Prior to this report, cryopreservation of the human oocyte was relatively unsuccessful and inefficient compared with cryopreservation of the human cleavage and blastocyst embryo (Cobo et al. 2008a; Brambillasca et al. 2013). This observation was similar to the different stages of the human oocyte. The initial slow freezing method of oocyte cryopreservation was associated with suboptimal post-thaw survival rates and clinical outcomes. Following this consistently low outcome over a decade it became apparent that applying the same protocol used in cleavage stage embryo freezing was inadequate for successful oocyte freezing, due to its unique physiology and structure (Almodin et al. 2015). Hence, the slow freezing procedure for oocyte cryopreservation was subsequently modified (Gook et al. 2016). Marginal improvement in post-thaw survival rates and clinical outcomes were observed following these modifications. A large multicentre observational study which compared clinical outcomes with slow frozen–warmed oocytes indicated that oocyte slow freezing may be associated with reduced efficacy as a result

of lower clinical pregnancy per thaw oocyte (4.3%) and an implantation rate of 3.3%, (Borini et al. 2010). Regardless of these modifications, the fertilization, clinical pregnancy, implantation, and live birth rates were still considered very low relative to those obtained in treatment cycles involving fresh oocytes (Fabbri et al. 2001; De Santis et al. 2007). The application of this slow freezing method of oocyte cryopreservation was routine practice in Italy due to the legal restriction on cryopreservation of human oocytes between 2004 and 2009 (Borini et al. 2010; Levi Setti et al. 2014).

The high water content of the oocyte, low surface area to volume ratio, the suspension of temperature sensitive cellular organelles (e.g. meiotic spindle) within the cytoplasm, and the delicate plasma membrane of the human oocyte are some of the unique features of the oocyte which presented initial challenges to successful cryopreservation of oocytes (Konc et al. 2014). This initial challenge seems to have been significantly overcome with the advent of open and closed systems of vitrification (Bagchi et al. 2008; Arav and Natan 2013). Kuleshova et al. (1999) reported the first successful birth following the application of vitrification methods of cryopreservation in ART.

Oocyte cryopreservation offers a very unique and significant benefit compared with those associated with embryo cryopreservation. It allows cryopreservation of oocytes which otherwise would have been discarded due to lack of a semen sample from the male patient following successful controlled ovarian stimulation and egg retrieval from the female patient. Similarly, cryopreserved oocytes can be thawed–warmed and used in cases of an absentee husband and in some extreme cases it facilitates the posthumous use of cryopreserved oocytes. Importantly, cryopreservation of oocytes offers female reproductive autonomy, in addition to avoiding possible ethical or religious challenges associated with embryo cryopreservation or disposal after the consented period of storage. The benefits and applications of oocyte cryopreservation remain critical in modern reproductive science and management of female infertility, such as fertility preservation and delayed childbearing. Hence, increasing numbers of babies are being born from the application of the procedure. To date, over 1500 babies are reported to have been born worldwide following the application of vitrification methods of cryopreservation in ART. Some investigators argue that this figure is an underestimate, as significantly higher numbers of babies are reported to have been born from the application of both slow and vitrification methods of cryopreservation in Italy alone (Herrero et al. 2011). A related retrospective study which includes data from the Italian Birth Registry by Levi Setti et al. (2014) reported the live births of 1338 babies with 778 and 556 arising from the application of slow freezing and vitrification procedures, respectively, between 2007 and 2011. This live birth data was associated with 14 328 frozen–thawed–warm oocyte treatment cycles in which a total of 11 599 patients had at least one embryo transferred. Similar live birth data following the application of oocyte cryopreservation has been reported in other studies (Cobo and Diaz 2011). In the UK, the Human Fertilisation and Embryology Authority (HFEA) (2013 and 2015) report indicated that an estimated 60 babies have been born from the application of both slow frozen–thawed and vitrified–warmed oocytes. Whilst this data may indicate that application of oocyte cryopreservation may not be routine in the UK, some treatment-licenced centres have reported a surge in the application of the procedure for medical or nonmedical reasons (HFEA Trends and Figures, 2015 report).

A prospective randomized sibling study involving fresh and vitrified–warmed MII oocytes by Rienzi et al. (2017) did not report any statistical differences in fertilization rate, pronuclei morphology, embryo development, and quality between the two different study groups. Also, similar ongoing clinical pregnancy per transfer and implantation rate per cycle of 30.8 and 20.8% versus 30.0 and 17.0% were reported in the vitrified–warmed and fresh treatment groups, respectively. This data suggest that treatment outcomes following oocyte vitrification are not inferior to those obtained in fresh treatment cycles. These findings were largely in agreement with a systematic review and meta-analysis of randomized controlled trials involving the clinical application of oocyte vitrification in ART by Cobo and Diaz (2011). However, the later study seems to suggest that vitrification methods are a more efficient means of oocyte cryopreservation.

Different protocols have been reported with successful oocyte and embryo cryopreservation

procedures in ART (Edgar and Gook 2012). These protocols are unique in terms of the concentration and type of cryoprotecting agent, the duration of exposure, and the type of carrier (straw) device used. Regardless of these variations or similarities in the procedure, cryopreservation procedures in ART equilibrium (slow freezing) and nonequilibrium (vitrification) are both established on the same basic principles of cryopreservation. These procedures involve initial cellular dehydration using a combination of CPA at different concentrations followed by exposures to appropriate cooling temperatures and subsequent storage in liquid nitrogen (LN) (Rienzi et al. 2017). Either of these two different methods of cryopreservation can be safely applied in ART for cryopreservation of human MII oocytes.

The slow method of cryopreservation was first described by Whittingham et al. (1972) and it is associated with appropriate cellular dehydration to mitigate the risks of ice crystal formation during the cooling stages of cryopreservation. The cooling rate employed by Whittingham et al. was reported to be in the region of -1 °C per minute until a temperature of -70 °C is attained before plunging in LN. This protocol provided the critical foundation for subsequent improvements in the slow freezing methods currently used for cryopreserving the human MII. As described by Borini et al. (2010), denuded MII oocytes are initially equilibrated using two different concentrations of cryoprotectants for 7 min 30 s in each solution, prior to further dehydration in a solution containing a combination of permeating and nonpermeating cryoprotectants at slightly higher concentration for 5 min. The latter stages of dehydration are arguably critical to gametes survival as several studies (De Santis et al. 2007; Edgar et al. 2009; Bianchi et al. 2012; Balaban et al. 2012) have reported increased survival rates of oocytes following the use of a higher concentration of cryoprotectant (e.g. sucrose) prior to exposures to cooling temperatures.

Oocytes are subsequently aspirated into appropriately labelled straws and sealed at both ends before loading into a LN controlled rate slow freezing unit at room temperature (20 °C). The temperature is subsequently reduced to -8 °C at the rate of 2 °C per minute and seeded at -8 °C. The temperature range of -50 °C and -80 °C is thought to be a relatively safe zone for initiation of ice in a controlled manner.

The temperature is held at -8°C for 10 min soaking before the temperature is further reduced to -30°C at a rate of 0.3°C per minute and subsequently to -150°C at a rate of -50°C followed by another round of soaking for 10 min before plunging into LN at -196°C for final storage.

Oocyte Thawing Procedure

Briefly, oocyte thawing procedures are routinely performed at room temperature. Straws are rapidly thawed in air for 30 s and plunged into a water bath at 30°C for 40 s. Recovered oocytes are subsequently exposed to varying concentrations of thawing solutions in the following order: solution 1 for 5 min; solution 2 for 5 min; solution 3 for 10 min; solution 4 for 10 min initially at room temperature and another 10 min at 37°C before transferring into the incubator for use in treatment (Bianchi et al. 2007; Bianchi et al. 2012; Parmegiani et al. 2014).

Sperm Cryopreservation

Human sperm cryopreservation procedures in ART involve the use of CPA that are predominantly sucrose or glycerol based (ethylene glycol or propylene glycol) or dimethyl sulfoxide (DMSO) based. The process involves diluting ejaculated and liquefied or processed sperm cells with CPA for equilibration. Subsequently, the equilibrated mixture is exposed to LN vapour for at least 10 min before being plunged in LN at a temperature of -196°C for final storage (Figure 29.2). Despite this arguably

simple procedure for sperm cryopreservation, the potential risks of intracellular or extracellular ice crystal formation, CPA, osmotic and/or thermal shock, and cooling rate are important factors that may affect the freeze–thaw outcomes of cryopreserved sperm cells (Polcz et al. 1998; Gonzalez-Marin et al. 2012).

The impact of these physical and chemical challenges may possibly explain the increase in the number of nonmotile sperm occasionally observed in frozen–thawed sperm samples. Therefore, permeating or nonpermeating CPA are routinely added to sperm cryopreservation media used in ART to reduce the impact of cryopreservation. In fact, cryopreservation procedures in ART have been observed to yield post-thaw semen parameters that are comparable to those of the prefreeze sample with the use of cryopreservation media supplemented with CPA and a buffer to stabilize the pH of the media (Medeiros et al. 2002; Montagut et al. 2015). The original discovery of the role of glycerol as a cryoprotectant by Polge et al. (1949) is now deeply entrenched in modern protocols for semen cryopreservation in ART. Cryoprotecting agents are groups of compounds that either prevent or mitigate the potential problems of cryodamage to sperm cells during cryopreservation. Despite the efficacy of these compounds and current protocols, the spontaneous removal of water molecules from within the sperm cell may cause osmotic shock, which is detrimental to sperm survival. Furthermore, excessive dehydration of sperm cells may also force an

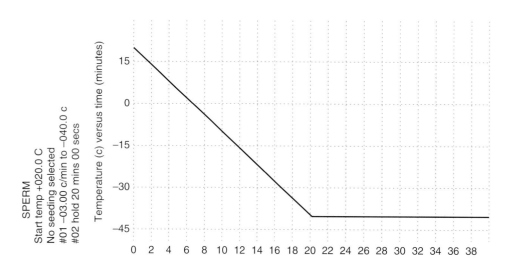

Figure 29.2 Slow freezing programme for sperm.

increase in the intracellular concentration of solutes above physiologically safe levels. These levels of solutes are thought to be highly toxic to sperm survival; therefore, the exposure of sperm cells to appropriate concentrations of CPA at optimum temperatures is essential for a successful cryopreservation outcome (Medeiros et al. 2002; Silva and Gadella 2006; Saravia et al. 2007; Elliott et al. 2017). Similarly, the progressive or slow thawing of samples and subsequent removal of cryoprotectants by washing with appropriate sperm preparation media prior to use in treatment is essential for optimum sperm freeze–thaw outcomes.

Vitrification of sperm is another viable method of sperm freezing which is thought to produce better freeze–thaw outcomes than the conventional slow freezing methods. This method is faster, cheaper, and often involves less expensive laboratory equipment compared with slow freezing procedures. Several authors have reported a better yield of motile sperm with fewer nonmotile sperm cells seen following vitrification procedures (Silva and Gadella 2006; Saravia et al. 2007; Endo et al. 2011; Vutyavanich et al. 2012). Moreover, these authors showed that vitrification can increase the likelihood of obtaining morphologically normal sperm for better fertilization outcomes, especially for ICSI procedures. However, only a very small volume of semen can be vitrified in any given instance. This may become a very important procedure when considering the cryopreservation of surgically recovered sperm cells that are often very fragile, precious, and limited in concentration and motility.

Regardless of the method of sperm cryopreservation, it has been established that cryopreservation procedures certainly create stressful conditions for sperm cells, which could be detrimental to their survival (Gomez-Torres et al. 2017). However, the advantages of sperm cryopreservation in ART arguably outweigh the risks by producing significantly better results and improving patient management (Horne et al. 1997; Horne et al. 2004; Kably-Ambe et al. 2016).

Embryo Cryopreservation

Exploring viable methods of preserving surplus good quality embryos became paramount following the birth of the world's first *in vitro* fertilization (IVF) baby (Louise Brown) in 1978. The first successful human pregnancy following cryopreservation and thawing of a Day 3 eight-cell embryo followed in 1983 (Trounson and Mohr 1983).

The emergence of this viable means of cryopreserving top quality human embryos at different stages of development has immensely contributed to the progressive increase in clinical pregnancy and live birth rates in ART. Savage et al. (2011) showed that approximately 25% of all ART babies were conceived from cryopreserved-thawed oocytes and embryos. This figure indicates a significant increase in the application of cryopreservation procedures during assisted conception treatment procedures. Similarly, the International Committee for Monitoring Assisted Reproductive Technologies (ICMART) reported that cryopreservation procedures are now routinely performed in over 2500 clinics in more than 58 countries around the world (Dyer et al. 2016).

Controlled ovarian stimulation in ART involves the development and recruitment of a cohort of multiple follicles from which matured MII oocytes can be recovered, fertilized with sperm, and several embryos created for subsequent use in treatment or storage for future use by the patient. In view of this, it is essential to anticipate the availability of surplus good to top quality embryos, which can be cryopreserved for future use or extended storage following the genetic screening of embryos, for donation to another couple, or for quarantine in treatment cycles involving the use of a surrogate. The availability of cryopreservation facilities and competently trained staff is regarded as good laboratory practice and a regulatory requirement for all treatment-licenced centres in the UK and several other countries around the world (De los Santos et al. 2016). Gamete and embryo cryopreservation services remain an essential contingency procedure for managing unforeseen circumstances such as an absentee husband, sudden hospital admission, difficulty with semen production, and complications arising from ovarian hyperstimulation syndrome (OHSS) (Mohamed et al. 2011; Davenport et al. 2017). The risk of OHSS presents a major safety challenge in ART, as the patient becomes very unwell and embryo transfer can be deferred in severe cases of OHSS (Massart et al. 2013; Youssef et al. 2014).

Embryo cryopreservation procedures have been identified as a valuable and efficient means of optimizing the cumulative clinical pregnancy rate following a single IVF/ICSI treatment cycle in which surplus top quality embryos can be cryopreserved and transferred in a frozen treatment cycle (Horne et al. 1997; Surrey et al. 2010; Mohamed et al. 2011; Harbottle et al. 2015). According to Damario et al. (2000), cryopreserved embryos at the pronuclear stage offers clinical pregnancy and implantation rates similar to those obtained in the fresh treatment cycle. Furthermore, other studies suggest this approach ensures that all normal fertilized oocytes (zygotes) are frozen, thus avoiding the potential risks of discarding these embryos if unsuitable for freezing at the cleavage stage. Also, these embryos can be thawed out conservatively, providing a significant economic saving to patients. Further studies have shown a post-thaw survival rate of 68%, and a clinical pregnancy rate and live birth rate of 41.8 and 36.9%, respectively.

Clinical data obtained from the optimized slow freezing methods of cryopreservation have continued to be reassuring and several clinicians and researchers are now advocating that all embryos created in a fresh cycle should be cryopreserved and replaced in a frozen cycle. This argument is motivated by the availability of superior post-thaw survival rates, and clinical pregnancy and live birth rates associated with the optimized slow freezing and vitrification methods of cryopreservation, in combination with a better endometrial environment (Surrey et al. 2010; Maheshwari et al. 2012; Maheshwari and Bhattacharya 2013).

Cryopreservation of cleavage and blastocyst stage embryos by vitrification have continued to emerge as an efficient procedure yielding significantly higher post-thaw survival, clinical pregnancy, and live birth rates (Van Landuyt et al. 2011; Rienzi et al. 2017). Recent evidence from a meta-analysis by Rienzi et al. (2017) indicated the superiority of vitrification methods for cleavage and blastocyst stage embryos. This observation follows from evidence obtained from seven randomized controlled trials which indicated significantly higher survival rates with vitrification compared with slow freezing (RR = 1.59, 95% CI: 1.30–1.93; $P < 0.001$; I2 = 93%). Also, significantly higher clinical pregnancy and live birth rates were also reported with vitrification. However, this increase did not reach statistical significance. Nonetheless, the authors argued that IVF clinics currently performing slow freezing methods of cryopreservation for cleavage stage and blastocyst embryos should consider a transition from slow freezing to vitrification methods for cleavage stage and blastocyst embryos.

Cryopreservation of Blastocyst Embryos

Initial success with slow freezing of blastocyst embryos using glycerol as the cryoprotectant was arguably suboptimal (Behr and Shu 2010). Although the post-thaw survival rate was 98%, only 50% of the inner cell mass and trophectoderm cells actually survived the procedure, yielding an implantation rate of 16%. Modifications to this protocol (Gardner et al. 2003) resulted in a marginal increase in post-thaw survival rate (69%) and implantation rate of 30%. However, methods of blastocyst vitrification have been shown to be reliable and consistent, yielding post-thaw survival rates between 85 and 99% with an implantation rate of 29.4% (Liebermann 2009). In this report, greater clinical outcomes were found to be associated with the quality of the blastocysts and the age of the patient with a higher number of pregnancies reported in young patients (<33 years of age). Findings from other clinical studies also supported these observations (Mukaida et al. 2003).

A large population-based study conducted by Li et al. (2014) involving vitrified, fresh (unfrozen), and slow frozen blastocysts demonstrated that the transfer of vitrified–warmed blastocyst resulted in the highest clinical pregnancy and live birth rates. Results obtained from vitrified–warmed blastocyst were associated with the highest proportion of single embryo transfer procedures relative to fresh and slow frozen–thawed blastocyst transfers. This reassuring clinical report indicates that vitrification procedures are essential for oocyte, cleavage stage embryo, and blastocyst embryo cryopreservation (Ybussry et al. 2008; Herrero et al. 2011; Desai et al. 2013).

Slow Freezing Techniques for Human Embryos

As part of the two-step slow freezing techniques, cleavage stage and pronuclear embryos are initially exposed to an equilibration solution, made up of a combination of permeating and nonpermeating CPA at low concentration for approximately 10 min at room temperature. Subsequently, embryos are transferred into a second freezing solution with the appropriate concentration of CPA for another

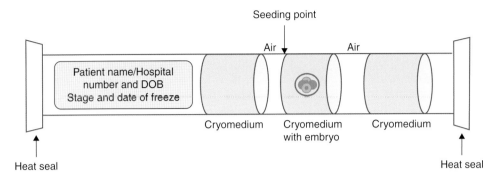

Figure 29.3 Loading the cryostraw for embryo freeze. Embryos are aspirated in to the cryostraw and heat sealed at both ends. Each straw contains the patient identification details, the stage of embryo development, and date of freeze. These straws can be then stored long-term in liquid nitrogen.

10 min and embryos are aspirated into appropriately labelled straws and sealed at both ends of the straw (Figure 29.3). All labelled straws are then loaded into the freezing chamber and cooled slowly from room temperature to –6 °C at a cooling rate of –0.3 °C per minute. The initiation of ice crystals (seeding) is manually induced at –7 °C using forceps previously cooled in LN. This is a critical step, which enhances further cell dehydration, thus reducing the risks of intracellular ice crystal formation within the embryo. Next, straws are gradually cooled to –30 °C at a rate of –0.3 °C per minute, followed by another round of cooling to –150 °C at the rate of –50 °C per minute, after which the straws can be removed from the freezing chamber and plunged into LN prior to final storage in LN at –196 °C (Edgar and Gook 2012). The entire duration of slow freezing is approximately 1 h and 45 min (Figure 29.4).

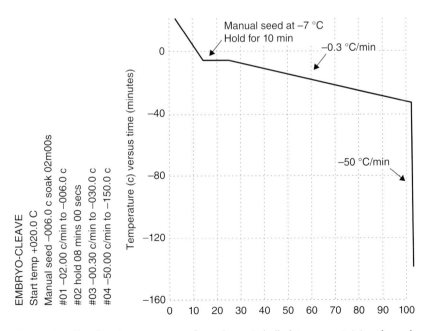

Figure 29.4 Slow freezing programme for embryos. Labelled straws containing the embryos are loaded into the freezing chamber and cooled slowly from room temperature to -6 °C at a cooling rate of -0.3 °C per minute. Manual seeding (initiating of ice crystal formation) is induced at -6 °C. The straws are gradually cooled to –30 °C at a rate of -0.3 °C per minute, followed by another round of cooling to -150 °C at the rate of -50 °C per minute, after which the straws can be removed from the freezing chamber and plunged into liquid nitrogen prior to final storage in liquid nitrogen at -196 °C.

Embryo Thawing Procedure

In contrast, thawing procedures are relatively quick, involving a very simple and rapid process of initial thawing in air for 30 s before being held in a water bath for 45 s. Upon thawing all embryos are transferred into thawing solutions 1 and 2, and equilibration solutions for 5 min in each of the solutions. Post-thaw survival rates between 65 and 75% have been reported with pronuclear and cleavage stage embryos (Van Landuyt et al. 2011; Debrock et al. 2015; Rienzi et al. 2017).

Vitrification

Contrary to slow freezing, vitrification methods of cryopreservation involves the use of high concentrations of cryoprotectants (permeating >4 M, and nonpermeating cryoprotectant >0.5 M) for optimum dehydration necessary for establishing a vitrified and thermodynamically stable glass-like solid state (Fahy et al. 1987; Kuwayama, 2007; Cobo et al. 2008a). Vitrification methods of cryopreservation are associated with an extremely high cooling rate (Antinori et al. 2007; De Munck et al. 2016). The procedure is thought to have evolved following decades of research studies focused on reducing the risks of ice crystal formation associated with cryopreservation procedures, particularly oocyte cryopreservation. Vitrification procedures are associated with the use of high concentrations of cryoprotectants. This presents a potential risk of cryoprotectant cytotoxicity to oocytes and embryos. This potential detrimental impact of cryoprotectants can be minimized with the use of a combination of permeating and nonpermeating cryoprotectants and the use of an extremely high cooling rate.

In practice, the initial stage of vitrification involves equilibration of the oocyte/embryo in a solution containing a combination of permeating and nonpermeating cryoprotectants for 10–15 min prior to exposure to a relatively higher concentration of cryoprotectants (Bonetti et al. 2011; Chen et al. 2013). The duration of exposure to the cryoprotectants used during the second stage of vitrification is routinely limited to between 45 and 90 s during which time the oocyte or embryo is loaded with minimal volume (~1 μL) of cryoprotectant solution onto an appropriate carrier device (open or closed) and plunged into LN (Balaban et al. 2012) (Figure 29.5).

Vitrification carrier devices in ART are unique and may either be a closed (Cobo and Diaz 2011) or open system/device (De Munck et al. 2016). Closed systems of vitrification involve the use of a simple barrier system (an outer straw) that prevents direct contact with LN (Desai et al. 2013), whereas open systems (Cobo et al. 2016b) provide direct contact with LN. This direct contact has been argued to provide an extremely high cooling rate of vitrification, which has been linked to the efficiency of open systems of vitrification (Cobo et al. 2016a). Unfortunately, the potential risk of cross-contamination as a result of this contact with LN remains a major concern in ART (Bielansk 2012). A related study by Craido et al. showed that closed systems of vitrification provide adequate solution to the potential risk of contamination that may arise from exposures to potentially contaminated LN in open devices (Criado et al. 2011). Similarly, an experimental study by Bonetti et al. (2011) argued that closed systems of vitrification may

(a)　　　　　　　(b)　　　　　　　(c)

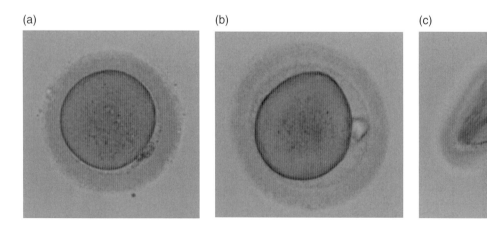

Figure 29.5 Vitrification of human metaphase II (MII) oocyte. (a) Human metaphase II (MII) oocyte prior to exposure to equilibration solution. (b) Oocyte gradually collapsing in equilibration solution after 1 min. (c) Oocyte fully collapsed in vitrification solution, prior to plunging in liquid nitrogen at -196 °C.

not completely preserve the ultrastructure of the human MII oocyte relative to the open system which confers the temperature of LN on the gamete during vitrification (Bonetti et al. 2011). However, increased survival rates, improved post-thaw embryo development, and improved clinical pregnancy and implantation rates have been reported with both open and closed devices of vitrification (Kuleshova and Lopata 2002; Chian et al. 2008; Chen et al. 2013). Similarly, no clinical evidence of cross-contamination has been reported in ART following the use of either closed or open devices of vitrification; nonetheless, safety of cryopreservation procedures, particularly open systems of vitrification, remains a critical subject of debate in ART (Cutting et al. 2009; Harper et al. 2012; Brison et al. 2012; Brison et al. 2013).

Warming procedures following successful vitrification are often associated with extremely high warming rate regardless of the device used. This is essential towards reducing the potential risks of ice crystal recrystallization that could become lethal to gamete survival and subsequent embryo development post-warming (Kuwayama et al. 2005; Mazur 2010; Vanderzwalmen et al. 2013). Oocytes and embryos intended for warming are directly warmed in warming solution at 37 °C for 3 min, followed by another 3 min in dilution solution 1 and 2, and finally in washing solutions 1 and 2 (3 min in each) after which the oocyte/embryo can be equilibrated in the incubator.

Conclusion

Cryopreservation of gametes and embryos is an important part of the treatment plan for IVF patients. This is especially true for fertility preservation in patients undergoing chemotherapy or radiotherapy as part of their cancer treatment. Gametes and embryo cryopreservation in ART offer IVF patients and young reproductive age women diagnosed with cancer the opportunities of achieving a successful pregnancy and live-birth. Furthermore, cancer treatment and survival rates have continued to improve in the UK and several high-income countries; such as Germany, Belgium, Sweden, and the U.S.A. Indeed, gamete cryopreservation arguably provides a valuable means of fertility preservation for potential future use (post-chemotherapy). A comparison between slow freezing and vitrification methods of cryopreservation in ART is displayed in Table 29.1.

Table 29.1 Differences between slow freezing and vitrification methods of cryopreservation in assisted reproductive technology.

Differences	Slow Freezing	Vitrification
Cryoprotectant concentration	Low concentration of cryoprotectants with minimal risks of cytotoxicity	High concentration of cryoprotectants with greater risks of cytotoxicity
Cooling rate	Low cooling rate in progressive manner with a high risk of ice crystal formation	Extremely high cooling rate usually between 1200 °C and 30 000 °C per minute providing a reduced risk of ice crystal formation
Thawing/warming rate	Low thawing rates	Extremely high warming rates
Survival rates	Associated with low survival rates relative to vitrification procedures	Associated with high survival rates usually between 75 and 95% for reproductive gametes and human embryos
Duration of procedure	A protracted procedure which could last up to 105 minutes (1 h 45 min)	A relatively quick procedure which takes between 15 and 20 min. However, the procedure may become protracted with several gametes of embryos often associated with fertility preservation or freeze-all due to ovarian hyperstimulation syndrome
Related equipment	A controlled rate programmable freezer is required and this is the single most expensive equipment used in slow freezing procedures	Less expensive equipment is required for the procedure

Cryopreservation in ART has expanded beyond the gametes and embryos. Ovarian tissue cryopreservation and transplantation have demonstrated some promising means of fertility preservation for women who have survived cancer, with live births being reported from this technique.

References

Aflatoonian, A., Oskouian, H., Ahmadi, S. et al. (2010). Can fresh embryo transfers be replaced by cryopreserved-thawed embryo transfers in assisted reproductive cycles? A randomized controlled trial. Hum Reprod 25: I99–I100.

Agarwal, A., Durairajanayagam, D. and du Plessis, S.S. (2014). Utility of antioxidants during assisted reproductive techniques: an evidence based review. Reprod Biol Endocrinol 12: 112.

Almodin, C.G., Ceschin, A., Nakano, R.E. et al. (2015). Vitrification of human oocytes and its contribution to in vitro fertilization programs. JBRA Assist Reprod 19: 135–140.

Amidi, F., Pazhohan, A., Nashtaei, M.S. et al. (2016). The role of antioxidants in sperm freezing: a review.Cell Tissue Banking 17: 745–756.

Antinori, M., Licata, E., Dani, G. et al. (2007). Cryotop vitrification of human oocytes results in high survival rate and healthy deliveries. Reprod Biomed Online 14: 72–79.

Arav, A. and Natan, Y. (2013). Vitrification of oocytes: from basic science to clinical application. Adv Exp Med Biol 761: 69–83.

Arcarons, N., Morato, R., Spricigo, J.F.W. et al. (2016). Spindle configuration and developmental competence of in vitro-matured bovine oocytes exposed to NaCl or sucrose prior to Cryotop vitrification. Reprod Fertil Dev 28: 1560–1569.

Argyle, C.E., Harper, J.C. and Davies, M.C. (2016). Oocyte cryopreservation: where are we now? Hum Reprod Update 22: 440–449.

Aye, M., Di Giorgio, C., De Mo, M. et al. (2010). Assessment of the genotoxicity of three cryoprotectants used for human oocyte vitrification: dimethyl sulfoxide, ethylene glycol and propylene glycol. Food Chem Toxicol 48: 1905–1912.

Bagchi, A., Woods, E.J. and Critser, J.K. (2008). Cryopreservation and vitrification: recent advances in fertility preservation technologies. Expert Rev Med Devices 5: 359–370.

Balaban, B., Bianchi, V., Bolton, V. et al. and Alpha Scientists (2012). The Alpha consensus meeting on cryopreservation key performance indicators and benchmarks: proceedings of an expert meeting. Reprod Biomed Online 25: 146–167.

Behr, B. and Shu, Y.M. (2010). Cryopreservation of human oocytes and embryos. In: (D. Carrell and C. Peterson C., eds) *Reproductive Endocrinology and Infertility*. New York: Springer.

Bianchi, V., Coticchio, G., Distratis, V. et al. (2007). Differential sucrose concentration during dehydration (0.2 mol/l) and rehydration (0.3 mol/l) increases the implantation rate of frozen human oocytes. Reprod Biomed Online 14: 64–71.

Bianchi, V., Lappi, M., Bonu, M.A. et al. (2012). Oocyte slow freezing using a 0.2–0.3 M sucrose concentration protocol: is it really the time to trash the cryopreservation machine? Fertil Steril 97: 1101–1107.

Bielanski, A. (2012). A review of the risk of contamination of semen and embryos during cryopreservation and measures to limit cross-contamination during banking to prevent disease transmission in ET practices. Theriogenology 77: 467–482.

Boldt, J. (2011). Current results with slow freezing and vitrification of the human oocyte. Reprod Biomed Online 23: 314–322.

Bonetti, A., Cervi, M., Tomei, F. et al. (2011). Ultrastructural evaluation of human metaphase II oocytes after vitrification: closed versus open devices. Fertil Steril 95: 928–935.

Borini, A., Levi Setti, P.E., Anserini, P. et al. (2010). Multicenter observational study on slow-cooling oocyte cryopreservation: clinical outcome. Fertil Steril 94: 1662–1668.

Brambillasca, F., Guglielmo, M.C., Coticchio, G. et al. (2013). The current challenges to efficient immature oocyte cryopreservation. J Assist Reprod Genet 30: 1531–1539.

Brison, D., Cuting, R., Clarke, H. et al. (2012). ACE consensus meeting report: oocyte and embryo cryopreservation Sheffield 17.05.11. Hum Fertil 15: 69–74.

Brison, D.R., Roberts, S.A. and Kimber, S.J. (2013). How should we assess the safety of IVF technologies? Reprod Biomed Online 27: 710–721.

Bromfield, J.J., Coticchio, G., Hutt, K. et al. (2009). Meiotic spindle dynamics in human oocytes following slow-cooling cryopreservation. Hum Reprod 24: 2114–2123.

Bunge, R.G., Keettel, W.C. and Sherman, J.K. (1954). Clinical use of frozen semen – report of 4 cases. Fertil Steril 5: 520–529.

Chen, C. (1986). Pregnancy after human oocyte cryopreservation. Lancet 1(8486), 884–886.

Chen, Y., Zheng, X., Yan, J. et al. (2013). Neonatal outcomes after the transfer of vitrified blastocysts: closed versus open vitrification system. Reprod Biol Endocrinol 11: 107.

Chian, R.C., Huang, J.Y.J., Tan, S.L. et al. (2008). Obstetric and perinatal outcome in 200 infants conceived from vitrified oocytes. Reprod Biomed Online 16: 608–610.

Cobo, A. and Diaz, C. (2011). Clinical application of oocyte vitrification: a systematic review and meta-analysis of randomized controlled trials. Fertil Steril 96: 277–285.

Cobo, A., Garcia-Velasco, J.A., Coello, A. et al. (2016a). Oocyte vitrification as an efficient option for elective fertility preservation. Fertil Steril 105: 755–764.e8.

Cobo, A., Garcia-Velasco, J.A., Coello, A. et al. (2016b). Oocyte vitrification as an efficient option for elective fertility preservation. Fertil Steril 105: 755–764.

Cobo, A., Kuwayama, M., Perez, S. et al. (2008a). Comparison of concomitant outcome achieved with fresh and cryopreserved donor oocytes vitrified by the Cryotop method. Fertil Steril 89: 1657–1664.

Cobo, A., Perez, S., De los Santos, M.J. et al. (2008c). Effect of different cryopreservation protocols on the metaphase II spindle in human oocytes. Reprod Biomed Online 17: 350–359.

Cobo, A., Serra, V., Garrido, N. et al. (2014). Obstetric and perinatal outcome of babies born from vitrified oocytes. Fertil Steril 102: 1006–U485.

Criado, E., Moalli, F., Polentarutti, N. et al. (2011). Experimental contamination assessment of a novel closed ultravitrification device. Fertil Steril 95: 1777–1779.

Cutting, R., Barlow, S., Anderson, R. et al. (2009). Human oocyte cryopreservation: evidence for practice. Hum Fertil 12: 125–136.

Damario, M.A., Hammitt, D.G., Session, D.R. et al. (2000). Embryo cryopreservation at the pronuclear stage and efficient embryo use optimizes the chance for a liveborn infant from a single oocyte retrieval. Fertil Steril 73: 767–773.

Davenport, M.J., Vollenhoven, B. and Talmor, A.J. (2017). Gonadotropin-releasing hormone-agonist triggering and a freeze-all approach: the final step in eliminating ovarian hyperstimulation syndrome? Obstet Gynecol Surv 72: 296–308.

De los Santos, M.J., Apter, S., Coticchio, G. et al. (2016). Revised guidelines for good practice in IVF laboratories (2015). Hum Reprod 31: 685–686.

de Menorval, M.A., Mir, L.M., Fernandez, M.L. et al. (2012). Effects of dimethyl sulfoxide in cholesterol-containing lipid membranes: a comparative study of experiments in silico and with cells. Plos One, 7.

De Munck, N., Santos-Ribeiro, S., Stoop, D. et al. (2016). Open versus closed oocyte vitrification in an oocyte donation programme: a prospective randomized sibling oocyte study. Hum Reprod 31: 377–384.

De Santis, L., Cino, I., Rabellotti, E. et al. (2007). Oocyte cryo preservation: clinical outcome of slow-cooling protocols differing in sucrose concentration. Reprod Biomed Online 14: 57–63.

Debrock, S., Peeraer, K., Gallardo, E.F. et al. (2015). Vitrification of cleavage stage day 3 embryos results in higher live birth rates than conventional slow freezing: a RCT. Hum Reprod 30: 1820–1830.

Desai, N.N., Goldberg, J.M., Austin, C. et al. (2013). The new Rapid-i carrier is an effective system for human embryo vitrification at both the blastocyst and cleavage stage. Reprod Biol Endocrinol 11: 41.

Ducibella, T., Huneau, D., Angelichio, E. et al. (2002). Egg-to-embryo transition is driven by differential responses to Ca2+ oscillation number. Dev Biol 250: 280–291.

Dyer, S., Chambers, G.M., de Mouzon, J. et al. (2016). International Committee for Monitoring Assisted Reproductive Technologies world report: Assisted Reproductive Technology 2008, 2009 and 2010. Hum Reprod 31: 1588–1609.

Edgar, D.H. and Gook, D.A. (2012). A critical appraisal of cryopreservation (slow cooling versus vitrification) of human oocytes and embryos. Hum Reprod Update 18: 536–554.

Edgar, D.H., Karani, J. and Gook, D.A. (2009). Increasing dehydration of human cleavage-stage embryos prior to slow cooling significantly increases cryosurvival. Reprod Biomed Online 19: 521–525.

Endo Y., Fujii Y., Shintani, K. et al., (2011). Single spermatozoon freezing using cryotop. J Mammal Ova Res 28: 47–52.

Elliott, G.D., Wang, S.P. and Fuller, B.J. (2017). Cryoprotectants: A review of the actions and applications of cryoprotective solutes that modulate cell recovery from ultra-low temperatures. Cryobiology 76: 74–91.

Fabbri, R., Porcu, E., Marsella, T. et al. (2001). Human oocyte cryopreservation: new perspectives regarding oocyte survival. Hum Reprod 16: 411–416.

Fahy, G.M., Levy, D.I. and Ali, S.E. (1987). Some emerging principles underlying the physical-properties, biological actions, and utility of vitrification solutions. Cryobiology 24: 196–213.

Garcia-Velasco, J.A., Domingo, J., Cobo, A. et al. (2013). Five years' experience using oocyte vitrification to preserve fertility for medical and nonmedical indications. Fertil Steril 99: 1994–1999.

Gardner, D.K., Lane, M., Stevens, J. et al. (2003). Changing the start temperature and cooling rate in a slow-freezing protocol increases human blastocyst viability. Fertil Steril 79: 407–410.

Gardner, D.K., Sheehan, C.B., Rienzi, L. et al. (2007). Analysis of oocyte physiology to improve cryopreservation procedures. Theriogenology 67: 64–72.

Gómez-Torres, M.J., Medrano, L., Romero, A. et al. (2017). Effectiveness of human spermatozoa biomarkers as indicators of structural damage during cryopreservation. Cryobiology 78: 90–94.

Gonzalez-Marin, C., Gosalvez, J. and Roy, R. (2012). Types, causes, detection and repair of dna fragmentation in animal and human sperm cells. Int J Mol Sci 13: 14026–14052.

Gook, D.A., Choo, B., Bourne, H. et al. (2016). Closed vitrification of human oocytes and blastocysts: outcomes from a series of clinical cases. J Assist Reprod Genet 33: 1247–1252.

Harbottle, S., Hughes, C., Cutting, R. et al. (2015). Elective single embryo transfer: an update to UK Best Practice Guidelines. Hum Fertil 18: 165–183.

Harper, J., Magli, M.C., Lundin, K. et al. (2012). When and how should new technology be introduced into the IVF laboratory? Hum Reprod 27: 303–313.

Herrero, L., Martinez, M. and Garcia-Velasco, J.A. (2011). Current status of human oocyte and embryo cryopreservation. Curr Opin Obstet Gynecol 23: 245–250.

Horne, G., Atkinson, A.D., Pease, E.H.E. et al. (2004). Live birth with sperm cryopreserved for 21 years prior to cancer treatment: case report. Hum Reprod 19: 1448–1449.

Horne, G., Critchlow, J.D., Newman, M.C. et al. (1997). A prospective evaluation of cryopreservation strategies in a two-embryo transfer programme. Hum Reprod 12: 542–547.

Kably-Ambe, A., Carballo-Mondragón, E., Roque-Sánchez A.M. et al. (2016). Evaluation of semen parameters in long term cryopreserved samples for over 10 years. Ginecol Obstet Mex 84:1–6.

Katz-Jaffe, M.G., Larman, M.G., Sheehan, C.B. et al. (2008). Exposure of mouse oocytes to 1,2-propanediol during slow freezing alters the proteome. Fertil Steril 89: 1441–1447.

Konc, J., Kanyo, K., Kriston, R. et al. (2014). Cryopreservation of embryos and oocytes in human assisted reproduction. Biomed Res Int 2014: 307268.

Kopeika, J., Thornhill, A. and Khalaf, Y. (2015). The effect of cryopreservation on the genome of gametes and embryos: principles of cryobiology and critical appraisal of the evidence. Hum Reprod Update 21: 209–227.

Kuleshova, L.L. and Lopata, A. (2002). Vitrification can be more favorable than slow cooling. Fertil Steril 78: 449–454.

Kuwayama, M. (2007). Highly efficient vitrification for cryopreservation of human oocytes and embryos: the Cryotop method. Theriogenology 67: 73–80.

Kuwayama, M., Vajta, G., Kato, O. et al. (2005). Highly efficient vitrification method for cryopreservation of human oocytes. Reprod Biomed Online 11: 300–308.

Lane, M., Maybach, J.M. and Gardner, D.K. (2002). Addition of ascorbate during cryopreservation stimulates subsequent embryo development. Hum Reprod 17: 2686–2693.

Larman, M.G., Katz-Jaffe, M.G., McCallie, B. et al. (2011). Analysis of global gene expression following mouse blastocyst cryopreservation. Hum Reprod 26: 2672–2680.

Larman, M.G., Katz-Jaffe, M.G., Sheehan, C.B. et al. (2007a). 1,2-propanediol and the type of cryopreservation procedure adversely affect mouse oocyte physiology. Hum Reprod 22: 250–259.

Larman, M.G., Minasi, M.G., Rienzi, L. et al. (2007b). Maintenance of the meiotic spindle during vitrification in human and mouse oocytes. Reprod Biomed Online 15: 692–700.

Larman, M.G., Saunders, C.M., Carroll, J. et al. (2004). Cell cycle-dependent Ca(2+) oscillations in mouse embryos are regulated by nuclear targeting of PLC zeta. J Cell Sci 117: 2513–2521.

Larman, M.G., Sheehan, C.B. and Gardner, D.K. (2006). Calcium-free vitrification reduces cryoprotectant-induced zona pellucida hardening and increases fertilization rates in mouse oocytes. Reproduction 131: 53–61.

Leibo, S.P. (1984). A one-step method for direct nonsurgical transfer of frozen-thawed bovine embryos. Theriogenology 21: 767–790.

Leibo, S.P., McGrath, J.J. and Cravalho, E.G. (1978). Microscopic observation of intracellular ice formation in unfertilized mouse ova as a function of cooling rate. Cryobiology 15: 257–271.

Levi Setti, P.E., Porcu, E., Patrizio, P. et al. (2014). Human oocyte cryopreservation with slow freezing versus vitrification. Results from the National Italian Registry data, 2007–2011. Fertil Steril 102: 90–95.e2.

Liebermann, J. (2009). Vitrification of human blastocyst: an update. Reprod Biomed Online 19(Suppl 4):4328.

Li, Z., Wang, Y.A., Ledger, W., Edgar, D.H. et al. (2014). Clinical outcomes following cryopreservation of blastocysts by vitrification or slow freezing: a population-based cohort study. Hum Reprod 29: 2794–2801.

Lin, L., Du, Y.T., Liu, Y. et al. (2009). Elevated NaCl concentration improves cryotolerance and developmental competence of porcine oocytes. Reprod Biomed Online 18: 360–366.

Lovelock, J.E. (1953). The mechanism of the protective action of glycerol against haemolysis by freezing and thawing. Biochim Biophys Acta 11: 28–36.

Lovelock, J.E. and Polge, C. (1954). The immobilization of spermatozoa by freezing and thawing and the protective action of glycerol. Biochemical J 58: 618–622.

Mackenzie, A.P. and Luyet, B.J. (1967). Freeze-drying and protein denaturation in muscle tissue – losses in protein solubility. Nature 215(5096): 83–84.

Magli, M.C., Van den Abbeel, E., Lundin, K. et al. and Committee of the Special Interest Group on Embryology (2008). Revised guidelines for good practice in IVF laboratories. Hum Reprod 23: 1253–1262.

Maheshwari, A. and Bhattacharya, S. (2013). Elective frozen replacement cycles for all: ready for prime time? Hum Reprod 28: 6–9.

Maheshwari, A., Pandey, S., Shetty, A. et al. (2012). Obstetric and perinatal outcomes in singleton pregnancies resulting from the transfer of frozen thawed versus fresh embryos generated through in vitro fertilization treatment: a systematic review and meta-analysis. Fertil Steril 98: 368–377.

Martinez-Burgos, M., Herrero, L., Megias, D. et al. (2011). Vitrification versus slow freezing of oocytes: effects on morphologic appearance, meiotic spindle configuration, and DNA damage. Fertil Steril 95: 374–377.

Massart, P., Sermondade, N., Dupont, C. et al. (2013). Elective cryopreservation of all embryos in women at risk of ovarian hyperstimulation syndrome: prevention and efficiency. Gynecol Obstet Fertil 41: 365–371.

Mazur, P. (1963). Kinetics of water loss from cells at subzero temperatures and likelihood of intracellular freezing. J Gen Physiol 47: 347–369.

Mazur, P. (1990). Equilibrium, quasi-equilibrium, and nonequilibrium freezing of mammalian embryos. Cell Biophys 17: 53–92.

Mazur, P. (2010). A biologist's view of the relevance of thermodynamics and physical chemistry to cryobiology. Cryobiology 60: 4–10.

Mazur, P. and Kleinhans, F.W. (2008). Relationship between intracellular ice formation in oocytes of the mouse and Xenopus and the physical state of the external medium – a revisit. Cryobiology 56: 22–27.

Medeiros, C.M.O., Forell, F., Oliveira, A.T.D. et al. (2002). Current status of sperm cryopreservation: why isn't it better? Theriogenology 57: 327–344.

Mohamed, A.M.F., Chouliaras, S., Jones, C.J.P. et al. (2011). Live birth rate in fresh and frozen embryo transfer cycles in women with endometriosis. Eur J Obstet Gynecol Reprod Biol 156: 177–180.

Montagut, M., Gatimel, N., Bourdet-Loubere, S. et al. (2015). Sperm freezing to address the risk of azoospermia on the day of ICSI. Hum Reprod 30: 2486–2492.

Mukaida, T., Nakumura, S., Tomiyama, T. et al. (2003). Vitrification of human blastocysts using cryoloops: clinical outcome of 223 cycles. Hum Reprod 18: 384–391.

Nagy, Z.P., Cobo, A. and Chang, C.C. (2016). Oocyte vitrification: donor "egg banking". In: (ed. M. J. Tucker and J. Liebermann) *Vitrification in Assisted Reproduction*, 2nd edn. Boca Raton: CRC Press.

Ozil, J.P., Markoulaki, S., Toth, S. et al. (2005). Egg activation events are regulated by the duration of a sustained Ca2+ (cyt) signal in the mouse. Dev Biol 282: 39–54.

Parmegiani, L., Tatone, C., Cognigni, G.E. et al. (2014). Rapid warming increases survival of slow-frozen sibling oocytes: a step towards a single warming procedure irrespective of the freezing protocol? Reprod Biomed Online 28: 614–623.

Polcz, T.E., Stronk, J., Xiong, C. et al. (1998). Optimal utilization of cryopreserved human semen for assisted reproduction: recovery and maintenance of sperm motility and viability. J Assist Reprod Genet 15: 504–512.

Polge, C., Smith, A.U. and Parkes, A.S. (1949). Revival of spermatozoa after vitrification and dehydration at low temperatures. Nature 164(4172): 666.

Quintans, C.J., Donaldson, M.J., Bertolino, M.V. et al. (2002). Birth of two babies using oocytes that were cryopreserved in a choline-based freezing medium. Hum Reprod 17: 3149–3152.

Rienzi, L., Gracia, C., Maggiulli, R. et al. (2017). Oocyte, embryo and blastocyst cryopreservation in ART: systematic review and meta-analysis comparing slow-freezing versus vitrification to produce evidence for the development of global guidance. Hum Reprod Update 23: 139–155.

Said, T.M., Gaglani, A. and Agarwal, A. (2010). Implication of apoptosis in sperm cryoinjury. Reprod Biomed Online 21: 456–462.

Saravia, F., Hernández, M., Wallgren, et al. (2007) Controlled cooling during semen cryopreservation does not induce capacitation of spermatozoa from two portions of the boar ejaculate. Int J Androl 30:485–499.

Savage, T., Peek, J., Hofman, P.L. et al. (2011). Childhood outcomes of assisted reproductive technology. Hum Reprod 26: 2392–2400.

Sherman, J.K. (1954). Freezing and freeze-drying of human spermatozoa. Fertil Steril 5: 357–371.

Sherman, J.K. (1963). Improved methods of preservation of human spermatozoa by freezing and freeze-drying. Fertil Steril 14: 49–64.

Silva, P.F. and Gadella B.M. (2006) Detection of damage in mammalian sperm cells. Theriogenology 65: 958–978.

Stachecki, J.J., Cohen, J. and Willadsen, S. (1998). Detrimental effects of sodium during mouse oocyte cryopreservation. Biol Reprod 59: 395–400.

Sunde, A. and Balaban, B. (2013). The assisted reproductive technology laboratory: toward evidence-based practice? Fertil Steril 100: 310–318.

Surrey, E., Keller, J., Stevens, J. et al. (2010). Freeze-all: enhanced outcomes with cryopreservation at the blastocyst stage versus pronuclear stage using slow-freeze techniques. Reprod Biomed Online 21: 411–417.

Szurek, E.A. and Eroglu, A. (2011). Comparison and avoidance of toxicity of penetrating cryoprotectants. Plos One 6(11).

Taylor, K., Roberts, P., Sanders, K. et al. (2009). Effect of antioxidant supplementation of cryopreservation medium on post-thaw integrity of human spermatozoa. Reprod Biomed Online 18: 184–189.

Toner, M., Cravalho, E.G. and Karel, M. (1993). Cellular-response of mouse oocytes to freezing stress - prediction of intracellular ice formation. J Biomech Eng Trans ASME 115: 169–174.

Trounson, A. and Mohr, L. (1983). Human-pregnancy following cryopreservation, thawing and transfer of an 8-cell embryo. Nature 305(5936): 707–709.

Van Landuyt, L., Stoop, D., Verheyen, G. et al. (2011). Outcome of closed blastocyst vitrification in relation to blastocyst quality: evaluation of 759 warming cycles in a single-embryo transfer policy. Hum Reprod 26: 527–534.

Vanderzwalmen, P., Connan, D., Grobet, L. et al. (2013). Lower intracellular concentration of cryoprotectants after vitrification than after slow freezing despite exposure to higher concentration of cryoprotectant solutions. Hum Reprod 28: 2101–2110.

Vutyavanich, T. Lattiwongsakorn, W. Piromlertamorn, W. et al. (2012). Repeated vitrification/warming of human sperm gives better results than repeated slow programmable freezing. Asian J Androl 14: 850–854.

Wennerholm, U.B., Henningsen, A.K.A., Romundstad, L.B. et al. (2013). Perinatal outcomes of children born after frozen-thawed embryo transfer: a Nordic cohort study from the CoNARTaS group. Hum Reprod 28: 2545–2553.

Wennerholm, U.B., Soderstrom-Anttila, V., Bergh, C. et al. (2009). Children born after cryopreservation of embryos or oocytes: a systematic review of outcome data. Hum Reprod 24: 2158–2172.

Will, M.A., Clark, N.A. and Swain, J.E. (2011). Biological pH buffers in IVF: help or hindrance to success. J Assist Reprod Genet 28: 711–724.

Whittingham, D.G., Leibo, S.P. and Mazur, P. (1972). Survival of mouse embryos frozen to K196 8C and K269 8C, Science 178: 411–414.

Ybussry, M., Ozmen, B., Zohni, K. et al. (2008). Current aspects of blastocyst cryopreservation. Reprod Biomed Online 16: 311–320.

Youssef, M., Van der Veen, F., Al-Inany, H.G. et al. (2014). Gonadotropin-releasing hormone agonist versus HCG for oocyte triggering in antagonist-assisted reproductive technology. Cochrane Database Syst Rev 10: CD008046.

30

Preimplantation Genetic Diagnosis and Screening

Colleen Lynch and Brendan Ball

Introduction

Preimplantation testing of embryos is seen by many, especially the general public, as a new and experimental technology. However, the first babies were born following this treatment little over 10 years following the birth of the first *in* vitro fertilization (IVF) baby (Handyside et al. 1990). In fact, Robert Edwards, a pioneer of both IVF and preimplantation testing, performed sexing of rabbit blastocysts (Edwards and Gardner 1967) 10 years before the world's first IVF birth, that would eventually lead to his Nobel prize.

Preimplantation testing of embryos requires IVF technologies, given that couples have to undergo IVF treatment to produce embryos for testing. Recent advances in both IVF technologies, molecular genetics, and cytogenetics have opened the door to offering such treatments to a much wider range of patients. There are two main categories of preimplantation testing: (i) preimplantation genetic diagnosis (PGD) involving testing for monogenic disease, tissue type, gender, and chromosome rearrangements, and (ii) preimplantation genetic screening (PGS) for the identification of chromosomally normal, or euploid, embryos in IVF treatment cycles (this is also known as PGD-AS, where AS stands for aneuploidy screening).

In recent years, PGD has garnered wider acceptance as a feasible reproductive option for couples at risk of passing a heritable condition to their children. The selection and use of unaffected embryos is, for most, an acceptable alternative to prenatal diagnosis and selective termination. For some,

however, there is still the issue of what happens to affected embryos and the message it sends to affected individuals. PGS remains more controversial, even within the scientific and medical communities, given different practices and technologies have shown conflicting results, for example decreasing pregnancy rates, providing no benefit, and increasing pregnancy rates (Mastenbroek et al. 2011). The theory behind the intervention – the high percentage of aneuploidy in human embryos – remains sound, however, and recent studies involving blastocyst biopsy and comprehensive chromosome screening are proving promising.

Preimplantation Genetic Diagnosis

PGD was developed in response to couples at risk of passing heritable conditions to their children. The diagnosis of affected embryos prior to implantation and conception circumvents the need for prenatal testing and selective termination. PGD is used in the following situations:

- Monogenic disorders inherited from a parent (dominant condition, e.g. Huntington's disease, achondroplasia, myotonic dystrophy).
- Monogenic disorders where neither parent is affected, but there may be a background of a wider family history or the birth of an affected child (recessive condition, e.g. cystic fibrosis, sickle cell anaemia, or X-linked conditions, e.g. Duchenne muscular dystrophy, haemophilia).

- Chromosome rearrangements where a parent has a balanced chromosome rearrangement such as a translocation or inversion.
- Medically indicated gender selection, where a genetic condition only affects one gender, or affects one gender more severely.
- Human leukocyte antigen (HLA) tissue matching, to enable the conception of a child who is HLA compatible with an existing child requiring a bone marrow or stem cell transplant (often performed in conjunction with testing for a recessive monogenic disorder).

PGD Technologies

The first PGD cases were performed in 1989 for X-linked monogenic disorders (Handyside et al. 1990). At this time, the specific genes and mutations involved in many conditions were unknown. Thus, in the situation of X-linked monogenic disorders, couples were offered prenatal diagnosis via chorionic villus sampling or amniocentesis with cytogenetic analysis to determine the gender of the fetus. Although only 50% of male fetuses would be affected, in some cases the inability to perform specific disease testing meant that to avoid the condition, selective termination of male pregnancies was the only option. PGD was developed as an alternative for couples who had already undergone previous terminations or had trouble conceiving naturally.

PGD was performed as a clinical treatment for the first time at Hammersmith Hospital in the UK. Couples at risk of having children with the X-linked conditions Lesch-Nyhan syndrome, adrenoleukodystrophy, Duchenne muscular dystrophy, and X-linked mental retardation underwent IVF cycles with embryo biopsy at the Day 3 stage. Analysis was performed by amplification of a Y chromosome specific repeat sequence detected via gel electrophoresis – in the absence of amplification the embryo was inferred to be female. This was made possible by the development of the polymerase chain reaction (PCR), allowing exponential amplification of specific DNA targets. The short amount of time required for the analysis protocol meant that embryos could be transferred on the same day as biopsy, as blastocyst culture would not be robust or routine for a number of years. Later, the technique was improved by amplification of both X- and Y-linked sequences and then the use of

fluorescent *in situ* hybridization (FISH) allowing for the visualization of both sex chromosomes, XX or XY, and reducing the possibility of misdiagnosis.

The introduction of FISH to single-cell work opened up the possibility of PGD to couples where one carried a chromosome rearrangement – a reciprocal or robertsonian translocation or an inversion. This was first applied in the mid-1990s, using FISH probes specific to the chromosomal breakpoints and enabling the detection of different unbalanced segregation patterns (Munne et al. 1998), although it had already been applied to general aneuploidy screening. The use of PGD for chromosome rearrangements remained more controversial as some groups showed that couples would be successful in the same time frame naturally when compared with multiple PGD cycles (Scriven et al. 2013). However, this failed to consider the emotional impact of recurrent miscarriage for couples. The advent of array-based comparative genomic hybridization (aCGH), then next generation sequencing (NGS), allowed off-the-shelf PGD testing for patients with chromosome rearrangements which would identify not only unbalanced segregants, but also any other aneuploidy present in the sample (Fiorentino et al. 2011; Zhang et al. 2016) (Figure 30.1). This has contributed to higher pregnancy rates and reduced miscarriage rates, and a wider application of the treatment.

In 1992, the molecular techniques that first allowed the gender determination of embryos were extended to look at specific disease-causing genetic mutations. Whilst the majority of groups continued to focus on blastomere biopsy, some undertook a combination of polar body and blastomere analysis – a position that was as much to do with legal implications as science. The first monogenic condition for which PGD was undertaken to detect a specific disease-causing mutation in human embryos was cystic fibrosis (Handyside et al. 1992) – previously, much research had taken place on mouse embryos. The deltaF508 mutation is the highest frequency cystic fibrosis transmembrane conductance regulator (*CFTR*) mutation and is a 3 base pair deletion. Thus a nested PCR of the region and gel electrophoresis allowed the detection of DNA homo- and heteroduplexes and the identification of affected, unaffected, and carrier embryos. However, this technique was vulnerable to failed amplification of a specific allele, as the first gender

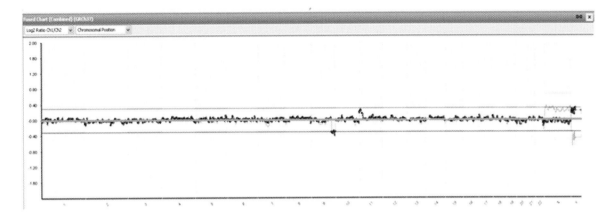

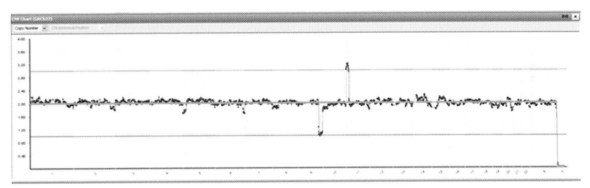

Figure 30.1 Preimplantation genetic diagnosis for a reciprocal translocation between the long arm chromosome 9 and the short arm of chromosome 11. The top and bottom images show analysis of the same trophectoderm sample via array-based comparative genomic hybridization and next generation sequencing respectively, revealing an unbalanced female karyotype. Reproduced with permission of Cooper Genomics.

selection cases had been. The introduction of multiplexing protocols allowed multiple linked markers to be used to follow disease inheritance (Dreesen et al. 2000) and then robust and accurate methods of whole genome amplification negated the need for multiplexing and greatly increased the number of linked markers that could be run and improved the reliability of testing (Spits et al. 2006). This also allowed more than one genetic condition to be tested for, or more commonly, to test for both disease and HLA type in embryos. For many years, these technologies were employed with little change to the diagnosis of monogenic disorders. However, the advent of single nucleotide polymorphism (SNP) arrays promises to be the biggest paradigm shift in the field since its introduction (Natesan et al. 2014) and potentially allows the tandem identification of meiotic aneuploidy. Karyomapping involves using

DNA samples from the couple requesting treatment and a reference (e.g. an affected child) to identify the parental origin at all SNP loci. This can be related to embryo samples to see if they have inherited the parental SNPs associated with the genetic condition (Figure 30.2). The genome wide coverage of this technique means that it can be used for the majority of single gene disorders and removes the need for the development of patient-specific tests.

Regulation and Guidelines

Regulation of PGD and PGS differs from country to country– whilst there may be no regulation in one country, it may be outlawed entirely in another. In addition to offering treatment in line with local regulatory requirements and accrediting or licensing bodies, IVF clinics should have their own guidelines

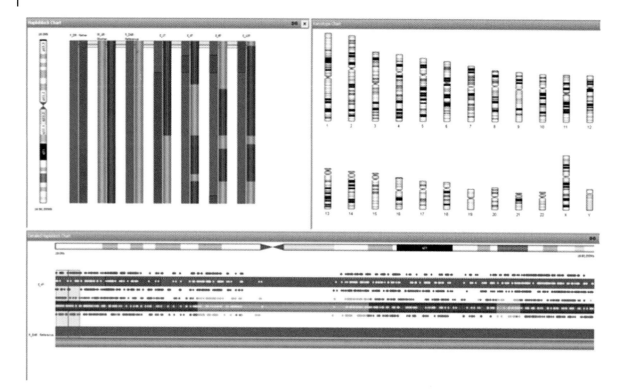

Figure 30.2 Software analysis of karyomapping data (Illumina). Preimplantation genetic diagnosis for a genetic mutation at 16p13.3. In the case of a recessive genetic condition where the reference was an affected child, embryo 8 would be affected, embryos 1 and 4 would be paternal carriers, and embryo 10 would be a maternal carrier. In the case of a paternally inherited dominant condition, where the reference was an affected child, embryos 1, 4, and 8 would be affected and embryo 10 would be unaffected. The detailed haploblock chart shows the single nucleotide polymorphism calling along chromosome 16 for embryo 4. Reproduced with permission of Cooper Genomics.

for staff, especially if offering PGD (Harton et al. 2011a). These may include stipulating which conditions PGD can be offered for and consideration of:

- Penetrance and variability
- Age of onset
- Symptoms.

For each case, the clinic may also wish to consider the reliability of the test available, likelihood of success, and safety (including any medical contraindications where an individual is affected by the condition for which testing is being performed). The clinic should also be able to provide or access appropriate counselling for couples seeking treatment including:

- Genetic risk assessment
- Reproductive options
- IVF-related counselling
- PGD counselling.

Preimplantation Genetic Screening

The introduction of FISH to single cell PGD was only subsequent to chromosome screening and PGS (Munne et al. 1993). The age-related decline in natural and IVF birth rates is linked to increased aneuploidy rates (Figure 30.3), which contribute to failed implantation, miscarriage, and increased rates of Down, Edwards, and Patau syndromes. Theoretically, the identification and negative selection of chromosomally abnormal embryos should mitigate the age effect in IVF and increase implantation and reduce miscarriage rates in patients of advanced maternal age. Thus, PGS was generally indicated in patients with advanced maternal age, recurrent miscarriage, and recurrent implantation failure and was reported to improve success rates (Munne 2002). However,

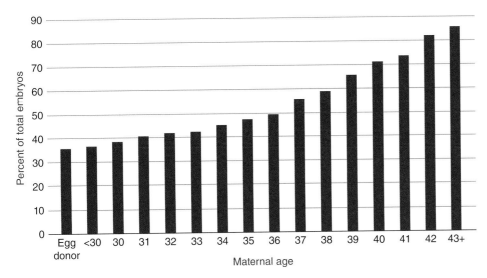

Figure 30.3 Data collected by Cooper Genomics showing the percentage of aneuploid embryos by maternal age. Reproduced with permission of Cooper Genomics.

there were a number of issues with this strategy. Firstly, FISH could only test a limited number of chromosomes– generally between five and eight. The chromosomes tested were those associated with miscarriage and live birth, meaning many abnormalities that would result in failed implantation were undetected. Secondly, there were a number of technical artefacts affecting the reliability of the testing: loss of micronuclei during cell fixing, split signals, and overlapping signals. Thirdly, the incidence and impact of mosaicism was not fully understood. Thus, when randomized clinical trials (RCTs) were published it was demonstrated that PGS in fact gave no advantage, or even reduced success rates (Mastenbroek et al. 2011). This was controversial at the time and hotly contended by the initial pioneers of the treatment who continued to evidence improved success rates (Munne et al. 2007). However, it did lead to many changes in practice, most notably the introduction of comprehensive chromosome screening (CCS). Despite more recent RCTs and systematic reviews supporting the use of PGS when CCS is employed, the majority of the scientific community seems to remain skeptical (Gleicher and Orvieto 2017).

Human reproduction is characteristic among mammalian species for the high rate of chromosomally abnormal gametes and embryos produced. Ten to fifteen percent of clinically recognized pregnancies end in first trimester miscarriage, which does not include occult or missed abortions. Transient implantation may occur with minimal disruption to the menstrual cycle and an individual might never realize that it has occurred. More than half of these events, 60–80%, are a result of aneuploidy in the embryo. Additionally, an even higher rate of aneuploidy exists at the embryo stage than detected in pregnancy given that many chromosomally abnormal embryos will simply fail to implant. Thus, the rationale behind PGS remains sound and the advent of CCS has led to evidence for it to be best employed as a method of embryo selection in patients with a good prognosis.

Unlike PGD, PGS has seen vast and regular changes in the technologies employed – from the advent of PGS via FISH looking at a single data point on a limited number of chromosomes, to quantitative PCR (qPCR) looking at two to four data points per chromosome, array-based comparative hybridization looking at hundreds of points per chromosome, and NGS looking at tens of thousands of data points per chromosome (Handyside 2013).

PGS Technologies

Most laboratories performing PGS now offer testing via technologies allowing CCS, usually aCGH, qPCR, or NGS. NGS is likely to become the most common technology as it is a quantitative technology with accurate detection of mosaicism and segmental changes, although this has also raised issues with respect to clinical management of patients (Capalbo et al. 2017; Sachdev et al. 2017). NGS also has high scalability, which means a significant reduction in cost per sample at higher volumes.

NGS involves creating tagged DNA fragments of 100–200 bp which are sequenced in parallel. These are compared to a reference genome and the read depth within each chromosome can be compared across the genome. The read depth is proportional to the copy number, and so trisomy or monosomy results in a greater or lesser read depth respectively (Figure 30.4). These results can be generated with genome coverage of only 5% (Handyside 2013). Whilst aCGH and NGS can both be used in single cells (i.e. can be used for polar body, blastomere or trophectoderm testing), qPCR requires multiple cells (i.e. trophectoderm). It continues to be used by clinics requiring a quick turnaround and fresh embryo transfer. It is also used by some who do not wish to know about segmental changes of mosaicism within the sample. A high-order multiplex PCR reaction is used to amplify markers on each chromosome – usually a minimum of two per arm – followed by a rapid quantification of each product (Handyside 2013).

The Embryology Laboratory

An absolute prerequisite to preimplantation genetic testing is the availability of a proficient embryology laboratory and access to a specialist genetics testing centre. Ideally, the genetics laboratory would be located with the IVF centre, but this is not always an option. The majority of IVF clinics work with an

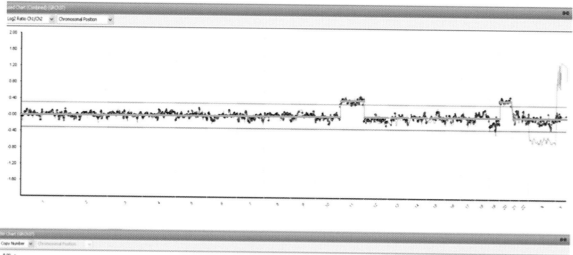

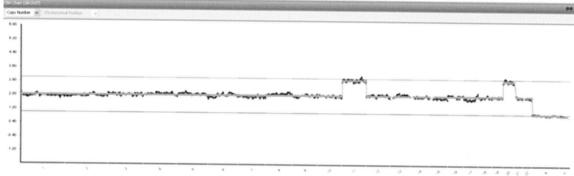

Figure 30.4 Preimplantation genetic screening for chromosome aneuploidy. The top and bottom images show analysis of the same trophectoderm sample via array-based comparative genomic hybridization and next generation sequencing respectively, revealing a male karyotype with trisomy of chromosomes 11 and 20. Reproduced with permission of Cooper Genomics.

independent specialist genetics laboratory. Whilst this requires coordination between laboratories, the transport of samples, and a service level agreement covering legal, insurance, and accountability issues it is an increasingly common arrangement that is usually very successful.

Beyond the training and validation of embryologists in biopsy and the tubing of samples, the embryology laboratory needs to consider other factors that will impact upon the success of patient treatment cycles:

- Air handling: all laboratories should operate within their regulatory requirements for air quality. Positive air pressure and class II hoods minimize the risk of contamination in the biopsy and tubing procedures.
- Incubation: biopsy necessitates multiple movements and door openings of incubators. An incubation system with quick recovery rates is an advantage.
- Culture system: with most laboratories moving to trophectoderm biopsy and freezing at the blastocyst stage, a robust culture system supporting embryos to Day 6 of development with good blastocyst formation rates is essential.
- Vitrification: the combination of trophectoderm biopsy with newer technologies such as karyomapping and NGS necessitates the freezing of embryos pending the return of results. Thus a robust vitrification system and successful clinical frozen embryo replacement programme is required.

Approaches to Biopsy

As a result of differences in local and national regulation, differences in practice for preimplantation testing will remain, but should not preclude best practice within that setting (Harton et al. 2011a). Historically, it has been recommended that insemination is via intracytoplasmic sperm injection (ICSI) prior to PCR-based testing (Harton et al. 2011b) primarily due to the risk of contamination from extraneous bound sperm (Wilton et al. 2009). However, research involving amplification of sperm DNA uses modified protocols to those used in preimplantation testing as the condensed nature of sperm DNA

makes it difficult to amplify (Patassini et al. 2013). Biopsy is generally performed at one of three stages:

- Polar body biopsy on Day 0 and 1
- Blastomere biopsy on Day 3
- Trophectoderm biopsy on Day 5 and 6.

However, some laboratories have performed sequential biopsies, for example polar bodies followed by blastomere biopsy, some have performed biopsy on Day 4 at the morula stage, and some continue culture for potential biopsy at Day 7.

A pH stable medium should be used to support the handling and manipulation of oocytes and embryos outside the incubator. For all techniques a microscope equipped with an ICSI rig and laser are also preferred (Figure 30.5). It is possible to breach the zona pellucida (ZP) mechanically using needles, or chemically with acid tyrodes or pronase, but these techniques have become less popular with the advent of the laser. It is very important for the embryologist to understand the operation of the laser to avoid damage to the embryo. Lasers can be fixed (the embryo/dish must be moved to the laser target) or directional (the laser target can be moved to a specific area on the embryo). Additionally, the power of different commercially available lasers may differ. When selecting a hole size on the laser software, the embryologist is, in fact, selecting the pulse length. A more powerful laser requires a shorter pulse length to create the desired hole size. The longer the pulse length, the bigger the hole created and the larger the field affected by the energy from the laser. Thus, it is always best practice to use a lower pulse length and multiple small holes, rather than fewer larger holes.

Regardless of the stage at which the biopsy is performed, the sampled cell(s), must be washed and placed in PCR tubes for transport to the genetic testing laboratory. This is the stage of the process most vulnerable to contamination. It is recommended that this is performed in a laminar flow or class II hood. The embryologist should also be wearing sterile gloves, sleeves, and a surgical mask. The biopsied sample is usually washed, using a narrow diameter denudation pipette, through a number of drops of buffer (usually phosphate-buffered saline), as provided by the genetic testing laboratory, and then placed into a PCR tube containing a specified volume of buffer. This should then be spun down in

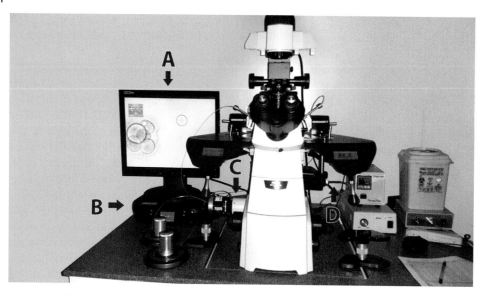

Figure 30.5 Typical embryology laboratory set up for biopsy including microscope, intracytoplasmic sperm injection holdings and syringes, laser, and PC with laser and biopsy software. Biopsy rig: A, video monitor; B, laser; C, video camera; D, laser fibre optic cable. Reproduced with permission of Bourn Hall Clinics IVF.

a microfuge before being frozen and stored to await transport to the genetic testing laboratory.

Polar Body Biopsy

The benefit of this approach is that no essential cellular material is removed for testing but it can only be used for maternally inherited genetic conditions and will not detect postmeiotic errors. The biggest advantage of polar body biopsy is that the ploidy of polar bodies I and II accurately predicts the ploidy of the zygote as shown through ESHRE's ESTEEM trial (Geraedts et al. 2011). It is often used where there are legal or ethical contraindications to embryo biopsy. For an accurate result both polar bodies must be removed and tested, either sequentially or simultaneously, the advantage of the former being the greater ease in differentiating them. The timing of the removal of the second polar body is important in terms of the completion of anaphase II, complete cleavage from the oocyte (reducing the risk of the presence of spindle remnants in the cytoplasmic bridge and removal of chromatids from the oocyte), and maximizing amplification rates (Magli et al. 2011). The process can be labour intensive, especially if the biopsies are performed sequentially, and given that not all oocytes will fertilize.

If performing sequential biopsy, the first polar body should be removed 36–42 h post-human chorionic gonadotropin administration (Verklinsky et al. 1990). The oocytes should be held in individual drops of buffered culture medium overlayed with oil during the biopsy procedure. With the polar body at the 12 o'clock position a slit of 15–20 μm is made at 1–2 o'clock (Figure 30.6). The first polar body is removed and then the oocytes are inseminated using ICSI. The second polar body can then be removed from fertilized oocytes at least 9 h after ICSI (Magli et al. 2011) using the same procedure and same ZP breach. Where simultaneous biopsy of both polar bodies is performed, the same procedures are followed and biopsy is performed at least 9–22 h after ICSI (Verlinsky et al. 1997).

Cleavage Stage Biopsy

Historically, cleavage stage was the most common embryo biopsy approach (De Ryke et al. 2015), although trophectoderm biopsy is now being more widely adopted. The technique is less labour intensive than polar body biopsy, as only embryos that have reached the requisite cell number and are of sufficient quality are biopsied. Using older PGD and PGS technologies, it allowed the return of results for

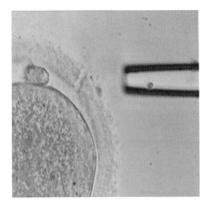 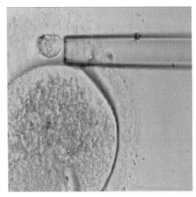 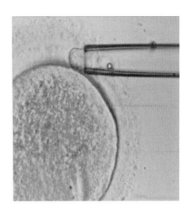

Figure 30.6 First polar body biopsy with polar body in 12 o'clock position and zona pellucida breach at 1–2 o'clock. With the oocyte and polar body on the same plane of focus, the biopsy needle can be inserted through the breach with light suction used to remove the polar body. Reproduced with permission of CARE Fertility.

fresh embryo transfer at the blastocyst stage. Newer technologies require embryo freezing and many clinics are moving towards frozen transfers to optimize outcomes (Coates et al. 2017). The biopsy is normally performed on the morning of Day 3, but may vary according to laboratory procedures. Criteria for embryos to be considered suitable for biopsy should be in place, with those having fewer than five cells, multinucleation/anucleation, or high levels of fragmentations, normally being excluded. The recent preference for trophectoderm biopsy over cleavage stage biopsy is mainly due to concerns relating to a possible reduction of implantation potential (Scott et al. 2013) and false positive/negative results relating to mosaicism (Baart et al. 2006; Hansen et al. 2009). Cleavage stage biopsy can be used to test for maternal and paternally inherited conditions, as well as meiotic and mitotic errors, but may miss some mitotic errors depending on the stage they arise at or the cell selected for testing.

Embryos should be held in individual drops of buffered Ca^{2+}/Mg^{2+}-free medium overlaid with oil. The Ca^{2+}/Mg^{2+}-free medium disrupts cadherin bonds between blastomeres, meaning individual blastomeres are more easily removed from the embryo. Time in Ca^{2+}/Mg^{2+}-free medium should be limited as much as possible and the embryo should be washed through multiple wash drops of culture medium before being returned to culture. The blastomere selected for biopsy should be of average size and have a visible nucleus. The embryo should be held with the selected blastomere at around the

3 o'clock position and the ZP breached nearby, where there are no blastomeres in contact with it where possible, making an opening of 30–40 μm (Figure 30.7). Ideally, only a single blastomere shoud be removed, as the removal of additional cells impacts on the embryo's implantation potential (Goosens et al. 2008). The most common practice is to aspirate the chosen blastomere with a biopsy pipette. The blastomere may also be removed by extrusion (where the blastomere is squeezed through the opening in the ZP by pushing against the exterior of the embryo with the biopsy pipette) or displacement (where medium is gently injected into the embryo to displace the blastomere through the ZP breach).

Trophectoderm Biopsy

Trophectoderm biopsy was first reported in 2004 (De Boer et al. 2004) but is now becoming widely adopted. The procedure is proposed to be safer than cleavage stage biopsy in that it is reported to have little to no impact on implantation (Scott et al. 2013), while the cells removed are destined to form placental rather than fetal tissue. Additionally, although multiple cells are removed, improving the robustness of the testing performed, they form a smaller proportion of the cellular volume of the embryo. Trophectoderm biopsy can be used for testing in the same scenarios as cleavage stage and may pick up additional meiotic errors occurring after Day 3. Mosaicism still exists at the blastocyst stage, but

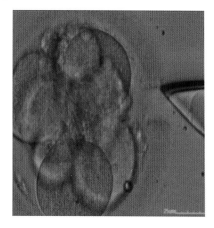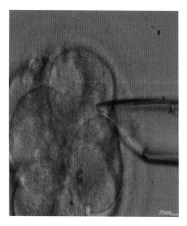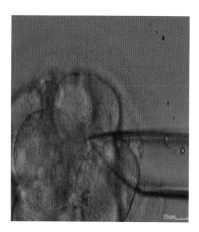

Figure 30.7 Blastomere biopsy with selected blastomere and zona pellucida breach at around 3 o'clock. With the zona pellucida and blastomere on the same plane of focus, the biopsy needle can be inserted through the breach with light suction used to remove the blastomere. Reproduced with permission of CARE Fertility.

technologies like NGS allow samples to be categorized as aneuploid, euploid, or aneuploid mosaic. However, this requires limits for each of these categorizations to be set, and to an extent it supposes that the levels of aneuploidy within the sampled cells is mirrored by the rest of the embryo. Nonetheless, some clinics are adopting the transfer of mosaic embryos in the absence of the availability of euploids, and achieving live births, albeit at a reduced rate (Greco et al. 2015; Munne et al. 2016). Whilst trophectoderm biopsy may initially appear the least labour intensive of the biopsy approaches, given the lower number of items being biopsied, the fact that embryos will reach blastocyst stage at different times over Days 5, 6, and 7 can make the biopsy logistically difficult for the laboratory in the initial stages of offering the procedure. The additional need to vitrify each biopsied blastocyst is also a consideration.

Blastocysts can be biopsied once they have cavitated and the inner cell mass (ICM) and trophectoderm can be differentiated. It is common practice to hatch the embryos on Day 3 or late on Day 4 (when it may be possible to visualize the ICM) to encourage herniation of the trophectoderm and make the biopsy procedure easier on Day 5 or 6 (McArthur et al. 2005). However, it is also possible to hatch the embryo at the time of biopsy (Capalbo et al. 2014). Whenever hatching is performed, the breach created should be 10–20 μm. It is important to biopsy cells

as far from the ICM as possible. If the embryo has been hatched on Day 3 or 4, or has hatched naturally, the ICM may be in the portion of cells that is herniating. In such cases the hole can be enlarged to take cells further away from the ICM, or a second breach can be created further away from the ICM. Where a second breach is created it may be advisable to perform a partial or total ZP dissection prior to embryo transfer to encourage normal hatching.

The blastocysts should be held in individual drops of buffered culture medium overlaid with oil. The blastocyst should be held with the herniating trophectoderm cells to be biopsied at the 3 o'clock position. The biopsy can be performed using a number of techniques (Figure 30.8):

- Laser: trophectoderm cells are aspirated into the biopsy pipette. With the embryo attached firmly to the holding, the laser is fired at cell junctions adjacent to the biopsy pipette, while the biopsy pipette is simultaneously drawn away. This should be continued, taking care not to fire the laser repeatedly in the same spot, until the sample of cells separates from the embryo.
- Mechanical: trophectoderm cells are aspirated into the biopsy pipette. The embryo is released from the holding and the embryo and biopsy pipette are positioned above the holding in the dish. The biopsy pipette is drawn down sharply across the holding, shearing the cells from the embryo.

(a) (b) (c)

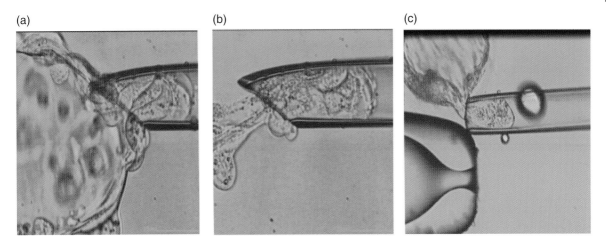

Figure 30.8 Trophectoderm biopsy with zona pellucida breach at around 3 o'clock. (a) Cells are aspirated into the biopsy pipette. (b) The laser is fired continually at different points on cell junctions as the biopsy pipette is drawn away, until the cells become detached. (c) The biopsy pipette is drawn sharply down across the holding pipette shearing the cells from the embryo. The laser can be used prior to this to create a weakness. Reproduced with permission of CARE Fertility.

- Laser and mechanical: trophectoderm cells are aspirated into the biopsy pipette. With the embryo attached firmly to the holding, the laser is fired at cell junctions adjacent to the biopsy pipette. The embryo is released from the holding and the embryo and biopsy pipette are positioned above the holding in the dish. The biopsy pipette is drawn down sharply across the holding, shearing the cells from the embryo.

It is important to try and avoid firing directly at cells and causing cell lysis. For reliable detection of mosaicism a minimum of five cells should be taken with care, as described, to minimize damage to cellular DNA.

Adverse Outcomes and Misdiagnosis

The true incidence of misdiagnosis using PGD and PGS is difficult to gauge. Many will go undetected, where a pregnancy or live birth does not occur, where there is no adverse indication (i.e. unaffected versus carrier), or where embryos are discarded without confirmatory diagnosis. Conversely, misdiagnosis may be incorrectly presumed in place of a natural conception. The ESHRE PGD consortium aims to collect and publish such data, although not all clinics offering the treatment report to the consortium. Between 1997 and 2010 they have reported 21 misdiagnoses via FISH for PGD or PGS and 13 via PCR-based approaches for PGD. This represents less than a 0.5% risk of misdiagnosis and is almost certainly lower than the actual figure (Harper et al. 2011; Moutou et al. 2014; De Ryke et al. 2015).

The causes of misdiagnosis can be categorized as human error, technical, or biological. In addition to this, the cause may be intrinsic (a known phenomenon or limitation) or extrinsic (introduced to the process) (Wilton et al. 2009). It is important to identify the specific root cause of the misdiagnosis to implement effective preventive or corrective action to prevent recurrence. For example, human errors may result from inadequate training, inadequate staff levels, or a failure of the standard operating procedure to fully or correctly describe the procedure.

Quality management is an essential part of preimplantation genetic testing. Identification and analysis of the likelihood and seriousness of risk and the implementation of preventive action is a necessity given the potential level of severity of adverse incidents in this field. Robust staff training, competency assessment, and comfirmatory diagnosis of untransferred embryos are vital parts of the embryology aspect of PGD and PGS programmes.

Conclusion

Since its inception in the late 1980s, PGD has become a widely accepted reproductive option to present to couples at risk of passing on hereditary genetic disease, although it does remain controversial and is against the law in some countries. Ethical arguments will always surround what conditions should be tested for, with testing of cancer susceptibility genes and adult onset disorders used as evidence by opponents of the treatment as a 'slippery slope' towards future eugenics. This highlights the importance of self-regulation and centralized regulation to ensure continued confidence in the industry and support for an important treatment option.

PGS remains a more controversial treatment option. The basic tenet of selecting against chromosome aneuploidy in embryos is sound but much remains to be understood about the biology of the early human embryo in this respect. Again, the onus is on the industry to research and investigate chromosome lineage in embryos and conduct large scale RCTs in an effort to negate charges of commercialism and profiteering in the field.

Future technologies may involve less invasive testing of embryos, using spent culture medium and blastocoele fluid to see if the same level of information can be obtained accurately and reliably, negating the need for biopsy of the oocyte or embryo.

References

Baart, E.B., Martini, E., van den Berg, I. et al. (2006). Preimplantation genetic screening reveals a high incidence of aneuploidy and mosaicism in embryos from young women undergoing IVF. Hum Reprod 21: 223–233.

Capalbo, A., Rienzi, L., Cimadomo, D. et al. (2014). Correlation between standard blastocyst morphology, euploidy adn implantation: an observational study in two centres involving 956 screened blastocysts. Human Reprod 29: 1173–1181.

Capalbo, A., Rienzi, L. and Maria Ubaldi, F. (2017). Diagnosis and clinical management of duplications and deletions. Fertil Steril 107: 12–18.

Coates, A., Kung, A., Mounts, E. et al. (2017). Optimal euploid embryo transfer strategy, fresh versus frozen, after preimplantation genetic screening with next generation sequencing: a randomized controlled trial. Ferti Steril 107: 723–730.

De Boer, K.A, Catt, J.W, Jansen, R.P.S et al. (2004). Moving to blastocyst biopsy for preimplantation genetic diagnosis and single embryo transfer at Sydney IVF. Fertil Steril 82: 295–298.

De Ryke, M., Belva, F., Goosens, V. et al. (2015). ESHRE PGD Consortium data collection XIII: cycles from January to December 2010 with pregnancy follow up to October 2011. Hum Reprod 30: 1763–1789.

Dreesen, J.C., Jacobs, I.J., Bras, M. et al. (2000). Multiplex PCR of polymorphic markers flanking the CFTR gene; a general approach for preimplantation genetic diagnosis of cystic fibrosis. Mol Hum Reprod 6: 391–396.

Edwards, R.G. and Gardner, R.L. (1967). Sexing of live rabbit blastocysts. Nature 214(5088): 576–577.

Fiorentino, F., Spizzichino, L., Bono, S. et al. (2011). PGD for reciprocal and Robertsonian translocations using array comparative genomic hybridization. Hum Reprod 26: 1925–1935.

Geraedts, J., Montag, M., Magli,M.C et al. (2011). Polar body array CGH for prediction of the status of the corresponding oocyte. Part I: clinical results. Hum Reprod 26: 3173–3180.

Gleicher, N. and Orvieto, R. (2017). Is the hypothesis of preimplantation genetic screening (PGS) still supportable? A review. J Ovar Res 10: 21.

Goosens, V., De Ryke, M., De Vos, A. et al. (2008). Diagnostic efficiency, embryonic development and clinical outcome after the biopsy of one or two blastomeres for preimplantation genetic diagnosis. Hum Reprod 23: 481–492.

Greco, E., Minasi, M.G. and Fiorentino, F. (2015). Healthy babies after intrauterine transfer of mosaic aneuploid blastocysts. N Engl J Med 373: 2089–2090.

Handyside, A.H. (2013). 24-chromsome copy number analysis: a comparison of available technologies. Fertil Steril 100: 595–602.

Handyside, A.H., Kontogianni, E.H., Hardy, K. et al. (1990). Pregnancies from biopsied preimplantation embryos sexed by Y-specific DNA amplification. Nature 344: 768–770.

Handyside, A.H., Lesko, J.G., Tarin, J.J. et al. (1992). Birth of a normal girl after in vitro fertilization and preimplantation diagnostic testing for cystic fibrosis. N Engl J Med 2327: 905–909.

Hanson, C., Hardarson, T., Lundin, K. et al. (2009). Re-analysis of 166 embryos not transferred after PGS with advanced reproductive maternal age as indication. Hum Reprod 11: 2960–2964.

Harper, J.C, Wilton, L., Traeger-Synodinos, J., et al. (2011). The ESHRE PGD Consortium: 10 years of data collection. Hum Reprod Update 18: 234–247.

Harton, G., Braude,P., Lashwood, A. et al. (2011a). ESHRE PGD consortium best practice guidelines for optimisation of a PGD centre for PGD/preimplantation genetics screening. Hum Reprod 26: 14–24.

Harton, G., Magli, M.C., Lundin, K., et al. (2011b). ESHRE PGD Consortium/Embryology Special Interest Group – best practice guidelines for polar body and embryo biopsy for preimplantation genetics diagnosis/screening. Hum Reprod 26: 41–46.

McArthur, S.J, Leigh, D., Marshall, J.T. et al. (2005). Pregnancies and live births after trophectoderm biopsy and preimplantation genetic testing of human blastocysts. Fertil Steril 84: 1628–1636.

Magli, M.C., Montag, M., Koster M., et al (2011). Polar body aCGH for prediction of the status of the corresponding oocyte. Part II: technical aspects. Hum Reprod 26: 3181–3185.

Mastenbroek, S., Twisk, M., van der Veen, F. et al. (2011). Preimplantation genetic screening: a systematic review and meta-analysis of RCTs. Hum Reprod Update 17: 454–466.

Moutou, C., Goosens, V., Coonen, E. et al. (2014). ESHRE PGD Consortium data collection XII: cycles from January to December (2009) with pregnancy follow up to October 2010. Hum Reprod 29: 880–903.

Munne, S. (2002). Preimplantation genetic diagnosis of numerical and structural chromosome abnormalities. Reprod BioMed Online 4: 183–196.

Munne, S., Gianaroli, L., Tur-Kaspa, I., et al. (2007). Substandard application of preimplantation genetic screening may interfere with its clinical success. Fertil Steril 88: 781–784.

Munné, S., Grifo, J., Wells, D. (2016). Mosaicism: 'survival of the fittest' versus 'no embryo left behind'. Fertil Steril 105: 1146–1149.

Munne, S., Lee, A., Rosenwaks, Z. et al. (1993). Diagnosis of major chromosome aneuploidies in human preimplantation embryos. Hum Reprod 8: 2185–2191.

Munne, S., Scott, R., Sable, D. et al. (1998). First pregnancies after preconception diagnosis of translocations of maternal origin. Fertil Steril 69: 675–681.

Natesan, S.A., Handyside, A.H., Thornhill, A.R. et al. (2014). Live birth after PGD with confirmation by a comprehensive approach (karyomapping) for simultaneous detection of monogenic and chromosomal disorders. Reprod Biomed Online 29: 600–6005.

Patassini, C., Garolla, A., Bottacin, A. et al. (2013). Molecular karyotyping of human single sperm by array-comparative genomic hybridisation. PLoS One 8: e60922.

Sachdev, N.M., Maxwell, S.M., Besser, A.G. et al. (2017). Diagnosis and clinical management of embryonic mosaicism. Fertil Steril 107: 6–11.

Scott, R.T, Upham, K.M, Forman, E.J et al. (2013). Cleavage-stage biopsy significantly impairs human embryonic implantation potential while blastocyst biopsy does not: a randomized and paired clinical trial. Fertil Steril 100: 624–630.

Scriven, P.N., Flinter, F.A., Khalaf, Y. et al. (2013). Benefits and drawbacks of preimplantation genetic diagnosis (PGD) for reciprocal translocations: lessons from a prospective cohort study. Eur J Hum Genet 21: 1035–1041.

Spits, C., Le Caignec, C., De Rycke, M., et al. (2006). Optimization and evaluation of single-cell whole-genome multiple displacement amplification. Hum Mutat 27: 496–503.

Verlinsky, Y., Ginsberg, N., Lifchez, A. et al. (1990). Analysis of the first polar body: preconception genetic diagnosis. Hum Reprod 5: 826–829.

Verlinsky, Y., Rechitsky, S., Cieslak, J. et al. (1997). Preimplantation diagnosis of single gene disorders by two-step oocyte genetic analysis using first and second polar body. Biochem Mol Med 62: 182–187.

Wilton, L., Thornhill, A., Traeger-Synodinos, J. et al. (2009). The causes of misdiagnosis and adverse outcomes in PGD. Hum Reprod 24: 1221–1228.

Zhang, W., Liu, Y., Wang, L. et al. (2016). Clinical application of next-generation sequencing in preimplantation genetic diagnosis cycles for Robertsonian and reciprocal translocations. J Assist Reprod Genet 33: 899–906.

31

Long-Term Follow-Up of Children Conceived Through *In Vitro* Fertilization

Omar Abdel-Mannan and Alastair G. Sutcliffe

Introduction

The population of children born after *in vitro* fertilization (IVF) has grown substantially over the last two decades following the birth in 1978 of the first child conceived by IVF (Louise Brown). Since then, more than six million children have been conceived through assisted reproductive technologies (ART) (Adamson et al. 2012; Focus on Reproduction 2016). Whilst these techniques are generally considered safe, there has been a need to study the long-term outcomes of ART, especially with the introduction of new technologies including cryopreservation and intracytoplasmic sperm injection (ICSI). The prevalence of major malformations following ART has ranged from 5.6 to 9.0% in comparison to 4.2 to 5% in the general population (Hansen et al. 2002; Merlob et al. 2005). There are various reasons why ART-conceived children may be exposed to greater health risks than their naturally conceived (NC) counterparts. ART carries a significantly increased risk of multiple pregnancies, which are associated with a higher rate of prematurity and low birth weight. These, in turn, carry well-established risks of morbidity for the child (Fauser et al. 2005). Subfertile couples have a unique background biology, which may be a risk factor for complications during gestation and birth (Gray and Wu 2000). Procedural factors such as artificial induction of ovulation, and freezing and manipulation of oocytes may also confer health risks on ART children.

The interpretation of data from epidemiological studies of ART is challenging due to differences in data collection and a lack of uniformity of clinical definitions. Nevertheless, it is crucial to follow up outcomes post ART, particularly as new techniques are constantly being introduced. This chapter will focus on summarizing the range of health outcomes being studied in ART children and providing insight into the long-term health threats for children conceived using ART. We will discuss the prognosis for various risks including congenital malformations, neurodisability, neurodevelopmental outcomes, malignancy, and future fertility.

Perinatal Risks

The higher frequency of multiple births in assisted reproduction has largely been attributed to a higher risk of prematurity and low birth weight in this cohort. Thus, multiple birth rates of between 22 and 32% have been reported in European and American studies following ART compared to 1–2% of all births in the general population (Fauser et al. 2005). Multiple pregnancy is a well-established risk factor for numerous adverse outcomes including neonatal mortality, congenital malformation, and disability amongst survivors (Koivisto et al. 1975). There has been a recent trend to limit the number of embryos transferred into the uterus per IVF cycle (single-embryo transfer, SET), for example in Sweden, where multiple birth rates have fallen to 5% while maintaining pregnancy rates of 30–40% per transfer (Bergh 2005). Nevertheless, numerous meta-analyses have shown increased risk of complications including intensive care admission in singleton SET babies compared with NC singleton controls (Helmerhost et al. 2004).

Clinical Reproductive Science, First Edition. Edited by Michael Carroll.
© 2019 John Wiley & Sons Ltd. Published 2019 by John Wiley & Sons Ltd.
Companion website: www.wiley.com/go/carroll/clinicalreproductivescience

With regard to prematurity, a meta-analysis in 2004 showed a doubling in relative risk of preterm birth in ART singletons compared with NC singletons and an even greater risk of prematurity (less than 32 weeks) in the ART group (McGovern et al. 2004). Numerous studies have shown that infertility itself is an independent risk factor of preterm birth. Henriksen et al. demonstrated that women conceiving after 7 months of trying for a baby had a 1.3 times greater risk of preterm delivery compared with women who conceived in the first 6 months (Henriksen et al. 1997). Admission to neonatal intensive care units, and neonatal morbidity and mortality are higher in infertile couples undergoing ovarian stimulation (without IVF) compared with NC couples (Ombelet et al. 2006). These increased complications associated with ART have led to a greater risk of perinatal mortality and admission to a neonatal intensive care unit.

Congenital Defects

The relationship between ART and increased risk of congenital anomalies has been well established through several meta-analyses after concerns were raised in the early 1980s and intensified following the introduction of ICSI (Rimm et al. 2004; Hansen et al. 2005). The increased risk remained only for singletons in subanalysis of the data. In their study, Hansen et al. established a twofold increased risk of major birth defects in children conceived by ART, including cardiovascular, urogenital, musculoskeletal, and chromosomal anomalies. However, a study by Davis et al. showed that IVF treatment did not confer an increased risk of congenital abnormalities as compared with ICSI, suggesting that the risk was more related to couples requiring fertility treatment generally (Davies et al. 2012). In contrast, a large Swedish study of over 32 000 IVF children demonstrated that the absolute risk of severe malformations was significantly higher in the IVF group compared with the NC group (3.7% IVF group; 3% NC group) (Orstavik et al. 2003).

There are also reports in the literature reporting an association between imprinting disorders including Russell–Silver syndrome, Angelman syndrome, Beckwith–Wiedemann syndrome and ART (Sutcliffe et al. 1995; Lidegaard et al. 2005; Cocchi et al. 2013). These exceedingly rare disorders result from abnormal methylation patterns on inherited genes, and have serious consequences for the children affected. However, it is important to note that many of these studies have significant methodological limitations, as reviewed by Sutcliffe and Ludwig (2007), for example, imprecise definition and classification of congenital abnormalities, differences in methods used to assess malformations, and differences in length of follow-up between groups. However, it is important that couples using ART be made aware of the increased risk of these major congenital abnormalities and that genetic testing is available in advance.

Neurological Outcome

Cerebral palsy (CP) is the most prevalent physical disability in childhood and affects around two children per 1000 live births. Various Scandinavian registry-based cohort studies have reported a significantly increased risk of CP diagnosis and hospitalizations with CP in ART children compared with NC children, with risk estimates between 1.6 and 3.7 fold (Ericson et al. 2002; Stromberg et al. 2002; Hvidtjorn et al. 2009). The risk can partly be explained by the increased proportion of preterm births and higher order pregnancies in ART children. A study using the Swedish Medical Birth Registry showed a fivefold increased risk of CP for singleton IVF children compared with NC children (Ericson et al. 2002). A meta-analysis by Hvidtjorn et al. (2009) with a total of 12 191 IVF singletons found an odds ratio (OR) for cerebral palsy of 1.8. No significant difference was found for IVF twins and NC twins (OR 1.0). The increased risk of CP in IVF singletons may be a consequence of the phenomenon of 'vanishing twins' in ART pregnancies, with the surviving co-twin having a higher incidence of CP (Glinianaia et al. 2002). Pinborg et al. (2005) reported that 10% of all singletons born from IVF originated from twin pregnancies with the surviving twin having an increased risk of low birth weight and prematurity. There was no significant difference in risk of CP or neurological sequelae between IVF twins and NC twins in this study.

The risk of epilepsy has been shown to be moderately elevated in some studies of ART children. For example, an investigation using the Danish national birth cohort found an increased risk of hospital admission due to epilepsy in singleton children born to subfertile couples, regardless of the use of ART (Sun et al. 2007). However, the results lost statistical significance when preterm deliveries were controlled for. Ericson et al. (2002) used the Swedish national register of IVF pregnancies and confirmed these findings with an increased risk of hospital admission due to epilepsy in IVF children.

An increased risk of neuropsychiatric disorders such autism and attention deficit hyperactivity disorder (ADHD) has been suggested for children born after IVF (Hvidtjorn et al. 2009; Källén et al. 2010). Autism spectrum disorders (ASD) are a group of conditions defined by stereotyped behaviours, communication defects, and social deficiencies. There is a clear shortage of studies investigating the association between ART and ASD, and the few that exist show conflicting results. High maternal age, high maternal educational level, and hormonal disturbances are three potential risk factors that may be predictive of an association. For instance, a Danish population study showed an increased risk of ASD diagnosis in children born after IVF or ovarian induction (Cederblad et al. 1996). After adjusting for maternal age, educational level, and birth weight, the risk however disappeared. It is important to note that the aetiology of ADHD is clearly very complex and many confounders may exist in studies investigating the relationship between ART and ADHD. Källén et al. (2011) investigated the risk of ADHD in 28 158 IVF children compared with 2 417 886 NC children and showed a small increase in the odds of drug-treated ADHD in the IVF group. In summary, it should be noted that there is currently no plausible hypothesis to link ADHD or autism with ART.

Neurodevelopmental Outcome

Several studies have investigated the neurodevelopmental outcome of children born by IVF and ICSI. Their findings have largely been consistent, with little evidence of any difference in neurodevelopmental outcome between ART and NC children.

Large-scale multicentre studies have investigated the long-term effects of ICSI in terms of development of preschool to school-aged children. For example, Ponjaert-Kristoffersen et al. (2005) found no significant differences in cognitive and motor development between 5-year-old ICSI and NC children. A prospective study by Sutcliffe et al. compared 208 ICSI conceived singleton children and 221 NC singleton children aged between 1 and 2, using the Griffiths Mental Development Scales (Sutcliffe et al, 2001). No difference was found between the study children and NC children in mean neurodevelopmental scores nor in any of the subscales of the Griffiths scales (Sutcliffe et al. 2003).

No evidence of limitations in educational performance at primary and secondary school level has been shown in IVF children compared with NC children (Ceelen et al. 2008a). Only a few studies have reported potential concerns regarding neurocognitive development in ART children. Bowen et al. (1998) reported delayed development in ART children at 13 months of age compared with NC children using the Bayley Scales of Infant Development. However, this study has been criticized for being statistically underpowered and using insufficient adjustment for demographic differences between groups.

Use of Health Services and Physical Health

ART children seem to have greater medical needs than their NC counterparts, although the evidence is somewhat inconsistent. In a large multicentre cohort study comparing the physical health of 5-year-old IVF and ICSI children with NC controls, Bonduelle et al. (2005) found a significantly higher rate of childhood illness in the former group. In addition, the use of medical therapy, hospital admissions, and surgical procedures (especially urogenital operations) were also increased. These findings are supported by a prospective, controlled, single-blinded study of ICSI children at 5.5 years old (Ludwig et al. 2008), which also found an increase in urogenital surgery and an increase in hospitalization. In a Swedish registry study with 16 000 IVF children, it was found that IVF children were hospitalized more often than non-IVF children for conditions such as asthma, infections, and accidents (Källén et al. 2005). It is important to note that certain factors need to be considered when healthcare utilization by ART children is discussed. For instance, the increased risk of cerebral palsy may account for such findings and there may be a degree of heightened parental anxiety regarding the health of these children (Ericson et al. 2002).

The majority of studies analysing growth of IVF children from birth to teen years have not found differences between ART and NC children (Ceelen et al. 2008a). Various parameters including weight, height, and head circumference of IVF and ICSI children at ages ranging from 6 months to 12 years in various studies have been reported to be normal. In addition, studies involving detailed physical examinations have not revealed significant differences between the two groups (Sutcliffe 2000; Källén et al. 2005). However, in a study of 299 IVF and 558 NC children, IVF singletons were significantly lighter in weight than NC controls up to 3 years of age (Koivurova et al. 2003) and a New Zealand-based cohort of 69 ART children were reported to be significantly taller than their NC counterparts, and also had higher serum levels of insulin-like growth factors I and II (Miles et al. 2007).

Certain studies have demonstrated that 8–18-year-old IVF children have higher blood pressure and blood glucose levels compared with age-matched controls (Ceelen et al. 2008b). Belva et al. (2007) showed that pubertal ICSI females have significantly increased central, peripheral, and total adiposity compared with NC controls, and ICSI-conceived males in later pubertal stages were also found to have increased peripheral adiposity.

Whilst many of these studies are methodologically flawed, these findings may be significant, if corroborated by population data, as it is well established via the Barker hypothesis that prenatal growth is associated with the development of cardiovascular diseases in adulthood (Barker 1995). The Barker hypothesis, more recently known as the 'developmental origins of health and disease hypothesis' (DOHaD), suggests that exposure to an adverse environment at key stages of development will cause adaptive changes, with subsequent medical sequelae in adult life, such as diabetes and cardiovascular disease.

Psychological Outcome

There have been theoretical concerns about the possibility of negative psychological effects of ART, especially with the invasive nature of the procedure and the need for repeated treatment causing extra stress for couples (Sutcliffe 2000). A study conducted in three countries using psychological testing of the cognitive, motor, and emotional behaviour aspects of 5-year olds reported minimal differences between ICSI children and NC children (Ponjaert-Kristoffersen et al. 2004). Interestingly, in this study the ICSI children had fewer behavioural problems and their parents had reduced stress compared with the control group. These findings were supported by a literature review showing no difference in the incidence of behavioural and socioemotional problems in IVF children compared with NC controls up to 8 years of age (Wagenaar et al. 2008).

Golombok et al. (1996) studied a cohort of 116 IVF children (compared with NC controls) initially between 4 and 8 years of age, and followed them up to the age of 12 years. The incidence of behavioural problems and psychiatric disorders was similar in both groups and maternal stress was lower in the IVF group. A Danish study analysed the emotional, social, and behavioural functioning of a cohort of 7–21-year-old children born with or without fertility assistance. Parental and self-reported emotional and hyperactivity scores were similar for both groups (Zhu et al. 2011). In summary, the idea that ART children experience negative psychological outcomes compared with their NC peers is not supported by the literature, with some studies actually reporting more positive relationships with their parents in ART children.

Fertility

The future fertility of ART offspring is a major concern for parents; parents treated by ICSI are 2.5 times more likely to question their child's future fertility (Fisher-Jeffes et al. 2006). There is a risk of Y microdeletions in the father being inherited by male offspring when ICSI is used since this technique is more commonly used for cases of male subfertility (Kurinczuk 2003). In a longitudinal cohort study of ICSI children, various markers of early testicular development (including testicular size, serum inhibin-B, anti-Müllerian hormone levels), were within the normal range, showing that fertility was unaffected by ART (De Schepper et al. 2009). Similarly, a study by Belva et al. (2007) demonstrated there was no significant difference in salivary testosterone levels between ICSI children and NC controls at 14 years of age, including those whose fathers had severe oligozoospermia. Nevertheless, female causes of infertility such as polycystic ovarian syndrome and endometriosis may have a heritable component, which may put a female offspring at increased risk of infertility (Frackiewicz et al. 2000). The fertility of children conceived by ART needs further assessment to ascertain the risk to these children and the effect of different techniques.

Cancer Risk

A limited number of studies have documented the risk of cancer in offspring conceived via IVF and ICSI. A large Danish study which included over 50 000 children followed for 10 years on average showed a standardized incidence ratio of 1.14 but no significant risk (Brinton et al. 2004). Previous registry-based studies gave similar reassuring results, with only smaller studies reporting links with retinoblastoma (Imhof et al. 2003) and hematopoietic malignancies (Brinton et al. 2004). In their comprehensive population-based linkage study, no increased risk of cancer was detected among children born after assisted conception (Williams et al. 2013) nor of leukaemia, neuroblastoma, retinoblastoma, central nervous system, renal or germ cell tumours. This conclusion is supported by a retro- spective cohort study comprising all children born after ART in Sweden, Denmark, Finland, and Norway between 1982 and 2007, which showed similar results (Sundhi et al. 2014). This is reassuring for both couples considering ART and for the children conceived in this manner.

Conclusion and Future Directions

In conclusion, the main risks for the health of ART children remain perinatal, such as multiple pregnancies and low birth weight, which can have longer term sequelae such as cerebral palsy. The evidence of risk for longer-term outcome of singletons born at term following ART compared with their NC peers is generally reassuring. However, future studies are needed to assess the health of ART children in later life. To date, most studies have followed ART children into early teenage years and many of the chronic health conditions such as cardiovascular disease and malignancies do not manifest until later. Low birth weight has previously been shown to be associated with increased risk of diabetes mellitus, hypertension, and cardiovascular disease in adult life. Given the increased risk of low birth weight in ART-conceived children, this group may well have an increased cardiovascular risk as they enter adulthood. An additional area of concern for ART children in adulthood is that of infertility, especially in boys conceived to infertile fathers through ICSI. Furthermore, it is crucial that follow-up of children conceived through newer technologies continues especially with the continuing rapid advances in invasive techniques in ART.

References

Adamson, G., Zegers-Hochschild, F., Ishihara, O. et al. (2012). ICMART world report: preliminary Data. Hum Reprod 27(Suppl 2): ii38–ii39.

Barker, D.J. (1995). Fetal origin of coronary heart disease. BMJ 311: 171–174.

Belva, F., Henriet, S., Liebaers, I. et al. (2007). Medical outcome of 8-year-old singleton ICSI children (born ≥32 weeks' gestation) and a spontaneously conceived comparison group. Hum Reprod 22: 506–515.

Bergh, C. (2005). Single embryo transfer: a mini-review. Hum Reprod 20: 323–327.

Bonduelle, M., Wennerholm, U.B., Loft, A. et al. (2005). A multi-centre cohort study of the physical health of 5-year-old children conceived after intracytoplasmic sperm injection, in vitro fertilization and natural conception. Hum Reprod 20: 413–419.

Bowen, J.R., Gibson, F.L., Leslie, G.I. et al. (1998). Medical and developmental outcome at 1 year for children conceived by intracytoplasmic sperm injection. Lancet 351: 1529–1534.

Brinton, L.A., Kruger Kjaer, S., Thomsen, B. L. et al. (2004). Childhood tumor risk after treatment with ovulation-stimulating drugs. Fertil Steril 81: 1083–1091.

Cederblad, M., Friberg B., Ploman F. et al. (1996). Intelligence and behaviour in children born after invitro fertilization treatment. Hum Reprod 11: 2052–2057.

Ceelen, M., vanWeissenbruch, M.M., Vermeiden, J.P. et al. (2008a). Growth and development of children born after in vitro fertilization. Fertil Steril 90: 1662–1673.

Ceelen, M., van Weissenbruch, M.M., Vermeiden, J.P. et al. (2008b). Cardiometabolic differences in children born after in vitro fertilization: follow-up study. J Clin Endocrinol Metab 93: 1682–1688.

Cocchi, G., Marsico, C., Cosentino, A. et al. (2013). Silver-Russell syndrome due to paternal H19/IGF2 hypomethylation in a twin girl born after in vitro fertilization. Am J Med Genet 161: 2652–2655.

Davies, M.J., Moore, V.M., Willson, K.J. et al. (2012). Reproductive technologies and the risk of birth defects. N Engl J Med 366: 1803–1813.

De Schepper, J., Belva, F., Schiettecatte, J. et al. (2009). Testicular growth and tubular function in prepubertal boys conceived by intracytoplasmic sperm injection. Horm Res 71: 359–363.

Ericson, A., Nygren, K.G., Olausson, P.O. et al. (2002). Hospital care utilization of infants born after IVF. Hum Reprod 17: 929–932.

Fauser, B.C., Devroey, P. and Macklon, N.S. (2005). Multiple birth resulting from ovarian stimulation for subfertility treatment. Lancet 365: 1807–1816.

Fisher-Jeffes, L.J., Banerjee, I. and Sutcliffe, A.G. (2006). Parents' concerns regarding their ART children. Reproduction 131: 389–394.

Focus on Reproduction (2016). https://focusonreproduction.eu/2016/07/05/6-5-million-ivf-babies-since-louise-brown/ (accessed 22 February 2018).

Frackiewicz, E.J. (2000). Endometriosis: an overview of the disease and its treatment. J Am Pharm Assoc 40: 645–657.

Glinianaia, S.V., Pharoah, P., Wright, C. et al. (2002). Northern Region Perinatal Mortality Survey Steering Group. Fetal or infant death in twin pregnancy: neurodevelopmental consequences for the survivor. Arch Dis Child Fetal Neonatal Ed 86: F9–F15.

Golombok, S., Brewaeys, A., Cook, R. et al. (1996). The European study of assisted reproduction families: family functioning and child development. Hum Reprod 11: 2324–2331.

Gray, R.H. and Wu L.Y. (2000). Subfertility and risk of spontaneous abortion. Am J Public Health 90: 1452–1454.

Hansen, M., Bower, C., Milne, E. et al. (2005). Assisted reproductive technologies and the risk of birth defects – a systematic review. Hum Reprod 20: 328–338.

Hansen, M., Kurinczuk, J.J., Bower, C. et al. (2002). The risk of major birth defects after intracytoplasmatic sperm injection and in vitro fertilization. N Engl J Med 346: 725–730.

Helmerhorst, F.M., Perquin, D.A., Donker, D. et al. (2004). Perinatal outcome of singletons and twins after assisted conception: a systematic review of controlled studies. BMJ 328: 261.

Henriksen, T.B., Baird, D.D., Olsen, J. et al. (1997). Time to pregnancy and preterm delivery. Obstet Gynecol 89: 594–599

Hvidtjorn, D., Schieve, L., Schendel, D. et al. (2009). Cerebral palsy, autism spectrum disorders, and developmental delay in children born after assisted conception: a systematic review and meta-analysis. Arch Pediatr Adolesc Med 163: 72–83.

Imhof, S.M., Cruysberg, J.R., Schouten-van Meeteren, A.Y. et al. (2003). Incidence of retinoblastoma in children born after in vitro fertilisation. Lancet 361: 309–310.

Källén, A.J., Finnström, O.O., Lindam, A.P. et al. (2010) Cerebral palsy in children born after in vitro fertilization. Eur J Paediatr Neurol 14: 526–530.

Källén, A.J., Finnström, O.O., Lindam, A.P. et al. (2011). Is there an increased risk for drug treated attention deficit/hyperactivity disorder in children born after in vitro fertilization? Eur J Paediatr Neurol 15: 247–253.

Källén, B., Finnström, O., Nygren, K.G. et al. (2005). In vitro fertilization in Sweden: child morbidity including cancer risk. Fertil Steril 84: 605–610.

Koivisto, M., Jouppila, P., Kauppila, A. et al. (1975). Twin pregnancy: neonatal morbidity and mortality. Acta Obstet Gynecol Scand Suppl, 21–29.

Koivurova, S., Hartikainen, A.L., Sovio, U. et al. (2003). Growth, psychomotor development and morbidity up to 3 years of age in children born after IVF. Hum Reprod 18: 2328–2336.

Kurinczuk, J.J. (2003). Safety issues in assisted reproduction technology. From theory to reality – just what are the data telling us about ICSI offspring health and future fertility and should we be concerned? Hum Reprod 18: 925–931.

Lidegaard, O., Pinborg, A. and Andersen, A.N (2005). Imprinting diseases and IVF: Danish National IVF cohort study. Hum Reprod 20: 950–954.

Ludwig, A.K., Katalinic, A., Thyen, U. et al. (2008). Physical health at 5.5 years of age of term-born singletons after intracytoplasmic sperm injection: results of a prospective, controlled, single-blinded study. Fertil Steril 91: 115–124.

McGovern, P.G., Llorens, A.J., Skurnick, J.H. et al. (2004). Increased risk of preterm birth in singleton pregnancies resulting from in vitro fertilization – embryo transfer or gamete intrafallopian transfer: a metaanalysis. Fertil Steril 82: 1514–1520.

Merlob, P., Sapir, O., Sulkes, J. et al. (2005). The prevalence of major congenital malformations during two periods of time, 1986–1994 and 1995–2002, in newborns conceived by assisted reproduction technology. Eur J Med Genet 48: 5–11.

Miles, H.L., Hofman, P.L., Peek, J. et al. (2007). In vitro fertilization improves childhood growth and metabolism. J Clin Endocrinol Metab 92: 3441–3445.

Ombelet, W., Martens, G., De Sutter, P. et al. (2006). Perinatal outcome of 12,021 singleton and 3108 twin births after non-IVF-assisted reproduction: a cohort study. Hum Reprod 21: 1025–1032.

Orstavik, K.H., Eiklid, K., Van der Hagen, C.B. et al. (2003). Another case of imprinting defect in a girl with Angelaman's syndrome who was conceived by intracytoplasmic sperm injection. Am J Hum Genet 72: 218–219.

Pinborg, A., Lidegaard, O., la Cour Freiesleben, N. et al. (2005). Consequences of vanishing twins in IVF/ICSI pregnancies. Hum Reprod 20: 2821–2829.

Ponjaert-Kristoffersen, I., Bonduelle, M., Barnes, J. et al. (2005). International collaborative study of intracytoplasmic sperm injection-conceived, in vitro fertilization-conceived, and naturally conceived 5-year-old child outcomes: cognitive and motor assessments. Pediatrics 115: e283–9.

Ponjaert-Kristoffersen I., Tjus T., Nekkebroeck J. et al. (2004). Psychological follow-up study of 5-year-old ICSI children. Hum Reprod 19: 2791.

Rimm, A.A., Katayama, A.C., Diaz, M. et al. (2004). A meta-analysis of controlled studies comparing major malformation rates in IVF and ICSI infants

with naturally conceived children. J Assist Reprod Genet 21: 437–443.

Stromberg, B., Dahlquist, G., Ericson, A. et al. (2002). Neurological sequelae in children born after in-vitro fertilisation: a population-based study. Lancet 359: 461–465.

Sun, Y., Vestergaard, M., Christensen, J. et al. (2007). Epilepsy and febrile seizures in children of treated and untreated subfertile couples. Hum Reprod 22: 215–220.

Sundh, K.J., Henningsen, A.K., Källen, K. et al. (2014). Cancer in children and young adults born after assisted reproductive technology: a Nordic cohort study from the Committee of Nordic ART and Safety (CoNARTaS). Hum Reprod 29: 2050–2057.

Sutcliffe, A.G. (2000). Intracyctoplasmic sperm injection and other aspects of new reproductive technologies. Arch Dis Child 83: 98–101.

Sutcliffe, A.G., D'Souza, S.W., Cadman, J. et al. (1995). Minor congenital anomalies, major congenital malformations and development in children conceived from cryopreserved embryos. Hum Reprod 10: 3332–3337.

Sutcliffe, A.G. and Ludwig, M. (2007). Outcome of assisted reproduction. Lancet 370: 351–359

Sutcliffe, A.G., Saunders, K., McLachlan, R. et al. (2003). A retrospective case-control study of developmental and other outcomes in a cohort of Australian children conceived by intracytoplasmic sperm injection compared with a similar group in the United Kingdom. Fertil Steril 79: 512–516.

Sutcliffe, A.G., Taylor, B., Saunders, K. et al. (2001). Outcome in the second year of life after in-vitro fertilisation by intracytoplasmic sperm injection: a UK case-control study. Lancet 357: 2080–2084.

Wagenaar, K., Huisman, J., Cohen-Kettenis, P.T. et al. (2008). An overview of studies on early development, cognition, and psychosocial well-being in children born after in vitro fertilization. J Dev Behav Pediatr 29: 219–230.

Williams, C.L., Bunch, K.J., Stiller, C.A. et al. (2003). Cancer risk among children born after assisted conception. N. Engl J Med 69: 1819–1827.

Zhu, J.L., Obel, C., Basso, O. et al. (2011). Infertility, infertility treatment and behavioural problems in the offspring. Paediatr Perinat Epidemiol 25: 466–477.

Index

Clinical Reproductive Science, First Edition. Edited by Michael Carroll.
© 2019 John Wiley & Sons Ltd. Published 2019 by John Wiley & Sons Ltd.
Companion website: www.wiley.com/go/carroll/clinicalreproductivescience